THE PRACTICAL PLAYBOOK III

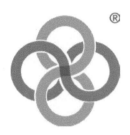

THE PRACTICAL PLAYBOOK III

Working Together to Improve Maternal Health

Edited by

**DOROTHY CILENTI,
ALISAHAH JACKSON,
NATALIE D. HERNANDEZ,
LINDSEY YATES,
SARAH VERBIEST,
J. LLOYD MICHENER,
AND BRIAN C. CASTRUCCI**

Managing Editors

BRITTANY HINNANT AND TAMALA GRISSETT

de Beaumont

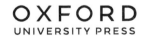

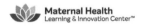

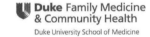

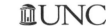

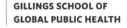

OXFORD
UNIVERSITY PRESS

Oxford University Press is a department of the University of Oxford. It furthers
the University's objective of excellence in research, scholarship, and education
by publishing worldwide. Oxford is a registered trade mark of Oxford University
Press in the UK and certain other countries.

Published in the United States of America by Oxford University Press
198 Madison Avenue, New York, NY 10016, United States of America.

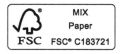
CIP data is on file at the Library of Congress

ISBN 978–0–19–766298–4

DOI: 10.1093/oso/9780197662984.001.0001

Printed by Integrated Books International, United States of America

MIX
Paper
FSC FSC® C183721

This book is dedicated to all the mothers and birthing people who lost their lives or experienced physical or emotional trauma because of pregnancy or childbirth. We also dedicate this book to all current and future mothers and birthing people, and to all the people who care and work tirelessly to ensure that all mothers, birthing people, and families can thrive and be healthy.

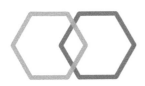

Contents

Foreword   **xiii**
Acknowledgments   **xvii**
Contributors   **xix**

SECTION I   **Introduction**

1   **Why a Practical Playbook about Working Together to Improve Maternal Health?**   3
Alisahah Jackson, Dorothy Cilenti, Lindsey Yates, Sarah Verbiest, J. Lloyd Michener, and Natalie D. Hernandez

2   **Promoting Federal Partnerships for Effective Program Implementation**   9
Clara E. Busse, Sandra J. Lloyd, Ashley Wilkes, and Catherine J. Vladutiu

3   **How Academic Centers Can Accelerate Partnerships and Progress in Maternal Health**   19
Alison M. Stuebe

4   **Transformational Maternal and Child Health through Expanded Healthcare Coordination and Community Engagement**   37
Ahmed V. Calvo, Lyndsey Stadtmueller, Anita Isama, Erica O'Neill, and Mark Loafman

5   **Improving Maternal and Child Health Outcomes: An Opportunity for Expanded Primary Healthcare Teams**   47
Mark Loafman, Kenya Thomas-Allen, Anita Isama, and Ahmed V. Calvo

6   **It's Not a Flip of the Switch: One Healthcare System's Collaborative Approach to Engaging External Partners to Support the Maternity Journey**   57
Brisa Urquieta de Hernandez, Christine Brocato, Manoja Ratnayake Lecamwasam, and Anuradhika Anuradhika

SECTION II	**Collaboration**	
7	**Collaborations to Improve Maternal Health** *Dorothy Cilenti and Ruth S. Buzi*	73
8	**Extending the Reach of Maternal Health Practice into New Zones of Transformation with the Framework for Aligning Sectors** *Daniel Lanford, Karen Minyard, Leigh Alderman, Japera Hemming, Christopher Parker, and Tanisa Foxworth Adimu*	77
9	**An Approach for Whole-Person Health: Oral Healthcare Integration for Improved Maternal Outcomes** *Timothy L. Ricks and Zachary A. Brian*	93
10	**What It Really Takes to Succeed: Practical Tips for Maternal Health Collaboration** *Piia Hanson and Kimberly Sherman*	107
11	**Bringing Together Clinical and Community Partners for Better Patient Care: Bootheel Perinatal Network** *Barbara Gleason, Rebecca Burger, Morgan Nesselrodt, Susan Kendig, and Tanisa Foxworth Adimu*	119
12	**A Community Approach to Addressing Inequities in Maternal Health** *Deidre McDaniel, Valerie Newsome Garcia, Karen Chustz, Saanie Sulley, Deborah Frazier, and Haywood Brown*	133
13	**The Broward Healthy Start Program: Cross-Sector Collaboration—Improving Pregnancy Outcomes and Birth Equity Using a Collective-Impact Framework** *Marci Ronik, Monica Figueroa King, Sharetta Remikie, and Roneé Wilson*	139
14	**Impacting Maternal and Prenatal Care Together: A Harris County/Houston Collaborative** *June Hanke, Jamie Freeny, and Ruth S. Buzi*	153

15 Activating Our Village in Los Angeles County:
    Birth Equity and Black Families   165
    Brandi Sims Desjolais, Melissa Franklin, Helen O'Connor, Kaci
    Patterson, Sonya Young Aadam, Deborah Allen, Adjoa Jones,
    and Sylvia Swilley

SECTION III   Equity

16 Centering Equity: Systemic Racism and Social
    Determinants of Maternal Health   187
    Natalie D. Hernandez and Tamaron A. Johnson

17 Historical Context Matters: Structural Racism,
    Maternal Health, and Reproductive Justice   191
    Christine M. Velez and Maria Mercedes Ávila

18 Equity and Systemic Racism   201
    Jonathan Webb

19 Introduction to Maternal Health Equity:
    A Consensus-Driven Definition and Research Priorities   213
    Elizabeth A. Mosley

20 Redesigning Systems with Black Women to Improve
    Maternal Health in Atlanta   227
    Jemea Dorsey and Kaprice Welsh

21 Doulas and Incarcerated Populations   237
    Crystal Hayes and Marisa Pizii

22 Environmental Impacts on Maternal Health   247
    Michele Okoh

23 Reimagining Prenatal Care: Designing a
    Justice-Conscious Approach to Reproductive Health,
    Pregnancy, and Early Parenthood   259
    Keegan D. Warren and Daphne McGee

SECTION IV   Data

24 Using and Improving Maternal Health Data to
    Achieve Equity   273
    Lindsey Yates

25 Democratizing Data: Understanding the Challenges and Opportunities for Community-Based Utilization of Maternal Mortality Data and Maternal Health Interventions   277
    Athena Cross and Pam Silberman

26 Decolonizing Maternal Health Research: An Introduction to Indigenous Research Methods and a Decolonial Framework for Indigenous Maternal Health Research   289
    Alayah Johnson-Jennings

27 Garbage In, Garbage Out: Examining How Maternal Health Data Tools Misuse Race   301
    Marie V. Plaisime

28 Maternal Health and Gathering Evidence of Structural Racism   309
    Lauri Andress

29 Using Narrative Medicine and Longitudinal Qualitative Research to Examine Maternal Health Outcomes   319
    Burcu Bozkurt

30 Culturally Responsive Evaluation   327
    Kimberley Broomfield-Massey, Rakiah Anderson, Calondra Tibbs, and Christine Tucker

SECTION V **Innovations**

31 Innovations to Improve Maternal Health   345
    Sarah Verbiest and Monica Beltran

32 Respectful Care and Reproductive Justice as Foundations for Maternal Health Innovation   349
    Aja Clark, Phoebe Wescott, Amy Ushry, Kiara Cruz, Christie Allen, and Inas-Khalidah Mahdi

33 Women's Health Before, Between, Beyond, and Regardless of Pregnancy   363
    Sarah Verbiest, Suzanne Woodward, and Lindsey Yates

34   Innovation in Systems of Postpartum Care   379
      Kimberly D. Harper, Nkechi U. Charles, Amelia N. Gibson,
      and Kristin P. Tully

35   The Integral Role of Community-Based Doulas in
      Supporting Birth Equity   391
      Twylla Dillion and Zainab Sulaiman

36   From Grassroots to Telecommunication Innovation:
      Bridging the Gap in Perinatal Mental Health   405
      Chris Raines and Wendy Davis

37   Using a Learning Community Model to Address
      Substance Misuse and Co-Occurring Mental Health
      Challenges among MCH Populations   415
      Sanaa Akbarali, Ramya Dronamraju, Katrin Patterson, Ellen
      Pliska, and Christine Mackie

38   Innovations in Virtual Care   427
      Leslie deRosset, Halle Neeley, and Aunchalee Palmquist

SECTION VI   **Systems and Scalability**

39   Scaling Up and Sustaining Improvements in
      Maternal Health Equity   447
      J. Lloyd Michener

40   The Role of the Maternal and Child Health Bureau
      in Supporting States and Communities to Advance
      Maternal Health Equity   451
      Michael D. Warren, Kathy K. Best, Erin Patton, and
      Belinda Pettiford

41   Driving Access, Health Equity, and Innovation in
      Maternal Healthcare through Medicaid   463
      Jessica C. Smith, Emily Heberlein, Angela Snyder, and
      Karen Minyard

42   Role of Academic Health Systems in Improving
      and Sustaining Maternal Health   477
      Olufunmilayo Makinde Chinekezi, Karey M. Sutton, Crista E.
      Johnson-Agbakwu, and Yhenneko J. Taylor

43   Building a Maternal Health Workforce to Advance
      Equity, Partnerships, and Healthy Communities   491
      Amy J. Mullenix and M. Kathryn Menard

44   The Role of the Family Physician in Pregnancy Care:
      Striving for Birth Equity and Reducing Maternal
      Morbidity and Mortality   513
      Julie K. Wood

45   Employing Policy and Advocacy for Sustainable Reduction
      of Maternal Mortality and Maternal Health Inequities   523
      Anna Kheyfets, Maria Gabriela Ruiz, Keri Carvalho,
      Candace Stewart, and Ndidiamaka Amutah-Onukagha

46   Sustainability and Finance: The Role of State and
      Territorial Health Agencies   539
      Ellen Pliska, Britta Cedergren, Kristin Sullivan, Melissa Touma,
      Karl Ensign, Sowmya Kuruganti, Deborah Backman,
      Alex Wheatley, Heather Pangelinan, Marijane Carey,
      Shannon Vance, and Sanaa Akbarali

47   How State-Based Foundations Can Leverage
      Collaboration to Improve Maternal Health:
      A Case Study from California   555
      Dana G. Smith and Stephanie S. Teleki

48   The Role of the Area Health Education Center in
      Improving Maternal Health   567
      Adam J. Zolotor, Jill M. Forcina, Tara Owens Shuler, and
      Hugh H. Tilson, Jr.

49   The Role of Local Health Departments in Women's
      Health and the Opportunity to Improve Rural
      Maternal Health Outcomes   579
      Lisa Macon Harrison and Abigail Kenney

SECTION VII   **Conclusion**

50   **The Journey Forward**   593
      Dorothy Cilenti, Alisahah Jackson, Natalie D. Hernandez,
      Lindsey Yates, Sarah Verbiest, and J. Lloyd Michener

Index   **595**

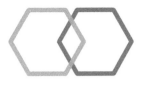

Foreword

This book marks the third in the Practical Playbook series, following *The Practical Playbook: Public Health and Primary Care Together* (2015) and *The Practical Playbook II: Building Multisector Partnerships That Work* (2019). The theme of the first two volumes was not to coalesce and repackage existing research, but to provide a timely core resource for more effective engagement and action for pressing frontline challenges. This third volume applies the same lens to one of our society's most pressing issues—the health of women and birthing people, infants, and children. While it differs from the previous playbooks by focusing on a specific population, the spirit of what is included is completely aligned: across all three volumes, the need for partnership and collaboration between different sectors, systems change to realize true impact, and continued innovation remain constant themes.

Improving the health of women and birthing people and their infants and children is an increasingly complex and nuanced challenge. The mid-20th-century Norman Rockwell paintings that suggested our health was confined to treatments and procedures in a physician's office seem almost fictional given the complex web of factors and influences shaping health outcomes now. The nation and the health of women and people who birth are at a unique crossroads. The United States is the eleventh richest nation on Earth, with the highest maternal mortality rate of any industrialized country.[1] And it's not even close. In 2020, in the United States, nearly 24 women die per 100,000 live births, compared to about nine maternal deaths in France and Canada and seven maternal deaths in the United Kingdom.[2] There are fewer than five maternal deaths per 100,000 live births in all other industrialized nations.[2] The rate of maternal mortality in the United States stands as a glaring example of the American healthcare paradox—spending more than any other nation on healthcare but not seeing the expected improvements in outcomes. America continues to search for medical answers to a question that is deliberately and single-mindedly medicalized.

Like the other books in *The Practical Playbook* series, this book was written by contributors who believe and understand that solutions to critical health problems cannot be found solely within clinic walls. Solutions will require communities, healthcare professionals, elected leaders, business leaders, and many others working together, through a shared understanding and commitment to aligned action, to actively confront and dismantle the complexities and inequities driving poor outcomes.

The refrain that more research is needed must be replaced with more action is needed, more results are needed, and more people surviving and thriving through their birthing experiences must be demanded. The present availability of knowledge and the ability to access it are unprecedented in human history. Additional research and further accumulation of knowledge will continue to fail us until our knowledge is operationalized to make the changes needed to improve outcomes. This book seeks to encourage, catalyze, and spur these necessary actions, and to spread the required thinking to evolve our society to one that prioritizes health and stands strongly against the unacceptable number of infant and maternal deaths that the nation continues to experience.

This third playbook provides the necessary grounding and practical tools and examples to achieve a shared goal of improved health specifically for women, mothers, all birthing people, infants, and children. Each chapter offers insights and the blueprints necessary to drive action that can be implemented in clinics or communities. The "plays" provided in the book are the paths through which we can achieve the necessary improvements in health.

Everyone involved in *The Practical Playbook III* has collectively produced a guide to positive, aligned action for improved maternal and child health. Like the other playbooks, it is not meant to be placed on a shelf or simply read cover to cover. It is meant to be used and applied. The factors and parameters that define the health journey for women and birthing people are not constant throughout the United States. Resources, healthcare access, environmental factors, economic opportunities, and other factors vary significantly from place to place. The sections, chapters, and concrete examples provided can be adapted, implemented, revised, and updated to the specific parameters of your communities and situations and as lessons are gathered. The goal of this book and its eventual success depend on its driving you to act and serving as an effective companion on your journey to achieve the outcomes and improvements you know are so critically needed in your communities and populations.

Brian C. Castrucci, DrPH
President and Chief Executive Officer
de Beaumont Foundation

REFERENCES

1. Worlddata.info. The Richest Countries in the World. N.d. https://www.worlddata. info/richest-countries.php.

2. Taylor J, Bernstein A, Waldrop T, Smith-Ramakrishnan V. The Worsening U.S. Maternal Health Crisis in Three Graphs. March 2, 2022. https://tcf.org/content/ commentary/worsening-u-s-maternal-health-crisis-three-graphs/.

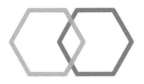

Acknowledgments

The genesis and chapters of this book are the result of the contributions of many, including and extending beyond the authors listed with each chapter. We are grateful for the support of the de Beaumont Foundation, Oxford University Press, *Practical Playbook* teams, and Maternal Health Learning and Innovation Center,* who were all instrumental in bringing this book to life. We are especially grateful for the individuals who worked alongside us to make this publication possible: Ariel Lewis, Grace Castillo, Diane Lazarus, Jessica Dixon, Tamaron A. Johnson, Mieasha Harris, Nalini Padmanabhan, Julia Haskins, Joseph Parsons, Dena Afrasiabi, and Christine Bixiones. We also thank The Illinois Maternal Health Digital Storytelling Project for allowing us to share some of the stories they collected. We hope this book highlights and reflects the ongoing work of people and partnerships that are involved in shaping maternal health efforts. Together, we can help reduce end the unnecessary deaths of mothers and birthing people and the devastating effects those losses have on us all.

With deep gratitude and appreciation,

The Editors

* The Maternal Health Learning and Innovation Center is supported by the Health Resources and Services Administration (HRSA) of the US Department of Health and Human Services (HHS) under grant number U7CMC33636 State Maternal Health Innovation Support and Implementation Program Cooperative Agreement. This information or content and conclusions are those of the author and should not be construed as the official position or policy of, nor should any endorsements be inferred by HRSA, HHS, or the US government.

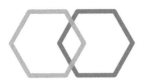

Contributors

Sonya Young Aadam
CEO, California Black Women's Health Project

Tanisa Foxworth Adimu
RMOMS HRSA Grant Coach, Georgia Health Policy Center/Maternal Health Learning and Innovation Center

Sanaa Akbarali
Senior Director, Maternal and Infant Health, Association of State and Territorial Health Officials

Leigh Alderman
Assistant Project Director, Georgia Health Policy Center, Andrew Young School of Policy Studies, Georgia State University

Christie Allen
Senior Director, American College of Obstetricians and Gynecologists

Deborah Allen
Deputy Director for Health Promotion, Los Angeles County Department of Public Health

Mary Beth Allen
Health Policy Specialist, Kentucky Perinatal Quality Collaborative

Ndidiamaka Amutah-Onukagha
Associate Professor, Julia A. Okoro Professor of Black Maternal Health, Department of Public Health and Community Medicine, Tufts University School of Medicine; Director and Founder of the Center for Black Maternal Health and Reproductive Justice

Rakiah Anderson
Evaluation Manager, Maternal Health Learning and Innovation Center, Department of Maternal and Child Health, University of North Carolina at Chapel Hill

Lauri Andress
Associate Dean, College of Population Health, University of New Mexico; Principal, Andress & Associates, Bridging the Health Gap Consultants, LLC

Anuradhika Anuradhika
System Vice President, Strategic Partnerships & Ventures, CommonSpirit Health

Maria Mercedes Ávila
Professor of Pediatrics, University of Vermont Larner College of Medicine

Deborah Backman
Maternal and Infant Health Senior Analyst, Association of State and Territorial Health Officials

Monica Beltran
Program Officer, W.K. Kellogg Foundation

Kathy K. Best
Public Health Analyst, Maternal and Child Health Bureau, Health Resources and Services Administration, US Department of Health and Human Services

Burcu Bozkurt
Department of Health Policy and Management, Gillings School of Global Public Health, University of North Carolina at Chapel Hill

Zachary A. Brian
Clinical Associate Professor, Director, Dentistry in Service to Community (DISC), Division of Pediatric and Public Health, Adams School of Dentistry, University of North Carolina at Chapel Hill

Christine Brocato
System Vice President Strategy Innovation, CommonSpirit Health

Kimberley Broomfield-Massey
Principal Research and Evaluation Consultant, Urban Metrics Consultants, LLC

Haywood Brown
Senior Associate Vice President of Academic Affairs for University of South Florida Health and the Vice Dean of Faculty Affairs for the Morsani College of Medicine

Rebecca Burger
System Care Coordinator, RMOMS HRSA Grant, Bootheel Perinatal Network

Clara Busse
Oak Ridge Institute for Science and Education Fellow, Maternal and Child Health Bureau, Health Resources and Services Administration

Ruth S. Buzi
Consultant (formerly Associate Professor and Director of Social Services, Baylor College of Medicine Teen Health Clinic)

Ahmed V. Calvo
Director of National Leadership Fellowship on Health Policy and Public Service, Stanford University Haas Center for Public Service

Marijane Carey
Consultant, Carey Consulting

Keri Carvalho
Tufts University

Britta Cedergren
Program Director, The University of Alabama at Birmingham School of Public Health

Nkechi U. Charles
Gillings School of Global Public Health

Olufunmilayo Makinde Chinekezi
Program Officer, National Academy of Medicine

Heidi Christensen
Maternal Health Innovation Program Manager, Bureau of Women's & Children's Health, Arizona Department of Health Services

Karen Chustz
Senior Program Manager, National Healthy Start Association

Dorothy Cilenti
Clinical Professor, Director, National MCH Workforce Development Center; Director, Maternal Health Learning and Innovation Center, Department of Maternal and Child Health, Gillings School of Global Public Health, University of North Carolina at Chapel Hill

Aja Clark
Senior Birth Equity Evaluation Analyst, National Birth Equity Collaborative

Monica Clouse
Program Manager, Kentucky Perinatal Quality Collaborative

Andreea A. Creanga
Associate Professor, Department of International Health & Department of Gynecology and Obstetrics, Director, Maryland Maternal Health Innovation Program, Associate Director, International Center for Maternal and Newborn Health, Johns Hopkins University

Athena Cross
Chief Program Officer, AIDS United

Kiara Cruz
Senior Research Analyst, National Birth Equity Collaborative

Wendy Davis
Executive Director, Postpartum Support International

Brisa Urquieta de Hernandez
System Director Operations, Lloyd H. Dean Institute for Humankindness & Health Justice, CommonSpirit Health

Leslie deRosset
Research Investigator, Implementation Specialist, Department of Maternal and Child Health, Gillings School of Global Public Health, University of North Carolina at Chapel Hill

Brandi Sims Desjolais
Director, Charles R. Drew University of Medicine and Science, Black Maternal Health Center of Excellence

Twylla Dillion
Executive Director, HealthConnect One

Jemea Dorsey
Chief Executive Officer, Center for Black Women's Wellness

Ramya Dronamraju
Director of Maternal and Infant Health, Association of State and Territorial Health Officials

Amanda Roccabruna Eby
Program Specialist Family and Community Health Bureau, Montana Department of Public Health and Human Services

Karl Ensign
Vice President for Island Support, Association of State and Territorial Health Officials

Stephanie Fitch
MOMS Grant Manager, Billings Clinic

Jill M. Forcina
Director of Education & Nursing, North Carolina Area Health Education Center

Melissa Franklin
CEO of Growth Mindset Communications

Deborah Frazier
CEO, National Healthy Start Association

Jamie Freeny
Director, Center for School Behavioral Health, Mental Health America of Greater Houston

Valerie Newsome Garcia
Community Transformation Strategist, National Healthy Start Association, Alliance for Innovation on Maternal Health Community Care Initiative

Amelia N. Gibson
Associate Professor, University of Maryland College of Information Studies

Anne Elizabeth Glassgow
Research Assistant Professor of Medicine and Pediatrics, College of Medicine, University of Illinois at Chicago; Executive Director, Illinois Maternal Health Innovation Program (I PROMOTE-IL); Medical Director, UI Health Two-Generation Clinic

Barbara Gleason
Project Director RMOMS HRSA Grant, Bootheel Perinatal Network

June Hanke
(formerly) Strategic Analyst, Harris Health System

Piia Hanson
President and Principal Consultant, Ph Solutions, LLC

Kimberly D. Harper
Perinatal/Neonatal Outreach Coordinator, Collaborative for Maternal and Infant Health, OBGYN-Division of Research, University of North Carolina at Chapel Hill

Lisa Macon Harrison
Local Health Director, Granville Vance Public Health

Crystal Hayes
Clinical Assistant Professor, Sacred Heart University

Emily Heberlein
Assistant Project Director, Georgia Health Policy Center, Andrew Young School of Policy Studies, Georgia State University

Japera Hemming
Assistant Project Director, Georgia Health Policy Center, Georgia State University

Natalie D. Hernandez
Associate Professor, Department of Obstetrics and Gynecology; Executive Director, Center for Maternal Health Equity, Morehouse School of Medicine

Anita Isama
Resident Physician, Family and Community Medicine, Cook County Health; GE-NMF Primary Care Leadership Program Scholar

Alisahah Jackson
President, Lloyd H. Dean Institute for Humankindness & Health Justice

Alayah Johnson-Jennings

Tamaron A. Johnson
Administrative Assistant, Morehouse School of Medicine, Center for Maternal Health Equity

Crista E. Johnson-Agbakwu
Executive Director, Collaborative in Health Equity, Office of Health Equity; Professor, Obstetrics & Gynecology, UMass Memorial Health; Professor, Population & Quantitative Health Sciences Division, Preventive and Behavioral Medicine, University of Massachusetts T.H. Chan Medical School

Adjoa Jones
Los Angeles County Department of Public Health

Susan Kendig
Women's Health Integration Specialist, SSM Health Maternal Services

Abigail Kenney
Nurse Practitioner

Anna Kheyfets
Medical Student, Tufts University School of Medicine

Monica Figueroa King
CEO, Broward Healthy Start Coalition

Sowmya Kuruganti
Public Health Analyst, Association of State and Territorial Health Officials

Lynn Lane
Tribal Maternal Health Innovation Program Manager, Bureau of Women's & Children's Health, Arizona Department of Health Services

Daniel Lanford
Senior Research Associate, Georgia Health Policy Center, Georgia State University

Manoja Ratnayake Lecamwasam
System Vice President, Intellectual Property and Life Sciences Innovation, CommonSpirit Health

Sandra J. Lloyd (formerly)
Public Health Analyst, Maternal and Child Health Bureau, Health Resources and Services Administration

Mark Loafman
System Chair, Family and Community Medicine, Cook County Health

Christine Mackie
Vice President, Association of State and Territorial Health Officials

Inas-Khalidah Mahdi
Vice President of Equity-Centered Capacity Building, Director of Training, Praxis and Evaluation, National Birth Equity Collaborative

Joyce Marshall
Director, Maternal & Child Health Service, Oklahoma State Department of Health

Deidre McDaniel
Alliance for Innovation on Maternal Health Community Care Initiative Clinical-Community Bundle Integration Specialist; President & Founder, Health Equity Resources & Strategies

Daphne McGee
Public Health Attorney

M. Kathryn Menard
Distinguished Professor, Maternal Fetal Medicine, Department of Obstetrics and Gynecology, University of North Carolina School of Medicine

J. Lloyd Michener
Professor Emeritus, Department of Family Medicine & Community Health, Duke School of Medicine; Adjunct Professor, Public Health Leadership, UNC Gillings School of Global Public Health

Karen Minyard
Georgia Health Policy Center, Georgia State University

Elizabeth A. Mosley
Assistant Professor, University of Pittsburgh School of Medicine; Affiliated Faculty, Emory University Center for Reproductive Health Research in the Southeast (RISE)

Amy J. Mullenix
Deputy Director, Maternal Health Learning and Innovation Center, National MCH Workforce Development Center, Department of Maternal and Child Health, Gillings School of Global Public Health, University of North Carolina at Chapel Hill

Jordan Murphy
Epidemiologist, Kentucky Perinatal Quality Collaborative

Halle Neeley
Development Director, Reaching our Sisters Everywhere (ROSE)

Morgan Nesselrodt
Project Coordinator, RMOMS HRSA Grant, Bootheel Perinatal Network

Jill Nobles-Botkin
Administrative Program Manager, Maternal and Child Health Service, Perinatal & Reproductive Health Division, Oklahoma State Department of Health

Helen O'Connor
Health Program Analyst, Division of Maternal, Child, & Adolescent Health, Health Promotion Bureau, Los Angeles County Department of Public Health

Michele Okoh
Assistant Professor, Lewis & Clark Law School

Erica O'Neill
Academic Lead in Medical Education, Department of Obstetrics and Gynecology, Cook County Health; Assistant Professor, Northwestern University Feinberg School of Medicine

Reena Oza-Frank
Data and Surveillance Administrator, Bureau of Maternal, Child and Family Health, Ohio Department of Health

Aunchalee Palmquist
Assistant Professor, Department of Maternal and Child Health, Gillings School of Global Public Health, University of North Carolina at Chapel Hill

Heather Pangelinan
Director, Public Health Services, Commonwealth Healthcare Corporation, Commonwealth of the Northern Mariana Islands

Christopher Parker
Director, Population and Global Health/ Assistant Research Professor, Georgia Health Policy Center, Georgia State University

Kaci Patterson
Senior Director, Los Angeles Partnership for Early Childhood Investment; Founder, Social Good Solutions

Katrin Patterson
Program Manager, Indigenous Health, American College of Obstetricians and Gynecologists

Erin Patton
Public Health Analyst, Maternal and Child Health Bureau, Health Resources and Services Administration, US Department of Health and Human Services

Belinda Pettiford
Chief, Women, Infant, and Community Wellness Section, North Carolina Department of Health and Human Services

Marisa Pizii
Deputy Director of Programs and Policy, Collective Power for Reproductive Justice

Marie V. Plaisime
Center for Health and Human Rights, Harvard T.H. Chan School of Public Health; Penn Program on Race, Science & Society Center for Africana Studies, University of Pennsylvania

Ellen Pliska
Senior Director, Family and Child Health, Association of State and Territorial Health Officials

Chris Raines
CEO/founder, Chris Raines Consulting PC; Board Chair Emeritus, Postpartum Support International; Adjunct Professor, University of North Carolina Women's Mood Disorder Program, Department of Psychiatry, University of North Carolina at Chapel Hill

Sharetta Remikie
Chief Equity and Community Engagement Officer, Children's Services Council of Broward County

Timothy L. Ricks

Marci Ronik
University of South Florida; M2M Counseling, Coaching, and Consulting, LLC

Maria Gabriela Ruiz
Tufts University School of Medicine

Rebecca Severin
Maternal Health Innovation Program Supervisor, Maternal Health Innovation Program, Maternal Health Branch, Women, Infant, and Community Wellness Section, Division of Public Health, North Carolina Department of Health and Human Services

Kimberly Sherman
Branch Chief for Maternal & Women's Health, Health Resources and Services Administration

Tara Owens Shuler
Branch Head, Maternal Health Branch, Women, Infant, and Community Wellness Section; Division of Public Health, North Carolina Department of Health and Human Services (formerly Director of Operations and Diversity, North Carolina Area Health Education Center)

Pam Silberman
Professor of the Practice Emerita, Department of Health Policy and Management, Gillings School of Global Public Health, University of North Carolina at Chapel Hill

Dana G. Smith
Independent writer

Jessica C. Smith
Clinical Assistant Professor, Department of Health Policy and Management, University of Georgia

Angela Snyder
Research Associate Professor, Georgia Health Policy Center, Georgia State University

Lyndsey Stadtmueller
Family Medicine Faculty Physician, Family Health Center of Worcester

Candace Stewart
Tufts University School of Medicine

Alison M. Stuebe
Professor, School of Medicine and Gillings School of Global Public Health, University of North Carolina at Chapel Hill

Zainab Sulaiman
VP of Impact & Advocacy, HealthConnect One

Saanie Sulley
Data Manager, National Healthy Start Association

Kristin Sullivan
Director, Public Health Systems Improvement and Infrastructure, Association of State and Territorial Health Officials

Karey M. Sutton
Scientific Director, Health Equity Research, MedStar Health Research Institute

Sylvia Swilley
Association of Black Women Physicians

Yhenneko J. Taylor
Assistant Vice President, Center for Outcomes Research and Evaluation, Atrium Health

Stephanie S. Teleki
Director, Learning & Impact, California Health Care Foundation

Kenya Thomas-Allen
Fellow, Preventive Medicine, Cook County Health

Calondra Tibbs
CEO and Principal Consultant, Trifecta Advising, LLC

Hugh H. Tilson, Jr.
Director, North Carolina Area Health Education Center

Melissa Touma
Senior Analyst, Public Health Systems and Improvement, Association of State and Territorial Health Officials

Christine Tucker
Evaluator, Maternal Health Learning and Innovation Center, Department of Maternal and Child Health, University of North Carolina at Chapel Hill

Kristin P. Tully
Research Assistant Professor, University of North Carolina at Chapel Hill

Amy Ushry
Senior Nurse Special Project Manager, American College of Obstetricians and Gynecologists

Shannon Vance
Family and Child Health Senior Analyst, Association of State and Territorial Health Officials

Christine M. Velez
Assistant Professor in Social Work at the University of Vermont

Sarah Verbiest
Clinical Professor and Executive Director, School of Medicine and School of Social Work, University of North Carolina at Chapel Hill

Catherine J. Vladutiu
Senior Epidemiologist, Maternal and Child Health Bureau, Health Resources and Services Administration, US Department of Health and Human Services

Keegan D. Warren
Executive Director, Institute on for Healthcare Access, Texas A&M University

Michael D. Warren
Associate Administrator, Maternal and Child Health Bureau, Health Resources and Services Administration, US Department of Health and Human Services

Jonathan Webb
CEO Association for Women's Health, Obstetric and Neonatal Nurses

Kaprice Welsh
Certified Nurse Midwife

Phoebe Wescott
Senior Birth Equity Analyst, National Birth Equity Collaborative

Alex Wheatley
Senior Analyst, Island Support, Association of State and Territorial Health Officials

Connie White
Medical Advisor, Kentucky Perinatal Quality Collaborative

Ashley Wilkes
Supervisory Public Health Analyst, Maternal and Child Health Bureau, Health Resources and Services Administration, US Department of Health and Human Services

Roneé Wilson
Assistant Professor, University of South Florida College of Public Health

Julie K. Wood
Senior Vice President, Research, Science, and Health of the Public, American Academy of Family Physicians

Suzanne Woodward
Communications Director, University of North Carolina Collaborative for Maternal and Infant Health

Lindsey Yates
Postdoctoral Trainee, Center of Excellence, Department of Maternal and Child Health, Gillings School of Global Public Health, University of North Carolina at Chapel Hill

Adam J. Zolotor
Associate Director for Medical Education, North Carolina Area Health Education Center

Introduction

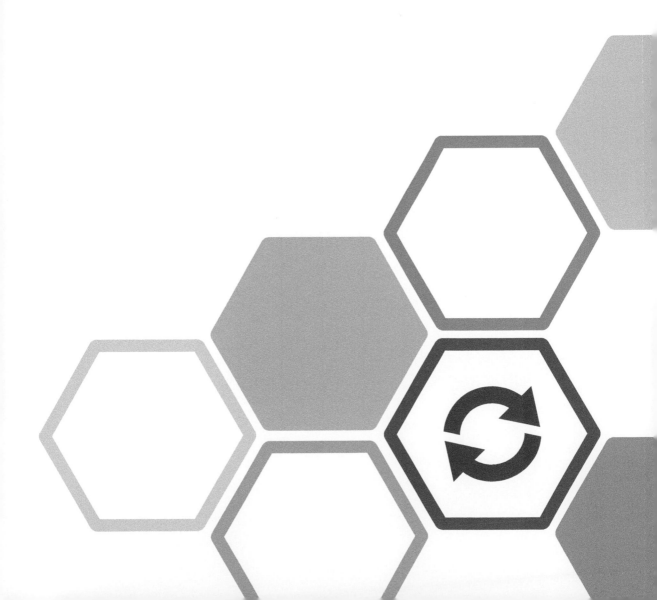

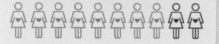

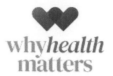

Source: Trost SL, Beauregard J, Njie F, et al. Pregnancy-Related Deaths: Data from Maternal Mortality Review Committees in 36 US States, 2017–2019. Atlanta, GA: Centers for Disease Control and Prevention, US Department of Health and Human Services; 2022.

Infographic Created By: Why Health Matters and Imaginari

Chapter 1

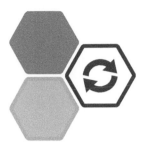

Why a Practical Playbook about Working Together to Improve Maternal Health?

ALISAHAH JACKSON, DOROTHY CILENTI, LINDSEY YATES,
SARAH VERBIEST, J. LLOYD MICHENER, AND NATALIE D. HERNANDEZ

Each day in the United States, more than 10,000 women and birthing people give birth.[1] While most parents and infants remain healthy through this experience, each day about 136 people will have some severe complication, such as cardiac arrest, acute renal failure, sepsis, the need for a blood transfusion, or respiratory distress syndrome,[2] and three people will die.[3] In the United States, more birthing people die because of pregnancy and childbirth than in other comparable countries.[4] Black, Indigenous, and Hispanic/Latina women have the highest rates of childbirth and pregnancy complications[5] and are more likely to die than white women.[3,6] These disparities are rooted at the intersection of racism, sexism, poverty, and other systems of oppression that lead to fewer opportunities, less access to resources and protections, increased stress, and poorer-quality care. At one of the most vulnerable times in their lives, women and birthing people face inequities that perpetuate illness and disease. This is unacceptable.

We demand change. This book is a response to the urgent matter of maternal health and health disparities in the United States. The book aims to:

- Highlight examples of multidisciplinary partnerships that leverage new ideas and resources, including innovative approaches to gathering and using data
- Demonstrate policies and practices that are improving the health and well-being of birthing people and children across the country

Alisahah Jackson, Dorothy Cilenti, Lindsey Yates, Sarah Verbiest, J. Lloyd Michener, and Natalie D. Hernandez, *Why a Practical Playbook about Working Together to Improve Maternal Health?* In: *The Practical Playbook III.* Edited by: Dorothy Cilenti, Alisahah Jackson, Natalie D. Hernandez, Lindsey Yates, Sarah Verbiest, J. Lloyd Michener, and Brian C. Castrucci, Oxford University Press. © de Beaumont Foundation 2024. DOI: 10.1093/oso/9780197662984.003.0001

- Identify strategies for scaling up and sustaining successful coalitions and programs
- Describe existing or promising tools and strategies to improve maternal health

BACKGROUND: THE CURRENT PROBLEM

The World Health Organization defines maternal death as "the death of a woman while pregnant or within 42 days of termination of pregnancy, irrespective of the duration and the site of pregnancy, from any cause related to or aggravated by the pregnancy or its management, but not from accidental or incidental causes."[7] Among wealthy countries, the rate of maternal deaths has been on the rise for the past 20 years, with the United States experiencing the highest number of maternal deaths.[4]

This increase is most apparent among non-Hispanic Black women. The numbers are both striking and increasing: In 2019, just over 20 mothers died per 100,000 live births[3]; in 2020, almost 24 mothers died per 100,000 live births[3]; and in 2021, nearly 32 mothers died per 100,000 live births.[3] The rates were two to three times higher among non-Hispanic Black women and American Indian and Alaska Native women.[3,8] In addition, maternal mortality rates rapidly increase with maternal age, with the rate for women age 40 and over being almost seven times higher than the rate for women under age 25.[3] The most alarming statistic is that 80% of maternal deaths are preventable.[9]

Reasons for the worsening death rate among pregnant and birthing people are multiple and intersectional. A chain is only as strong as its weakest link, and services and care for pregnant people have multiple weak and failing links. One issue is the lack of access to high-quality care. There have been federal and state efforts to increase access to good healthcare; however, variations in state laws and regulations, as well as widespread attacks on reproductive rights, mean that there is uneven access to important health services that are key for pregnant people. A 2022 March of Dimes report showed that 36% of US counties were considered maternity care deserts,[10] defined as any county without a hospital or birth center offering obstetric care and without any obstetric providers. In addition, approximately 12% of births occur in counties with limited or no access to maternity care.[10] This is a systemic issue that requires urgent solutions.

Access to healthcare is essential but is insufficient in addressing maternal mortality. Other weak links in the chain include lack of access to mental health and substance use disorder services,[9] untreated chronic conditions,[9] interpersonal violence in the home,[11] and stress caused by inequitable pay,[12,13] climate change,[14] and racism.[12,13]

The costs of poor maternal health are high. One study estimated that the societal costs of maternal morbidity through five years postpartum was $32.3 billion.[15] Moreover, when a birthing person experiences a severe pregnancy-related health issue or there is a maternal death, the costs are not just financial. Women and birthing people who experience a severe maternal health complication may experience temporary or permanent disability, including changes to their physical and mental health. If a person dies, a family and community lose that person's contributions and presence—and a child loses a parent. These losses to individuals, families, and our communities are avoidable, but addressing them requires us to work together in new ways.

The complex systems that are responsible for supporting women face multiple challenges, but we have the opportunity to make critical investments in emerging solutions, all along the chain.

OVERVIEW OF THE BOOK

This book and its authors are part of the growing chorus of vision sharers in the United States who are determined to bring attention to, and advance innovative ideas to address, the unacceptable rate of maternal deaths.

People may ask, "Why a playbook?" We use the playbook metaphor because such a complex issue requires collaboration among multiple actors and an intentional, comprehensive game plan. This playbook is not meant to be a rule book or to provide rigid recommendations. It is practical and inclusive of real-life interventions and partnerships that are accelerating evidence-based guidelines into widespread use. Earlier books in the Practical Playbook series discussed partnerships between public health and primary care (*The Practical Playbook: Public Health and Primary Care Together*) and building multisector partnerships (*The Practical Playbook II*). Improving maternal health builds on that work and requires coordinated efforts that are centered on the experiences, needs, and strengths of women and birthing people across diverse communities. Given this imperative, the key audiences for this playbook include anyone with an interest in improving maternal health outcomes, including public health professionals, healthcare providers, women's health advocates, policymakers, hospital and healthcare system administrators, community leaders, doulas, and others. Each of the 50 chapters in this book offers different "plays" or perspectives that readers can apply. What unifies all chapters is the thread that this problem can be solved and we can reach maternal health equity by working together to support birthing people in achieving health for themselves, their families, and their communities.

The Practical Playbook III is divided into six main sections. The Introduction establishes why the book is needed and introduces the multiple actors and sectors needed to implement solutions. The Collaborations section highlights collective efforts that are driving changes at the community and state levels. The Equity section describes the importance of working with historically underserved populations to address inequities and provides examples of how applying an antiracist lens can improve interventions. The Data section gives an overview of available maternal health data and outlines opportunities for improving maternal health data collection. The Innovations section explores innovations that advance maternal health and equity through novel, multisector approaches. Finally, the Systems and Scalability section discusses methods and tools that can be, and are being, used to transform systems of maternal health for individuals and communities. While each section includes unique content, similar chapter topics may appear in more than one section, but they are presented from a slightly different perspective.

The contributors to the book are from a variety of backgrounds and identities. They are practitioners, researchers, clinicians, and advocates. They work in federal and state agencies, academia, hospitals, and community settings. They offer distinct viewpoints on the maternal health challenge we face, and they are united in their passion and pursuit of solutions to achieve maternal health equity and well-being. We honor each author's unique approach and the experiences they bring to the issue.

Throughout the book there are infographics that illustrate recent statistics about maternal health in the United States. They are included to make information and data about maternal health accessible to everyone. But numbers and images are not enough. Also included are stories of people with lived experience. In partnership with, and with permission from, the Illinois Maternal Health Digital Storytelling Project, we include stories from women who describe select physical and emotional challenges of pregnancy and childbirth. Including these stories underlines who and what are at risk when our healthcare system fails to take care of birthing people.

The authors have aimed to use language inclusive of all genders, with the recognition that full equity and inclusiveness have not yet been achieved. To promote inclusivity, and out of respect for the diversity of identities of pregnant and birthing people, the book uses the terms *birthing person*, *mother*, *pregnant woman*, *pregnant person*, *woman*, *women*, and *maternal health*. Some chapters refer specifically to fathers because of continued efforts to achieve greater involvement of men in reproductive healthcare and childcare. These efforts should be inclusive of coparents and caregivers regardless of gender identity.

We recognize that the terminology may be limiting for some and essential to others. For some—specifically transgender men and nonbinary people who can get pregnant and give birth—the focus on maternal health may feel exclusive. But for others, including racialized populations who were perpetually denied rights because they were not considered human, let alone honored as mothers, the right to be called "woman" or "mother" is important and key to their identity.

The authors of each chapter carefully considered the language they used for their topics. Accordingly, terminology varies among chapters and sections.

SUMMARY

While *The Practical Playbook III* is meant to be informative and inspirational, we hope that it also drives some important, and possibly uncomfortable, conversations about maternal health in this country. By having these conversations, we mobilize individuals, organizations, and communities to continue demanding change.

We are deeply grateful for all those who have shared their stories and lessons learned through their contributions to this book. We trust it will assist the wide range of partners working to improve maternal health so that they may support thriving, diverse communities in which women, birthing people, and children are valued and supported. We have a long way to go, but we also have wonderful examples from which to learn and build.

REFERENCES

1. Martin JA, Hamilton BE, Osterman MJK. *Births in the United States, 2021*. NCHS Data Brief No. 442. https://www.cdc.gov/nchs/data/databriefs/db442.pdf. Published online August 2022. Accessed January 28, 2023.

2. Callaghan WM, Creanga AA, Kuklina EV. Severe maternal morbidity among delivery and postpartum hospitalizations in the United States. *Obstet Gynecol*. 2012;120(5):1029–1036. https://journals.lww.com/greenjournal/Fulltext/2012/11000/Severe_Maternal_Morbidity_Among_Delivery_and.8.aspx.

3. Hoyert DL. *Maternal Mortality Rates in the United States, 2021*. NCHS Health E-Stats. 2023. doi:https://dx.doi.org/10.15620/cdc:124678.

4. Munira Z, Gunja ED, Gumas RD, Williams II. The U.S. maternal mortality crisis continues to worsen: an international comparison. https://www.commonwealthfund.org/blog/2022/us-maternal-mortality-crisis-continues-worsen-international-comparison#:~:text=In%202020%2C%20the%20maternal%20mortality,exceptionally%20high%20for%20Black%20women. Published online December 1, 2022. Accessed January 28, 2023.

5. Admon LK, Winkelman TNA, Zivin K, Terplan M, Mhyre JM, Dalton VK. Racial and ethnic disparities in the incidence of severe maternal morbidity in the United States, 2012–2015. *Obstet Gynecol*. 2018;132(5):1158–1166. https://journals.lww.com/greenjournal/Fulltext/2018/11000/Racial_and_Ethnic_Disparities_in_the_Incidence_of.11.aspx

6. Petersen EE, Davis NL, Goodman D, et al. Racial/Ethnic Disparities in Pregnancy-Related Deaths—United States, 2007–2016. *MMWR Morb Mortal Wkly Rep*. 2019;68(35):762–765. doi:http://dx.doi.org/10.15585/mmwr.mm6835a3.

7. World Health Organization. *International Statistical Classification of Diseases and Related Health Problems*, 10th Revision. World Health Organization. 2009.

8. Petersen EE, Davis NL, Goodman D, et al. Racial/Ethnic Disparities in Pregnancy-Related Deaths—United States, 2007–2016. *MMWR Morb Mortal Wkly Rep*.

2019;68(35):762–765. https://www.cdc.gov/mmwr/volumes/68/wr/mm6835a3. htm?s_cid=mm6835a3_w#suggestedcitation.

9. Trost S, Beauregard J, Chandra G, et al. Pregnancy-related deaths: data from Maternal Mortality Review Committees in 36 states, 2017–2019. *Education (Chula Vista)*. 2022;45(10):1. https://www.cdc.gov/reproductivehealth/maternal-mortality/docs/pdf/Pregnancy-Related-Deaths-Data-MMRCs-2017-2019-H.pdf. Accessed January 28, 2023.

10. Brigance C, Lucas R., Jones E, et al. Nowhere to go: maternity care deserts across the U.S. (Report No. 3). March of Dimes. 2022. https://www.marchofdimes.org/maternity-care-deserts-report. Accessed January 12, 2023.

11. Campbell J, Matoff-Stepp S, Velez ML, Cox HH, Laughon K. Pregnancy-associated deaths from homicide, suicide, and drug overdose: review of research and the intersection with intimate partner violence. *J Womens Health*. 2021;30(2):236–244.

12. Hill L, Artiga S, Ranji U. Racial disparities in maternal and infant health: current status and efforts to address them. *KFF*. https://www.kff.org/racial-equity-and-health-policy/issue-brief/racial-disparities-in-maternal-and-infant-health-current-status-and-efforts-to-address-them/. Published online November 1, 2022. Accessed January 28, 2023.

13. Katon JG, Enquobahrie DA, Jacobsen K, Zephyrin L. Policies for reducing maternal morbidity and mortality and enhancing equity in maternal health: a review of the evidence. The Commonwealth Fund. https://www.commonwealthfund.org/publications/fund-reports/2021/nov/policies-reducing-maternal-morbidity-mortality-enhancing-equity#15. Published online November 2021. Accessed January 28, 2023.

14. US Environmental Protection Agency. Climate change and the health of pregnant, breastfeeding, and postpartum women. https://www.epa.gov/climateimpacts/climate-change-and-health-pregnant-breastfeeding-and-postpartum-women. Published December 13, 2022. Accessed January 28, 2023.

15. O'Neil SS, Platt I, Vohra D, et al. Societal cost of nine selected maternal morbidities in the United States. *PLOS One*. 2022;17(10):e0275656. https://doi.org/10.1371/journal.pone.0275656.

Chapter 2

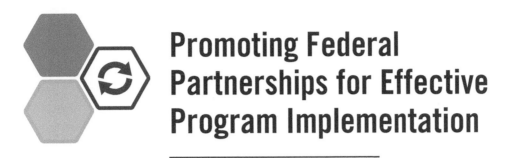

Promoting Federal Partnerships for Effective Program Implementation

CLARA E. BUSSE, SANDRA J. LLOYD, ASHLEY WILKES,
AND CATHERINE J. VLADUTIU

THE ROLE OF THE HEALTH RESOURCES AND SERVICES ADMINISTRATION IN IMPROVING MATERNAL HEALTH

Adverse maternal health outcomes in the United States are far too common. Each year, approximately 700 women die from pregnancy or delivery complications[1] and approximately 30,000 women experience severe pregnancy complications (severe maternal morbidity).[2] There are meaningful differences in rates of pregnancy-related mortality and severe maternal morbidity by sociodemographic factors, such as race and ethnicity, education, and rurality.[2,3] Recognizing that, according to the CDC, more than 80 percent of pregnancy-related deaths are considered preventable,[4] federal agencies have made considerable efforts to address this critical issue.

Situated within the US Department of Health and Human Services (HHS), the Health Resources and Services Administration (HRSA) aims to improve the health outcomes of underserved populations, including women, children, and families, and to support programs and initiatives critical to the achievement of maternal health equity. HRSA is the primary federal agency responsible for increasing access to healthcare for people who are geographically isolated and/or medically or economically vulnerable, and for strengthening the systems of care that serve them. HRSA's mission is "to improve health outcomes and achieve health equity through access to quality services, a skilled health workforce, and innovative, high-value programs."[5] To accomplish this mission, HRSA invests in programs and initiatives that foster health equity and improve access to high-quality health services. Specific to maternal health, HRSA also

Clara E. Busse, Sandra J. Lloyd, Ashley Wilkes, and Catherine J. Vladutiu, *Promoting Federal Partnerships for Effective Program Implementation* In: *The Practical Playbook III*. Edited by: Dorothy Cilenti, Alisahah Jackson, Natalie D. Hernandez, Lindsey Yates, Sarah Verbiest, J. Lloyd Michener, and Brian C. Castrucci, Oxford University Press. © de Beaumont Foundation 2024. DOI: 10.1093/oso/9780197662984.003.0002

focuses on strengthening service-delivery systems to improve maternal health at the population level, particularly among those who are at highest risk for adverse perinatal outcomes. This focus aligns with HHS's *Healthy People 2030* goal of preventing pregnancy complications and maternal deaths and improving women's health before, during, and after pregnancy.[6]

Several programs across HRSA's 11 Offices and seven Bureaus promote the health of birthing people and their pregnancies, including those that address women's preventive services, interconception care, family planning, mental health, and child/adolescent health.[5] Within HRSA, the Maternal and Child Health Bureau (MCHB) aims to improve the health and well-being of America's mothers, children, and families. In pursuit of this mission, MCHB administers programs, bolsters research, and supports workforce training.[5] Selected MCHB programs that address maternal health are described in Table 2.1.

HRSA and MCHB take a life-course approach to maternal and child health by supporting these populations across each life stage, from infancy through adulthood.[5] Life-course theory informs and motivates interventions that affect early or upstream determinants of health and the development of integrated health-service delivery systems designed to promote lifelong health.[7]

DEVELOPMENT OF GOVERNMENT-FUNDED PROGRAMS

Federal Budget and Appropriations

In recent years, there has been growing interest and support from Congress for development and enhancement of new and existing maternal health programs and activities. As a result, MCHB has received increased funding to extend current activities and to establish new investments to support maternal health. Consistent with this additional funding, MCHB also has fielded a rising number of maternal-health-focused Congressional inquiries. MCHB responds to member questions regarding specific programs, provides technical assistance on draft legislation, and delivers topical and/or programmatic briefings. These activities may inform ongoing or future legislative efforts and may improve constituent services and supports through member and staff education.

MCHB's maternal health programs are established through authorization laws passed by Congress that outline the terms and conditions under which the programs operate and authorize enactment of appropriations. (Before authorized maternal health programs can be implemented, Congress must first appropriate funding.) In most cases, appropriations are provided through the annual appropriations process (discretionary spending), although in some cases authorization law may also provide for spending directly (mandatory spending).

Table 2.1 MCHB Investments in Maternal Health*

Title V Maternal and Child Health Block Grant (Title V)	Partners with states to support the health and well-being of all mothers, children, and families and reduce maternal morbidity and mortality
Maternal, Infant, and Early Childhood Home Visiting (MIECHV)	Funds states, territories, and Tribal entities to develop and implement voluntary evidence-based home visiting programs for pregnant people and parents with young children
Healthy Start Initiative: Eliminating Disparities in Perinatal Health	Advances community-based approaches for improving health before, during, and after pregnancy and reducing racial and ethnic disparities in perinatal health
Alliance for Innovation on Maternal Health (AIM)	Develops and implements maternal safety bundles of evidence-based practices for use in hospitals and other types of birthing facility settings to reduce severe maternal illness and deaths
AIM Community Care Initiative (AIM-CCI)	Develops and implements maternal safety bundles of evidence-based practices for use in nonhospital settings to improve maternal health and address systemic inequities
State Maternal Health Innovation (State MHI)	Establishes state-focused maternal health task forces, improves state-level data surveillance on maternal mortality and severe maternal morbidity, and promotes and executes innovation in maternal health service delivery
Maternal Health Learning and Innovation Center (MHLIC)	Established a resource center that provides national guidance to HRSA award recipients, states, and key stakeholders to improve maternal health and that provides capacity-building assistance to HRSA maternal health award recipients
Screening and Treatment for Maternal Depression and Related Behavioral Disorders	Funds states to provide training and tools to frontline healthcare providers to integrate behavioral healthcare into their routine maternal healthcare through telehealth services, including real-time psychiatric consultation and care coordination
National Maternal Mental Health Hotline	Provides free, confidential support, resources, and referrals to pregnant and postpartum people and their loved ones 24/7 via phone and text
Rural Maternity and Obstetrics Management Strategies (RMOMS)**	Improves access to, and continuity of, maternal and obstetrical care in rural communities through network models
Secretary's Advisory Committee on Infant and Maternal Mortality (ACIMM)	Advises the Secretary of HHS and the Administrator of HRSA about HHS programs that are directed at reducing infant mortality and improving the health status of pregnant people and infants

*This information is current as of May 2022. For more information, visit https://mchb.hrsa.gov/programs-imp act/programs.
**The initial cohort of RMOMS grantees were funded in part by MCHB with the Federal Office of Rural Health Policy.

Administration policy is reflected in the President's budget (also called the Congressional Budget Justification), which outlines proposed funding and policies for the fiscal year. This document is presented to Congress at the beginning of the Congressional appropriations process and can influence the direction of appropriations decisions, including what programs are included and at what level of funding. For the last few years, the President's budget has included proposed increases in maternal health programs.

Conceptualizing and Designing Programs

Program Design

Designing government-funded programs and initiatives to support health across the life course is an iterative process. It often begins during the legislative and budget to provide, when MCHB may be asked technical assistance or subject matter expertise on a maternal or child health subject.

Program Purpose

Whether beginning program design as part of the budget proposal process or in follow-up to an appropriation or legislative directive, it is important to understand the primary purpose or goal of the program, which should be informed by evidence, such as data from scientific research and program evaluations. For example, a program may aim to reduce maternal mortality by increasing access to doulas, by increasing bias and antidiscrimination training among maternal healthcare providers, or by improving access to prenatal care. The purpose of a particular program is often grounded in the authorization law that establishes the program and can also be informed by language in the appropriations report.

Evidence-Informed Programs

When developing and implementing programs to promote maternal health, it is important to understand existing evidence and to identify areas of high need to inform the specific approach of a program and to achieve its purpose. This can be accomplished through extensive review and analysis of peer-reviewed literature and gray literature sources to identify promising practices. It is also important to identify target populations and geographic priority areas. HRSA has engaged in analytic efforts to identify need and geographic priority for program resources, including an interactive mapping application and a pilot initiative to develop a methodology to better target resources to populations and geographic areas with high need for maternal health services. These efforts rely on a variety of data sources, including state- and county-level data, as well as program service areas and resources. HRSA recently finalized criteria for identifying shortages of maternity care services within Health Professional Shortage

Areas.[8] The identification of these Maternity Care Health Professional Target Areas informs the placement of maternity care professionals in areas that lack access to maternal care providers.

Program Funding

Determining the appropriate level of funding and the funding structure for a program is critical to ensuring that a program can meet the identified needs. It may be reasonable to invest in more awards of fewer dollars each to expand the reach of a program depending on the program purpose, program needs, existing evidence, and target population. Alternatively, investing more dollars in a few larger awards may maximize impact in a particular area or within a target population. Assessing impact may also require funds to support data infrastructure for measuring key indicators and program evaluation for reporting on the program's progress and accomplishments. It is also important to consider costs related to program administration, including whether federal staff are needed to implement, monitor, and/or evaluate the program.

Performance Measurement

Performance measurement tracks how programs are doing over time and assesses program impact on key indicators of maternal and child health (see Figure 2.1). In the same way that understanding the evidence is one of the initial considerations in program design, selecting program performance measures that are aligned with, and representative of, the purpose and goals of a program

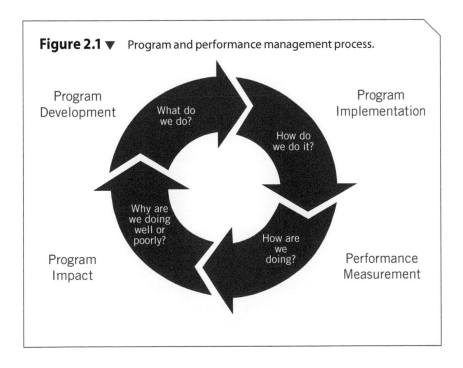

Figure 2.1 ▼ Program and performance management process.

Program Development

What do we do?

Program Implementation

How do we do it?

Why are we doing well or poorly?

How are we doing?

Program Impact

Performance Measurement

helps to ensure that the program is accomplishing its goals and contributing to the evidence base. MCHB uses different types of performance measures, such as process measures, which assess the implementation of a program, and outcome measures, which assess the impact or results of program processes. These two types of measures drive program improvement by marking progress and guiding shifts to program activities if the intended impacts are not observed.

Barriers and Challenges

There are several barriers and challenges in the development and implementation of government-funded programs, including those related to time constraints, budget cycle and appropriations, legislative authority, communication, and data limitations.

Another challenge in developing and implementing government-funded programs is the nature of the budget process and resulting appropriations. Budget formulation, appropriations, and budget execution cycles can become misaligned. The process is intended to flow in a predictably cyclical manner, with budget formulation occurring from approximately May to January, appropriations occurring February into summer, and execution beginning in October, at the start of the next fiscal year. This cycle is not often realized, however. Delays in release of the President's budget (due to a change in administration, for example) or in the appropriations decisions for a fiscal year can hinder budget execution and program implementation and thus add challenges to program planning.

The legal authority to operate a program, while necessary, can pose challenges in adapting programs over time. The legislative authority is the blueprint for a program and must be passed into law by Congress before a program can operate. These laws are typically enacted for a certain period (FY 2018 to FY 2022, for example). Over that time, Congress may modify or update the law. This often occurs as program authority nears expiration, although there are exceptions. Legislative authorities are the North Star for program development, as they often outline some of the core parameters of a program, such as the program's purpose, individuals eligible to receive funds, target population(s), and types of awards that can be used to implement the program. Until a law changes, program design must reflect this legislative language. The legislative authority can therefore limit a program's ability to adapt to changing needs in the field or populations served. For example, to support health and wellness across the life course, a program may consider modifications to address social determinants of health, including housing and transportation, to improve health outcomes at the community level. However, if the legislative authority includes limitations on the use of funds, such as prohibiting support of temporary housing for a pregnant person, then the program design is limited by those legal components. In addition, if there is an emerging need in the field but an existing legislative authority to support activities that address the need are lacking, then it may be difficult to design an appropriate program until Congress enacts a new law.

Data availability, quality, and timeliness can impede program development, especially for programs that seek to address emerging issues. HRSA and its partners may identify a new need or issue among a particular population but lack current data to support a proposal for a new program or action to address the issue. Paradoxically, the ability to gather high-quality data in a timely manner can be limited if there is not a program or system funded for collecting that data.

FEDERAL PARTNERSHIPS

Overview and Importance

A key element to effective development and implementation of HRSA programs is the establishment of federal partnerships. Through these critical connections, HRSA strengthens support of mission activities, increases program effectiveness, and maximizes impact. Partnerships can increase investment in, and support for, evidence-based interventions by sharing knowledge, experience, subject-matter expertise, and resources. Following program conceptualization and development, collaborative relationships can provide opportunities to enhance communication, strengthen efficiency, identify possible solutions to challenges encountered during implementation, and strengthen organizational capacity.

Each of HRSA's Offices and Bureaus partners with other federal entities both within and outside of HRSA's to strengthen the administration's efforts to implement more than 90 programs and support more than 3,000 grantees[6] that help tens of millions of Americans to receive high-quality, affordable healthcare and related services. Based on HRSA's mission to improve health outcomes and achieve health equity through access to high-quality services, a skilled health workforce, and innovative, high-value programs, most HRSA-funded organizations are multifaceted and may receive funding from several different federal agencies, offices, and/or Bureaus to support the programs they manage. Therefore, many of these federal entities share the same grantees.

For federally funded programs to be most effective, collaboration among partners, through either informal or formal partnerships, is essential. Federally funded grantees often work collaboratively with other grantees within the same state, region, or community. HRSA supports the establishment of partnerships among federally funded grantees and often includes collaboration as an expectation of funding to foster information- and resource-sharing and to contribute to program success.

Example of a Strong Federal Partnership

The partnership between MCHB's Division of Healthy Start and Perinatal Services and the Centers for Disease Control and Prevention's (CDC) Division of Reproductive Health to support HRSA's State Maternal Health Innovation (State MHI) program[9] and the CDC's Enhancing Reviews and Surveillance to

Eliminate Maternal Mortality (ERASE MM)[10] demonstrates the benefit of federal partnerships. Eight of the nine states that receive funding from HRSA for the State MHI program are also recipients of an ERASE MM award and share the overarching goal of reducing maternal mortality and severe maternal morbidity. The programs' activities are synergistic and a natural fit for partnership. According to the CDC, funding for ERASE MM awardees directly supports agencies and organizations that coordinate and manage maternal mortality review committees (MMRCs) to identify, review, and characterize maternal deaths and to inform development of recommendations for preventing future deaths. Each State MHI grantee has been tasked with developing a maternal health strategic plan that outlines actionable recommendations based on state-level maternal health data, including information obtained from the MMRC. They are also responsible for promoting and executing innovative strategies to address disparities in maternal health and to improve outcomes. Federal staff within both entities work closely to share ideas, resources, and technical assistance in support of the State MHI and ERASE MM programs. They are joined by staff from the Maternal Health Learning and Innovation Center, which is also a recipient of HRSA funding and provides direct capacity-building assistance to State MHI grantees.

Additional Considerations for Partnerships

Federal partnerships are most beneficial when initiated at the point of program conceptualization. Forming partnerships early in the creation of new programs can minimize the potential for duplicative, conflicting, or competitive program activities and can avoid overburdening grantees who already experience the challenges of meeting funding expectations. Early collaboration also provides opportunities, when applicable, for federal entities to incorporate expectations within funding opportunities for recipients to establish collaborative relationships with the federal partner's grantees.

Federal partners also can collaborate to provide capacity-building technical assistance for grantees throughout program implementation. Federal agencies and their grantees can benefit from networking, participating in joint technical assistance activities, copresenting at national conferences, and potentially cohosting grantee meetings. In addition, sharing evaluation findings and best practices among federal partners and their grantees may strengthen opportunities for new program development through the expansion of existing concepts and may intensify sustainability efforts of effective programs, which are successes for all those involved.

CONCLUSION

HRSA invests in programs and initiatives that increase access to healthcare and strengthen systems of care for people who are geographically isolated and medically or economically vulnerable. Improving maternal health outcomes and achieving maternal health equity are directly aligned with HRSA's mission and are at the core of MCHB's work.

Congressional interest in maternal health has grown in recent years. To support legislative efforts related to maternal health, MCHB has conducted briefings on maternal health, responded to congressional inquiries, and provided technical assistance on draft legislation to create or to amend laws authorizing maternal health programs as well as laws to appropriate funding for such programs. Program design must always begin with an understanding of the primary purpose or goal of the program as informed by evidence, followed by careful consideration of the target population and geographic priority areas for the program. MCHB then designs and implements a performance measurement strategy aligned with the program's goals.

Once Congress has authorized and funded maternal health programs, federal partnerships are critical to program development and implementation. Strong partnerships can create efficiencies across complementary programs to ease burden on grantees and strengthen organizational capacity. Ongoing partnerships between the CDC and HRSA showcase the power of collaboration and complementary maternal health programming.

DISCLAIMER

The views expressed in this publication are solely the opinions of the authors and do not necessarily reflect the official policies of the US Department of Health and Human Services or the Health Resources and Services Administration, nor does mention of the department or agency names imply endorsement by the US Government.

REFERENCES

1. Petersen EE, Davis NL, Goodman D, et al. Vital signs: pregnancy-related deaths, United States, 2011–2015, and strategies for prevention, 13 states, 2013–2017. *MMWR*. 2019;68:423–429.

2. HCUP Fast Stats. Severe maternal morbidity (SMM) among in-hospital deliveries. https://www.hcup-us.ahrq.gov/faststats/SMMServlet. Accessed March 20, 2022.

3. US Department of Health and Human Services. *Healthy Women, Healthy Pregnancies, Healthy Futures: The U.S. Department of Health and Human Services' Action Plan to Improve Maternal Health in America*. 2020. https://aspe.hhs.gov/system/files/aspe-files/264076/healthy-women-healthy-pregnancies-healthy-future-action-plan_0.pdf. Accessed April 2, 2022.

4. Trost SL, Beauregard J, Njie F, et al. *Pregnancy-Related Deaths: Data from Maternal Mortality Review Committees in 36 US States, 2017–2019*. Atlanta, GA: Centers for Disease Control and Prevention, US Department of Health and Human Services; 2022. Accessed October 2023.

5. Health Resources and Services Administration. About HRSA. https://www.hrsa.gov/about/index.html. Accessed March 20, 2022.

6. US Department of Health and Human Services. *Healthy People 2030: Pregnancy and Childbirth*. https://health.gov/healthypeople/objectives-and-data/browse-objectives/pregnancy-and-childbirth. Accessed March 20, 2022.

7. Fine A, Kotelchuck M. Rethinking MCH: the life course model as an organizing framework. https://unnaturalcauses.org/assets/uploads/file/Rethinking%20MCH%20-Fine.pdf. Published November 2010. Accessed October 23, 2023.

8. Federal Register Notice. Criteria for Determining Maternity Care Health Professional Target Areas. https://mchb.hrsa.gov/programs-impact/programs/state-mhi. Accessed October 23, 2023.

9. Health Resources and Services Administration. State maternal health innovation program. https://www.hrsa.gov/grants/find-funding/hrsa-19-107. Accessed March 20, 2022.

10. Centers for Disease Control and Prevention. *Enhancing Reviews and Surveillance to Eliminate Maternal Mortality (ERASE MM)*. Atlanta, GA: Centers for Disease Control and Prevention. https://www.cdc.gov/reproductivehealth/maternal-mortality/erase-mm/index.html. Accessed October 23, 2023.

Chapter 3

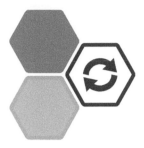

How Academic Centers Can Accelerate Partnerships and Progress in Maternal Health

ALISON M. STUEBE

Maternal health encompasses the lived experience of each of us—many of us have been parents, many more have been aunts, uncles, siblings, and friends of birthing people, and all of us have been babies. The communities we create (or disrupt) determine whether birthing people suffer, survive, or thrive. Thus, to the extent that colleges, universities, and academic centers seek to understand and improve the human condition, they seek to understand and improve maternal health.

The Society for Maternal-Fetal Medicine has created an infographic to illustrate the differences between equality, equity, and justice (Figure 3.1). When equal care is provided, the person who is standing on higher ground can see over the fence, but the person standing on lower ground cannot. Importantly, it is the structure—the ground—that differs, not the people, because it is social position and circumstances, not inherent characteristics, that produce disparate outcomes. In the second panel, equity is provided by tailored supports—extra blocks—that allow the people on lower ground to see over the fence. However, the ultimate goal is not equity, but justice, where each individual is able to achieve their full potential.

Justice in maternal health is manifested in reproductive justice. The concept of reproductive justice was conceived by a group of Black women in 1994,[1] and it comprises: The right to bodily autonomy, the right not to have a child, the right to have a child, and the right to raise that child in a safe and healthy environment.

Academic centers can advance reproductive justice, and thereby maternal health, on multiple levels, from clinical care of individuals to scholarship that critiques and creates cultural norms. This chapter applies a socioecological

Alison M. Stuebe, *How Academic Centers Can Accelerate Partnerships and Progress in Maternal Health* In: *The Practical Playbook III*. Edited by: Dorothy Cilenti, Alisahah Jackson, Natalie D. Hernandez, Lindsey Yates, Sarah Verbiest, J. Lloyd Michener, and Brian C. Castrucci, Oxford University Press. © de Beaumont Foundation 2024. DOI: 10.1093/oso/9780197662984.003.0003

Figure 3.1 ▼
Health equity, defined.

Source: Society for Maternal-Fetal Medicine and National Birth Equity Collaborative. Used with permission.

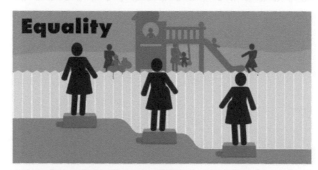

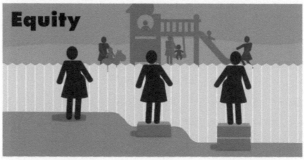

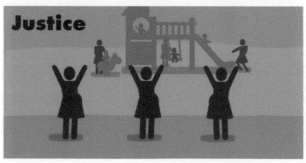

model (Figure 3.2) to outline the many ways that academic centers can accelerate progress in maternal health, from individual-level patient care to scholarship and society, and the discussion includes examples of innovative programs and policies at multiple institutions.

Figure 3.2 ▼

A socioecological model for the role of academic centers in advancing reproductive justice.

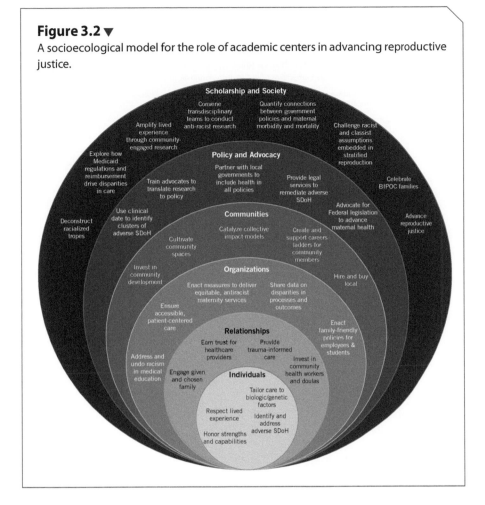

ACADEMIC MEDICAL CENTERS AND COMMUNITY BENEFITS

Currently, the community role of academic medical centers (AMCs) is changing. Nonprofit hospitals are required to provide specific community benefits in exchange for their tax-exempt status (Figure 3.3); however, community benefits are not explicitly defined, and a recent GAO report called for congressional legislation to clarify what activities constitute community benefits.[2]

Providing care for uninsured patients is a required community benefit, but there is wide variation among centers. A Health Affairs analysis found that nonprofit hospitals spent only $2.30 of every $100 in total expenses on charity care, compared to $4.10 spent by government hospitals and $3.80 spent by for-profit hospitals.[3]

More fundamentally, there is a growing appreciation that solutions to intractable problems of racism, inequality, and preventable morbidity and mortality require more than provision of acute care for the underinsured. For

Figure 3.3 ▼

Requirements for nonprofit hospitals to obtain and maintain a tax exemption.

Source: US Government Accountability Office. Tax Administration: Opportunities Exist to Improve Oversight of Hospitals' Tax-Exempt Status. GAO-20-679. Public domain.

Requirements for Nonprofit Hospitals to Obtain and Maintain a Tax Exemption
ORGANIZATIONAL AND OPERATIONAL REQUIREMENTS A hospital must be organized and operate to achieve a charitable purpose—the promotion of health for the benefit of the community.
COMMUNITY BENEFITS Internal Revenue Service has identified six factors that demonstrate community benefit: • Operate an emergency room open to all, regardless of ability to pay • Maintain a board of directors drawn from the community • Maintain an open medical staff policy • Provide care to all patients able to pay, including those who do so through Medicare and Medicaid • Use surplus funds to improve facilities, equipment, and patient care • Use surplus funds to advance medical training, education, and research
PATIENT PROTECTION AND AFFORDABLE CARE ACT (PPACA) REQUIREMENTS Hospitals must: • Conduct a community health needs assessment   • Set a limit on charges • Maintain a written financial assistance policy   • Set billing and collection limits
IRS must review each tax-exempt hospital's community benefit activities at least once every 3 years.

AMCs to address these issues, they will need to move beyond their traditional community-service role to engage communities as partners. As Wilkins and Alberti wrote:

> An enterprise-wide approach to community engagement will require reconsideration of communities, moving from viewing them as people or groups in need of service to seeing them as assets who can help AHCs better understand and address social determinants of health, enhance students' and trainees' ability to provide care, and increase the relevance and potential impact of research discoveries.[4]

By engaging community members and other stakeholders as partners with unique strengths, wisdom, and lived experience, AMCs can be part of transformative solutions to improve health and well-being for every birthing person.

INDIVIDUALS

Teaching hospitals care for 43% of the people who give birth each year in the United States.[5] The care provided shapes a family's experience during a pivotal life event. Ideally, maternity providers center care on the birthing person, honoring their strengths and capabilities, respecting lived experience, and identifying and addressing biological and social vulnerabilities. For many birthing people, pregnancy and childbirth are their first significant interaction with the healthcare system, making this a powerful opportunity to build trust. If birthing people feel seen, heard, and valued, they will carry that sense of agency with them to their own care, as well as the care of their children and their extended family. Conversely, if they experience marginalization and institutional betrayal, pregnancy and birth will estrange them from the healthcare system, to the detriment of their community, their families, and the healthcare system.

RELATIONSHIPS

Adverse lived experiences have caused many individuals to distrust the healthcare system. To remediate these adverse experiences, academic centers can invest in proven strategies to foster positive relationships and to earn trust during maternity care. Pregnancy and birth grow families, underscoring the importance of including given and chosen family members in prenatal care, birth, and postpartum services. Training in trauma-informed care and emotional support[6] enables team members to build rapport with patients. In addition, academic centers can fund community health workers and doulas on maternity care teams, approaches that have been shown to improve pregnancy outcomes.[7-9] Academic centers can foster these relationships by ensuring that birthing and postpartum rooms include comfortable spaces for given and chosen family, by funding staff time and costs for trauma-informed training, and by financing living wage salaries and benefits for doulas and community health workers as integral members of the healthcare team.

ORGANIZATIONS

Academic centers provide clinical care and education, and they are also major employers and purchasers in their communities. They can affect maternal health through all of these roles.

Clinical Care

As organizations, academic centers make decisions that can foster or derail conditions for trustworthy care. In many academic centers, Medicaid-insured patients are cared for in prenatal clinics staffed by physicians-in-training. This stratified care exists in part due to differences in billing for hospital-based clinics: in hospital-based clinics, Medicaid pays a facility fee, in addition to a professional fee, which increases reimbursement for prenatal care. For commercially insured patients, the facility fee is an additional out-of-pocket cost, so commercially insured patients typically prefer to be seen in separate, physician-based clinics. Writing in the *New England Journal of Medicine*, Kavita Vinekar challenged this model[10]:

> If our academic institutions and hospital systems truly support Black Lives—if they seek to be antiracist and to address implicit biases, and if they are serious about addressing racial healthcare inequities—they will start by desegregating their own training hospitals. Segregation is not a billing thing. It's a systemic racism thing.

Medicaid-regulated care also creates intrusions into women's privacy and autonomy, as anthropologist and lawyer Khiara Bridges wrote in *Reproducing Race: An Ethnography of Pregnancy as a Site of Racialization*.[11] She described the lengthy, inefficient experience of initiating prenatal care at "Alpha Women's Health Clinic," a pseudonym for a New York City public hospital:

> It communicates to women that their time is not highly valued; the exorbitant length of the PCAP [Prenatal Care Assistance Program] day, and the excessive waiting periods that can be expected more generally within the Alpha WHC, abundantly demonstrate the state's conception of their time as being something utterly negligible.

Desegregating clinical care is necessary, but not sufficient, to provide trustworthy care. Zoë Julian and colleagues contrasted physician-centered models of perinatal and reproductive healthcare delivery with community-centered informed models,[12] which shift the goal of care from clinical health risk mitigation to the pursuit of social justice, liberation, and collective autonomy and self-determination in care experiences. Group prenatal care is one promising model for community-centered care: in their article on the EleVATE group prenatal care model, physician Ebony Carter and colleagues describe how interactions between centering patients and providers build empathy and diminish bias.[13] To improve maternal health outcomes, academic centers can invest in accessible, person-first models of maternity care.

Centers can also build trust by partnering with community-led organizations to evaluate patient experiences and to enact measures to deliver equitable, antiracist maternity services.

- In Cincinnati, Ohio, a community-developed initiative, Mama Certified, has engaged with health systems in Hamilton County. Participating systems will be assessed on infant care, maternal care, staff care, and community care, and progress and results disaggregated by race will be made publicly available to the community.
- Birthing Cultural Rigor, LLC, offers a measurement, monitoring, and accountability program, working with institutions to recognize and mitigate obstetric racism (https://www.phi.org/our-work/programs/birthing-cultural-rigor-llc/).

- "Irth, Birth, but we dropped the B for Bias," is a "Yelp-like" platform that invites reviews of providers, hospitals, and health systems. The team works with institutions to respond to qualitative reviews with actionable strategies for providing more respectful and equitable care to birthing people of color (https://irthapp.com).

Education and Training

Progress in maternal health requires inclusive, antiracist medical education and training. Structural racism and classism have long been embedded in obstetrics and gynecology, and intentional strategies are needed to address and undo racism in medical education. A team of medical educators at the Icahn School of Medicine at Mount Sinai led a multiyear change management process to "become a health system and health professions school with the most diverse workforce, providing healthcare and education that is free of racism and bias."[14] This work has grown into a three-year collaborative for antiracist transformation in medical education, including 11 medical schools in the United States and Canada.[15] The scope of this work underscores the need for academic centers to support transformative efforts in undergraduate and graduate medical education.

The Icahn School of Medicine initiative includes multiple strategies to recruit and retain groups that are underrepresented in medicine (URiM). For postgraduate training, a recent survey of residency program directors in obstetrics and gynecology found that more concrete support from medical schools and hospitals was needed to recruit and retain URiMs.[16]

Human Resources for Health Equity

As major employers in their communities, academic centers impact health and well-being for thousands of workers. To improve maternal health and enable safe transitions to parenthood, it will be essential for human resource policies and practice to include paid sick days, paid parental leave, flexible work conditions, and affordable, accessible child care.[17] For example, Vanderbilt University Medical Center's Racial Equity Task Force identified multiple opportunities to advance equity through investment in employee career development, health, and well-being.[18]

COMMUNITY

The major drivers of maternal health outcomes are social circumstances (15%), environmental exposures (5%), and behavioral patterns (40%).[19] To improve maternal health, academic centers must extend their work outside of the health system to engage communities in transformative solutions.

Economic Development

Because healthcare organizations are often anchor employers in their communities, their employment and procurement policies are powerful levers for community development. The Build Healthy Places Network and the National Alliance of Community Economic Development Associations (NACEDA) have identified five collaborative strategies for community–healthcare partnerships[20]: training and career pathways, support for local entrepreneurs, health facility development and financing, healthy food access and food sovereignty, and leveraging assets from health institutions.

For example, in the Clark-Fulton neighborhood of Cleveland, Ohio, MetroHealth partnered with MetroWest, a community economic development organization, and the Cleveland Foundation to codevelop a master plan, using the EcoDistrict protocol for sustainable development. MetroHealth has partnered with a local community college to offer free education and career planning. This career development work complements the existing partnership with Lincoln-West School of Science and Health at MetroHealth, which complements a traditional curriculum with interactive learning in a healthcare setting.[15]

Major academic centers in urban areas have implemented anchor institution strategies to hire and buy local. In 2015, Johns Hopkins University in Baltimore launched HopkinsLocal, a commitment to purchase from local minority and woman-owned business enterprises (MWBE), to recruit from focus areas in Baltimore, and to hire justice-involved individuals.[21] From FY 2019 to FY 2021, the institution committed $41.8 million to contractors who were minority-owned, women-owned, or disadvantaged business enterprises, hired 1,448 people living in focus ZIP Codes, and spent $406.8 million at local businesses. In San Francisco, the University of California, San Francisco Anchor Institution Initiative sought to determine how the University might leverage workforce development, procurement, and community investment, with the goal of advancing health equity in San Francisco.[22]

Nationally, the Healthcare Anchor Network "convenes health systems in order to share best practices for advancing an anchor mission approach within their health institutions, address common challenges, codevelop new tools, and identify areas where collaborative efforts may be possible." For example, 12 health systems in the Network pledged to increase spending with MWBE by $1 billion by 2025 as part of a commitment to supplier diversity, sustainability, and community wealth-building.[23]

These anchor institution programs have the potential to build a more diverse workforce with lived experience in the surrounding community, as well as to increase wealth and economic security, addressing a root cause of adverse maternal health outcomes.

Collective Impact Models

Growing evidence supports collective impact models as a highly effective strategy for addressing complex social problems. Collective impact is defined as "a network of community members, organizations, and institutions that advance equity by learning together, aligning and integrating their actions to achieve population and systems-level change."[24] In a recent paper in the *Stanford Social Innovation Review*, John Kania and colleagues described key strategies to center equity in collective impact work:

1. Ground the work in data and context, and target solutions.
2. Focus on systems change, in addition to programs and services.
3. Shift power within the collaborative.
4. Listen to, and act with, the community.
5. Build equity leadership and accountability.

Academic centers are uniquely situated to accelerate partnerships and progress in maternal health by enabling collective impact work. For example, Cradle Cincinnati[25,26] uses a collective impact framework to engage community, academic, and healthcare stakeholders in Hamilton County to reduce infant mortality. In the past five years, infant deaths have declined 15%, including a 17% reduction in extreme preterm births and a 25% decline in sleep-related deaths. The collaborative's "About Us" Web page outlines these accomplishments, and it also includes a section called "Our Failures," candidly sharing lessons learned through their decade of work.

Cradle Cincinnati is changing the narrative through initiatives like Queens Village.[27] Queens Village is "a supportive community of powerful Black women who come together to relax, repower and take care of ourselves and each other." Organized around a theoretical framework of fostering a sense of community, Queens Village holds village meetings, wellness workshops, and neighborhood gatherings. Their work actively transforms narratives: In a collaborative empowerment art project, ten artists shared their stories at the Contemporary Arts Center in an exhibit titled "FIERCE: Black MotHERstory."[28]

Moreover, Queens Village "has been intentional about giving power to Black women where power did not exist." When Ohio Medicaid sought to fund community agencies to address infant mortality, Queens Village convened an advisory board to determine how best to allocate funds. Queens Village's work has coincided with a 24% reduction in the infant mortality rate (IMR) in Hamilton County. Knox-Kazimierczuk et al noted, "While there are numerous factors that impact IMR, community building can be an effective approach to address intractable multidimensional sociocultural problems."

POLICY AND ADVOCACY

Along with community-engaged innovations, academic centers can leverage clinical data to identify clusters of adverse health outcomes and use the data to advocate for solutions. In 2015, Dr. Mona Hanna-Attisha, a pediatrician at Hurley Hospital in Flint, Michigan, used the health system's electronic health record (EHR) data to detect a marked increase in elevated lead levels in children less than 5 years old after the city switched its water supply from Detroit to the Flint River.[29] In an interview with NPR,[30] Hanna-Attisha said, "We also know that it's a form of environmental racism. . . . The burden of lead does not fall equally on our nation's children. Poor kids, Black and brown kids, communities of color are disproportionately shouldering the burden of lead poisoning and other environmental contaminants."

Hanna-Attisha's work demonstrates how AMCs can aggregate individual-level data to identify and address community-level drivers of disease. Routine screening for social determinants of health can also inform advocacy and policy. In Cincinnati, a medical-legal partnership used pediatric clinic screening data to identify patterns of housing risk associated with a single developer and successfully advocated for mitigation of pest infestation.[31] Embedding legal advocacy in a pediatric clinic reduced asthma hospitalizations by 69.7%.[32]

In maternity care, legal advocacy is a promising strategy for navigating employment, particularly in high-risk pregnancies that may require multiple appointments and accommodations. Sarahn Wheeler and colleagues found that employed women described "negative situations that ranged from challenging to potentially unlawful." Based on these findings, the team is collaborating with the Duke Health Justice Clinic to develop training and educational materials.[33] Embedded legal services can address individual patient needs, and they can also identify patterns of unjust practice for remediation.

Academic centers can partner with local government to address systems-level drivers of health inequity. In Richmond, California, a Health in All Policies ordinance was enacted in 2014. Berkeley's Center for Global Healthy Cities[34] has partnered with Richmond to evaluate outcomes and codevelop future strategies,[35] demonstrating how academic–community partnerships can improve health.

More broadly, academic centers can train advocates to translate research to policy. At UCSF, the Program on Reproductive Health and the Environment conducts translational research, and from 2010 to 2016, the program ran the Reach the Decision Makers program, a year-long fellowship that trained 152 fellows in environmental policy and advocacy.[36] A recommendation from the first Reach cohort to install particulate monitors near roadways with heavy traffic was incorporated into new National Ambient Air Quality Standard rules. The program illustrates how academic centers can facilitate translation of research on systemic risk factors for poor health outcomes into lasting policy change.

Academic centers can also advocate for national policies that support maternal health.

The Momnibus[37] is a package of key legislation to improve maternal health that has been endorsed by more than 250 organizations, including America's Essential Hospitals, the Federation of American Hospitals, and the Illinois Health and Hospital Association. Academic centers can play a key role in advancing this legislation by advocating for these measures with their members of Congress.

SOCIETY AND SCHOLARSHIP

Through scholarship and education, academic centers shape crucial narratives around maternal roles and responsibilities in public health, social work, law, sociology, anthropology, literature, and more. These narratives can celebrate the diversity of ways that families form and grow, or they can contribute to the hierarchy of human value that is currently embodied in unjust health and social policies (Box 3.1).

To spur reproductive justice, colleges, universities, and academic centers can create spaces to convene scholars who are actively rewriting the narrative. For example, at the University of Minnesota, Rachel Hardeman leads the Center for Antiracism Research for Health Equity. The Center aims to move from racist research questions (such as "What's wrong with people of color that makes them die younger and at higher rates, and suffer more illness?") to antiracist questions that ask, "How do systems, policies, and social structures combine to create the conditions for poor health?"[37]

Academic centers can advance maternal health by convening scholars from multiple disciplines. Across the country, scholars in law, anthropology, government, urban studies, and literature are engaged in formative work to transform maternal health. Box 3.2 gives examples of scholarship that illustrate how a pandisciplinary approach can complement and strengthen partnerships to advance maternal health and reproductive justice.

The movement for reproductive justice requires a rethinking of our roles and responsibilities in the human community. At Berkeley, The Othering & Belonging Institute frames health equity within the structural formations of society. The Institute notes that othering excludes some groups from the circle of human concern. The remedy, argues Institute director john a. powell, is targeted universalism.[38] Targeted universalism sets an overarching goal and recognizes that different groups will need different interventions to reach that goal, depending on their position and lived experience. As john a. powell and Eloy Toppin wrote:

Box 3.1 | How a Case Series Created the Crack Baby Panic and Fueled Mass Incarceration

A 1985 study in the *New England Journal of Medicine* described 23 pregnancies affected by cocaine use[i] and introduced the concept of "crack babies" into social discourse.[ii] Media coverage vilified women with substance use disorder, leading to punitive policies with long-lasting adverse effects on birthing people. Subsequent research debunked the concept that cocaine caused long-term harm. In an essay in *The Atlantic*, journalist Vann R. Newkirk II outlined how the downstream effects of the "crack baby" panic contributed to the 1994 crime bill and mass incarceration:

> Even in 1990, legal reviews and lawsuits found that state and local prosecutors were basically inventing statues [statutes] and offenses out of whole cloth in order to imprison mothers who gave birth while addicted to drugs. Authorities in most states, instead of crafting public-health interventions and bolstering safety nets to combat drugs, simply leveraged the threat of incarceration or child removal against mothers. And, of course, lingering fears about the coming crack baby and "super predator" generation gave the country laws that disproportionately incarcerated Black people, like the 1994 Crime Bill, which passed with massive margins, public approval, and bipartisan support.[iii]

As Oritz and Briggs explained,[iv] the crack baby panic reflects decades of discussion about intergenerational poverty:

> We argue that through these discourses, a biologically suspect and racialized US "underclass" was produced through a description of kinds of reproduction and childhood in a way that rendered its members— and particularly its children—intrinsically pathological and completely irredeemable.

The crack baby panic underscores the need for academic centers to frame research findings with care and to partner with communities to craft solutions.

References

i. Chasnoff IJ, Burns WJ, Schnoll SH, Burns KA. Cocaine use in pregnancy. *N Engl J Med*. 1985;313(11):666–669. doi:10.1056/NEJM198509123131105.

ii. *Retro Report. Crack Babies: A Tale From the Drug Wars* [video]. *New York Times*. https://www.nytimes.com/video/booming/100000002226828/crack-babies-a-tale-from-the-drug-wars.html. Accessed February 17, 2022.

iii. Newkirk VR. What the 'crack baby' panic reveals about the opioid epidemic. *The Atlantic*. 2017.

iv. Ortiz AT, Briggs L. The culture of poverty, crack babies, and welfare cheats: the making of the "healthy white baby crisis." *Soc Text*. 2003;21(3):39–57.

Box 3.2 | Pan-Disciplinary Scholarship in Maternal Health and Reproductive Justice

Khiara Bridges, professor of law at the University of California, Berkeley, has dual training in anthropology and law. Her dissertation, "Reproducing Race: An Ethnography of Pregnancy as a Site of Racialization," analyzes the marginalizing experiences of publicly funded maternity care. More recently, she criticized the Preventing Maternal Deaths Act, noting that the word *race* does not appear in the text of the statute, and that the legislation is limited to gathering more information about pregnancy-related deaths. She wrote, "We already know why women are dying, and we already know how to save them. In this way, the tragedy of maternal mortality in the United States is not a problem of information; it is a problem of political will."[i]

Dorothy Roberts, George A. Weiss University Professor of Law and Sociology and the Raymond Pace and Sadie Tanner Mossell Alexander Professor of Civil Rights at the University of Pennsylvania, introduced stratified reproduction into public discourse with her 1997 book, *Killing the Black Body: Race, Reproduction, and the Meaning of Liberty.*[ii]

Jamila Michener, associate professor of government at Cornell University and codirector of the Cornell Center for Health Equity, studies the politics, causes, and consequences of poverty and racial inequity and recently published an issue brief, "A Racial Equity Framework for Assessing Health Policy,"[iii] a framework that can inform actors working to improve maternal health.

Tina Sacks, associate professor at UC Berkeley's School of Social Welfare, studies racial inequities in health, social determinants of health, and poverty and inequality. Her book, *Invisible Visits: Black Middle-Class Women in the American Healthcare System,*[iv] describes the persistent and pernicious stereotypes that women of color navigate when they access healthcare.

Dána-Ain Davis is a professor of urban studies at Queens College and director of the Center for the Study of Women and Society at the Graduate Center. In her book, *Reproductive Injustice: Racism, Pregnancy and Prematurity,*[v] she noted that "there has never been a time when Black women's reproduction was treated respectfully in the United States," and she described how mythologies of "strong Black babies" contribute to inferior care.

Loretta Ross is one of co-creators of reproductive justice and an associate professor of the study of women and gender at Smith College. Her book, *Reproductive Justice: An Introduction,*[vi] is a powerful primer for academic center leaders, faculty, and staff seeking to advance maternal health.

Kimberly C. Harper is an associate professor of English at North Carolina Agricultural and Technical State University who researches Black maternal health and ethos. Her book, *The Ethos of Black Motherhood in America: Only White Women Get Pregnant,*[vii] places the current Black maternal health crises within the disregard for Black reproduction that dates back to chattel slavery.

Box 3.2 | Continued

References

i.   Bridges KMB. Racial disparities in maternal mortality. *N Y Univ Law Rev.* 2020;95(5):1229–1318.

ii. Roberts DE. *Killing the Black Body: Race, Reproduction, and the Meaning of Liberty.* New York, NY: Pantheon Books; 1997.

iii. Michener J. A racial equity framework for assessing health policy. 2022. https://doi.org/10.26099/ej0b-6g71.

iv. Sacks TK. *Invisible Visits: Black Middle-Class Women in the American Healthcare System.* New York, NY: Oxford University Press; 2019.

v.   Davis D. *Reproductive Injustice: Racism, Pregnancy, and Premature Birth.* New York, NY: NYU Press; 2019.

v.   Ross L, Solinger R. *Reproductive Justice: An Introduction.* Oakland: University of California Press; 2017.

vi. Harper KC. *The Ethos of Black Motherhood in America: Only White Women Get Pregnant.* Lanham, MD: Lexington Books; 2020.

Targeted universalism also shifts the narrative of othering and belonging away from a disparities-based strategy for extending the boundary of human concern. When a disparities-based approach is taken, groups are measured against a normalized group—generally whites in the US context. A disparities-based approach also tends to stigmatize othered groups because the underlying issue of a lack of belonging for certain populations goes unaddressed. When groups do not belong and are seen as the other, a sense of undeservingness is associated with them.[38]

Academic centers can improve health and well-being for birthing families by actively working to extend the boundary of concern with strategies that span the continuum from individuals to scholarship and society.

CONCLUSION

AMCs, universities, and colleges are uniquely positioned to engage with communities to transform the lived experience of pregnancy, birth, and parenting. Such transformation requires the academy to rethink long-standing patterns. As Park and colleagues wrote,

> Current approaches to academic–community partnerships traditionally focus on service and outreach opportunities (e.g., patient advisory councils, temporary grant-funded programs) that could disproportionately benefit Academic Health Centers (AHCs), and these approaches have not consistently yielded sustainable or replicable solutions. Our strategies for

building academic–community health systems restore bidirectional benefits for AHCs and communities, minimizing the perpetuation of existing disparities through inclusive hiring practices, learning and applying inequity-responsive mindsets, and incorporating community agendas in research.[19]

By engaging communities as true partners, with humility and deep respect for individual lived experience, academic centers can improve health across generations.

REFERENCES

1. Ross L, Solinger R. *Reproductive Justice: An Introduction*. Oakland: University of California Press; 2017.

2. Lucas-Judy J. Tax Administration: Opportunities Exist to Improve Oversight of Hospitals' *Tax-Exempt Status*. Washington, DC: US Government Accountability Office; 2020:35. https://www.gao.gov/products/gao-20-679.

3. Bai G, Zare H, Eisenberg MD, Polsky D, Anderson GF. Analysis suggests government and nonprofit hospitals' charity care is not aligned with their favorable tax treatment. *Health Aff (Millwood)*. 2021;40(4):629–636. doi:10.1377/hlthaff.2020.01627.

4. Wilkins CH, Alberti PM. Shifting academic health centers from a culture of community service to community engagement and integration. *Acad Med*. 2019;94(6):763–767. doi:10.1097/ACM.0000000000002711.

5. Handley SC, Passarella M, Herrick HM, et al. Birth volume and geographic distribution of US hospitals with obstetric services from 2010 to 2018. *JAMA Netw Open*. 2021;4(10):e2125373. doi:10.1001/jamanetworkopen.2021.25373.

6. Hall S, White A, Ballas J, Saxton SN, Dempsey A, Saxer K. Education in trauma-informed care in maternity settings can promote mental health during the COVID-19 pandemic. *J Obstet Gynecol Neonatal Nurs*. 2021;50(3):340–351. doi:10.1016/j.jogn.2020.12.005.

7. Thomas MP, Ammann G, Brazier E, Noyes P, Maybank A. Doula services within a Healthy Start program: increasing access for an underserved population. *Matern Child Health J*. 2017;21(suppl 1):59–64. doi:10.1007/s10995-017-2402-0.

8. Attanasio LB, DaCosta M, Kleppel R, Govantes T, Sankey HZ, Goff SL. Community perspectives on the creation of a hospital-based doula program. *Health Equity*. 2021;5(1):545–553. doi:10.1089/heq.2020.0096.

9. Mottl-Santiago J, Herr K, Rodrigues D, Walker C, Walker C, Feinberg E. The Birth Sisters Program: a model of hospital-based doula support to promote health equity. *J Health Care Poor Underserved*. 2020;31(1):43–55. doi:10.1353/hpu.2020.0007.

10. Vinekar K. Pathology of racism—a call to desegregate teaching hospitals. *N Engl J Med*. 2021;385(13):e40. doi:10.1056/NEJMpv2113508.

11. Bridges KM. *Reproducing race: an ethnography of pregnancy as a site of racialization*. Berkeley: University of California Press; 2011.

12. Julian Z, Robles D, Whetstone S, et al. Community-informed models of perinatal and reproductive health services provision: a justice-centered paradigm toward equity among Black birthing communities. *Semin Perinatol*. 2020;44(5):151267. doi:10.1016/j.semperi.2020.151267.

13. Carter EB, Ele VWC, Mazzoni SE. A paradigm shift to address racial inequities in perinatal healthcare. *Am J Obstet Gynecol*. 2021;224(4):359–361. doi:10.1016/j.ajog.2020.11.040.

14. Hess L, Palermo AG, Muller D. Addressing and undoing racism and bias in the medical school learning and work environment. *Acad Med*. 2020;95(12S):S44–S50. doi:10.1097/ACM.0000000000003706.

15. Icahn School of Medicine at Mount Sinai. Anti-racist transformation in medical education. https://icahn.mssm.edu/education/medical/anti-racist-transformation. March 5, 2022.

16. Mendiola M, Modest AM, Huang GC. An inside look: qualitative study of underrepresented in medicine recruitment strategies used by OB-GYN program directors. *J Surg Educ*. 2022;79(2):383–388. doi:10.1016/j.jsurg.2021.10.013.

17. North Carolina Early Childhood Foundation. Family Forward NC. https://familyforwardnc.com.

18. Wilkins CH, Williams M, Kaur K, DeBaun MR. Academic medicine's journey toward racial equity must be grounded in history: recommendations for becoming an antiracist academic medical center. *Acad Med*. 2021;96(11):1507–1512. Doi:10.1097/ACM.0000000000004374.

19. Park H, Roubal AM, Jovaag A, Gennuso KP, Catlin BB. Relative contributions of a set of health factors to selected health outcomes. *Am J Prev Med*. 2015;49(6):961–969. doi:10.1016/j.amepre.2015.07.016.

20. Dailey C, Flynn C, Penfield S, Thomas-Squance R, Woodruff F. *Community Economic Development & Healthcare Playbook*. Build Healthy Places Network, based in San Francisco, CA; 2021. https://buildhealthyplaces.org/tools-resources/community-economic-development-healthcare-playbook/.

21. Johns Hopkins Health System. HopkinsLocal. https://hopkinslocal.jhu.edu. Accessed March 6, 2022.

22. Pinderhughes R, Bui A, Alexander B, King B, McCaffrey E, Onda T. *Advancing Health Equity in San Francisco: An Assessment of UCSF's Anchor Institution Capacity and Recommendations for Strategic Direction*. University of California, San Francisco based in San Francisco, CA; 2019. https://anchor.ucsf.edu/report.

23. Healthcare Anchor Network. Impact Purchasing Commitment. June 9, 2021. https://healthcareanchor.network/2021/06/impact-purchasing-commitment-ipc/. Accessed March 6, 2022.

24. Kania J, Williams J, Schmitz P, Brady S, Kramer M, Juster JS. Centering equity in collective impact. *Stanf Soc Innov Rev*. 2021;20(1):38–45. doi:10.48558/RN5M-CA77.

25. Cradle Cincinnati. https://www.cradlecincinnati.org/. Accessed February 17, 2022.

26. Healthy People 2020. Partnering to reduce infant mortality in Cincinnati. Stories from the Field [blog]. February 17, 2017. https://www.healthypeople.gov/2020/healthy-people-in-action/story/partnering-to-reduce-infant-mortality-in-cincinnati.

27. Knox-Kazimierczuk F, Andavarapu D, Shockley-Smith M. Addressing Black infant mortality through harnessing the power of community. *Health Promot Pract*. 2021:15248399211062246. doi:10.1177/15248399211062246.

28. FIERCE: Black MotHERstory. https://www.fierceblackmotherstory.com. Accessed February 17, 2022.

29. Hanna-Attisha M, LaChance J, Sadler RC, Champney Schnepp A. Elevated blood lead levels in children associated with the Flint drinking water crisis: a spatial analysis of risk and public health response. *Am J Public Health*. 2016;106(2):283–290. doi:10.2105/AJPH.2015.303003.

30. Shapiro A, Venkat M, Caldwell N, Jarenwattananon P. Billions of federal dollars could replace lead pipes. Flint has history to share. *NPR*. https://www.npr.org/2021/11/30/1037897216/billions-of-federal-dollars-could-replace-lead-pipes-flint-has-history-to-share. Accessed April 26, 2022.

31. Beck AF, Klein MD, Schaffzin JK, Tallent V, Gillam M, Kahn RS. Identifying and treating a substandard housing cluster using a medical-legal partnership. *Pediatrics*. 2012;130(5):831–838. doi:10.1542/peds.2012-0769.

32. Mainardi AS, Harris D, Rosenthal A, Redlich CA, Hu B, Fenick AM. Reducing asthma exacerbations in vulnerable children through a medical-legal partnership. *J Asthma*. 2022;60(2):1–11. doi:10.1080/02770903.2022.2045307.

33. Wheeler SM, Massengale KEC, Adewumi K, et al. Pregnancy vs. paycheck: a qualitative study of patient's experience with employment during pregnancy at high risk for preterm birth. *BMC Pregnancy Childbirth*. 2020;20(1):565. doi:10.1186/s12884-020-03246-7.

34. Corburn J. Center for Global Healthy Cities. http://healthycities.berkeley.edu. Accessed March 7, 2022.

35. Coburn J, Fukutome A, Asari M. *Health in All Policies, Richmond CA: 2020 Progress Report*. Richmond, CA; 2020:58. https://www.ci.richmond.ca.us/DocumentCenter/View/57209/HiAP-Report-2020.

36. Heft-Neal S, Driscoll A, Yang W, Shaw G, Burke M. Associations between wildfire smoke exposure during pregnancy and risk of preterm birth in California. *Environ Res*. 2022;203:111872. doi:10.1016/j.envres.2021.111872.

37. Black Maternal Health Caucus. Momnibus. https://blackmaternalhealthcaucus-underwood.house.gov/Momnibus. Accessed March 6, 2022.

38. Powell JA, Toppin E. Health equity and the circle of human concern. *AMA J Ethics*. 2021;23(2):E166–E174. doi:10.1001/amajethics.2021.166.

Chapter 4

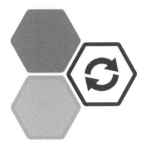

Transformational Maternal and Child Health through Expanded Healthcare Coordination and Community Engagement

AHMED V. CALVO, LYNDSEY STADTMUELLER, ANITA ISAMA, ERICA O'NEILL, AND MARK LOAFMAN*

Health disparities in maternal and child health (MCH) persist despite remarkable investment and advancements in traditional prenatal and newborn care, neonatal intensive care units, and monitoring technologies, staffing, and protocols deployed in labor and delivery units. This chapter builds on the evidence from several decades of epidemiology that improving MCH outcomes calls for a transformational approach, one that includes a life-course perspective that extends far beyond the limited time frame of the very best perinatal care currently available. By applying lessons learned from population and public health, we can incorporate a longer, broader, and more comprehensive scope for MCH that leverages community collaboration and an expanded healthcare team.

Understanding the evolution of a more comprehensive, longitudinal approach to MCH starts with recognizing the relevance and applicability of healthcare's quality-improvement endeavors that have focused on care of chronic conditions. In 1998, for example, the Health Disparities Collaboratives (HDC) of the Health Resources and Services Administration (HRSA) began scaling to the national level a commitment to team-based care, achieving significant advances in treating multiple chronic illnesses. The HDC process for improving care drew on the framework of the Wagner Chronic Care Model,

---

* This writing was conducted by the authors and is not to be construed as representing the opinions of the federal government or any of its agencies. The opinions are solely those of the authors.

Ahmed V. Calvo, Lyndsey Stadtmueller, Anita Isama, Erica O'Neill, and Mark Loafman, *Transformational Maternal and Child Health through Expanded Healthcare Coordination and Community Engagement* In: *The Practical Playbook III*. Edited by: Dorothy Cilenti, Alisahah Jackson, Natalie D. Hernandez, Lindsey Yates, Sarah Verbiest, J. Lloyd Michener, and Brian C. Castrucci, Oxford University Press. © de Beaumont Foundation 2024.
DOI: 10.1093/oso/9780197662984.003.0004

which includes integration of six essential elements of a healthcare system. The HDC was launched with a focus on improving diabetes care at five federally qualified health centers (FQHCs). By building on a history of community-oriented primary care, a founding principle in the genesis of FQHCs, the HDC process ultimately reached over 86% of existing FQHCs to improve care in conditions like diabetes, cardiovascular disease, asthma, and depression, as well as cancer screening.[1,2] The HDC was the largest ambulatory care effort of its kind in the United States at the time.

In 2004, as persistence of racial MCH disparities became more and more evident, and the role FQHCs were taking in serving affected populations expanded, HRSA launched the Perinatal and Patient Safety Collaborative (PPSC). Focused on MCH, the PPSC brought together five FQHCs in a national learning community. Given the epidemiology in communities with historical racial and ethnic disparities, the HDC national director and faculty considered the Wagner Chronic Care Model to be insufficient to address MCH equity outcomes. The timeline for traditional prenatal care begins only after a pregnancy is established and many subsequent perinatal outcomes already have been set in motion. While traditional perinatal healthcare services provide remarkable access to genetic diagnostic testing, fetal imaging, and world-class medical care for pregnant persons and premature or ill infants, the ability to alter the trajectory of social determinants of health influenced by structural racism, toxic stress, and adverse life events has been limited. Improving MCH outcomes calls for a more longitudinal, comprehensive approach that recognizes and addresses the impact of social disparities and structural racism and uses an expanded care team. When deployed with solid community engagement in a transformational manner, this approach is known as the expanded care model.[3,4]

As applied to MCH, the expanded care model is more comprehensive than the care that traditional clinical teams and services provided. It is more comprehensive in terms of the scope of health factors addressed and more inclusive of the longitudinal timeline that influences MCH outcomes. Ideally, the expanded scope and timeline are informed by data and analytics in the population health domain from local and regional public health departments, managed care organizations, and other stakeholders, and by local community organizations, with their health data and insights from lived experience. Perhaps most importantly, this approach requires decision-making that includes and engages the pregnant person at the center of the expanded care team.

Upstream, prevention-oriented engagement by the pregnant person needs to begin long before pregnancy is established. This allows time for risks to be identified—and to determine which risks can be mitigated by the person with help from the expanded care team and other key community and family resources, and which risks require local societal investments, policy change, and structural reforms. For example, although well beyond the scope of the clinical practice of medicine, stress and ill health can stem from structural racism that affects individuals and communities, and communities and healthcare systems must confront this risk. The social, clinical, mental health, dietary, and lifestyle factors associated with MCH outcomes simply cannot be adequately addressed by traditional prenatal care inside the four walls of a typical medical practice. Therefore, this chapter calls for a systemic approach to the expanded care model, with a call for action that focuses on more than improving clinical practice.

Conceptually, the expanded care model is an evolution of the Patient-Centered Medical Home (PCMH) model, pushing beyond provision of medical care to individuals during relatively brief office visits.[5] Adding a population and public health approach on a more comprehensive level can be understood as a combination of PCMH elements with those of a Community-Centered Health Home model.[6,7] As shown in Figure 4.1, leveraging the strengths of these two models to yield better health data analysis and interoperability has the potential to produce better outcomes—at both the individual and the community levels—and can be understood as a Comprehensive Health Home model.[4]

Applied to the MCH field, this Comprehensive Health Home framework has transformational implications for the healthcare team, especially if linked with modern data platforms and data systems for improved data analytics and leveraging new composite metrics of tremendous practical potential. This conceptual model was used during creation of the PPSC. The PPSC selected five FQHCs based on their innovation in previous HDC participation and specific

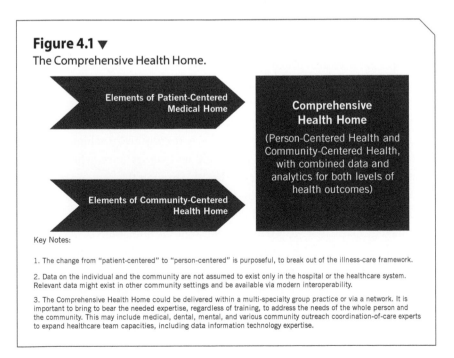

Figure 4.1 ▼
The Comprehensive Health Home.

Elements of Patient-Centered Medical Home

Elements of Community-Centered Health Home

Comprehensive Health Home

(Person-Centered Health and Community-Centered Health, with combined data and analytics for both levels of health outcomes)

Key Notes:

1. The change from "patient-centered" to "person-centered" is purposeful, to break out of the illness-care framework.

2. Data on the individual and the community are not assumed to exist only in the hospital or the healthcare system. Relevant data might exist in other community settings and be available via modern interoperability.

3. The Comprehensive Health Home could be delivered within a multi-specialty group practice or via a network. It is important to bring to bear the needed expertise, regardless of training, to address the needs of the whole person and the community. This may include medical, dental, mental, and various community outreach coordination-of-care experts to expand healthcare team capacities, including data information technology expertise.

interest in providing MCH care to African American populations who were experiencing some of the nation's most disparate MCH outcomes. The PPSC was led by a core national faculty charged with (1) connecting improved teams-based prenatal care with labor-and-delivery care in their affiliated hospitals and (2) fostering a network-driven approach to identify and promote better connections with community resource organizations from local partners of the involved FQHCs.[8]

At the outset, a new and foundational perspective for the PPSC was a focus on more comprehensive and longitudinal risks and interventions, and the associated care and care coordination that appeared to be required to improve MCH health equity. This called for a departure from historically siloed efforts to advance individual aspects of prenatal care, labor and delivery, and care coordination, all of which focused solely on traditional maternal care provided within an isolated pregnancy. The expanded care model applies regardless of whether clinical care is provided by an obstetrician, nurse midwife, family medicine physician, or advanced practice provider. Because the clinical approach is a tactical approach to pregnancy that uses a "go-at-it-alone" medical framework, none of these practitioners by themselves has the skills or practice setting to address racial and ethnic health disparities in birth outcomes.

MCH strategic care coordination improvements require context and understanding of the additional types of focused engagement needed from other staff, such as nurse educators, social workers, behavioral health providers, community health workers, care coordinators, and others who can bring critical insights from outside the traditional healthcare setting, especially when working and collaborating with other community resources and organizations outside traditional healthcare entities. The impact that this more comprehensive and longitudinal view has on MCH outcomes is depicted in the life-course perspective, which has been articulated by Michael Lu and others.[9] Figure 4.2 is adapted from Lu's initial contextual framing, represented here in a feedback loop that is helpful in conveying the true scope of preconception and interconceptual care for pregnant persons. We now know that the MCH-outcome life-course trajectory is influenced beginning with fetal life—where epigenetic "volume controls" are turned up or down—through childhood and adolescence, where adverse events alter future physical and mental health, through the preconception period and eventually the pregnancy itself.

The life-course perspective and the current understanding of the associated epidemiology in terms of MCH outcomes illustrate the limitations of waiting until a pregnancy is established to initiate outcome-improving care. They also show that improvements in prenatal and delivery-related clinical care alone cannot be expected to address many of the preexisting and subsequent issues faced by the pregnant person, in terms of both other pregnancies and the care of a child.

Initial work within the PPSC drew from evidence-based clinical practice in team-based coordination of care, with the goal of scaling up and spreading

Figure 4.2 ▼
Maternal and child health implications of action in a Comprehensive Health Home (seen from a life-course perspective).

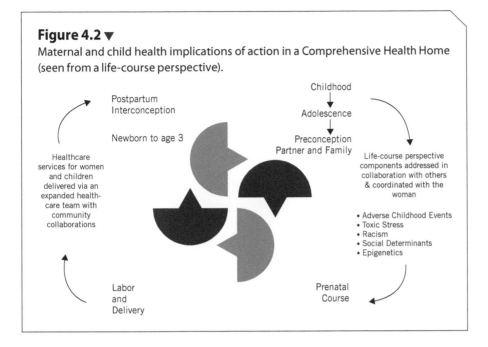

Childhood

Adolescence

Preconception
Partner and Family

Postpartum
Interconception

Newborn to age 3

Healthcare
services for women
and children
delivered via an
expanded health-
care team with
community
collaborations

Life-course perspective
components addressed in
collaboration with others
& coordinated with the
woman

- Adverse Childhood Events
- Toxic Stress
- Racism
- Social Determinants
- Epigenetics

Labor
and
Delivery

Prenatal
Course

models that work. These generally involve expanding the care team, whose members do not have the time or often the skills needed to address social, behavioral health, and related factors—which in some cases present the most significant risks to the pregnant person, future child, and family. The ability to implement these changes was challenged by lack of reimbursement for work outside the scope of facility-based clinical care by licensed providers. Additional resources were required, in some cases through collaboration within or beyond healthcare settings—with social work staff, care coordinators, and so on. This reinforced the critical need to have local community partners from a variety of other organizations, at both the individual and community levels of intervention.

Adapting the life-course perspective to advance MCH outcomes challenged the PPSC to consider a broader framework—moving from healthcare to health, from illness care to healthcare, and from medical care to a more collaborative framework that expanded the traditional medical team and deliberately involved multiple other disciplines and resources as members of the expanded healthcare team. Recognizing the impact that social and structural factors have on health outcomes, and then envisioning how healthcare systems can and should adapt, required broadening the "medical home" concept to that of a "health neighborhood." Using the home and neighborhood construct, consider the following analogy: Imagine a community where the goal is to maintain health and to avoid injury. The emphasis is mainly on safety and wellness in the home, and tremendous investment and scientific advancements are made to help make homes safe and healthy. Meanwhile, injuries and illnesses can occur due to lapses in traffic and workplace safety, episodic violence, and paucity of access to healthy food and activities, with some populations in the community disproportionately affected. In this example, the state-of-the-art home cannot on its own insulate populations from factors that arise in the surrounding neighborhood.

Similarly, it is essential for healthcare systems, and for those who practice in them, to expand the scope of the work that is done and the members of the team who do that work, and at the same time to recognize the factors beyond the scope of the expanded care team that call for system-level intervention. In this context, the Comprehensive Health Home includes medical, dental, and behavioral health practitioners and adds a variety of people and resources that can reach deep into the community to deliver connectivity, education, and assistance beyond the care typically delivered by a medical practice, even if it is a multispecialty medical group.

Since the PPSC approach required reaching beyond traditional medical care (in an illness-care sense) to a framework where medical, dental, mental health, and population health prevention were concretely addressed, there was a need initially to approach the effort via contracted networks and networks of influence, rather than hiring additional staff for an organization. PPSC explored a variety of relationships with multiple agencies to do the work and proactively improve some outcomes. Relationships included linkages with local and national medical-legal partnerships, linkages with community faith-based organizations, and expansion of health promoter jobs, either directly in an FQHC or within its networks, as economic and educational opportunities.

In this way, the PPSC involved a broader sense of engagement at the family level, at the community level, and at network levels, with the pregnant person at the center of the effort. Interoperability for data exchange and analytics is not the hindrance it once was, and the technical and communication issues of expanding relationships were manageable. What is most necessary is the will to do this work and a commitment to collaboration at community network levels, as opposed to the traditional healthcare framing within the walls of a clinical facility.

The PPSC ultimately showed that the approach of a Comprehensive Health Home can be delivered via a network—the expanded healthcare team does not have to work for a single organization. With solid collaboration based on good communication and good exchange of data, a well-run network can reach population health goals of better health at the community level—proactively and inclusive of prevention and components that address social and ethnic concerns.

Partly based on the lessons learned from the HDC, in many parts of the country FQHCs practice as a single organization and at the same time use a community network approach—with a mix of medical, dental, and mental health practitioners as well as community outreach staff operating different programs of emphasis in the local community. This level of clinical engagement for the whole person, as well as community engagement, begins to reach

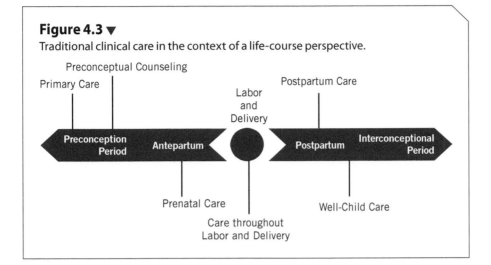

Figure 4.3 ▼
Traditional clinical care in the context of a life-course perspective.

the level of health equity engagement called for by the National Academy of Medicine (NAM) in its 2022 commentary on advancing health equity through transformed systems for health.[10]

The PPSC elected to leverage the six dimensions of quality healthcare from the Institute of Medicine (now known as NAM). The STEEEP elements (safe, timely, effective, efficient, equitable, and patient-centered) clearly require care coordination. The PPSC undertook this not merely as care coordination in a traditional medical practice, in the sense of being responsible for care only within a single clinical practice. Applying the life-course perspective required engaging a new approach to a network methodology—that of collaborating with practitioners from the community. The PPSC deliberately required expanded care coordination across a continuum—involving interconceptual care, prevention care, and addressing the social determinants of health—both for the pregnant person and the child, delivered via collaboration with whomever had the expertise to influence and truly affect population health outcomes.

The practical experience of the PPSC resulted in insights about clinical practice and led to the realization that mere improvements in the clinical delivery of care typically taught in family medicine and obstetrics training programs (pediatrics, nurse midwives, and behavioral health, for example) are insufficient to address current health equity outcomes. Figure 4.3 illustrates that a life-course perspective, as explored in the PPSC, requires interventions in other ways than just clinical activity in a medical practice.

Long-term components, which address lifestyle, stressors, and stress response, for example, could not be easily addressed by a medical practice during prenatal care only; neither could educational and economic support services be provided. Those efforts required the collaboration of other community entities, perhaps coordinated via a network approach. Figure 4.4 illustrates how the PPSC accomplished this. For example, PPSC collaborated with medical-legal

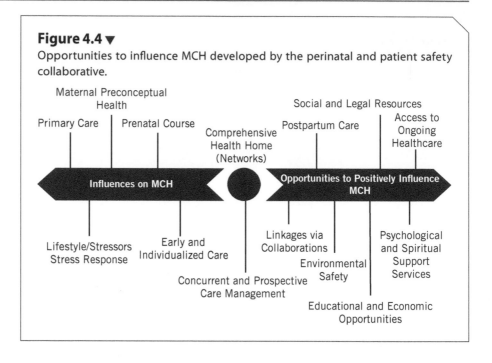

Figure 4.4 ▼

Opportunities to influence MCH developed by the perinatal and patient safety collaborative.

partnerships and other organizations both locally and nationally to bring to bear additional perspective beyond the clinical point of view. These expanded influence perspectives proved valuable to the individuals and communities involved.

Key lessons from these efforts converge in the discussions of transformational MCH through expanded care coordination that reaches beyond the traditional medical model. Therefore, encouraging the clinician to reach out to other organizations in the community (via facilitating processes and workflows, for example) becomes important as a way to evolve potential collaborations.

As an evolution of the PCMH model, an expanded healthcare team that is more comprehensive in both staffing and scope—as strongly advocated for in this chapter—requires increased collaboration and communication and improved facility with data use, analytics, and metrics. From the point of view of primary care alone, the perspective recommended by some is that primary care requires "the ten building blocks of high-performing primary care" articulated by Bodenheimer et al[11]:

> The building blocks include four foundational elements—engaged leadership, data-driven improvement, empanelment, and team-based care—that assist the implementation of the other six building blocks—patient–team partnership, population management, continuity of care, prompt access to care, comprehensiveness and care coordination, and a template of the future.[11]

With regard to system implications, beyond changes to delivery of healthcare, a broader system change is needed, so that support to clinicians, to pregnant persons, and to families comes from components of community organizations beyond healthcare. A more comprehensive aspirational model implies collaboration with organizations outside the medical practice alone—a network approach. In a sense, this harkens back to the community-oriented primary care model, which also challenged the narrow approach to primary care typically taught and practiced in the United States. As still is true today, the business of operating a primary care practice incentivizes a traditional, facility-based, licensed-provider approach because that is what healthcare insurance pays for. We suggest that, based on the experience of the PPSC, there may be hope in implementing a network approach to collaboration, as those elements would not have to be paid for by the clinical payment system.

KEY MESSAGES

In MCH, it is imperative to expand beyond the medical care/episodic illness care framework for an individual patient and the acute-care approach limited to prenatal care, labor/delivery, and a single postpartum encounter. This paradigm is insufficient to address today's MCH outcomes, which are affected by historical disparities—including racial and ethnic stressors—and issues of access to care. A life-course perspective is more constructive, enabling feedback processes that show promise.

MCH must evolve beyond the traditional medical care approach to include dental and mental health, both of which affect the clinical outcomes of the pregnant person and the child. Preventive care that includes all these aspects of health is important to consider for improving outcomes.

For better MCH outcomes, the strategic approach cannot be just illness care or acute care for an existing pregnancy. An expanded healthcare approach based on a life-course perspective is much more rational and, to truly go from healthcare to health, requires getting beyond the "medical care alone" point of view.

Using the Comprehensive Health Home model is a way to interrupt the lone-clinician mindset as well as the PCMH mindset of individual illness care by a single medical practice. Adding Community-Centered Health Home elements is important because this expertise broadens both the notion of medical home to health home and the notion of individual care to population health community care.

In MCH, it is important to evolve beyond individual-care thinking and the practice of traditional primary care. Adding insights from population and public health will be valuable in changing the outcomes achieved to date. Leveraging modern data systems and analytics promises to enhance clinical practices.

Many issues raised about this approach assumed more technological barriers than currently exist. Payment and reimbursement issues remain; however, COVID-19 has accelerated breakthroughs in the evolution of telehealth delivery.

Advancing health equity will require a pivot to engagement with communities that can result in a shift from sickness care to a true health framework of action by the person, by the team, by communities, and by the system. Satisfying community needs is what NAM is calling for. Although making changes within the traditional clinical team framework will better the clinical team experience, it will be insufficient for improving MCH outcomes.

REFERENCES

1. Harris Y, Kwon L, Berrian A, Calvo A. Redesigning the system from the bottom up: lessons learned from a decade of federal quality improvement collaboratives. *J Health Care Poor Underserved.* 2012;23:11–20.

2. Stevens DM. Health centers after fifty years: lessons from the Health Disparities Collaboratives. *J Health Care Poor Underserved.* 2016;27:4:1621–1631.

3. Calvo A. Taking collaboration to scale. In: Michener JL et al, eds. *The Practical Playbook II: Building Multisector Partnerships That Work.* New York, NY: Oxford University Press; 2019:125–136.

4. Calvo A, Calvo LR, Bezold C. Comprehensive Health Home: using the expanded care model of the collaboratives—implications of convergence of the Chronic Care Model, planned care model, and Patient-Centered Medical Home model. Alexandria, VA: Institute for Alternative Futures; 2008. Retrieved from: http://www. altfutures.org/draproject/pdfs/report_08_05_comprehensivehealthhome_using_ expandedcaremodelcollaboratives.pdf.

5. Kilo CM, Wasson JH. Practice redesign and the patient-centered medical home: history, promises, and challenges. *Health Aff.* 2010;5:773–778. doi:10/1377/ hlthaff.2010.0012 7.5.w328.

6. Prevention Institute. Community-Centered Health Homes: bridging the gap between healthcare services and community prevention. Oakland, CA: Prevention Institute; 2011.

7. Mikkelsen L, Panares R, Cohen L. Community-Centered Health Homes: bridging health care services and community prevention. In: Michener JL et al, eds. *The Practical Playbook II: Building Multisector Partnerships That Work.* New York, NY: Oxford University Press; 2019:291–299.

8. Loafman M, Calvo A, Wan S, Song S. Improving maternal and child health outcomes: family medicine obstetrics and the HRSA Perinatal Collaborative Project. *Am J Clin Med.* 2009; 6(2):48–52.

9. Lu MC, Halfon N. Racial and ethnic disparities in birth outcomes: a life-course perspective. *Matern Child Health J.* 2003;7(1):18.

10. Aguilar Axiola S., Ahmed SM, Anise A et al. Organizing Committee for Assessing Meaningful Community Engagement in Health & Health Care Programs & Policies. Assessing meaningful community engagement: a conceptual model to advance health equity through transformed systems for health. *NAM Perspect.* 2022. https:// doi.org/10.31478/202202c.

11. Bodenheimer T, Ghorob A, Willard-Grace R, Grumbach K. The 10 building blocks of high-performing primary care. *Ann Fam Med.* 2014;12(2):166–171. doi: 10.1370/ afm.1616.

Chapter 5

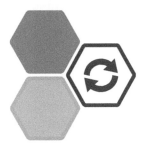

Improving Maternal and Child Health Outcomes: An Opportunity for Expanded Primary Healthcare Teams

MARK LOAFMAN, KENYA THOMAS-ALLEN, ANITA ISAMA, AND AHMED V. CALVO[*]

BACKGROUND AND OVERVIEW

The Maternal and Child Health Workforce: Numbers and Scope of Practice

There is a critical need for a more equitably distributed and resourced maternal and child health (MCH) workforce. This chapter discusses the acute need for family medicine physicians with a broad scope of practice, deployed in expanded care teams, in collaboration with obstetricians and others, to address overall MCH workforce needs.

Provider workforce challenges are most dramatic among maternity care providers. The shortage of OB-GYN physicians is projected to be 9,000 by 2030 and 30,000 by 2050, with more than 50% of US counties currently without a single obstetrician, yet there are no plans to increase the number of obstetricians in the United States. There are recommendations to expand the number of midwives, but they would not replace physicians prepared to manage perinatal complications, operative deliveries, newborn care, and primary care for pregnant persons and children.

In addition, decades of compelling evidence call for expanding the scope of MCH care to make it more comprehensive and longitudinal. An evidence-based response would organize the scope of this care around the life-course

---

[*] This writing was conducted by the authors and is not to be construed as representing the opinions of the federal government or any of its agencies. The opinions are solely those of the authors.

Mark Loafman, Kenya Thomas-Allen, Anita Isama, and Ahmed V. Calvo, *Improving Maternal and Child Health Outcomes*
In: *The Practical Playbook III*. Edited by: Dorothy Cilenti, Alisahah Jackson, Natalie D. Hernandez, Lindsey Yates, Sarah Verbiest, J. Lloyd Michener, and Brian C. Castrucci, Oxford University Press. © de Beaumont Foundation 2024.
DOI: 10.1093/oso/9780197662984.003.0005

perspective (see Chapter 4). The perinatal MCH life course begins with the epigenetic biopsychosocial influences on fetal life, extends through early childhood, adolescence, and an individual's pre- and interconception time, and ideally includes a pregnant person's partner and family, social supports, the social and physical environment, and the community itself.

The need to expand this comprehensive approach "upstream" has been recognized for some time. Disparities in MCH outcomes have persisted in the United States for the past four decades. This is despite significant advances in perinatal healthcare technology and large, multipronged public and private investments in expanding access to that care. As well described by Rosenblatt, the "perinatal paradox" reflects that the United States far exceeds all other developed high-income countries in expenditures for healthcare, yet experiences MCH outcomes that are worse than in every other developed high-income nation.[1] We also have known for decades that Black women and children suffer disproportionately poorer outcomes than white women and children. It is now clear that poorer MCH outcomes for Black women and children are not due to genetics, income, or level of education, but rather the biophysiologic impact of racism. In developing an effective strategy to address poor MCH outcomes, it is instructive to recognize the critical elements that underlie the perinatal paradox.

Content of Care

Perinatal care is largely organized and compartmentalized around the prenatal, labor and delivery (L&D), neonatal, and early childhood time frames. Advances in maternity care have largely been in areas of antenatal screening: genetic testing, sonographic imaging, and screening for medical conditions that may be associated with poorer outcomes. With few exceptions, these clinical tools are designed for use well after conception, by which time many perinatal outcomes are already "hardwired." Offering pregnant persons the option of continuing or not continuing the pregnancy has been a significant aspect of antenatal genetic and other diagnostic testing; recent actions to significantly limit these options will decrease the positive impact these clinical tools have on perinatal outcomes.

Changes in the approach to L&D include dedicated in-house laborists, safety drills and order sets, a lower threshold for induction of labor—both at term and when maternal/fetal well-being appears to be at risk—and an ongoing focus on the indications for, and approach to, operative delivery. Evidence supports the use of staff and techniques to support laboring women, although this is not routine, and access is not equally distributed.

Advancements in perinatal care over the past few decades have contributed to improved outcomes in several areas. The remarkable increase in survival for low-birth-weight (LBW) and particularly very low-birth-weight (VLBW) infants is among the most notable. The use of surfactant and antenatal steroids and optimal ventilator management in specialized neonatal ICUs are some of the more significant interventions.

Early childhood is a critical period, and access to quality healthcare during this time strongly influences future health outcomes. In 1967, Congress introduced the Medicaid benefit for children and adolescents known as the Early and Periodic Screening, Diagnostic and Treatment (EPSDT) benefit. The main goal of EPSDT services is to ensure that children insured under Medicaid receive proper treatment and interventions to prevent adverse childhood events (ACEs). The primary care provided by pediatricians, family physicians, and advanced practice providers (APPs) is pivotal in identifying ACEs. According to the description of EPSDT services on the Medicaid website, "States are required to provide comprehensive services and furnish all Medicaid coverable, appropriate, and medically necessary services needed to correct and ameliorate health conditions, based on certain federal guidelines." These interventions include essential newborn testing, developmental screenings, and appropriate vaccinations.

Despite these advancements in services and care delivery, maternal mortality for all women remains higher in the United States than in other wealthy nations, while it is roughly four times higher for Black women, and the rate of LBW, VLBW, and preterm birth remains largely unchanged, including persistent, and at times worsening, racial disparities. Four decades of ongoing perinatal paradox suggest the need for change.

TRANSFORMING THE MCH SCOPE OF WORK

Calls for action to address MCH outcomes have consistently encouraged a more comprehensive, longitudinal approach, beginning early in the preconception and interconception time frames before pregnancy occurs, and including a focus on identifying and then working to mitigate biological and psychosocial risk factors. This model is represented by the comprehensive, expanded primary healthcare team approach (see Chapter 4). Applying this model to MCH populations calls for a new era of engagement and collaboration among all stakeholders, centered on MCH outcomes.

The content of prenatal care continues to be organized around what has been described as the preeclampsia model, in which prenatal care starts near the end of the first trimester, followed by infrequent visits timed according to standard screening recommendations, with more frequent visits near term. This "back-loaded" approach was challenged in 1990 by the Center for Disease Control and Prevention's (CDC) expert panel on the content of prenatal care. The experts noted that pregnancy outcomes largely appear to be associated with psychosocial factors thought to be already determined for most women before the end of the first trimester, when traditional care is just starting. They called for care that is individualized, based on comprehensive risk factors, and "frontloaded" to mitigate risks before they have an impact. This necessarily includes preconception care, with the goal of helping to optimize the patient's outcome by controlling comorbidities prior to pregnancy.

Preconception Care

Nearly half of the pregnancies that occur in this country are unplanned. Preconception care for all reproductive-age persons can help identify and mitigate potential deleterious pregnancy outcomes. The CDC has developed a comprehensive list for preconception health that includes ten main points, each with action items. They include: a reproductive life plan for each person/couple, consumer awareness, preventive primary care visits, interventions for identified risks, interconception care, pre-pregnancy checkup, health insurance for women with low income, public health and program strategies, investments in research, and monitoring to guide further improvements. The NIH has preconception recommendations that align with the CDC's, further emphasizing the role of the family medicine physician in counseling patients prior to pregnancy. This includes managing chronic conditions and promoting healthy nutrition and weight. The NIH also recognizes that excessive (toxic) stress can result in adverse effects on the health of pregnant persons and their offspring. Ideally, preconception and early prenatal care include comprehensive screening and targeted interventions, resources, and support before irreversible consequences occur.[2-4]

Prenatal Care

Enrollment in prenatal care during the first trimester is associated with better outcomes. Approximately 77% of women in the United States receive prenatal care in the first trimester, but the percentage of Black women receiving care in the first trimester is 62%. According to a study conducted by Health Services Research, Medicaid expansion in several states between 1987 and 2011 increased the number of women who received prenatal care. The recipients were mostly lower income women who were previously unable to afford and/or access prenatal care. The positive impact of early individualized prenatal visits is gaining momentum as we recognize that earlier care allows us to identify potentially harmful risk factors, including those that are psychosocial, and to provide support that aims to mitigate adverse events as a pregnancy proceeds. In addition, more emphasis is being placed on incorporating partner and family support for women during pregnancy and thereafter, during the early childhood phase. Suboptimal support for mothers and families in the United States is one of the factors that causes the country to lead in infant mortality in the modernized world.

Primary Healthcare for Women

Primary healthcare for women is, and should be, more comprehensive than reproductive healthcare alone, calling for greater emphasis on treating the whole woman in the context of her social and community networks. Heart disease is the leading cause of death for women in the United States, and evidence supports more preventive care and earlier diagnosis and treatment at primary care visits for women. It is not uncommon for women to receive their primary care from an OB-GYN or reproductive health APP, practitioners who may not address the full scope of primary healthcare needs. Comprehensive primary healthcare for reproductive-age persons prior to conception is an essential component of addressing poor MCH outcomes, and the workforce and the healthcare delivery system should be organized accordingly.

THE MCH WORKFORCE: THE ONE WE HAVE, AND THE ONE WE NEED

The MCH workforce shortage has two key dimensions: the number of people needed to do the work as currently organized, and the people needed to provide the expanded scope of primary healthcare that the ongoing disparities in access and outcomes make necessary.

Staffing the Present Scope of Care

The maternity care workforce shortage is at a crisis level for obstetricians, and there are no formal plans to increase the number of OB resident slots. Meanwhile, an increasing number of OB-GYN grads choose to subspecialize in areas that do not include maternity or L&D care. There also is an increasing trend for senior obstetricians to stop providing maternity or L&D care and to focus on other aspects of their practice. These trends are aggravated by diminishing numbers of family medicine physicians who include L&D or any aspect of maternity care in their practice. Most OB-GYNs are located in urban and suburban areas, leaving some urban areas underserved and many rural areas in real crisis.

APPs (midwives in particular) play a vital and welcome role in maternity care, and expanding their numbers and geographical distribution will address some workforce needs. Most maternity care and L&D settings, however, require the ready availability of an obstetrician (or in some cases, a family physician or surgeon with operative delivery skills). There also is a need for clinicians with experience managing complex medical conditions that can arise during the prenatal course—and with experience providing care for newborns and children. There is a clear need for more family medicine clinicians to provide care across the full scope of perinatal care: maternity care, L&D, and child health. This is true for staffing the current scope of care and is essential if we are to attain a transformational scope of comprehensive care in our communities. This full-scope family medicine workforce is critically needed in many rural regions and some underserved urban areas.

Staffing an Expanded Scope of MCH Care via Evolution of Family Medicine

Key solutions for work scope and workforce that are within reach in the foreseeable future include training and deploying primary healthcare teams more effectively, particularly by leveraging family medicine.

The expanded primary healthcare team approach (including its practical aspects) aligns well with the ongoing evolution of family medicine and its residency training programs. Here, there is the opportunity to harness the energy and idealism of young physicians and their enthusiasm for more sophisticated teamwork as well as the potential impact primary healthcare teams (as opposed to narrower primary care) can have on health outcomes.

Comprehensive MCH care must engage the pregnant person as well as the entire family—all in the context of the community. This scope is unique to family medicine, a specialty designed to care for the family unit in everyday community practice and across the entire life course. Just as is commonly and effectively accomplished with primary healthcare, family medicine MCH services are best provided in collaboration with obstetrics, pediatrics, and other specialties as—and when—needed. This collaboration is also required for MCH training in family medicine in most settings.

In this context, there is a critical opportunity for family medicine to transform trainee education to actively engage qualitative models that help mitigate the impacts of structural and systemic racism on maternal outcomes, particularly Black maternal health outcomes.[5] The latter point was further informed by Green et al, who described their Cycle to Respectful Care framework as a practical tool and "an actionable guide toward respectful care for Black mothers, and eventually all birthing people."[6]

This is far more than a philosophical debate over the role of family medicine, because the maternity care workforce faces a real crisis that affects many rural and underserved urban settings.[7] Trends in the training and practice of obstetricians project that fewer and fewer will provide maternity care. While expanding the certified midwife and APP workforce is an essential, much-needed step, the scope of practice for these clinicians does not meet comprehensive MCH healthcare needs. This leaves family medicine as the only clinical discipline able to fill the maternity care workforce shortage and the one uniquely prepared to provide care across the life course.

Currently, less than 10% of family physicians provide maternity care that includes L&D. This downward trend is also associated with provision of less care in primary reproductive healthcare and care for children. There are several significant system and individual-level factors that affect MCH training and education, which must be malleable and evolve to respond to today's needs. Four different scopes of MCH practice have emerged in family medicine, ranging from practitioners who provide no pregnancy-related care at all (Tier 0) to those who have advanced training and practice maternity care and delivery (Tier 3) at a level comparable to obstetricians.

The four scopes of family medicine MCH practice, and defining competencies for each tier, are[8]:

- Tier 0: Clinicians defer most MCH care to other providers.
- Tier 1: Clinicians provide comprehensive, disparity-addressing healthcare for women and children and are linked to others who provide L&D care.
- Tier 2: Clinicians include L&D and newborn care in collaboration with OB-GYNs, family medicine Tier 3 physicians, and nurse midwives.
- Tier 3: Clinicians provide advanced MCH care, including operative delivery and care for pregnancies at higher risk.

Family medicine training varies widely in terms of access to skill development in the various scopes of MCH practice. Graduate medical education requirements continue to be adjusted in response to the widespread barriers faculty and residents face in developing needed skills. A few nonstandard OB and MCH fellowships have been a valued resource for family physicians who choose to practice at the more advanced tiers.

In practice, clinicians generally do what they feel called to do, are comfortable doing, and are trained to do with competency. Therefore, practical considerations for family medicine clinicians in terms of MCH include:

- Which MCH scope will I train for?
- Which community partners will I need to collaborate with?
- Will I do this on my own in a small or solo practice, or in a larger, group-practice setting?

Given projected shortages in the maternity care workforce, and the need to expand the scope of MCH practice to include far more emphasis on psychosocial determinants and a more comprehensive and longitudinal timeline for patients and their families, there is an opportunity to leverage family medicine as part of the expanded primary healthcare team model. This must be done in collaboration with the essential care provided by obstetricians, midwives, and many others. There are examples of successful local models, many of which work with vulnerable populations and workforce challenges that require innovation and collaboration. Replicating these models should be a priority, in a way that facilitates robust expansion of the clinical and community team, all deployed across the comprehensive and longitudinal timeline we now know is required.

Recent moves in several states to extend healthcare coverage for pregnant persons well beyond the six-week postpartum follow-up visit create an interesting opportunity to make care more comprehensive and longitudinal. We can imagine, for example, well-person visits for parent(s) and families that coincide with traditional well-child visits during the critical newborn-to-age-3 time frame. Clinical content, in the comprehensive sense we advocate, could be developed—as has been done for well-child visits—with both prescribed aspects and individualized elements specific to the parent, family, and community. To accomplish more than providing another means for generating billable visits, this will require an unprecedented collaboration across the various medical, behavioral health, and social service disciplines.

Comprehensive reproductive health and maternity care has been, and should again become, an essential part of family medicine and the family medicine residency experience. However, in a time of maternal health crisis in our country, we must acknowledge some barriers to training and practice. There needs to be a more collaborative effort among practitioners in family medicine, nursing, and behavioral health, OB-GYNs, nurse midwives, and the health system itself to support the overall health of women and their children, partners, and families. Fewer family medicine graduates are choosing to offer obstetrical services at Tier 1 and Tier 2—the reasons are varied and require focus not just on training programs but on practice settings themselves. Providing adequate support for both practice and training is crucial for establishing outcome- and access-focused collaboration with obstetricians and other stakeholders.

Adopting models that work and additional program and service development in these areas can be expected to promote collaboration and partnership with community-based resources positioned to augment the favorable influence providers hope, and need, to have on the life-course trajectory. Ideally, these and many related opportunities will trigger the transformation process needed for primary care, as these examples are within the fiscal and practical abilities of many early adopters who are ready for change.

A well-trained and strategically deployed family medicine workforce is the most feasible and readily attainable approach to help address disparities in both access and outcomes. Workforce and scope-of-practice approaches are tangible, evidence-informed components that can help drive transformational shifts in training and practice.

REFERENCES

1. Rosenblatt RA. The perinatal paradox: doing more and accomplishing less. *Health Aff.* 1989;8(3):158–168.

2. Jack BW, Atrash H, Coonrod DV, et al. The clinical content of preconception care: an overview and preparation of this supplement. *Am J Obstet Gynecol.* 2008; 199(6 suppl 2):S266–S279.

3. Frieder A, Dunlop AL, Culpepper L, Bernstein PS. The clinical content of preconception care: women with psychiatric conditions. *Am J Obstet Gynecol.* 2008;199(6 suppl 2):S328–S332.

4. Johnson K, Posner SF, Biermann J, et al. Recommendations to improve preconception health and health care—United States: a report of the CDC/ATSDR Preconception Care Work Group and the Select Panel on Preconception Care. *MMWR.* 2006;55(RR06):1–23.

5. Magee SR, Eidson-Ton WS, Leeman L, et al. Family medicine maternity care call to action: moving toward national standards for training and competency assessment. *Fam Med.* 2017;49(3):210–217.

6. Green CL, Perez SL, Walker A, et al. The Cycle to Respectful Care: a qualitative approach to the creation of an actionable framework to address maternal outcome disparities. *Int J Environ Res Public Health.* 2021;18:4933. https://doi.org/10.3390/ijerph18094933.

7. Rayburn WF, Klagholz JC, Murray-Krezan C, Dowell LE, Strunk AL. Distribution of American Congress of Obstetricians and Gynecologists fellows and junior fellows in practice in the United States. *Obstet Gynecol.* 2012;119:1017–1022.

8. Coonrod R, Kelly BF, Ellert W, Loeliger SF, Rodney WM, Deutchman M. Tiered maternity care training in family medicine. *Fam Med.* 2011;43(9):631–637.

Chapter 6

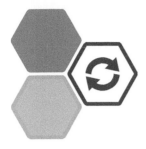

It's Not a Flip of the Switch: One Healthcare System's Collaborative Approach to Engaging External Partners to Support the Maternity Journey

BRISA URQUIETA DE HERNANDEZ, CHRISTINE BROCATO,
MANOJA RATNAYAKE LECAMWASAM, AND ANURADHIKA ANURADHIKA

INTRODUCTION

Today in the United States, how women experience care during their maternity journey is not equitable, as has been shown by both anecdotal and formal evidence.[1] Reiger and Morton[2] wrote:

> In the interest of increased accountability and quality in healthcare in recent decades, policymakers, professionals, and consumers have sought to standardize service provision. Yet in maternity care in particular, the resulting spread of evidence-based clinical guidelines and care protocols remains at odds with an alternative humanistic discourse stressing the importance of individualizing women's care. (p. 173)

This is especially significant as the United States undergoes dynamic demographic changes that are not expected to slow anytime soon.[3] As the cultural and ethnic diversity of our communities increases, guidelines and maternity care should also adapt to reflect the needs and preferences of the multifaceted patients who need maternal care—one size does not fit all.[4] Care needs to be culturally engaging and personalized, and to take individual needs into account as much as possible.[4] More important, the care provided needs to account for the

Brisa Urquieta de Hernandez, Christine Brocato, Manoja Ratnayake Lecamwasam, and Anuradhika Anuradhika,
It's Not a Flip of the Switch In: *The Practical Playbook III*. Edited by: Dorothy Cilenti, Alisahah Jackson,
Natalie D. Hernandez, Lindsey Yates, Sarah Verbiest, J. Lloyd Michener, and Brian C. Castrucci,
Oxford University Press. © de Beaumont Foundation 2024. DOI: 10.1093/oso/9780197662984.003.0006

birthing person's lived experience, preferences, and upstream factors, such as social determinants of health.[5]

There are many structural and systemic issues that affect how healthcare is provided, especially when it comes to personalized maternity care. Health systems traditionally have difficulty personalizing care due to the demands of caring for a high volume of patients with varying conditions and needs. Recently, more innovative health systems have engaged with external vendors to support some aspects of care delivery in novel ways that are not endemic to many traditional healthcare systems. Instead of journeying alone, healthcare systems and industry partners may have a prime opportunity to develop collaborative partnerships to enhance a patient's experience.

From a clinical perspective, a maternity journey focuses on the physical and hormonal changes that ensure growth and development of the baby. All the experiences that occur during pregnancy, from labor to birth to initiating breastfeeding, are critical to support the transition into motherhood.[6] As Kitzinger wrote, "Everything that happens once a baby is born is the outcome of all that has come before" (p. 82).[7] This is why it is critical to implement a patient-centered approach to supporting women during pregnancy. It should be a process that empowers mothers to be better advocates for themselves and that provides resources to support them beyond the clinical maternity journey into the journey of motherhood.[8]

Traditionally, obstetric practice and providers have viewed patient choice as secondary to their commitment to quality, evidence-based care, and the policies of the organizational structures in which they practice. Although safety and quality remain the primary lens, patient choice is increasingly coming to the fore, mainly due to increasing demand from patients, who have diverse opinions about how they want to engage in their maternity journey.[9] This is especially relevant because vulnerable mothers may choose not to seek care if they feel they will be judged, if they feel they cannot afford it, or if they do not understand the information being conveyed to them. In recent years, health systems have adopted processes and facilitators that support implementation of patient-centered care, including, but not limited to, strong engagement of patients and families throughout the healthcare system continuum, active processes for patients to report on their experiences, personalized care delivery design, improved staff capacity and training/education, and a strong commitment from senior leadership to support such efforts.[10] Even with these resources, it is important to acknowledge the limitations of healthcare systems and to recognize that engaging with external partners to supplement the maternity care journey and patient experience is a real opportunity. In these collaborations, the clinician implements established clinical workflows while the external partner serves as an extension of the care team, focusing on the nonclinical and low-acuity care aspects of the patient journey that also are important (social determinants of health, for example). Healthcare systems need to identify external partners who can work hand in hand with clinicians to make it easy for patients to advocate for themselves and create broader access to resources that go beyond clinical needs.

Programs implemented by external partners (third-party vendors) have had a positive effect on maternal health outcomes, but these organizations do not do it alone. Healthcare systems and private partners should recognize the opportunity to leverage collective impact to pull together the various resources that will engage and empower the patients in their care. In other words, technological or virtual solutions provide the opportunity to augment, elevate, and integrate into existing systems and infrastructures to build stronger support systems for patients. Healthcare systems, both clinicians and administrative leadership, respond well to evidence-based solutions (as opposed to generalizable metrics), so it is important to have collaboration and consensus between health-system and private-sector partners about defining success metrics and how to measure them.

This chapter explores how CommonSpirit Health's commitment to health equity, population health outcomes, and patient experience led to implementation of a novel approach to address gaps in maternity care. It describes the process of identifying external partners by developing criteria, assessing key capabilities, and aligning the effort with organizational values and operations; it also identifies ways to codify the relationship by aligning objectives, metrics, and targets.

GETTING TO POTENTIAL SOLUTIONS

Motherhood can be an intense and intimidating experience for a first-time birthing person. When asked, many birthing persons report that it is very important to have their questions answered and to feel heard. To ensure that patients feel that their voice is respected, health systems are rethinking communication methods and solutions to engage patients throughout the maternity journey. Much of this journey traditionally has been through physical visits, emails, and telephone calls, when a patient interacts with clinicians and staff. This type of engagement, however, is costly and hard to scale with a high degree of customization for a large and diverse population. Given the bleak maternal mortality rates in this country, health systems know the urgency of rethinking the way they care for their maternity patients, but because of staff shortages and financial challenges, taking on full responsibility for initiating a new program is overly time-consuming and fiscally unfeasible. As an alternative, health systems are innovating beyond their four walls and developing external partnerships with smaller companies and start-ups to improve the patient experience by including the patient's voice in their service design. If health systems and external partners are mindful about creating partnerships that integrate care, safety, quality, and patient experience, the impact can be fruitful for all parties.

CommonSpirit Health, one of the nation's largest nonprofit health systems, serves diverse communities across 21 states and is committed to health equity and addressing disparities in maternal health. Interdepartmental efforts have been implemented over time and many lessons have been learned along the way, allowing the development of a framework of vendor engagement. In developing a collaboration with external partners, CommonSpirit Health can serve as a case study that highlights seven key steps for health systems to follow.

Step 1: Understanding What to Solve

Organizations need to evaluate and map all aspects of the patient's journey to understand and document the key issues that cause communication and/or care gaps. Beyond examining data on delivery outcomes, performing patient and staff focus groups and surveys can help identify areas for improvement. This process must ensure that a diverse patient population is engaged.

Key Questions during This Phase

- Which areas are most problematic in the journey?
- What type of clinical outcomes does our current process achieve?
- What do our patients tell us about their experience that they wish could be improved?
- Should multiple journeys be designed based on diversity of ethnicity, religion, and socioeconomic status of mothers?

Box 6.1 | Case Study: One Health System's Approach— CommonSpirit Health

Over the last four years, as CommonSpirit Health worked to improve its maternity offerings, internal data and external research revealed two areas for improving patient care:

Frequent two-way communication. Patients expressed the desire to have frequent communication touchpoints and informal check-ins to understand how to adhere to their care plan and to share their preferences for their childbirth experience.

Access for the vulnerable. Assessing maternal care at CommonSpirit also highlighted the need for a cost-effective clinical model that could increase maternity access for vulnerable populations.

Step 2: Identifying and Confirming Sponsors and Stakeholders

While Step 1 involves mapping the many aspects of the patient's journey, the second step involves mapping all the critical stakeholders along this journey. This is an internal process that must be completed prior to engaging external partners. In determining the types of solutions to consider, perspectives from a diverse set of CommonSpirit Health stakeholders were gathered, including team members from the women's service line, obstetric clinicians, midwife experts, managed care experts, health equity leaders, IT leaders, and population health leaders. Using a roles-and-responsibilities charting process, the head of the women's service line was identified as a key decision maker, while other accountable and influential stakeholders were also identified.[11] A core working team was responsible for developing initial criteria, researching solutions, seeking feedback from accountable stakeholders, filtering potential solutions, and proposing a final recommendation.

Key Questions during This Phase

- Who/what plays a significant role in the outcomes of a pregnant person's maternal journey?
- Who/what plays a significant role in the experience of a pregnant person's maternal journey?

Step 3: Defining the Mission and the Vision

Once an organization understands the key issues, it is helpful to develop a document that describes the prioritized issues to address, the mission of an ideal program, and the vision and objectives to be achieved for clinicians and patients. Again, this is an internal process to be completed prior to engaging an external partner. The document should describe key clinical, operational, and financial metrics the organization is looking to affect and the timeline in which it aims to create the change.

Key Questions during This Phase

- What do we want this program to look like today and in three to five years? How will it be effective for patients?
- What metrics will be measured and what targets do we want to achieve one year into the program?
- What budget do we have to solve this problem, both start-up and ongoing capital?
- What would we want patients to say about this program when they describe it?

Step 4: Developing Criteria to Select a Partner

The core team must be clear on key criteria required from the ideal partner, separating aspects that are "must have" from "nice to have." CommonSpirit Health recognizes that every partner/program has different factors that are important, but common criteria may include: (1) established health-system clients, (2) historical patient satisfaction scores, (3) appropriate financial backing, (4) leadership-team experience, (5) mission orientation and fit, and (6) sustainable pricing model. It is tempting to have a long list of criteria to capture every aspect of a program. For the sake of managing the project, however, we recommend no more than 10 must-have criteria.

Key Questions to Align Your Stakeholders during This Phase

- What is the immediate effect that we are envisioning by addressing this problem?
- What are the other important facets/capabilities that are needed but could wait, if necessary, until phase two or the next iteration of the solution?
- What attributes, capabilities, and customizations are we seeking in a solution?
- Do we need a product that is turnkey for easy implementation? Can we contribute some of our resources and know-how to codevelop a solution with a partner?
- What kinds of experience must a partner have to serve the target patient population?
- Are we willing to be an early adopter of a solution, or do we need a vetted solution with ample proof of concept in place?
- How does the company/product philosophy align with our core values and mission to provide equitable, accessible, high-quality care to our patients and communities?

Step 5: Identifying a Partner

Once the criteria have been established, the organization will have a better sense of the type of company they should evaluate. Companies can be discovered by tapping networks that include other health systems partners, membership organizations committed to innovation (such as the Health Management Academy or the Scottsdale Institute), the venture capital community, the start-up accelerator community, existing community partners, and nonprofit organizations. Each company identified should be evaluated and rated against established criteria using a scoring methodology. In addition to performance against criteria, other factors the CommonSpirit Health team considered—such as a company's commitment to health equity and sustainability, observed partnership orientation and flexibility, and past experience with the company's leadership team—can be equally important. Interviewing clients of the top five

Box 6.2 | Case Study—*continued*: Improving Maternal Care and Access for the Vulnerable

Two problems with CommonSpirit's maternal care were initially identified by the core team, and one—access for the vulnerable—was prioritized. In seeking a partner to provide maternity solutions that increased access for vulnerable patient populations, the CommonSpirit team aligned around the following must-have criteria:

Access: Ability to significantly increase maternity care access for the vulnerable, including prenatal care, postnatal care, and care coordination.

Equity: Ability to engage diverse patient populations who may not seek traditional medical care, especially those on Medicaid or the uninsured. Ability to provide services in Spanish. Diverse representation among staff who interact with patients. Commitment to provide a diversity, equity, and inclusion (DEI) statement describing the potential partner's position on DEI as it relates to hiring, company culture, product building, and serving customers. Demonstration of a formalized process to assess social needs and active referral to community organizations to address needs.

Sustainability: Ability to be accretive or cost-neutral to operate over time. Not dependent on grants or philanthropy to sustain.

Start-up inertia: Low resource/staff lift to implement. Low cost to implement.

Usability: Easy for patients to use, especially those with low tech literacy. Easy for CommonSpirit staff to use and to refer patients. Solution must not require the patient to have Internet access.

Viability: Evidence-based medical model. Partner must have an established track record with other US-based health systems.

Robustness/service levels: Ability to service multiple CommonSpirit facilities at once with high service levels.

Quality improvement: Ability to support and improve quality metrics that are important to CommonSpirit.

companies being considered will help attain a pragmatic perspective on the company's performance.

Key Questions during This Phase

- Which networks can we tap to attain a diverse set of solutions?
- What maturity level of solution are we seeking—in inception, early, or enterprise level? (The answer to this question will determine how widely to cast the net in the search.)
- What scoring methodology will we deploy to rate solutions?
- Does the organization currently deploy a similar solution in one of its divisions or hospitals?

Box 6.3 | Case Study—*continued*: Access for the Vulnerable

The CommonSpirit team evaluated several novel clinical models as they considered ways to increase maternity access for the vulnerable. In the present environment of well-capitalized healthcare companies, there are many robust, evidence-based maternity solutions for serving vulnerable populations.

Extensive studies demonstrate that midwifery-led care supports better birth outcomes. Births attended by certified nurse midwives have lower rates of labor induction,[12] operative birth,[13] cesarean section,[13] preterm birth,[14] and newborn death.[15] While only 8% of US births are attended by midwives, there are many more low-risk births that could be supported by a midwife. The midwifery model's whole-person approach, including its focus on addressing social needs, fills an unmet need in holistic pregnancy care. In addition, research shows that women who use a birth doula are less likely to need Pitocin, are less likely to have a cesarean birth, are less likely to use any pain medication, and are more likely to rate their childbirth experience positively. Doulas often are viewed as trusted guides for vulnerable women, because they often come from the communities they serve.[16] Hence, a clinical model that provides pregnant patients with access to both midwives and doulas has many potential advantages for vulnerable patients.

Given the evidence, the CommonSpirit team favored a novel midwifery–doula clinical model. While several CommonSpirit facilities employed midwives already, shortages existed and there was a limited budget for hiring the necessary number of full-time midwife employees across the organization. During Step 5, the team discovered that a CommonSpirit facility was piloting a similar solution effectively and was planning to expand based on early results.

In examining the potential of a midwifery–doula combination program, the core team and sponsors developed the following objectives:

1. To advance evidence-based midwifery-led care models for populations best suited for such care.
2. To create access to inclusive, compassionate, personalized prenatal care.
3. To enable seamless transitions across the pregnancy, labor, and postpartum periods.
4. To eliminate birth disparities by tailoring solutions to meet the needs of each demographic, with a focus on vulnerable and disadvantaged populations.
5. To support community-based navigation and referrals to meet vulnerable patients' social needs.

Step 6: Codifying the Partnership

Developing a new partnership and generating a successful vision document entails both parties' aligning on what success should look like and clearly articulating the road map and metrics that will help assess progress toward the established program goals. Typically, a partnership has an initiation or pilot period to evaluate its potential, which then can lead to an expanded, ongoing customer relationship. During the pilot phase, it is important to identify and agree on which qualitative and quantitative metrics to use. Equally important is to align on the source of each metric and the cadence at which each metric will be used. Compile a set of leading indicators that contribute to the core KPIs (key performance indicators) of the program and form a steering or oversight committee (composed of operational, executive, frontline, and champion stakeholders from both partners) to regularly review progress on metrics. The steering/oversight committee also serves as the core body that addresses any rollout challenges, with an eye toward successful deployment of the project. We recommend starting with three to five key metrics for measuring success that are aligned with the organization's strategy and capture ROI (return on investment). As a best practice, an organization should also consider the volume, hurdle rate, and target outcome for each success metric by the end of the pilot.

Key Questions during This Phase

- Which metrics that we currently use for our maternity programs are applicable to this partnership program?
- Which quality metrics should be tracked and aligned with our organization's quality initiatives?
- Which metrics are most important for defining the ROI for this relationship? Will the metrics chosen allow us to establish a direct correlation?

Step 7: Operationalizing the Partnership

Last, the preceding steps are meant to prepare and ease the way for operationalizing any type of partnership and program. Engaging the key clinical and administrative stakeholders from local markets is critical for successfully implementing a program. Special attention should be paid to the timing of implementation and potential for competing demands. Local facilities and clinics may have developed programming or interventions to support the needs of their patients within the constraints of their specific needs. In such cases, it is best to engage the local facilities and/or clinics to perform a gap analysis of workflows that adapt the chosen external partner's service design in a more intentional manner to support the needs of providers and patients.

Often, operational leaders worry about duplication of services or the cost of having to reduce numbers of staff, but as previously mentioned, this exercise can be an opportunity for healthcare systems and external partners to evaluate the collective impact of resources that can be made available to support patients. Once an external partnership is chosen according to the steps described above, a clear communication plan that ensures that the overall care team and support services (business development, marketing, and communications, for example) have bought into the implementation is vital for success.

Key Questions during This Phase

- Which facilities/clinics do we want to prioritize for engagement?
- Who are the operational leads for the local service line?
- What programming already exists?

Box 6.5 | Case Study—*continued*: Implementing a Virtual Patient Navigation Solution

When it came time for implementation, the CommonSpirit team identified business and operational leads to support and guide the implementation. These stakeholders were responsible for ensuring that the partnership was implemented in accordance with the contracted scope. They also were the key points of contact for the facilities, external partner, and senior leadership. Before going live with the program, the business and operational leads established a framework for engaging facilities that included:

1. Meeting with facility leadership (including CEO, CMO, CNE, CMIO, CFO, maternity director, community health director, clinical informatics, business development, and communications) to introduce the program. At this meeting, the site implementation team was identified and a timeline for implementation and concerns and/or questions were addressed.
2. Meeting with the site implementation team to discuss the existing maternity journey and programs/initiatives at the facility. Opportunities for supporting existing programming and adapting new solutions to fit needs were addressed.
3. Meeting with the site implementation team, including the external partner, to introduce and demonstrate how the solution would be implemented and how patients would be engaged. The site implementation team had the opportunity to adapt solutions by asking questions and reviewing existing programming. Planning for operational go-live occurred at this meeting.
4. Operational go-live meeting was the final opportunity to review and fine-tune the service and workflows for supporting patients and providers.

Monthly operations meetings brought together all operational leads from multiple sites to review key performance indicators and to discuss any issues with implementation of the program at the local market level.

CALL TO ACTION

Population demographics in the United States have evolved dramatically during the past few decades. With such change, an intensely personal process like a maternity journey must adapt to meet the needs and care preferences that usually are influenced by the ethnicity, socioeconomic status, and culture of the pregnant person. This type of personalization is not an easy task for a health system to take on by itself. Therefore, potential opportunities for health systems to partner with external healthcare companies to jointly leverage resources and skills can be vital when providing the pregnant person with an optimal maternity journey.

The key considerations described in this chapter for establishing multisector partnerships and the case study example of the innovative, structured approach taken by CommonSpirit Health are meant to provide guidance to a reader exploring a provider–industry partner relationship. The case study shows how a well-planned process not only allows for internal clinical and administrative alignment but also is helpful when choosing the external partner that best aligns with the mission and vision of the partnership. Collaborations between health systems and external partners will bring transformative innovation to healthcare and help address generations of disparities. Now is the time to bridge the access and information divides that have exacerbated health inequities in the United States and to be intentional about changing systems to provide a healthy and thriving space for generations to come.

REFERENCES

1. Wang E, Glazer KB, Sofaer S, Balbierz A, Howell EA. Racial and ethnic disparities in severe maternal morbidity: a qualitative study of women's experiences of peripartum care. *Womens Health Issues*. 2021;31(1):75–81.

2. Reiger K, Morton C. Standardizing or individualizing? A critical analysis of the 'discursive imaginaries' shaping maternity care reform. *Int J Childbirth*. 2012;2(3):173–186.

3. Vespa J, Armstrong DM, Medina L. *Demographic Turning Points for the United States: Population Projections for 2020 to 2060*. Washington, DC: US Department of Commerce, Economics and Statistics Administration, US Census Bureau. 2018.

4. Lally S, Lewis V. *Maternity Care Patient Engagement Strategies* (Issue Brief No. 12). Oakland, CA: Integrated Healthcare Association; 2014:1–12.

5. Wang E, Glazer KB, Howell EA, Janevic TM. Social determinants of pregnancy-related mortality and morbidity in the United States: a systematic review. *Obstet Gynecol*. 2020;135(4):896.

6. Rubin R. *Maternal Identity and Maternal Experience*. New York, NY: Springer; 1984.

7. Kitzinger S. *Ourselves as Mothers: The Universal Experience of Motherhood*. New York, NY: Addison-Wesley; 1992.

8. Lothian JA. The journey of becoming a mother. *J Perinat Educ*. 2008;17(4):43–47.

9. Diamond-Brown, L. "It can be challenging, it can be scary, it can be gratifying": obstetricians' narratives of negotiating patient choice, clinical experience, and standards of care in decision-making. *Soc Sci Med*. 2018;205:48–54.

10. Luxford K, Safran DG, Delbanco T. Promoting patient-centered care: a qualitative study of facilitators and barriers in healthcare organizations with a reputation for improving the patient experience. *Int J Qual Health Care*. 2011;23(5):510–515.

11. Smith ML, Erwin J, Diaferio S. Role & responsibility charting (RACI). In: *Project Management Forum (PMForum)*; 2005:5. https://par.nsf.gov/servlets/purl/10118958

12. Declercq ER, Belanoff C, Sakala C. Intrapartum care and experiences of women with midwives versus obstetricians in the Listening to Mothers in California Survey. *J Midwifery Womens Health*. 2020;65(1):45–55.

13. Souter V, Nethery E, Kopas ML, Wurz H, Sitcov K, Caughey AB. Comparison of midwifery and obstetric care in low-risk hospital births. *Obstet Gynecol*. 2019;134(5):1056–1065.

14. Loewenberg Weisband Y, Klebanoff M, Gallo MF, Shoben A, Norris AH. Birth outcomes of women using a midwife versus women using a physician for prenatal care. *J Midwifery Womens Health*. 2018;63(4):399–409.

15. Sandall J, Soltani H, Gates S, Shennan A, Devane D. Midwife-led continuity models versus other models of care for childbearing women. *Cochrane Database Syst Rev*. 2016;4:CD004667.

16. Maternal Health Learning and Innovation Center. *Doula Care in the United States*. https://maternalhealthlearning.org/wp-content/uploads/2021/08/MHLIC-Report_Doula-Care-in-the-United-States.pdf. Accessed September 12, 2023.

Collaboration

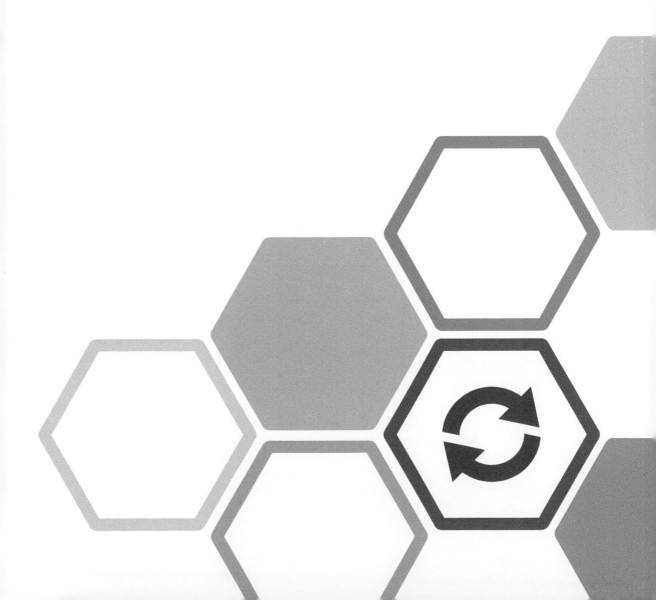

Angelica's Story

I felt sudden, severe abdominal pain. I was eight days post-partum and breastfeeding at the emergency department. The OB resident diagnosed me with a uterine infection, but I could barely tolerate the touch to my abdomen. I couldn't even sit up.

The resident said I shouldn't be experiencing that much pain. I had retained placenta after both of my previous deliveries, so I asked, "Could that be causing the pain?"

"It's a uterine infection," the resident and the attending OB told me.

"Then why am I in severe pain?"

But no one listened.

"I'll give you a prescription for Norco," she said, clearly annoyed.

I replied, "I'm not here for narcotics. I'm a nurse, and this pain is not consistent with a uterine infection."

Then the ED doctor admitted me to the hospital, against the attending OB's order. Later, my own OB examined me and said I had a uterine infection. After two days, I was discharged.

Three weeks later, I reached to pick up Elisa and I felt a gush. Within seconds, I was soaked in blood. I left a trail all the way to the bathroom. The discharge instructions after delivery say you should contact your provider if you saturate a pad within one hour. I filled one in ten seconds.

I grabbed towels to soak up the blood and lay on the floor next to Elisa. Finally, I reached 911. While I waited for the ambulance, I called my brother, Manny. "If I don't make it, tell Hector and the kids I love them. Tell them stories so they don't forget me."

Finally, the doctors did an ultrasound. There was still placenta in my uterus.

Then I had an emergency DNC and more complications. Finally, recovery.

The doctor said, "You're very lucky. Someone's watching over you."

At my five-week postpartum visit, I told my OB that my uterine infection became a life-threatening hemorrhage. I asked, "Knowing my history, why wasn't an ultrasound ordered?" I asked several times. "How did four doctors miss this?" My OB just looked at me after a few seconds. "Well, I'm glad you're okay."

I wasn't looking for sorry. I wanted my case to be a teachable moment. Use my case in grand rounds. "Show residents and doctors, so this doesn't happen to other women," I said, but my OB was noncommittal. I still felt like no one was listening to me.

Source: Illinois Maternal Health Digital Storytelling
Project. Angelica's Story. September 24, 2021.
https://www.youtube.com/watch?v=d-LjAk3D8H4.

Chapter 7

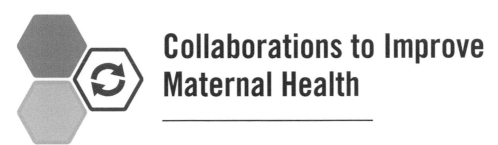

Collaborations to Improve Maternal Health

DOROTHY CILENTI AND RUTH S. BUZI

Cross-sector collaborations are needed to address root causes of persistent public health challenges. A cross-sector collaboration is an alliance among people and organizations from multiple sectors, such as health, education, and business, working together to achieve a common goal.[1] Such alliances are effective strategies for addressing complex social problems, such as mental health, environmental health justice, and health disparities. In an effective collaborative partnership, organizations coordinate and leverage resources to improve population health. Regardless of the cause for which the collaboration is formed, broad community engagement is fundamental in creating and sustaining conditions that promote and maintain behaviors associated with widespread health and well-being.[2]

Involving community members as active partners in addressing health and social concerns raises the potential to effect long-term change and alleviate persistent health disparities in historically underserved communities.[3] Community engagement is an essential aspect of many cross-sector collaborations, though specific approaches and the extent of engagement vary. Engagement strategies may be implemented across the spectrum from consultation to shared leadership within these relationships.

As described in previous chapters, maternal health in the United States remains a public health concern with major racial disparities. The factors that contribute to poor maternal health outcomes are multifaceted and include socioeconomic inequities, the health status of women, access to healthcare, and quality of care.[4] Addressing the complexity of poor maternal health outcomes thus requires new types of community responses. Cross-sector collaborations utilize various engagement strategies to address the complexities and disparities of maternal health. In this section, you will read about a range of successful

Dorothy Cilenti and Ruth S. Buzi, *Collaborations to Improve Maternal Health* In: *The Practical Playbook III*. Edited by: Dorothy Cilenti, Alisahah Jackson, Natalie D. Hernandez, Lindsey Yates, Sarah Verbiest, J. Lloyd Michener, and Brian C. Castrucci, Oxford University Press. © de Beaumont Foundation 2024. DOI: 10.1093/oso/9780197662984.003.0007 collaboration and engagement strategies to address maternal health inequities in various communities.

In Chapter 8, "Extending the Reach of Maternal Health Practice into New Zones of Transformation with the Framework for Aligning Sectors," Lanford et al identify four maternal health transformation zones that provide opportunities for practitioners to rethink their practice and extend their work into areas beyond traditional healthcare and public health services. Traditional healthcare and public health services must be augmented with changes based on a broader view of the factors that affect maternal health and health equity.

As an example of going beyond traditional healthcare, in Chapter 9 Ricks and Brian highlight the importance of maternal and child oral health and describe factors affecting the oral health of pregnant mothers. The authors look at how increased integration of oral healthcare services into primary care and other nondental settings can help improve maternal oral health and overall maternal health outcomes.

In Chapter 10, Hanson and Sherman discuss the State Maternal Health Innovation program, which assists states in strengthening their capacity to address disparities in maternal health and improve maternal health outcomes, including the prevention and reduction of maternal mortality and severe maternal morbidity. The authors describe the work of nine states that have been funded to strengthen partnerships and collaborations by establishing a state-focused Maternal Health Task Force, improving state-level data surveillance on maternal health outcomes, and promoting and executing innovation in maternal health service delivery. The chapter provides practical tips for collaboration and describes the core components of state maternal health innovation made possible through these collaborations.

Chapter 11 examines the Rural Maternal and Obstetrics Strategies Program, an initiative of HRSA's Federal Office of Rural Health Policy and the Maternal and Child Health Bureau. Using the Bootheel Perinatal Network as an example, the authors describe application of the clinical-community integration framework and provide insights and considerations for other organizations that deliver maternal health services in rural communities.

The Alliance for Innovation on Maternal Health Community Care Initiative is a community-based, data-driven quality improvement program aimed at decreasing maternal morbidity and preventable maternal mortality, particularly among Black and Indigenous women and birthing persons. In Chapter 12, McDaniel et al describe efforts to build a clinical–community integration model in one city through the infusion of community voices and collaborative leadership.

In their chapter on the Broward Healthy Start Program (Chapter 13), Ronik et al present a model for examining rates of maternal mortality and maternal characteristics that may lead to adverse birth outcomes at the micro level and demonstrate how a small group of community-invested stakeholders use data to develop strategic plans of action that are measurable, meaningful, and sustainable. Ingredients for success, as well as lessons learned, are included at the conclusion of the chapter.

The next chapter, by Hanke et al, focuses on a cross-sector collaboration in Harris County, Texas, that was started in 2010 to address worsening disparities in maternal and infant health outcomes. The Improving Maternal and Prenatal Care Together (IMPACT) Collaborative comprises action groups focused on service delivery/quality of care, public awareness, resource enrollment, and legislative advocacy. The work accomplished through the action groups and community-based programs reached a significant number of community residents through many initiatives. Obtaining input from community members and finding ways to compensate them for their contributions helped facilitate meaningful and consistent participation.

Finally, Chapter 15, "Activating Our Village in Los Angeles County: Birth Equity and Black Families," underscores the importance and the power of naming racism as the root cause of health disparities in maternal health outcomes. The authors of this chapter illuminate strategies to operationalize a collaborative antiracist agenda and highlight the benefits of a unified public-private-community partnership to effect large-scale change.

Together, the chapters of this section offer readers a better understanding of collective impact approaches and other collaboration models for addressing complex public health issues, such as maternal health outcomes. Descriptions of how these programs are initiated and maintained, and the roles of relationships and trust, will help readers assess readiness in their own communities to engage key partners to facilitate awareness and participation, receive feedback and input, and mobilize community leaders. The lessons, tools, and practices described in these chapters will help readers learn to facilitate true engagement and to share power and resources to build trust and belonging around the shared goal of ending inequities in maternal health.

REFERENCES

1. Roussos ST, Fawcett SB. A review of collaborative partnerships as a strategy for improving community health. *Annu Rev Public Health*. 2000;21:369–402.

2. Varda D, Shoup J, Miller S. A systematic review of collaboration and network research in public affairs literature: implications for public health practice and research. *Am J Public Health*. 2012;102(3): 564–571.

3. Butterfoss FD. Process evaluation for community participation. *Annu Rev Public Health*. 2006;27:323–340.

4. McCarthy J, Maine D. A framework for analyzing the determinants of maternal mortality. *Stud Fam Plan*. 1992;23:23–33.

Chapter 8

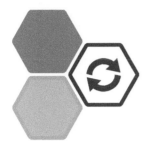

Extending the Reach of Maternal Health Practice into New Zones of Transformation with the Framework for Aligning Sectors

DANIEL LANFORD, KAREN MINYARD, LEIGH ALDERMAN, JAPERA HEMMING, CHRISTOPHER PARKER, AND TANISA FOXWORTH ADIMU

INTRODUCTION

The United States is unique among wealthy nations of the world for its rising maternal mortality rates. Despite the nation's having one of the most expensive healthcare systems in the world, there has been a steady upward trend in US maternal mortality for the past three decades.[1,2] These numbers represent a tragic loss of human life. They also represent untold suffering for families and for women who did not lose their lives but experienced largely preventable pain and illness. The burden of this tragedy falls more heavily on certain groups of women, with the mortality rate for non-Hispanic Black women greater than twice the overall rate.[3]

Many aspects of this situation call for improvement within the traditional parameters of healthcare and public health services. This is underscored by the Maternal and Child Health Bureau's ten essential services, which emphasize access to healthcare and public health services (see Figure 8.1). However, many problems have roots beyond these bounds. Factors like access to nutrition and healthy living environments are hard to address with traditional healthcare and public health service offerings, yet they are increasingly recognized as important contributors to maternal health outcomes and maternal health equity.

Accordingly, practitioners and researchers increasingly take a more holistic view of the factors that drive maternal health outcomes. Shortfalls in basic needs, like safe living environments, are now recognized as important factors in

Daniel Lanford, Karen Minyard, Leigh Alderman, Japera Hemming, Christopher Parker, and Tanisa Foxworth Adimu, *Extending the Reach of Maternal Health Practice into New Zones of Transformation with the Framework for Aligning Sectors* In: *The Practical Playbook III*. Edited by: Dorothy Cilenti, Alisahah Jackson, Natalie D. Hernandez, Lindsey Yates, Sarah Verbiest, J. Lloyd Michener, and Brian C. Castrucci, Oxford University Press. © de Beaumont Foundation 2024. DOI: 10.1093/oso/9780197662984.003.0008

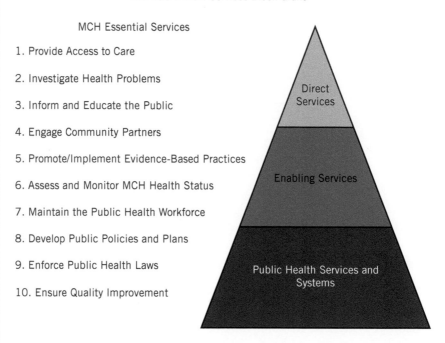

Figure 8.1 ▼

Public health services for maternal and child health (MCH) populations.

Source: US Department of Health and Human Services, Health Resources and Services Administration, Maternal and Child Health Bureau, Division of State and Community Health. *Guidance and Forms for the Title V Application/Annual Report: Appendix of Supporting Documents.* (n.d.).

Public Health Services for MCH Populations:
The Title V MCH Services Block Grant

MCH Essential Services

1. Provide Access to Care

2. Investigate Health Problems

3. Inform and Educate the Public

4. Engage Community Partners

5. Promote/Implement Evidence-Based Practices

6. Assess and Monitor MCH Health Status

7. Maintain the Public Health Workforce

8. Develop Public Policies and Plans

9. Enforce Public Health Laws

10. Ensure Quality Improvement

Direct Services

Enabling Services

Public Health Services and Systems

maternal health outcomes. Economic status, despair, and respect for diversity and cultural sensitivity are likewise now viewed as important maternal health concerns. At a broader level, our institutions and the social structures that flow through them—including racism, class inequality, and the marginalization of women, among others—are now understood as affecting inequalities in health.[4] To help practitioners rise to the challenges presented by this wider range of issues, this chapter concretely outlines ways to expand maternal health practice into a broader set of maternal health zones of transformation.

Aligning Across Sectors

The Georgia Health Policy Center, with the support of the Robert Wood Johnson Foundation, recently developed the Framework for Aligning Sectors (see Figure 8.2) to help change makers tackle an expanded range of challenges to community well-being, including maternal health. The framework encourages users to think beyond the traditional bounds of healthcare and public health services and is therefore helpful for thinking about new zones of maternal

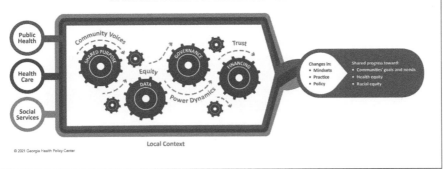

Figure 8.2 ▼

The Framework for Aligning Sectors.

Source: The Georgia Health Policy Center and the Robert Wood Johnson Foundation, Aligning Systems for Health Landers G, Minyard K, Heishman H. *How aligning sectors builds resilient, equitable communities. J Public Health Manage Pract.* 2022 Jul-Aug;28(4 Suppl 4):S118–S121.

health transformation. For example, it identifies the importance of making connections with social services. It also highlights the importance of looking within organizations, not just in traditional areas like governance and finance but also in areas like equity, trust, and power dynamics. The framework also emphasizes working directly with members of the community being served, for example, in developing effective processes and defining objectives. Finally, the framework encourages users to think about how changes in mindsets, practices, and policies affect health and equity outcomes.

The main point for maternal health practitioners is that, while healthcare and public health services are important in themselves, there is a much wider world of leverage points for making a positive impact. This chapter discusses new ways of thinking about extending the reach of maternal health practice by:

- Presenting the maternal health zones of transformation model
- Providing examples of opportunities for anyone wishing to extend maternal health practice into new zones of transformation
- Highlighting four case examples of maternal health practice that extend across zones of transformation

EXTENDING THE REACH OF MATERNAL HEALTH PRACTITIONERS

Healthcare and public health practitioners are working harder than ever in an era heavily affected by concerns related to COVID-19, and the prospect of extending the practice of maternal health work may seem daunting. Yet the challenges of COVID-19, especially those related to health and health inequities, highlight the need to incorporate new ways of working with each other and

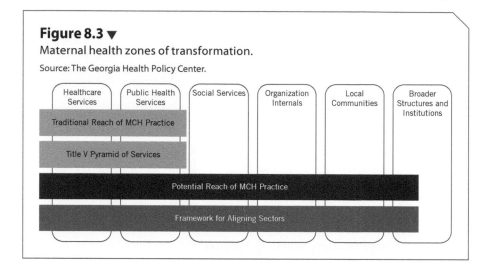

Figure 8.3 ▼

Maternal health zones of transformation.

Source: The Georgia Health Policy Center.

forming partnerships. Emerging research demonstrates that areas with greater service integration and with denser networks among organizational partners have better health outcomes.[5] Practitioners in such spaces also felt better prepared during the emergence of the pandemic.[6]

A first step in extending the reach of maternal health work is to develop a picture of the directions in which maternal health practice can be expanded. Figure 8.3 identifies several maternal health zones of transformation beyond the traditional bounds of healthcare and public health services: social services, organization internals, local communities, and broader structures and institutions. Note that Figure 8.3 can be read from left to right, but the zones of transformation can be addressed in any order and multiple zones of transformation can be addressed simultaneously.

Social Services

Social services that address needs like housing, nutrition, and economic status have long been understood as being related to maternal health, but where they once were considered distantly related, they are increasingly viewed as being central to improving maternal health. The range of social factors recognized as important has grown to include factors like transportation and physical access to care, the need for quality information on which to base decisions, the need for living wages and time off work to manage maternal health challenges, the need for more productive interactions with the medical and legal systems, and the need for respect and dignity—in short, whole-person care.

Organization Internals

Another place to look for new opportunities to improve maternal health is within organizations. Organization internals are systems, processes, and people that comprise organizations and form the groundwork from which organizational action emerges. While the services that organizations provide are important, how organizations provide services also matters, and organization internals are the "how" of their services. Consider an example of an organization internal involving people. Creating a leadership structure and staff that reflect the identities of the population being served is now recognized as an important factor in building trusting relationships between organizations and the communities they serve. Addressing organization internals by acknowledging, addressing, and mitigating the effects of personal biases or conflicting organizational priorities positions organizations to act with greater unity. Dedicating staff to coordination and whole-person care expends resources but may pay dividends when connections with new partners are made. Looking inward at organization internals may create uncomfortable moments or even challenge established power structures. Yet the potential payoff from acknowledging organization internals as an important potential zone of transformation may be significant, resulting in greater self-awareness, responsiveness to community needs, and improved clarity on how organizations present themselves to their own staff, organizational partners, and the people they serve.

Local Communities

Like social services and organization internals, increased connections with the community being served had once been a marginal concern, but these connections are increasingly recognized as a central issue. Traditional concerns around rapport and trust are still important,[7] but additional issues have risen to prominence. For example, many organizations are expanding their efforts to incorporate—and professionally compensate—members of the community on boards and decision-making committees. Staff might also be hired directly from the community being served. Support can be given to community groups that are self-organizing, forming research teams, or taking leadership roles in maternal health initiatives and programs themselves. Processes that promote accountability to the community being served can be written into mission statements, bylaws, contracts, and work procedures. Data can be shared and reported. Data processes in general might be designed and executed in collaboration with the very members of the community whose data is being collected and reported.

Broader Structures and Institutions

Across each zone of transformation, there is the underlying theme that today's social structures are creating significant health risks, that those risks are distributed in systematically unequal ways, and that the institutions forming the backdrop of maternal health work have, in recent decades, faced significant challenges in making continued progress on maternal health outcomes in the face of these risks. Maternal health outcomes in the United States are getting worse in many cases, and they are getting worse for some women more than others, as demonstrated by higher rates of maternal mortality among Black women.[3] In some cases, systems and institutions need more support. In other cases, they need to change. There are many systems and institutions that affect maternal health. Examples include healthcare systems, economic systems, educational systems, political systems, and social support systems, to name a few. Common challenges in these systems are that they often focus on treating severe issues when prevention might have been more effective, that they can be quite expensive, that they present more barriers to those with fewer resources, and that they create opportunities for widespread biases to negatively affect the people in the systems with the greatest need. Solutions include implementing proactive initiatives that prevent maternal health challenges from arising, working toward sustainable and effective financing, making access to maternal health services simpler and more comprehensive, and adjusting public and private policies using an explicit focus on reducing maternal health inequalities and improving maternal health outcomes.

EXTENDING MATERNAL HEALTH PRACTICE BEFORE, DURING, AND AFTER PREGNANCY

Like healthcare and public health services, the four added zones of transformation offer many opportunities for those looking to refocus their activities. Options for restructuring their maternal health practice extend to everyone from individual frontline workers to large organizations. New resources are likely to help when setting up new activities and developing new partnerships, but simple changes in practices and policy may themselves prove helpful in the larger effort to improve maternal health outcomes.

Table 8.1 presents concrete examples of opportunities for extending the reach of maternal health practice into the four added zones of transformation. To underscore the importance of holistic perspectives, the table includes opportunities that relate to all three phases of the maternal health cycle: before pregnancy, during pregnancy, and after pregnancy. It also gives examples of opportunities that extend across all three phases.

CASE EXAMPLES OF ALIGNING MATERNAL HEALTH PRACTICE ACROSS THE ZONES OF TRANSFORMATION

This section describes case examples in which maternal health practitioners extended their maternal health practice into one of the zones of transformation. Additional elements from the Framework for Aligning Sectors are highlighted when they appear in the case examples.

Table 8.1	Opportunities for Extending Maternal Health Practice across the Zones of Transformation
Before Pregnancy	• Social Services—Promote a healthy environment for women (for example, by helping women obtain safe living situations, economic security, and quality maternal health information). • Organization Internals—Create institutional bonds with organizations that promote women's health and well-being before pregnancy. • Local Communities—Work with community groups to promote high-quality, culturally sensitive family planning and maternal health information. • Broader Structures and Institutions—Promote policy that prevents maternal health challenges by addressing the social determinants of health before maternal health is negatively affected (for example, by helping women to stay out of economic difficulty or to manage substance use disorders).
During Pregnancy	• Social Services—Coordinate one-stop-shop services and wrap-around services with organizations across sectors to minimize stressors during pregnancy. • Organization Internals—Work with community members to bring in facilitators for helping care providers address the unique concerns of women who identify with marginalized racial and ethnic groups. • Local Communities—Offer prenatal services in settings that are familiar and accessible to community members. • Local Communities—Work with local community groups to establish culturally sensitive maternal health and delivery practices. • Broader Structures and Institutions—Balance the medicalization of childbirth with sensitivity to culture and individuality.
After Pregnancy	• Social Services—Integrate two-generation care for mothers and families alongside efforts to promote healthy child development. • Organization Internals—Create institutional bonds with organizations that support women's health and well-being after pregnancy. • Local Communities—Include local women, mothers who have experienced your systems, and representatives from community groups as decision makers for new projects. • Broader Structures and Institutions—Encourage policy that reduces stress for women in the postpartum period (for example, by promoting economic security and psychological well-being). • Broader Structures and Institutions—Help women with smooth transitions between services designed for the perinatal period and services designed to be helpful over a longer period.
Across Phases	• Social Services—Configure and coordinate services across organizations to minimize the burden women face in encountering multiple healthcare, public health, and social service systems. • Organization Internals—Reconfigure boards, committees, and staff to reflect the community of mothers being served. • Local Communities—Work with community groups to define maternal health priorities and monitor progress toward maternal health goals. • Broader Structures and Institutions—Reach out to women in the community instead of waiting for them to come to you. • Broader Structures and Institutions—Promote policy that holds institutions accountable to the women in the community being served. • Broader Structures and Institutions—Promote and coordinate access to quality information, preventive measures, and acute care services, especially in rural contexts.

Social Services

Practitioners and policymakers increasingly recognize the importance of the social determinants of health for improving maternal health outcomes. In response, maternal health practitioners are expanding their connections with social service providers and others working to address the social determinants of health. By collaborating, maternal health practitioners can prevent maternal health issues from arising in the first place and help women and mothers more holistically. The connections made through partnerships with social service providers also create opportunities to do things like identify new areas for change, share information, and simplify coordinated service delivery.

Networks and collaboratives involving social service providers are well positioned to address long-standing challenges in whole-person care and coordination that have plagued practitioners as well as the people they serve. These challenges exist at the population level, where jurisdictional differences and disconnected information systems can prevent efficient cooperation among service organizations. They also exist at the individual level, where women and mothers in need often spend prohibitive amounts of time navigating complex red tape to find help, if that help is available at all.

Efforts to address such challenges likewise exist at the population and individual level. At the population level, red tape can be identified and removed, information can be shared, and achievements can be measured. At the individual level, collaboratives can institute no-wrong-door programs that simplify access to care, offer comprehensive care coordination services that address the whole person, and offer outreach and wraparound services that increase prevention and reduce the burdens women and mothers may face when seeking help.

Illinois Family Case Management is an example of a collaborative program that operates at both the population and individual levels to improve maternal health outcomes. Family Case Management is a statewide program that provides multiservice coordination for low-income pregnant women, mothers, and infants. Its services address healthcare, social needs, educational needs, and developmental needs.[8]

At the population level, Family Case Management brings together Medicaid programming and funding, the Illinois Department of Human Services, and many other organizations, including social service organizations in the fields of education, childcare, housing, transportation, and nutrition.[9] Through the Family Case Management network, cross-sector relationships are strengthened and information is shared among agencies.

At the individual level, Family Case Management is achieved through case managers with backgrounds as social workers or registered nurses. Case managers work in local health departments and in other locations.[10] Practitioner activities in these locations include outreach and early identification of potential participants to aid with prevention. Other Family Case Management services include prenatal care, individually facilitated connections with healthcare providers, and individually facilitated connections with a wide range of social service providers.[9]

Illinois Family Case Management began in the 1980s with geographically limited prenatal care programs. It grew to include statewide reach and a wide range of service offerings in the mid-1990s. Studies of the program suggest that participation reduces the rate of low-birth-weight babies.[10,11] Since 1990, the infant mortality rate in Illinois has decreased by 23%, and nearly 90,000 women, infants, and children are seen annually through this program.[8]

Organization Internals

While many maternal health organizations are building external partnerships, others are creating change by looking inward. Examples of these internally focused initiatives include incentivizing patient-centered care, hosting trainings that focus on the unique needs of women of color, increasing provider diversity, improving data infrastructure, and integrating policies and practices to eliminate implicit bias and discrimination.[12,13]

Several of these internally focused initiatives are a response to the growing body of literature indicating that implicit bias and racism experienced by women of color in clinical practices and healthcare systems adversely impact maternal health outcomes.[14] Black, Latina, and Asian women are more likely than white non-Hispanic women to experience multiple illnesses during pregnancy,[15] to report unfair treatment in healthcare settings based on their race or ethnicity,[16] and to die during the perinatal period.[17] There is a wide and increasing maternal mortality gap between non-Hispanic Blacks and all other birthing persons in the United States. Delayed response to clinical warning signs and a lack of culturally competent and respectful quality care are among the factors commonly cited as contributors to racial and ethnic disparities in maternal death rates.[16] Despite these race-related outcomes, there is a shortage of resources and practices dedicated to assisting clinical practices and providers in recognizing and reducing biased practices and beliefs, and there is an ongoing need to change policies that perpetuate racism in the healthcare system, including those that tend to limit access to quality care for women in racial and ethnic minority groups.

Here, we highlight a training course designed to reduce bias and advance equity in maternity care. Supported by the California Health Care Foundation (see Chapter 47 for more information), the Dignity in Pregnancy and Childbirth Project is a course developed in accordance with training requirements outlined in a new California law, the California Dignity in Pregnancy and Childbirth Act (Senate Bill 464). This trailblazing law requires several types of organizations, including hospitals providing perinatal care, alternative birthing centers, and certain primary care clinics, to offer an evidence-based implicit bias program for all of their perinatal care providers, with a refresher course required every two years.[18]

The project trains staff in participating clinics and hospitals on ten specific topics through an online course. Topics include identifying unconscious biases and misinformation, power dynamics, the impact of historical oppression on minority communities, and local perspectives on provider–community relations.[19] Perinatal providers take a one-hour introductory course divided into short segments designed to accommodate clinicians with demanding schedules and to allow for greater uptake.

The training offers pragmatic approaches for immediate implementation in the delivery room and in the healthcare system more broadly. It includes three case examples of Black women whose stories illuminate experiences during childbirth, preventable deaths, and the various forms of racism that affect patients. Providers also learn about a positive story of a birth outcome that is rooted in reproductive justice and patient-centered care. Hospitals that use this online resource are also offered a toolkit of other resources and activities that serve to deepen understanding and support development of comprehensive strategies to improve healthcare environments.

Although the Dignity in Pregnancy and Childbirth Project covers all areas required by the California law, its creators caution that it alone will not result in the organizational change needed to eliminate implicit bias and racism in maternal care. Rather, the course is intended to be the start of a longer-term journey that clinical entities and maternal health practitioners must take to address systemic root causes and interpersonal biases.

Local Communities

Maternal health outcomes overall, and Black–white and rural–urban pregnancy-related outcome inequities specifically, are well documented, and they are linked to a variety of community-level factors. These factors include access to the social determinants of health (nutritious foods and safe and stable affordable homes, for example), a higher prevalence of preexisting health conditions (chronic disease, for example), less access to care generally, and specifically less access to respectful and high-quality care.[20] Because people in the communities most affected by these inequities have invaluable expertise in the form of lived experience with these and other factors that shape maternal health, researchers and practitioners increasingly recommend more community-driven approaches to maternal health and health equity.[21] Organizations and communities alike are expected to benefit when working together to implement community-based approaches to promoting equity and improving community-level factors that influence pregnancy-related outcomes.[22]

A variety of community-based approaches have been shown to improve pregnancy-related outcomes, promote positive patient experiences, and potentially reduce healthcare costs. These approaches are often designed to benefit people most at risk for poor outcomes, including people of color, people with low incomes, and people who live in rural areas.[23] Research indicates that these approaches can promote healthier and more equitable birth outcomes.[24]

One such community-based approach highlighted here is community-based maternal healthcare. This approach is designed specifically to address barriers to healthcare faced by those most at risk for poor outcomes by offering a variety of reproductive healthcare and childbirth services through midwives, doulas, and community birth workers, in addition to wraparound services and interventions to address the social factors that influence birth outcomes. "Tackling Maternal Health Disparities: A Look at Four Local Organizations with Innovative Approaches," a 2019 article from the National Partnership for should be Woman & Families, describes four examples where community-based maternal healthcare was implemented—in New Mexico, Texas, Florida, and Washington, DC.[24] This section presents an overview of the common elements of the four examples, with a focus on the community being served.

Community-based maternal healthcare in the four examples emphasizes reproductive social justice through culturally relevant and respectful care and services that emphasize autonomy and individual decision-making. The approach involves partnering with, and investing in, communities using an assets-based lens that emphasizes a community's existing assets and strengths. For example, all four organizations discussed in the article involved investing in workforce development by recruiting and training staff from the communities served; training staff to become midwives, perinatal birth workers, birth companions, or other care providers; and paying staff a living wage. Beyond short-term reproductive services, the highlighted organizations are building positive community change through community-informed strategies, capacity building, workforce and career development, well-paying jobs, and development of a more diverse pool of care providers who better reflect the characteristics of the communities they serve.

Promising community-based work focused on promoting equitable pregnancy-related outcomes is already underway in many communities. Organizations and others with similar goals may wish to identify such work in their communities and to reach out to explore partnership opportunities. Similarly, communities already engaged in such work may wish to consider and to seek out organizations and agencies to explore and expand partnerships. Such broader partnerships supporting community-driven approaches could lead to better-resourced and better-informed strategies that cross the zones of transformation, potentially expanding the number of communities served or types of services offered.

Broader Structures and Institutions

There are many ways that maternal health practitioners can expand the scope of their work to include systems transformation, and the Framework for Aligning

Table 8.2	Funding and Finance Strategies				
Funding			**Financing**		
Traditional Development Assistance	Conditional	Catalytic	Loans and Investments		
Categorical grants	Pay-for-performance; value-based payments; debt swaps	Seed funding; innovation awards	Impact investing	Socially responsible investing	Commercial investing

Adapted from USAID Center for Impact and Innovation, *Investing for Impact*. https://www.usaid.gov/cii/investing-impact.

Sectors identifies many areas where transformation can occur, for example through new forms of data-sharing or changes in governance structures. This section describes a form of systems transformation that itself underlies these types of systems transformation and many others: funding and finance reform.

For purposes of this discussion, *funding* is defined as money granted or awarded to an organization or agency, usually by a government sector or philanthropic organization, for a specific purpose, without any expectation of fiscal return. *Financing* is the process by which an organization receives capital or money to address a specific issue or to develop a product or set of products. It is usually provided by financial institutions, such as banks or other lending agencies that expect a return on the investment. Funding and finance reform happens when organizations adopt new strategies, such as those listed in Table 8.2.

This section describes structural transformation in maternal health practice through funding and finance changes in the form of pooled funds. Pooled funds are usually blended or braided. Blending involves mixing into a single pot funds that can be used to achieve a collaborative's goals. Braiding involves coordination of separate streams of money for the same ultimate goal: achieving the collaborative's objectives.

Community Health Access Project (CHAP) in Mansfield, Ohio,[25] is a Pathways Community HUB, meaning that the collaborative is certified as positioned to address social determinants of health, to work with community local members, and to link funding and finance directly to outcomes.[26]

Like many collaboratives engaged in funding and finance reform, CHAP involves changes in three areas: money sources, money uses, and money governance structures. In terms of money sources, CHAP uses a braided funding and finance model. Medicaid Managed Care Organizations (MCOs) finance care-coordination organizations that disburse payments to social service providers based on a series of formulas. Grants and philanthropic organizations provide start-up funding and fill gaps not covered by the MCOs. In terms of changes in money uses, performance-based payments are distributed upon successful completion of pathways. Pathways are checklists for addressing risk factors related to social determinants of health that, in partnership with community members, are identified as important. In terms of changes in governance structures, CHAP is special for both its incorporation of community voices in decision-making and for its emphasis on a central care-coordination organization that manages payment disbursement.

CHAP has demonstrated improved maternal health outcomes and reduced rates of low-birth-weight babies.[27] Much of this is credited to the Pathways Community HUB model it employs. CHAP and other Pathways Community HUBs demonstrate that systems transformation, and funding and finance transformation specifically, are ripe areas for action that can improve maternal health.

CONCLUSION

Reversing unwanted trends in maternal health requires new ways of thinking about maternal health practice. Traditional healthcare and public health services must be augmented with changes based on a broader view of the factors that affect maternal health and health equity.

As the four case examples discussed demonstrate, multiple zones of transformation can be addressed at the same time. For example, in the cases that focused on organization internals and finance systems transformation, both organizations—CHAP and the Dignity in Pregnancy and Childbirth Project—emphasized community partnerships, and the Illinois Family Case Management example that employed a community-driven initiative also emphasized social services.

Another opportunity is collaboration. Extending maternal health practice often involves partnerships that link maternal health practitioners, bring in resources, and promote coordinated service. Collaborations offer opportunities to formalize and streamline partnerships in intentional ways.

There are many ways practitioners can extend their maternal health practice beyond traditional services in healthcare and public health. In doing so, they will find opportunities to address a much wider range of maternal health challenges. By addressing this wider range of challenges, practitioners can find new strategies to help close maternal health equity gaps and send maternal health trends in a better direction.

REFERENCES

1. Centers for Disease Control and Prevention. Pregnancy Mortality Surveillance System. Atlanta, GA: Centers for Disease Control and Prevention. Accessed January 3, 2022, https://www.cdc.gov/reproductivehealth/maternal-mortality/pregnancy-mortality-surveillance-system.htm?CDC_AA_refVal=https%3A%2F%2Fwww.cdc.gov%2Freproductivehealth%2Fmaternalinfanthealth%2Fpregnancy-mortality-surveillance-system.htm.

2. Hill I, Benatar S, Garrett B, et al. *Strong Start for Mothers and Newborns Evaluation: Year 5 Project Synthesis, Volume 1: Cross-Cutting Findings*. Washington, DC: Urban Institute; 2018.

3. Bond RM, Gaither K, Nasser S, et al. Working agenda for Black mothers: a position paper from the Association of Black Cardiologists on solutions to improving Black maternal health. *Circ. Cardiovasc Qual Outcomes*. 2021;14(2):e007643.

4. Phelan JC, Link BG. Is racism a fundamental cause of inequalities in health? *Annu Rev Sociol*. 2015;41:311–330.

5. Mays GP, Mamaril CB, Timsina LR. Preventable death rates fell where communities expanded population health activities through multisector networks. *Health Aff*. 2016;35(11):2005–2013.

6. Mclean M, et al. Testing the theory of change: lessons from hospital-embedded social services in the Spring 2020 COVID-19 crisis. In: Health Aff, ed. *Aligning Systems for Health: Two Years of Learning*. Georgia Health Policy Center; 2021:320–338.

7. 10 Essential Public Health Services Futures Initiatives Task Force. *The 10 Essential Public Health Services: to protect and promote the health of all people in all communities*. Public Health Infrastructure Center; 2020.

8. Bureau of Maternal and Child Health. Family Case Management: history. Illinois Department of Human Services. Accessed April 1, 2022. https://www.dhs.state.il.us/page.aspx?item=31893.

9. Bureau of Maternal and Child Health. Family Case Management: frequently asked questions. Illinois Department of Human Services. Accessed April 1, 2022. https://www.dhs.state.il.us/page.aspx?item=30517.

10. Silva R, Thomas M, Caetano R, Aragaki C. Preventing low birth weight in Illinois: outcomes of the Family Case Management Program. *Matern Child Health J*. 2006;10:481–488. doi:10.1007/s10995-006-0133-8.

11. Keeton K, Saunders S, Koltun D. The effect of the Family Case Management Program on 1996 birth outcomes in Illinois. *J Womens Health*. 2004;13(2):207–215. doi:10.1089/154099904322966191.

12. National Partnership for Women and Families. Black women's maternal health: a multifaceted approach to addressing persistent and dire health disparities. 2018. https://www.nationalpartnership.org/our-work/resources/health-care/maternity/black-womens-maternal-health-issue-brief.pdf.

13 Chappel A, DeLew N, Grigorescu V, Smith SR. Addressing the maternal health crisis through improved data infrastructure: guiding principles for progress. Health Affairs Blog. 2021. Accessed April 1, 2022. https://www.healthaffairs.org/do/10.1377/forefront.20210729.265068/.

14. McLemore MR, Altman MR, Cooper N, Williams S, Rand L, Franck L. Health care experiences of pregnant, birthing and postnatal women of color at risk for preterm birth. *Soc Sci Med*. 2018;201:127–135. doi:10.1016/j.socscimed.2018.02.013.

15. Fridman M, Korst L, Chow J, Lawton E, Mitchell C, Gregory K. Trends in maternal morbidity before and during pregnancy in California. *Am J Public Health*. 2014;104(S1):S49–S57. doi:10.2105/AJPH.2013.301583.

16. Vedam S. The Giving Voice to Mothers study: inequity and mistreatment during pregnancy and childbirth in the United States. *Reprod Health*. 2019;16:77–94. doi:10.1186/s12978-019-0729-2.

17. Petersen EE. Racial/ethnic disparities in pregnancy-related deaths—United States, 2007–2016. *MMWR*. 2019;68:262–265. https://www.cdc.gov/mmwr/volumes/68/wr/pdfs/mm6835a3-H.pdf.

18. Hardeman R. Dignity in Pregnancy and Childbirth Project. Diversity Science. Accessed April 8, 2022. https://www.diversityscience.org/evidence-based-capacity-building/equal-perinatal-care/.

19. Teleki S. Challenging providers to look within themselves: a new tool to reduce bias in maternity care. *Health Affairs*. Accessed April 8, 2022. https://www.healthaffairs.org/do/10.1377/forefront.20210630.980773/.

20. Ogunwole SM, Bennett WL, Williams AN, Bower KM. Community-based doulas and COVID-19: addressing structural and institutional barriers to maternal health equity. *Perspect Sex Reprod Health*. 2020;52(4):199–204. doi:https://doi.org/10.1363/psrh.12169.

21. Tilsen N. Taking community action to promote health equity: the Thunder Valley Community Development Corporation. In: National Academies of Sciences, Engineering, and Medicine, ed. *Communities in Action: Pathways to Health Equity*. National Washington, DC: Academies Press; 2017:chap 4, 185–210.

22. National Academies of Sciences, Engineering, and Medicine. Partners in promoting health equity in communities. In: National Academies of Sciences Engineering, and Medicine, ed. *Communities in Action: Pathways to Health Equity*. National Washington, DC: Academies Press; 2017:chap 7, 383–446.

23. Zephyrin L, Seervai S, Lewis C, Katon JG. *Community-Based Models to Improve Maternal Health Outcomes and Promote Health Equity*. New York, NY: Commonwealth Fund; 2021.

24. Godbolt D, Glover S, Sakala C. *Tackling Maternal Health Disparities: A Look at Four Local Organizations with Innovative Approaches*. Washington, DC: National Partnership for Women and Families; 2019.

25. Community Health Access Project. About the HUB. Community Health Access Project. Accessed April 8, 2022. https://chap-ohio.com/about

26. Pathways Community HUB Institute. Pathways Community HUBs: identifying and addressing risks in a whole person approach. Pathways Community HUB Institute. Accessed April 8, 2022. https://pchi-hub.com/

27. Redding S, Conrey E, Porter K, Paulson J, Hughes K, Redding M. Pathways Community Care coordination in low birth weight prevention. *Matern Child Health J*. 2015;19:643–650.

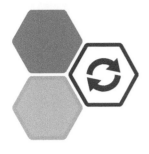

Chapter 9

An Approach for Whole-Person Health: Oral Healthcare Integration for Improved Maternal Outcomes

TIMOTHY L. RICKS AND ZACHARY A. BRIAN

INTRODUCTION

The late Dr. C. Everett Koop, US Surgeon General from 1982 to 1989, once said, "You're not healthy without good oral health."[1] This message was enhanced in 2000 with the release of *Oral Health in America,* the first-ever surgeon general's report on oral health. The report's primary message was that oral health means more than just healthy teeth and is integral to the general health and well-being of all Americans.[2] Oral disease is associated with multiple systemic conditions, including diabetes, adverse pregnancy outcomes, atherosclerotic cardiovascular disease, rheumatoid arthritis, Alzheimer's disease, chronic obstructive pulmonary disease, non-alcoholic fatty liver disease, and more.[3] The common link between oral diseases—specifically periodontal (gum) disease—and chronic diseases is the presence of bacterial toxins and inflammatory processes.

Oral health plays a very important role in maternal and child health. For example, pregnant mothers may be susceptible to gingivitis and dental caries (cavities) due to hormonal and nutritional issues.[4] Healthcare professionals sometimes do not provide oral health education to pregnant mothers; at the same time, many pregnant women may not seek or receive care from an oral health professional, further exacerbating oral health problems. But the impact of oral health neglect isn't confined to the mother. Evidence points to the fact that most infants and children acquire their oral microflora (bacteria) from their mothers, including caries-causing bacteria.[5] This affects young children, especially those

Timothy L. Ricks and Zachary A. Brian, *An Approach for Whole-Person Health* In: *The Practical Playbook III.* Edited by: Dorothy Cilenti, Alisahah Jackson, Natalie D. Hernandez, Lindsey Yates, Sarah Verbiest, J. Lloyd Michener, and Brian C. Castrucci, Oxford University Press. © de Beaumont Foundation 2024. DOI: 10.1093/oso/9780197662984.003.0009

in certain high-risk subgroups (those living in poverty and certain racial/ethnic groups), with a condition known as early childhood caries (ECC).

ECC is the presence of one or more decayed, missing (due to caries/decay), or filled teeth in any primary tooth in a child between birth and 71 months of age.[6] ECC is a multifactorial, infectious disease that can start as soon as an infant's teeth erupt. Besides the obvious pain and infection caused by dental caries progressing into the pulp of the teeth, ECC can also evoke a series of psychosocial, physical, and functional consequences, including sleep loss, irritability, eating difficulty, effects on overall nutrition and development, and even iron-deficiency anemia.[7] ECC can also affect speech development and communication, school performance later as a child enters school, and quality of life later into adulthood.[8] This cascade of adverse, systemic sequelae from ECC makes the disease much more than just a dental problem in baby teeth; ECC is a significant health problem and the most prevalent one in early childhood, even more common than childhood asthma. The prevalence of ECC may be as high as 70% in less developed countries and among disadvantaged groups in developed countries.[9]

ACHIEVING ORAL HEALTH EQUITY

Addressing ECC and all oral health issues across the life span among disadvantaged groups is a central tenet of oral health equity. Dental caries, which can lead to pain, infection, social stigmatization, missing teeth, eating difficulties (and resulting nutritional deficiencies), economic consequences from the cost of dental care, and even diminished hiring potential, affects people of certain ethnic backgrounds and incomes more than others. For example, the prevalence of dental caries experience—any history of decay (filled or missing teeth or active disease)—is 10% to 15% higher in Black non-Hispanic Americans and Mexican Americans across the life span compared with white non-Hispanic Americans. These same groups have as much as twice the amount of untreated dental caries (active disease) as white non-Hispanic Americans. Similarly, those living at or below 200% of the Federal Poverty Level (FPL) have double the prevalence of untreated caries across the life span compared with those living at or above 200% of the FPL and three times the prevalence of total tooth loss for those 65 years and over compared with those living at or above 200% of the FPL.[10]

Unfortunately, access to dental care continues to be a problem in the United States: Only 43% of the US population had a dental visit in 2015. Moreover, some segments of the population—certain racial/ethnic minority groups, people living in poverty, and people living in rural areas—have even less access to dental care. Overall, people of all ages living in rural America have about 8% (children age ≥ 2 years) to 10% (adults age 18 to 64 years) less access to dental services compared with their urban counterparts. Children in rural areas are 5% less likely to receive preventive dental care than children in urban areas, and adults in rural areas are 7% more likely to have missing teeth.[3] Medical professionals have a unique opportunity to inform patients about oral healthcare. In 2018, 121.2 million Americans visited both an oral health and medical professional at least once. Another 112.3 million visited only a medical professional, while 28.2 million visited only an oral health professional.[11]

Many factors contribute to the low rate of access to dental care in the United States. The cost of oral health is one barrier: While per capita oral health costs almost doubled from 1990 to 2018—from $232 to $413—the percentage of people who did not obtain oral health services during the previous 12 months due to cost was almost double that for people who did not seek prescription drugs, optometry, or medical care over the same period (8.9% versus 5.3%, 4.8%, and 5.0%, respectively).[12] An estimated 74 million Americans lack any dental coverage from employer-sponsored, government-sponsored, or private-sponsored insurance, as a direct result of the cost. For example, as of 2021, only 21 states provided extensive dental coverage for adults receiving Medicaid benefits.[13] Another factor is location, with over 60 million Americans residing in areas designated by the Health Resources and Services Administration as a dental health professional shortage area, denoting an insufficient number of oral health providers.

To address gaps in dental coverage across the country, various alternative dental workforce models have been implemented. These include a type of midlevel oral health provider, the dental therapist, a role that was developed in 2000 in the remote villages of Alaska and had extended as of 2021 to over a dozen states, with Minnesota being the first to legislate dental therapy, in 2009. Another model is the expansion of the scopes of practice for dental hygienists, with multiple states implementing independent practice, collaborative practice, and public health dental hygienist models. Community dental health coordinators, who are dental hygienists or dental assistants who specifically target patients from vulnerable and underserved populations and help coordinate care for them in community health centers and private practice dental programs, are another model. Finally, expanded function dental assistants, a model pioneered by the Indian Health Service in 1961, have been adopted in over a dozen states. These trained assistants can place restorations (dental fillings) and/or perform basic dental cleanings under indirect supervision of a dentist. Alternative dental workforce models like these can significantly increase access to dental care for vulnerable populations, including pregnant mothers, infants, and toddlers. In particular, they are effective in identifying and tracking patients who may have fallen through the cracks of continuity of care.

CURRENT SYSTEM DESIGN

Dentistry and medicine in the United States have long operated in silos. The dental–medical divide is a significant factor in the lack of the integrated care required to improve access to maternal and child oral health and achieve whole-person health. "The need for integration is increasingly apparent," according to Atchison et al.[14] Children are significantly affected: A report on integrated care for children's oral health noted that only 3% of children on Medicaid receive oral health services from their medical providers, despite having multiple well-child visits, and only 1% of children on Medicaid under age 1 have a dental visit.[15] A 2016 national survey found that only 63% of pregnant women saw a dentist during their pregnancy, making screening and referral of oral conditions in primary care even more important.[16] Dr. Lisa Simon, who became a physician after seeing the need for care integration firsthand while working as a dentist in a community health center, observed that the separation of dentistry and medicine "continues to have [a] lasting and meaningful impact on the lived experiences of millions of Americans, especially those from at-risk communities already poorly served by the medical system."[17] In recent years, many organizations have worked to remedy the dental–medical divide, issuing guidelines intended to improve maternal and child health by integrating oral health screenings and services in prenatal, pediatric, and primary care.

One of these organizations is the American Academy of Pediatrics (AAP). The AAP has been at the forefront of efforts to improve integration of oral health services into both prenatal and pediatric care. According to the organization's Bright Futures guidelines, "Even before the baby's birth, parents and other caregivers should make sure their own mouths are as healthy as possible to reduce transmission of caries-causing harmful bacteria from their saliva to the newborn's mouth."[18] Dr. J. Shahangian, a board-certified pediatric dentist and member of the AAP Section on Oral Health, observed, "A mom who cares for herself is also caring for her unborn child—that's especially true when it comes to oral health. . . . When you take care of your teeth and gums, it can potentially make a difference for your baby, both before and after birth."[19] Writing for the AAP's HealthyChildren.org, he recommended that pregnant individuals brush their teeth regularly with fluoridated toothpaste, floss regularly, adhere to a diet rich in calcium and low in acidity and sugar, and increase the frequency of dental cleanings.[19] AAP guidelines also encourage new parents to practice good oral hygiene; not to share cups, utensils, or toothbrushes with the infant; and not to place the infant's pacifier in their own mouth, but instead to clean it with mild soap and water.[18] The AAP also encourages breastfeeding when possible; research in the organization's *Pediatrics* journal determined that predominant breastfeeding was associated with a lower prevalence of malocclusion (misalignment of teeth).[20] At the center of all these recommendations are early detection, prevention, education, and, critically, integration of oral health services into prenatal, pediatric, and primary care. Oral health risk assessments for both pregnant individuals and infants are recommended: "To prevent caries in children, high-risk individuals must be identified at an early age (preferably high-risk [individuals] during prenatal care)"[21] and "since 2003, the American

Academy of Pediatrics has recommended that health professionals conduct an oral health risk assessment when an infant is 6 months of age."[18]

Similar calls for care integration to improve maternal and child oral health (and, by extension, overall health) have been made by other prominent organizations, including the National Interprofessional Initiative on Oral Health (NIIOH) and the American Public Health Association (APHA). NIIOH's Oral Health Delivery Framework—a series of guidelines for integrating oral health into primary care—has been endorsed by the AAP, the National Association of Pediatric Nurse Practitioners, and the American Academy of Family Physicians, among others.[22] Foremost among the framework's guidelines are recommendations for oral health screenings, preventive services, and referrals to dental homes.[22] NIIOH is also a lead supporter and promoter of Smiles for Life, a widely used curriculum for primary care clinicians on integration of oral healthcare services into primary care. APHA is similarly focused on advancing dental–medical integration, especially regarding maternal and child oral health. In the APHA's *American Journal of Public Health*, Dr. Stephen Martin, a physician, and Dr. Lisa Simon, a dentist, noted that "We are stymied by the historical vagaries of excluding dentistry from the medical system,"[23] and the APHA has taken a more prescriptive approach to health policy to address the problem. In a 2020 policy statement, for example, the APHA wrote, "State Medicaid programs should provide dental coverage during pregnancy through 1 year postpartum to maximize the window for dental care and provide reimbursement for oral health services delivered by prenatal providers to sustain the integration of oral health into primary care practice."[24]

PRACTICAL TIPS FOR MEDICAL PROFESSIONALS

Many credible organizations and researchers have issued guidelines intended to improve maternal and child oral health. These guidelines can be used by primary care physicians, pediatric physicians, obstetricians/gynecologists, behavioral health professionals, and others to integrate oral health into their regular workflows and improve their patients' overall health and well-being.

Oral Health Screenings

The AAP suggests that primary care physicians discuss oral health with parents and conduct an oral exam when the child's primary teeth first erupt (roughly six months after birth).[18] The guidance recommends that this and subsequent visits include "a risk history for caries [cavities], an oral exam, dental hygiene and diet advice, an assessment of the need for systemic fluoride, and a referral to the dentist, with the first dental visit before the child's first birthday."[25] As described in *Family Practice Management*, the journal of the American Academy of Family Physicians (AAFP), "Family physicians can start this discussion even earlier with women of childbearing age, as maternal oral health is a strong predictor of a child's oral health."[25] Research shows that physicians can easily acquire the skills needed to perform relatively accurate screenings for caries in infants and children. The pediatric primary care providers in one study "achieved an adequate level of accuracy identifying children with cavitated carious lesions" after just two hours of training.[26] The same study determined that dental screenings can easily be incorporated into a busy pediatrics practice.[26] Training sources for medical providers are readily available, including the Smiles for Life curriculum. Beyond pediatric practices, oral health risk assessments, preventive treatments, and education for children and pregnant individuals can be implemented in a variety of other nondental environments, including primary care practices, OB-GYN practices, behavioral health practices, community health centers, and WIC offices, to name a few.

Closing the Referral Loop

Oral health assessments to identify potential caries should result in referral to a dental home, and medical providers should also educate parents on the importance of regular dental visits and provide referrals accordingly. According to a 2021 report on integrating oral healthcare into primary care, "With early referral to an oral health professional, there is an opportunity to maintain good oral health, prevent oral disease, and treat oral disease early. Establishing collaborative relationships between PCPs and oral health professionals at the community level is essential."[27] A proactive referral to a dental home is also an opportunity for medical providers to divert patients from emergency departments, where treatment for dental problems does not address the root cause and often is not followed by a visit to a dentist. A 2015 study of Medicaid claims data in Iowa, for example, found that just 52% of patients who visited the emergency department for a dental problem saw a dentist within six months of that visit.[28]

When referring patients to a dental home, medical professionals should remember that the "traditional" dental home—a private practice—is not the only option. Dental "safety-net" clinics include community health centers and school-based health centers (SBHCs). These sites provide crucial access points for vulnerable and low-income populations in need of dental services.[29] These populations are concentrated in rural areas and urban centers, as most dentists' offices are located in suburban areas.[30] Dental "navigators" or community dental health coordinators are also increasingly used in nondental settings to address patients' barriers to access (often driven by the social determinants of health) and to close the referral loop, often connecting patients with safety-net clinics or SBHCs.

Technology and Teledentistry

There are many opportunities for medical providers to utilize technology to increase medical–dental integration and improve patients' oral health. Electronic health record (EHR) systems and teledentistry are two primary examples. The use of both is ideal and can further support the referral process, allowing integrated practices to transmit a patient's oral health data to a dentist for follow-up diagnosis and care. Intraoral cameras can be used in pediatric primary care offices and other settings, for example, as part of oral health assessments to capture evidence that a dentist can later evaluate. Dr. Paul Glassman, an innovator in the field of teledentistry, observed, "Using telehealth-connected teams to expand dental care and dental services into community locations and integrating dental care in community organizations has the potential to reach many people not reached currently and the ability to use prevention and early intervention strategies to keep them from developing advanced disease."[31] It's important to note that using teledentistry in a nondental setting does not necessarily require integrated EHR, provided that transmission of patient data between practices is HIPAA-compliant. On its own, medical–dental integration through EHR systems is relatively rare. A recent article noted that dentistry has been slow to adopt electronic dental records and that there is a lack of data standardization in the dental domain.[32]

Fluoride Varnish

The importance of the dental home notwithstanding, certain treatments can be administered by medical professionals themselves based on demographics and oral health risk assessments and are essential in promoting maternal and child oral health. The application of fluoride varnish is an easy-to-implement preventive treatment that medical providers can offer in the nondental settings outlined above. A 2013 systematic analysis determined that young people treated with fluoride varnish experienced on average a 43% reduction in decayed, missing, and filled tooth surfaces.[33] After an initial recommendation in 2014, the US Preventive Services Task Force issued guidance in 2021 that primary care clinicians apply fluoride varnish to the primary teeth of all infants and children.[34] A 2016 study also found that fluoride varnish could easily be incorporated into well-child visits.[35] Applying varnish is easily learned, and costs roughly $1 per application.[25] A clinical report published by the AAP recommends applying fluoride varnish at least once every six months, and preferably every three, starting at tooth eruption.[36] A recent article in the AAFP journal offers practical suggestions for medical providers, including that "the medical assistant or nurse can apply fluoride varnish . . . in follow-up to the exam. . . . This arrangement allows the physician or midlevel provider to move more quickly on to the next patient and helps to preserve productivity."[25] The authors also noted that to maintain office efficiency, practices should keep fluoride varnish supplies in exam rooms or in a toolbox that can be transported from a central location into the exam room.[25] Importantly, fluoride varnish application in primary care clinics is both easy to implement and financially sustainable: A how-to guide from Smiles for Life says that the treatment can be applied in less than two minutes[37] and the organization notes that all 50 state Medicaid programs offer reimbursement to primary care providers.[38]

Silver Diamine Fluoride

When caries is identified early enough by a medical provider, application of silver diamine fluoride (SDF) is a low-cost, nonsurgical intervention that can be administered to arrest decay. SDF has been determined to be more effective than other preventive management strategies for arresting caries in the primary dentition,[39] with various studies demonstrating that its application arrested caries in 30% to 70% of cases.[40] An article in the journal *Dimensions of Dental Hygiene* observed that SDF is particularly advantageous for the most vulnerable patient populations, including children."[41] Drs. Elise Sarvas and Jeffrey M. Karp advised in *AAP News* that pediatricians should identify and refer patients to a dental home when they could benefit from SDF therapy.[42] However, SDF application by nondental providers, such as pediatricians or primary care physicians, may also be an option, depending on state laws and regulations. A 2019 study reviewed a model for this integrated delivery system, concluding that it is feasible for physicians to treat ECC with SDF in a primary care setting.[43] The study also found that "partnership with an on-site hygienist is helpful, but physician-only sessions were still beneficial."[43] Nondental professionals interested in providing SDF treatments should review their state's medical practice act and associated legislation and regulations before pursuing this therapy. While 35 state Medicaid programs covered SDF application by a dental provider as of May 2021, as with other preventive treatments discussed in this chapter, reimbursement for application by a nondental provider may or may not be available.[44]

Interprofessional Practice

Beyond providing risk assessments, preventive treatments, patient education, and referrals themselves, medical providers can also integrate oral health through more innovative models. In some cases, it may be possible to place a dental hygienist or other dental professional (such as a dental navigator or community dental health coordinator) in nondental settings to improve integration, increase access to preventive care, and close the referral loop. While such interprofessional practice is increasingly happening in safety-net health centers (where dental and medical providers often are already located under one roof), it is uncommon in private practice settings. A 2019 report noted that in several states, dental hygienists and other allied dental personnel work in general healthcare environments, where they can engage patients and provide prevention services.[45] The American Dental Hygienists' Association offers a guide to states where legislation or regulatory rules allow dental hygienists to provide services in medical settings.[46] Nevertheless, scientific research on this degree of interprofessional practice remains relatively limited and needs future attention. Those interested in this degree of collaboration should keep in mind that hygienists' presence on the care team should not preclude primary care providers or other medical support staff from fully engaging in preventive oral healthcare.[47] Effectiveness of this strategy can be increased with teledentistry, in which embedded dental professionals connect with a remote dentist for a more full-service delivery system.[45]

Healthcare professionals not traditionally associated with oral healthcare can help improve maternal oral health as well. A study in 2010, for example, showed that pregnant patients demonstrated much better oral health practices in pregnancy and lower patient plaque index scores after receiving oral health and oral hygiene education from a trained midwife.[48] With midwife-attended births on the rise across the United States, such interprofessional practice may prove increasingly important in tackling disparities in maternal oral health.

Community Water Fluoridation

According to the Centers for Disease Control and Prevention (CDC), drinking fluoridated water reduces caries development by 25% in children and adults.[49] Despite its efficacy and research showing that water fluoridation offers significant cost savings for communities,[50] the CDC further reports that, as of 2018, just 73% of the US population on a community water system had access to fluoridated water.[51] For many women of reproductive age and pregnant women, this reality underscores the importance of the fluoride varnish applications discussed above. There also is a prime opportunity for medical providers to join their oral healthcare counterparts in policy advocacy to advance community water fluoridation across the country.

Payment Reform

Another opportunity for medical providers to promote maternal and child oral health is policy advocacy concerning payment reform. Private and public payers have often lagged behind providers in both interest and urgency when it comes to integrating oral healthcare in nondental settings. In most states, Medicaid offers reimbursement for medical providers who address oral health, but services covered and to what extent vary widely. As a result, reimbursement is a significant barrier to widespread availability of oral health services for children and maternal patients from medical providers. Going forward, payment reform will be a critical area of focus for dental and medical providers interested in expanding access to child and maternal oral health services in nondental settings.

CONCLUSION

For primary care and other medical providers interested in improving maternal oral health (and, by extension, overall health) among their patient populations, opportunities are widespread. It is important to note, however, that integration of oral health and overall health is bidirectional, and success relies upon dental, medical, and behavioral healthcare providers alike to educate and collaborate with each other. While oral healthcare professionals can, and should, for example, provide education to promote screening for dental disease and certain preventive procedures in primary care settings, medical professionals can likewise provide education to oral healthcare professionals to increase chronic disease screenings in dental settings. Both are critical in addressing "whole-body" maternal and child health and closing the referral loop that, when left unaddressed, may otherwise result in pregnant women and children falling through the cracks. Building relationships among dental, medical, and behavioral healthcare providers is key to the success of this effort, especially in consideration of the traditional silos discussed earlier.

Evidence supporting the relationship between oral health and overall health cannot be ignored, and there is both a moral and ethical imperative for medical providers to address the oral health of pregnant women and infants. With greater understanding of the relationship between periodontal disease and delivery of preterm, low-birth-weight babies, for example, a whole-body approach to maternal healthcare is necessary. Primary care and oral healthcare providers together should strive to educate pregnant women about these relationships, and primary care providers should make appropriate referrals to dentists to screen and treat pregnant women who may have periodontal disease. Only with such integration and interprofessional collaboration can maternal health be addressed as effectively and efficiently as possible. It is perhaps no exaggeration that when it comes to optimal outcomes in oral health and overall maternal health, neither can exist without the other.

REFERENCES

1. Allukian, M. The neglected epidemic and the surgeon general's report: a call to action for better oral health. *Am J Public Health*. 2008;98(suppl 1):S82–S85.

2. US Department of Health and Human Services. *Oral Health in America: A Report of the Surgeon General*. Rockville, MD: US Department of Health and Human Services, National Institute of Dental and Craniofacial Research, National Institutes of Health; 2000.

3. Hannan C, Ricks T, Espinoza L, Weintraub J. Addressing oral health inequities, access to care, knowledge, and behaviors. *Prev Chronic Dis*. 2021;18:210060. http://dx.doi.org/10.5888/pcd18.210060.

4. US Department of Health and Human Services. *The Surgeon General's Call to Action to Improve Maternal Health*. Rockville, MD: US Department of Health and Human Services; 2020.

5. Oral Health Care During Pregnancy Expert Workgroup. *Oral Health Care During Pregnancy: A National Consensus Statement—Summary of an Expert Workgroup Meeting*. Washington, DC: National Maternal and Child Oral Health Resource Center; 2012.

6. American Dental Association. *Statement on Early Childhood Caries, 2000*. https://www.ada.org/en/about-the-ada/ada-positions-policies-and-statements/statement-on-early-childhood-caries. Accessed November 8, 2021.

7. Collado V, Pichot H, Delfosse C, Eschevins C, Nicolas E, Hennequin M. Impact of early childhood caries and its treatment under general anesthesia on orofacial function and quality of life: a prospective comparative study. *Med Oral Patol Oral Cir Bucal*. 2017;22(3):e333–e341.

8. National Maternal and Child Oral Health Center, Georgetown University. Promoting Awareness, Preventing Pain: Facts on Early Childhood Caries (ECC). 2004. https://www.maineoralhealthcoalition.org/docs/ECCFactSheet.pdf. Accessed November 8, 2021.

9. Anil S, Anand P. Early childhood caries: prevalence, risk factors, and prevention. *Front Pediatr*. 2017;5:157.

10. Centers for Disease Control and Prevention. *Oral Health Surveillance Report: Trends in Dental Caries and Sealants, Tooth Retention, and Edentulism, United States, 1999–2004 to 2011–2016*. Atlanta, GA: Centers for Disease Control and Prevention; 2019.

11. Manski R, Rohde F, Ricks T. *Trends in the Number and Percentage of the Population with Any Dental or Medical Visits, 2003–2018*. Statistical Brief #537. October 2021. Rockville, MD: Agency for Healthcare Research and Quality. https://meps.ahrq.gov/data_files/publications/st537/stat537.pdf.

12. American Dental Association, Health Policy Institute. Cost Barriers to Dental Care in the U.S. 2016. https://www.ada.org/~/media/ADA/Science%20and%20Research/HPI/Files/HPIgraphic_1117_4.pdf?la=en.

13. DentaQuest. Adult dental benefit. https://dentaquest.com/oral-health-resources/adult-dental-benefit/. Accessed November 8, 2021.

14. Atchison KA, Rozier RG, Weintraub JA. Integration of oral health and primary care: communication, coordination and referral. *NAM Perspectives*. 2018;8(10):1–12. doi:10.31478/201810e.

15. Edelstein B, Rubin M. Improving children's oral health by crossing the medical-dental divide. Connecticut Health Foundation. January 2015. https://www.cthealth.org/wp-content/uploads/2015/02/Crossing-the-Medical-Dental-Divide-Final-2.pdf. Accessed February 7, 2022.

16. Delta Dental. Number of pregnant women in U.S. getting dental care on the rise. Delta Dental Plans Association; 2016. https://www.deltadental.com/us/en/about-us/press-center/2016/newsreleasepregnantwomenontherise201605.html.

17. Simon L. Inequity along the medical-dental divide. *AMA J Ethics*. 2022;24(1):E3–E5. doi:10.1001/amajethics.2022.3.

18. American Academy of Pediatrics. Bright futures guidelines for health supervision of infants, children, and adolescents. 2017. https://brightfutures.aap.org/Bright%20Futures%20Documents/BF4_OralHealth.pdf. Accessed February 7, 2022.

19. Shahangian, J. Brushing for two: how your oral health affects baby. American Academy of Pediatrics. November 19, 2019. https://www.healthychildren.org/English/ages-stages/prenatal/Pages/Brushing-for-Two-How-Your-Oral-Health-Effects-Baby.aspx. Accessed February 7, 2022.

20. Peres K, Cascaes A, Peres M, et al. Exclusive breastfeeding and risk of dental malocclusion. *Pediatrics*. 2015;136(1):e60–e67. doi:10.1542/peds.2014-3276.

21. Hale K. Oral health risk assessment timing and establishment of the dental home. *Pediatrics*. 2003;111(5):1113–1116. doi:10.1542/peds.111.5.1113.

22. National Interprofessional Initiative on Oral Health. Oral health integration implementation project. 2017. http://www.niioh.org/Implementation-Guide. Accessed February 7, 2022.

23. Martin S, Simon L. Oral health and medicine integration: overcoming historical artifact to relieve suffering. *Am J Public Health*. 2017;107(1):30–31. doi:10.2105/AJPH.2017.303683.

24. American Public Health Association. Improving access to dental care for pregnant women through education, integration of health services, insurance coverage, an appropriate dental workforce, and research. October 24, 2020. https://www.apha.org/policies-and-advocacy/public-health-policy-statements/policy-database/2021/01/12/improving-access-to-dental-care-for-pregnant-women. Accessed February 7, 2022.

25. Silk H, Deutchman M. Offering oral health services in your office. *Fam Pract Manage*. 2014;21(4):21–24. https://www.aafp.org/fpm/2014/0700/p21.html.

26. Pierce K, Rozier R, Vann W. Accuracy of pediatric primary care providers' screening and referral for early childhood caries. *Pediatrics*. 2002;109(5):e82–e82. doi:10.1542/peds.109.5.e82.

27. Battani K, Holt K. The partnership for integrating oral health care into primary care project 2019-2021: final report. National Maternal and Child Oral Health Resource Center. 2021. https://www.mchoralhealth.org/PDFs/piohcpc-final-report-2021.pdf. Accessed February 7, 2022.

28. Singhal A, Momany E, Jones M, Kuthy R, Buresh C, Damiano P. Dental care after an emergency department visit for dental problems among adults enrolled in Medicaid. *J Am Dent Assoc*. 2016;147(2):111–119. doi:10.1016/j.adaj.2015.08.012.

29. Yalowich R, Corso C. Enhancing oral health access through safety net partnerships: a primer and resource guide for Medicaid agencies. National Academy for State Health Policy. 2015. https://www.nashp.org/wp-content/uploads/2015/08/Enhancing-Oral-Health-Primer-for-Medicaid-Agencies.pdf.

30. National Oral Health Policy Center at Children's Dental Health Project. The dental home: summary from an MCHB expert meeting. 2008. https://www.mchoralhealth.org/PDFs/DentalHome_Report.pdf. Accessed February 7, 2022.

31. Glassman P. Teledentistry: improving oral health using telehealth-connected teams. University of the Pacific Arthur A. Dugoni School of Dentistry Pacific Center for Special Care. August 2016. https://www.americanteledentistry.org/wp-content/uploads/2018/02/UofP_WhitePaper_Telehealth.pdf. Accessed February 7, 2022.

32. Webb A, Sommers S. Medical and dental data integration: how can this become a reality? *Dental Econ*. February 1, 2021. https://www.dentaleconomics.com/macro-op-ed/technology-trends/article/14197059/medical-and-dental-data-integration-how-can-this-become-a-reality. Accessed February 7, 2022.

33. Marinho V, Worthington H, Walsh T, Clarkson J. Fluoride varnishes for preventing dental caries in children and adolescents. *Cochrane Database Syst Rev*. 2013;7:CD002279. doi:10.1002/14651858.CD002279.pub2.

34. US Preventive Services Task Force. Prevention of dental caries in children younger than 5 years: screening and interventions. December 7, 2021. https://www.uspreventiveservicestaskforce.org/uspstf/recommendation/prevention-of-dental-caries-in-children-younger-than-age-5-years-screening-and-interventions1. Accessed February 7, 2022.

35. Tellez M, Wolff M. The public health reach of high fluoride vehicles: examples of innovative approaches. *Caries Res.* 2016;50(1):61–67. doi:10.1159/000443186.

36. Clark M, Slayton R. Fluoride use in caries prevention in the primary care setting. *Pediatrics.* 2014;134(3):626–633. doi:10.1542/peds.2014-1699.

37. Smiles for Life. Fluoride varnish manual for medical clinicians. January 2009. https://www.smilesforlifeoralhealth.org/wp-content/uploads/2020/01/STFM_SFL_3_Fluoride_Varnish_Manual.pdf. Accessed February 7, 2022.

38. Smiles for Life. Fluoride varnish ordering and state specific information. 2022. https://www.smilesforlifeoralhealth.org/resources/practice-tools-and-resources/state-specific-fluoride-varnish-information/. Accessed February 7, 2022.

39. Contreras V, Toro M, Elias-Boneta A, Encarnacion-Burgos A. Effectiveness of silver diamine fluoride in caries prevention and arrest: a systematic literature review. *Gen Dent.* 2017;65(3):22–29. https://www.ncbi.nlm.nih.gov/pmc/articles/PMC5535266/#:~:text=A%20systematic%20review%20of%207,caries%20in%20th.

40. Janakiram C, Ramanarayanan V, Devan I. Effectiveness of silver diamine fluoride applications for dental caries cessation in tribal preschool children in India: study protocol for a randomized controlled trial. *Methods Protoc.* 2021;4(2):30. doi:10.3390/mps4020030.

41. MacLean J. Dimensions of dental hygiene: a practical guide to silver diamine fluoride. February 3, 2020. https://dimensionsofdentalhygiene.com/article/a-practical-guide-to-silver-diamine-fluoride/. Accessed February 7, 2022.

42. Sarvas E, Karp J. Silver diamine fluoride arrests untreated dental caries but has drawbacks. *AAP News.* August 5, 2016. https://publications.aap.org/aapnews/news/13524. Accessed February 7, 2022.

43. Bernstein R, Johnston B, Mackay K, Sanders J. Implementation of a primary care physician-led cavity clinic using silver diamine fluoride. *J Public Health Dent.* 2019;79(3):193–197. doi:10.1111/jphd.12331.

44. Caffrey E, Lu J, Wright R, Litch C, Casamassimo P. Are your kids covered? Medicaid coverage for the essential oral health benefits. American Academy of Pediatric Dentistry. May 2021. https://www.aapd.org/globalassets/media/policy-center/areyourkidscovered-ii-final.pdf. Accessed February 7, 2022.

45. Glassman P. Improving oral health using telehealth-connected teams and the virtual dental home system of care: program and policy considerations. DentaQuest Partnership for Oral Health Advancement. August 2019. https://www.utah.gov/pmn/files/556629.pdf. Accessed February 7, 2022.

46. Dental hygiene in medical settings and health clinics. American Dental Hygienists' Association. June 2019. https://www.adha.org/resources-docs/Dental_Hygiene_in_Medical_Settings.pdf. Accessed February 7, 2022.

47. Goldie M. Could the primary-care physician's office be the next non-traditional practice setting for dental hygienists? *DentistryIQ.* January 14, 2016. https://www.dentistryiq.com/dental-hygiene/clinical-hygiene/article/16352338/could-the-primarycare-physicians-office-be-the-next-nontraditional-practice-setting-for-dental-hygienists. Accessed February 7, 2022.

48. Mohebbi SZ, Yazdani R, Sargeran K, Tartar Z, Janeshin A. Midwifery students training in oral care of pregnant patients: an interventional study. *J Dent (Tehran).* 2014;11(5):587–595. https://www.ncbi.nlm.nih.gov/pmc/articles/PMC4290779/.

49. Centers for Disease Control and Prevention. Community water fluoridation. January 15, 2020. https://www.cdc.gov/fluoridation/index.html. Accessed February 7, 2022.

50. Griffin S, Jones K, Tomar S. An economic evaluation of community water fluoridation. *J Public Health Dent.* 2001;61(2):78–86. doi:10.1111/j.1752-7325.2001.tb03370.x.

51. Centers for Disease Control and Prevention. Water fluoridation data and statistics. August 28, 2020. https://www.cdc.gov/fluoridation/statistics/index.htm. Accessed February 7, 2022.

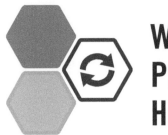

Chapter 10

What It Really Takes to Succeed: Practical Tips for Maternal Health Collaboration

PIIA HANSON AND KIMBERLY SHERMAN

The present focus on addressing maternal morbidity and mortality is long overdue. Rates of maternal death in the United States have been documented since the 1900s, yet the number and rate of deaths continue to escalate. With renewed attention to the issue, all facets of public, private, and nonprofit organizations have joined together to systematically improve maternal health outcomes.

This chapter is a resource for frontline public health practitioners who engage with the challenges of maternal morbidity and mortality at the state and community levels. It discusses nine states that work in and across various sectors to address this national crisis and what it takes to succeed in this work. Practitioners from each state describe successful cross-sector partnerships and identify the frameworks and tools that have been useful in building them; discuss the elements of authentic engagement; and highlight barriers to and facilitators of achieving equitable partnerships, including the importance of sharing power and resources.

STATE MATERNAL HEALTH INNOVATION PROGRAM: AN OVERVIEW

In June 2018, the Health Resources and Services Administration (HRSA) of the US Department of Health and Human Services convened maternal health stakeholders for a Maternal Mortality Summit. Development and implementation of the State Maternal Health Innovation Program (State MHI Program) was just one of the outcomes of this convening.

Piia Hanson and Kimberly Sherman, *What It Really Takes to Succeed* In: *The Practical Playbook III*. Edited by: Dorothy Cilenti, Alisahah Jackson, Natalie D. Hernandez, Lindsey Yates, Sarah Verbiest, J. Lloyd Michener, and Brian C. Castrucci, Oxford University Press. © de Beaumont Foundation 2024. DOI: 10.1093/oso/9780197662984.003.0010

The program began in September 2019, with nine award recipients that entered into five-year cooperative agreements. Funded states include Arizona, Illinois, Iowa, Maryland, Montana, New Jersey, North Carolina, Ohio, and Oklahoma. The purpose of the demonstration program is to assist states in strengthening their capacity to address disparities in maternal health and improve maternal health outcomes, including prevention and reduction of maternal mortality and severe maternal morbidity. Specifically, the funded states are tasked with strengthening partnerships and collaboration by establishing a state-focused maternal health task force, improving state-level data surveillance on maternal mortality and severe maternal morbidity, and promoting and executing innovation in maternal health service delivery.

The nine State MHI Program awardees address a variety of US maternal health challenges, each taking a unique approach to improving maternal health outcomes in their state. Across the program, awardees test various innovative approaches, collaborate with key stakeholders, and address and advance maternal health equity. As of this writing, the existing award recipients are in the third year of the funding opportunity and will continue with testing and evaluating innovative activities, enhancing maternal health data systems, and supporting each state's maternal health infrastructure through the leadership of its maternal health task force. Table 10.1 summarizes the target populations and program components of each state awardee.

BUILDING COLLABORATIONS: ESTABLISHING STATE-LED MATERNAL HEALTH TASK FORCES

The State MHI Program seeks to improve state capacity through coordination and collaboration using public health approaches, direct service delivery, and maternal health data to support the implementation of innovative maternal health strategies. Creation of a state-focused maternal health task force (MHTF) is a primary component of the program. While most states have a comprehensive task force to address a broad array of priorities, development of a task force specifically invested in maternal health ensures that these priorities can be moved forward effectively and efficiently.

Each MHTF is charged with creating and implementing a maternal health strategic plan that incorporates activities outlined in the state's most recent Title V needs assessment, improves state-level data surveillance on maternal mortality and severe maternal morbidity (SMM), and implements innovative strategies targeted at the state's leading causes of adverse maternal health outcomes.

There is a growing need for cross-sector partnerships that collaborate and innovate on key issues impacting maternal health outcomes, and implementation of innovations to improve those outcomes cannot be done in isolation.

Table 10.1	2019 State Maternal Health Innovation Program Award Recipients	
Award Recipient	**Target Population**	**Key Program Components**
Arizona Department of Health Services (Phoenix, AZ)	Pregnant and postpartum persons residing in Arizona, with a focus on African American, Indigenous, and rural communities	• Postpartum warning signs • Telehealth • Tribal maternal health
University of Illinois (Chicago, IL)	Pregnant and postpartum persons, as well as healthcare providers, including emergency departments and home visitors	• State data capacities • Provider trainings • Coordination of care • Telehealth
Iowa Department of Public Health (Des Moines, IA)	Birthing persons residing in Iowa	• Workforce development • Maternal transport • Telehealth • Mobile OB simulation
The Johns Hopkins University (Baltimore, MD)	Birthing persons, healthcare providers, hospitals, and home visiting programs in Maryland	• Maternal morbidity surveillance • Telemedicine • Postpartum warning signs education • Hospital provider trainings
Montana Department of Public Health and Human Services (Helena, MT)	Pregnant and postpartum persons and those planning to become pregnant; rural, remote populations; Native American populations; and healthcare providers offering prenatal care services	• Provider trainings • Telemedicine • Mental health/substance use disorders
New Jersey Department of Health (Trenton, NJ)	Prenatal and postpartum persons and providers in New Jersey	• Data and surveillance • Implicit bias training • Coordination of care
North Carolina Department of Health and Human Services (Raleigh, NC)	North Carolina perinatal care regions and providers, as well as pregnant and postpartum persons in North Carolina	• Provider trainings • Postpartum visits • Telehealth
Ohio Department of Health (Columbus, OH)	Pregnant and postpartum persons, women of reproductive age, providers, and WIC clinics in Ohio	• AIM bundle implementation • Urgent maternal warning signs • Workforce training efforts
Oklahoma State Health Department (Oklahoma City, OK)	Low-income, Native American, African American, Hispanic, uninsured, underinsured, and rural pregnant and postpartum women in Oklahoma	• Project ECHO (telehealth) • Substance use disorders • Expanded access to prenatal care • Mobile maternal health units

As such, all State MHI programs are committed to developing a diverse MHTF with both traditional and nontraditional stakeholders. Traditional partners, such as perinatal quality collaboratives, community action networks, and maternal mortality review committees, bring expertise, lessons learned, and key connections. Nontraditional partners, such as women's shelters, public safety organizations, refugee and immigration service providers, state hospital associations, payers (including state Medicaid agencies and health plan organizations), assistance agencies, and charitable donor organizations, bring innovation, diverse perspectives, and lived experience to improving maternal health. Using this strategy, the State MHI programs created a safe space for women, families, and communities to be heard.

Practical Tips for Collaboration

- Acknowledge existing statewide efforts that affect maternal health outcomes.
- Use existing tools and environmental scans to ensure the right infrastructure for your task force.
- Bring together multidisciplinary teams.
- Include the voice of people with lived experience in decision-making.
- Ensure buy-in from persons and groups affected by proposed policy and program changes.
- Use community-driven and culturally competent approaches to improving maternal health when providing k to birthing and parenting education.
- Leverage federal funds from grants, collaborate with state agencies working toward the same goals, and utilize staff from community partners to amplify your work.
- Enlist your local hospital association as a resource and partner.
- Create projects together with your partners to establish trust.
- Create space to brainstorm and innovate with a variety of thought leaders and partners.
- Be transparent in your efforts with partners and ensure regular and ongoing communication.
- Don't be afraid to bring voice to issues of equity, diversity, and inclusion in maternal health.
- Leverage existing funding to establish a learning management platform for your team and partners.
- Connect your providers to each other, and bring information, training, and education directly to them.
- Lean into the basics—patient education remains a critical strategy for improving maternal health outcomes.
- Use data and data dashboards to tell a compelling story about advancements in maternal health.

Tips from Arizona: Co-Creating Projects with Tribal Communities to Improve Maternal Health

Lynn Lane and Heidi Christensen

The Maternal Health Innovation Program (MHI) at the Arizona Department of Health Services collaborated with maternal health champions within Arizona's Tribal communities to identify activities to improve maternal health outcomes. The Maternal and Family Wellness From an Indigenous Perspective training series was built on these conversations.

Arizona is home to 22 Tribal Nations and to many other American Indian/Alaskan Native people living in both Tribal and urban settings; each Tribe has its own rich culture, language, and governance structure. Assets of Tribal communities include traditional values, practices, teachings, and stories that can create cultural protection and resiliency as well as community connections and support systems. Extended family, Tribal elders, traditional teachings, and cultural restoration of mentors, crafts, stories, and language are important strengths to build on.

Sessions of the Maternal and Family Wellness series were created by, and for, Tribal communities and Indigenous populations and were provided at no cost. It was important that the sessions were community-driven and incorporated culturally competent approaches to maternal health and traditional birthing and parenting education. Topics included an Indigenous breastfeeding counselor course, Indigenous doula trainings, culturally competent approaches to maternal health, and traditional birth education, among many others.

Because of past untrustworthy relationships and historical trauma related to state and government agencies, navigating conversations about this project was challenging, and it was important that the MHI team was transparent with its efforts and listened to and followed through on Tribal requests. Because creating a space exclusively for Tribal members was a priority for some communities, attendance at some sessions was restricted to Tribal members; others were open to all. Tribes that hosted sessions said that the cultural and community-based approach was welcome and was not often seen in program planning and implementation.

Tips from Illinois: Utilizing Interdisciplinary Care Teams to Address Maternal Health

Anne Elizabeth Glassgow

Innovations to ImPROve Maternal OuTcomEs in Illinois (I PROMOTE-IL), the state's MHI program, is led by a team of maternal health stakeholders at the University of Illinois Chicago (UIC) in partnership with the Illinois Department of Public Health (IDPH). UIC and IDPH implement a host of maternal health innovations to drive improvement throughout the state on maternal mortality and severe maternal morbidity and have garnered widespread support for their new Two-Generation Clinic, which provides wraparound care to postpartum families. The clinic addresses the issue of improving access to care and care coordination by combining well-child infant health visits with postpartum care services and education on postpartum warning signs into all components of the clinical care.

The Two-Generation Clinic launched in October 2020 and is co-located with the University of Illinois's Health Outpatient Care Center. The clinic provides direct service delivery to many of Chicago's most vulnerable communities that have limited access to medical, social, and behavioral health services. Services offered include care coordination, health coaching, lactation support services, and counseling and psychiatry services. The Two-Generation Clinic allows Illinois to bring together multidisciplinary care teams to meet the needs of families in Chicago and to provide a greater scope of care in one setting. During early phases of the clinic's development, the team reviewed and modified screening tools for trauma, substance use, and social determinants of health for use in the clinic setting. I PROMOTE-IL partners with a variety of providers to meet the needs of families, and the interdisciplinary care teams meet to review clinic processes and care delivery and to conduct visit planning as well as follow-up sessions with patients.

Tips from Iowa: Learning by Example—Iowa's OB-GYN Residency Training Program to Address Workforce Shortages
Stephanie Fitch

Iowa's Maternal Health Innovation program (Iowa MHI) is led by the Iowa Department of Public Health (IDPH) in collaboration with the University of Iowa Department of Obstetrics and Gynecology, with the goal of improving access to obstetrical care for all. Due to a high number of labor and delivery unit closures and decreasing numbers of practicing OB-GYNs in the state, Iowa MHI focuses particularly on underserved rural populations. The work of Iowa MHI is conducted by the Iowa Maternal Quality Care Collaborative, the state maternal health task force. Iowa MHI centers its efforts on increasing access through telehealth services, virtual training to hospitals, and enhancing workforce capabilities through a rural-track obstetrics residency and family-medicine obstetrics fellowship program.

Iowa has the fewest OB-GYN physicians per capita in the country. Maternal health outcomes will continue to be affected if providers are unable to deliver critical care, especially for high-risk pregnant and postpartum women. Iowa MHI's solution to workforce shortages is to provide enhanced training for family physicians through a fellowship program that includes learning how to perform cesarean deliveries, as well as to create a rural track and to implement a rural OB-GYN residency program at the University of Iowa.

Developing the residency track required strong collaboration and planning among the university, the state, and the hospitals in more rural areas of Iowa; working closely with the university's residency training program remains the focus for project implementation. While developing this activity, IDPH staff followed the University of Wisconsin's example, so that residents spend 75% of their time at the University of Iowa hospital and clinics and 25% off site at rural hospitals away from Iowa City. This model allows residents to experience community hospital practice. Iowa MHI also offers loan forgiveness for participants who plan to practice in rural areas of the state.

Tips from Maryland: One Size Does Not Fit All—Individualized Training and Support to Birthing Hospitals to Address Bias in Maternity Care

Andreea A. Creanga

Patient education about the signs of pregnancy and postpartum complications—and when to seek care—has been proposed as a critical strategy for improving maternal health outcomes.[1] Therefore, the Maryland Maternal Health Innovation Program (MDMOM) is addressing maternal health needs through a multipronged approach that includes data enhancements, workforce training, and patient education about the signs of pregnancy and postpartum complications. MDMOM's Hospital Equity Initiative aims to promote safety, equity, and respectful care through quality-improvement activities that address conditions that place Maryland mothers' lives at risk.[2] Instead of coordinating statewide quality improvement, MDMOM works with each of the 32 birthing hospitals in the state to meet its specific needs and to adapt to different care delivery models. Through monthly meetings with leaders of obstetric units, MDMOM develops a schedule and monitors implementation of new activities.

One such hospital-based activity includes an online implicit bias training developed by March of Dimes via MDMOM's learning management platform. This training meets the state mandate, which MDMOM leadership and other stakeholders advocated for with state legislators. After half of each hospital's obstetric providers complete this training, MDMOM schedules two skill-building sessions to offer opportunities for clinical application and facilitates practice changes that promote equitable and respectful maternity care.

Content for the sessions was developed by MDMOM staff in collaboration with specialists at Johns Hopkins Medicine's Office of Diversity, Inclusion and Health Equity; representatives from five community-based organizations; and a Baltimore-based, women-owned communications company. The sessions are delivered online or in person through grand rounds presentations, and they build on a series of videos that depict "good" versus "bad" provider practices (language, attitudes, care, for example) and feature women with various racial, ethnic, and cultural backgrounds.

Tips from Montana: Strengthening Partnerships to Improve Care
Amanda Roccabruna Eby

Montana Obstetrics and Maternal Support (MOMS) is a collaborative effort among diverse partners with a unified mission to improve maternal outcomes. The Montana Department of Public Health and Human Services, Billings Clinic, and the University of Montana successfully navigated the crosswalk among government, healthcare, and academia to develop partnerships that drive quality improvement in maternal healthcare. The partners trust each other, understand that each plays a critical role, and communicate regularly.

MOMS maintained engagement of Maternal Health Leadership Council members through regular communication, shared decision-making, celebrating the impact of their collective voice, and a semiannual member survey. The collaboration that the leadership council demonstrated to stakeholders as it nurtured new partnerships and shared information spurred participation of more partners in more maternal health projects.

In addition, MOMS partnered with the Montana Hospital Association (MHA) to achieve the commitment of 65% of birthing facilities to the maternal track of the Montana Perinatal Quality Collaborative. The collaborative improved communication among birthing facilities as they supported each other in improving management of obstetrical hemorrhage. The relationship with MHA and the leadership council's unanimous endorsement supported successful implementation of the Levels of Care Assessment Tool to inform stakeholder policy and program conversations on maternal and neonatal healthcare.

MOMS relied on the Montana Primary Care Association, the Montana Nurses Association, the Area Health Education Center, and others to build a reputation as a trusted source on maternal health and to disseminate information to recruit participants for corresponding grant procurement, simulation training, and Project ECHO. Partnerships were essential in getting critical training to rural providers, eliminating duplicative efforts, maximizing resources, creating communities of urban and rural providers that reduce isolation, and, most important, getting the right care at the right time in the right way to mothers.

Tips from New Jersey: Data Lead the Way

Acknowledgment: The authors thank the NJ Maternal Care Quality Collaborative for sharing their expertise about the efforts in New Jersey.

New Jersey's Maternal Health Innovation Program (MHI) is led by the New Jersey Department of Health (NJDOH) and seeks to provide quality care to New Jersey mothers by improving data collection through a statewide maternal data center, by creating and conducting implicit and explicit bias training programs for clinical providers, and by supporting hospital-specific maternal levels of care tools. Efforts in New Jersey have been directly affected by the governor's stance on reducing maternal mortality and severe maternal morbidity (SMM), with a particular emphasis on addressing the racial and ethnic disparities that persist in maternal health outcomes for residents.[3]

Access to maternal health data has been a driver of the state's ability to innovate and address the leading causes of maternal morbidity and mortality. From the program's inception, the state focused on enhancing its capacity for maternal health data analysis, with the understanding that it would be a key focus in moving innovations forward. The state's MHI program has revised its maternal mortality report card and launched hospital-level report cards from its maternal data center Web site. In July 2020, the New Jersey Maternal Health Hospital Report Card was published on the NJDOH Web site.[4] It included data by birth type (nulliparous, term, singleton, vertex cesarean, etc.), birthing facility, SMM with transfusion, and vaginal birth after cesarean (VBAC). Several changes have been made to the report cards since their launch, including the addition of new metrics on provision of care (VBAC rates and delivery method, for example).

New Jersey has used data and data dashboards to inform program implementation and to make progress on its maternal health strategic plan. The use of hospital-specific maternal health data highlights maternal health outcomes at the facility level to support innovations to include implicit and explicit bias training tailored to the population.

Tips from North Carolina: Better Together—Authentic Engagement with Multidisciplinary Partners

Rebecca Severin

Cross-sector partnership is essential to North Carolina's success in building a community of practice around improving maternal health. Multidisciplinary partnerships on maternal health have a long history in the state and can be traced to the creation of the North Carolina Perinatal Health Strategic Plan (NC PHSP). Cultivating partnerships among government agencies, hospital systems, private providers, payer systems, nonprofit organizations, public and private colleges and universities, and persons with lived experience is a key aspect of maintaining longevity and sustaining collaboration under this effort.

Two essential components of North Carolina's Maternal Health Innovation program (MHI) are the Maternal Health Task Force (MHTF) and the Statewide Provider Support Network (SPSN). The MHTF convenes diverse stakeholders, including persons with lived experience, which is essential in responding to the needs of pregnant and postpartum women. MHTF meetings culminated with the development of a maternal health strategic plan, which includes statewide policy-level recommendations on improving maternal health in the state.

The SPSN comprises family medicine physicians, obstetricians/gynecologists, pediatricians, and perinatal nurses, who champion quality service delivery to improve outcomes. The SPSN collaboration has resulted in close working relationships for its members, who provide evidence-based training to hundreds of clinicians in North Carolina's perinatal care regions, with a particular focus on rural and underserved areas. Providers in rural communities often face professional isolation and may be unable to collaborate with, or learn from, other clinicians as easily as their counterparts in more urban areas. The SPSN seeks to change that paradigm by connecting providers and bringing information, training, and education directly to them.

Partners from across North Carolina now have equal access to virtual meetings, resulting in providers being more easily able to collaborate. The reduced travel burden also has increased engagement with partners in more rural areas.

Tips from Ohio: Don't Reinvent the Wheel—Intentionality Is Essential to Improve Maternal Health
Reena Oza-Frank

The Ohio Maternal Health Innovation program (Ohio MHI), awarded to the Ohio Department of Health, established the Ohio Council to Advance Maternal Health (OH-CAMH). To build this statewide maternal health task force, the team used a multipronged approach.

First, Ohio MHI recognized long-standing efforts to address infant mortality. It is imperative to be aware of the organizations and individuals working together to address infant mortality, as these efforts inform maternal mortality. Next, Ohio MHI built on these established activities to organize OH-CAMH membership, which is based on the socioecological model.[5] This tool allowed Ohio MHI to differentiate between layers of partnership and highlight how individuals may be affected by their environment. OH-CAMH membership represents each of the layers, including the patient and family perspective, local organizations, state agencies and organizations, and national agencies.

Third, Ohio MHI gathered previously developed tools to identify Ohio's maternal health priorities. These resources included the State Health Improvement Plan,[6] the Title V needs assessment,[7] and the Ohio Pregnancy-Associated Mortality Review.[8] It was critical to also collect information directly from members. Through one-on-one interviews, OH-CAMH members shared professional and personal challenges to improving maternal health. Data from interviews and surveys helped identify state-specific gaps and themes, which resulted in a blueprint for working with the over 80 organizational members of OH-CAMH to design and begin to implement a state maternal health strategic plan.

In some ways, the strength of multilevel and multidisciplinary collaboration with organizations focused on maternal health comes naturally, thanks to the passionate and committed individuals who make up the organizations. To extend efforts for statewide impact, Ohio MHI learned that transparency, trust, and innovation are essential components to synergize efforts across partners with common goals. Further, collaboratively designing the collective effort facilitates and establishes trust among partners.

Tips from Oklahoma: Working Together to Improve Maternal Health in Oklahoma

Joyce Marshall and Jill Nobles-Botkin

 The Oklahoma Maternal Health Task Force (OMHTF) set out to address maternal and child health issues by developing the Oklahoma Maternal Health Task Force Strategic Profile and Plan. This includes four priority pillars that are addressed by four separate workgroups. The priority areas include improving access to care and maternal health programs, expanding mental health and substance use services, implementing innovative technology and data systems, and addressing racial disparities.

A key component to their success is ensuring participation in decision-making by persons and groups affected by proposed changes. Individuals and groups need to be valued and feel that their voices and concerns are heard. Accountability for follow-up is also critical. When action items are identified during meetings, appropriate partners are tasked with responsibility to ensure that follow-up is completed, which lends credibility and encourages partners to stay engaged. To overcome one potential barrier to success, OMHTF found that compromising on meeting times and hosting meetings virtually helped to ensure participation from as many partners as possible.

Funding and personnel can also create barriers to innovative ideas. Utilizing federal funds from grants, collaboration between state agencies working toward the same goals, and utilization of staff from community partners has resulted in various successful initiatives to improve outcomes in Oklahoma. These include establishment of a maternal–fetal medicine clinic in a Tribal facility, a high-risk obstetric Project ECHO, monthly provider and community partner learning opportunities, establishment of a substance use disorder clinic for pregnant women in an educational healthcare facility, gap-filling prenatal care clinics in mobile units and county health departments in rural areas of the state, and widened access to the CHESS Health e-intervention app for making behavioral and mental health referrals to all Oklahoma hospitals and county health departments.

REFERENCES

1. Centers for Disease Control and Prevention. Pregnancy-related deaths. https://www.cdc.gov/vitalsigns/maternal-deaths/.

2. Maryland Maternal Health Innovation Program. Hospital initiative. https://mdmom.org/hospitalInitiative.

3. PRAMS Racial Perception and Adverse Birth Outcomes. November 2019. https://nj.gov/health/fhs/maternalchild/documents/Racial%20Perception.pdf.

4. New Jersey Maternal Health Hospital Report Card. 2021. https://nj.gov/health/maternal/morbidity/mhh_reportcard/2018-2019/index.shtml.

5. McLeroy, KR, Bibeau D, Steckler A, Glanz K. An ecological perspective on health promotion programs. *Health Educ Q.* 1988;15(4):351–377.

6. Ohio Department of Health. State Health Improvement Plan (SHIP). 2020. https://odh.ohio.gov/wps/portal/gov/odh/about-us/sha-ship.

7. Ohio Department of Health. Title V Maternal and Child Health Block Grant summary. 2020. https://odh.ohio.gov/wps/portal/gov/odh/know-our-programs/title-v-maternal-and-child-health-block-grant/title-v.

8. Ohio Department of Health. Ohio Council to Advance Maternal Health Overview. https://odh.ohio.gov/wps/portal/gov/odh/know-our-programs/pregnancy-associated-mortality-review/oh-camh.

Chapter 11

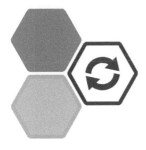

Bringing Together Clinical and Community Partners for Better Patient Care: Bootheel Perinatal Network

BARBARA GLEASON, REBECCA BURGER, MORGAN NESSELRODT, SUSAN KENDIG, AND TANISA FOXWORTH ADIMU

INTRODUCTION

People in rural communities face significant barriers to maternity care. Rural hospitals are closing at high rates and the hospitals that remain are closing their obstetric units, leaving nearly half of rural counties without maternal and obstetric services.[1] Lack of access to prenatal care increases the likelihood that women will die of a pregnancy-related complication and contributes to high rates of infant mortality.[2]

There is increasing recognition that clinical care is necessary but not sufficient to address inequitable and disparate health outcomes. Improving these outcomes requires making connections between traditional clinical practice and the sectors of communities that address barriers to good health, such as inadequate housing, lack of transportation, and economic hardship. The clinical community is only one part of the larger ecosystem necessary to achieve person-centered approaches for addressing the multiple factors that contribute to optimal perinatal outcomes. The clinical–community approach requires intentional strategies that connect traditional clinical structures with community-based organizations and programs. Integration of clinical and community-based providers, such as local health departments and social service agencies, with schools, community organizations, home visitors, the faith community, and other stakeholders offers a true wraparound approach to comprehensive care.[3-5]

Barbara Gleason, Rebecca Burger, Morgan Nesselrodt, Susan Kendig, and Tanisa Foxworth Adimu, *Bringing Together Clinical and Community Partners for Better Patient Care* In: *The Practical Playbook III*. Edited by: Dorothy Cilenti, Alisahah Jackson, Natalie D. Hernandez, Lindsey Yates, Sarah Verbiest, J. Lloyd Michener, and Brian C. Castrucci, Oxford University Press. © de Beaumont Foundation 2024. DOI: 10.1093/oso/9780197662984.003.0011

A clinical–community integration framework recognizes six critical stakeholder groups: clinicians, community members and organizations, spanning personnel and infrastructure, national and/or state leadership, local leaders, and funders.[4] The Maternal and Child Health Bureau's Rural Maternity and Obstetrics Management Strategies (RMOMS) program, piloted in 2019 by the Health Resources and Services Administration's (HRSA) Federal Office of Rural Health Policy, was designed to address the need to strengthen access to services and to improve maternal outcomes in rural areas. The initial Notice of Funding Opportunity (NOFO) required four partners, including a minimum of two rural or critical access hospitals, one federally qualified health center (FQHC) or FQHC lookalike, the state-funded home visiting agency or the Healthy Start program if available, and the state Medicaid agency.[6] These four required partners align with, and signal application of, a community–clinical integration framework.

The Bootheel Perinatal Network (BPN), one of the first three funded RMOMS programs, is built on the clinical–community integration framework. This chapter highlights the BPN program as a case example of clinical–community integration. The discussion offers insights and considerations for other organizations interested in advancing critical work in maternal health with clinical and community partners.

HISTORY OF THE BPN AND ITS RMOMS PROGRAM
Bootheel Babies Journey

Missouri's Bootheel region has a long history of collaboration. In 2013, the Missouri Foundation for Health funded a long-term, place-based collective-impact Infant Mortality Reduction Initiative (IMRI) to target the urban core of St. Louis, Missouri, and the six-county Bootheel region, communities with the highest infant mortality in the foundation's catchment area. This 10-year commitment, currently in year nine, established Bootheel Babies and Families (BBF), a coalition of healthcare providers, healthcare systems, social service and community wraparound agencies, community members, and other stakeholders, to identify the drivers of infant mortality and to develop a community-based approach for selecting priorities and developing interventions. BBF is a convener for health and social services providers, community stakeholders like businesses and the faith community, and community members to build consensus, set a common agenda of priorities, coordinate efforts, and measure success in reducing infant mortality and improving maternal health. Throughout the duration of the IMRI, BBF has convened multiple focus groups and regional meetings to gain input from community members in the six counties about access to care and other issues that affect maternal and infant health. The goal of decreasing infant mortality by 15% during the 10 years was met and exceeded by year eight. This established network of community-based organizations played a key role in developing the relationships currently in place to support BPN and laid the foundation for the Bootheel region's successful response to the RMOMS funding opportunity.

Purpose of the Federal RMOMS Program

To improve access to, and continuity of, maternal and obstetrics care in rural communities, HRSA's Federal Office of Rural Health Policy and its Maternal and Child Health Bureau funded RMOMS.[4] Goals of the program include:

- to improve maternal and neonatal outcomes in a rural region,
- to develop a sustainable network approach to increase the delivery of, and access to, preconception, prenatal, pregnancy, labor and delivery, and postpartum services,
- to develop a safe delivery environment with the support of, and access to, specialty care for perinatal patients and infants, and
- to develop sustainable financing models for the provision of maternal and obstetrics care in rural hospitals and communities.

RMOMS intends to demonstrate the impact on access to and continuity of maternal and obstetrics care in rural communities through testing models (a set of strategies or approaches) that address the following areas of focus:

- rural hospital obstetric service aggregation and approaches to risk-appropriate care
- network approach to coordinating a continuum of care
- leveraging telehealth and specialty care
- financial sustainability

RMOMS awardees are encouraged to propose innovative ways to achieve these goals through an established or formal regional network structure.

Expansion of Bootheel Babies through the BPN's RMOMS Program

Given the Bootheel's poor perinatal outcomes, high poverty, and disparate access to resources, maternal and child health leaders throughout the state are invested in supporting innovation and resource development in the area. When the RMOMS NOFO was released, the state Perinatal Learning Action Network (LAN), a precursor to Missouri's Perinatal Quality Collaborative, offered facilitation to support planning the Bootheel's response. BPN secured grant-writing support through the Missouri Foundation for Health's MO CAP program, which provides technical and grant-writing expertise to not-for-profit entities responding to federal funding opportunities.

With these resources in place, BPN was able to engage a wide range of community representatives and to leverage, rather than supplant, established work in the Bootheel region. During the planning phase of the BPN grant, the facilitator convened representatives of each core partner a minimum of four times. Most core partners already were engaged in the BBF network, which helped expedite gap analysis and contributions to project design. In addition, input was garnered via telephone interviews with other key stakeholders, such as the Missouri Home Visiting Coordination and Collaboration Project; others participated by email or conference call. Agencies provided information from their assessments, focus groups, and other activities to inform the process. BBF and its partners obtained comments from listening sessions, focus groups, agency interviews, and discussions with other key stakeholders to capture the lived experiences and voices of the target population.

Bootheel stakeholders involved in BPN planning identified a range of community-based organizations to include as partners, resulting in BPN's becoming the largest project in the first RMOMS cohort. Importantly, because they recognized the impact of mental health and substance use disorders on maternal mortality and morbidity, BPN stakeholders insisted that all three of the region's mental and behavioral health providers be included in the NOFO response, making BPN the only RMOMS project to designate behavioral and mental health providers in its network. BPN's application included 14 distinct organizations representing over 20 entities. Most BPN partners have collaborated over two decades in both formal and informal efforts that developed organically to ensure that all babies reach their first birthday, and all mothers live to celebrate this milestone.

Simultaneously with implementing BPN, BBF has moved to a community-driven model, in which community members and organizations guide the work of county-based hub partners. Community-based hub partners link BBF priorities to collective-impact efforts within their respective counties to support a systems approach to maternal-child health. Hubs link community-based resources to BPN's clinical components and provide a foundation for health equity work. Through a braided funding mechanism, BPN and BBF partnered to bring the Bootheel Resource Network (BoRN), a digitized resource and referral network, to the region in 2022, thus creating a Community Information Exchange (CIE) that will support closed-loop referrals between clinical and community partners and improve data-sharing. The CIE will provide the infrastructure needed to support the BPN's clinical–community integration framework.

BPN'S STORY OF COLLABORATION

BPN's Partners

The inner workings of rural partnerships are often based on social relationships. A person's words and a handshake can be as binding as an organizational

Figure 11.1 ▼
Expansion of all partners necessary for change.

Required RMOMS Partners	BPN Partners	Informal Partners
2 Rural Hospitals	2 Rural Hospitals	Prescription Drug Program
	2 Delivering Hospitals	Caring Councils
FQHC-Federally Qualified Health Center	FQHC-Federally Qualified Health Center	Parenting Education Programs
		Pregnancy Support Centers
Medicaid	Medicaid	Food Bank
		Domestic Violence Shelter
MIECHV Home Visiting	MIECHV Home Visiting	Suicide Hotline
	Healthy Start	Telehealth Pregnancy and Postpartum Depression Peer Support
Healthy Start	3 Behavioral Health	Sexual Violence Support
	6 Public Health Departments	Energy Assistance
		Initiative Network
	Perinatal Health System	Resource Center
		Homeless Shelter
		Child Development
		Warmlines
		Navigators
		Community Action Agencies
		Home Visiting

memorandum of understanding. Partnerships are all-inclusive, leaving no one out of the network. Figure 11.1 lists all partners in the BPN.

Creating strong, trusting relationships is vital to the strength of collaboration, and rural partners value honesty and transparency. BPN created a network of partners by identifying common goals, strategically engaging partners, and embracing the ebb and flow of relationships. Even when goals and missions seem aligned, organizational relationships can become messy. BPN leaned into the mess and embraced the lessons that came from those relationships. This was vital to moving the work forward.

BPN RMOMS Goals

Network core partners demonstrated a collective mission and vision to collaborate effectively in achieving the goals of the RMOMS program. BPN's goals for the RMOMS programs are listed in Figure 11.2.

BPN designed comprehensive surveys for each partner category—hospital, community-based clinical providers, mental health and substance use disorder providers, and home visitors/social service providers—to distribute among core partners. The surveys elicited comprehensive information about the types and

Figure 11.2 ▼
RMOMS goals.

> Improve maternal and neonatal outcomes within a rural region

> Develop a sustainable network approach to increase the delivery and access of preconception, prenatal, pregnancy, labor and delivery, and postpartum services

> Develop a safe delivery environment with the support and access to specialty care for perinatal patients and infants

> Develop sustainable financing models for the provision of maternal and obstetrics care in rural hospitals and communities

timing of clinical services, provider types, and patient education/support services available at each core partner site.

Program Approach to Care Coordination

The RMOMS approach to improving maternal outcomes emphasizes creating a strong community network that includes clinical, community, and behavioral health agencies. Using Kaizen methodology (*Kaizen* is the Japanese word for "improvement" or "change for the better"[5]), approximately 50 core partner representatives came together to identify gaps in the "system" of care for pregnant mothers in the Missouri Bootheel. All sectors identified navigation services as needing improvement. Partners that provide navigation services, however, said that existing services were currently underutilized and that they should be leveraged, rather than increasing the number of these programs.

To honor the request to improve navigation without adding service providers and programs, BPN created the role of system care coordinator (SCC). The SCC meets with pregnant mothers and uses standardized assessments to determine medical and social determinants of health needs. The SCC quickly discovered that the strong and resilient mothers of the Bootheel were resistant to many of the social programs designed to support them during, after, and between pregnancies. To increase the understanding of resources and their role, the BPN's team, particularly the SCC, had to shift the message. "You Matter, Your Voice Matters," BPN's care coordination campaign, asks mothers to share their stories of being pregnant in rural Southeast Missouri, where hospitals recently have closed and providers often are 60 to 90 minutes away. Showing mothers that BPN cares about their experiences has created an avenue for discussing resources and how the resources can support mothers and their families.

Care coordination aims to seamlessly bridge clinical care with community support programs. The clinical–community integration model focuses on improving pregnancy outcomes and quality of life.

Enhancing Telehealth Opportunities and Technologies

BPN identified the need for telehealth services and technologies in the rural service area and focused efforts to implement opportunities by utilizing work groups, clinical discussions, and partner-funded opportunities. The SCC process identified a gap in telehealth services when the need arose for a Level 2 obstetric ultrasound with transportation as a barrier. BPN used its budgeted financial resources to supply the rural clinic with telehealth equipment and to ensure that future clients would have access to needed care close to home. Concurrently, BPN's perinatal center partner, SSM Health, received USDA funding to partner with and equip two public health departments with telehealth services, thereby expanding services in areas where obstetric care is scarce.

Building a Sustainable System

BPN uses a combination of case studies and data collection on pregnancy outcomes to identify sustainability options. With Medicaid expansion, mothers will retain their medical coverage through the first year after pregnancy. Social determinants of health are "the conditions in the environments where people are born, live, learn, work, play, worship, and age that affect a wide range of health, functioning, and quality-of-life outcomes and risks,"[8] and active listening is key to identifying these conditions. Connecting mothers to resources is more than making a referral; its success comes in closing that referral and providing families the support they need to thrive. BPN is exploring the use of a Pathways Community HUB model, an example of which is the Pathways Community HUB Institute (PCHI) model. The PCHI process creates financial accountability from an outcomes-payment model. This model "encompasses community network development guidance, incentives for community-based organization collaboration, client and family risk assessments, Community Health Worker training (CHW), [and] Pathway's risk-mitigation workflows to confirm that outcomes are achieved, as well as billing and common reporting and benchmarks."[9] Creating a value-based model strengthens the entire network, increasing revenue streams that ensure sustainability for community agencies that depend on soft money (grants).

EXAMPLES OF SUCCESSFUL COLLABORATION IN ACTION: AREAS OF SUCCESS

To meet the needs of their patient population and to improve access to quality maternal and social services in the area, BPN partners set out to design services tailored to those they serve. Each partner plays a distinct and integral role in delivering services to patients in accessible and culturally appropriate ways. The success of the collaboration is rooted in the key elements of the clinical–community integration model. Clinical–community integration programs promote customization of clinical services to fit individuals' unique experiences and to address their unmet social needs. The five key elements of this model, from the Connecticut Health Foundation, are shown in Figure 11.3. BPN has achieved success in each of the five elements through its RMOMS program.

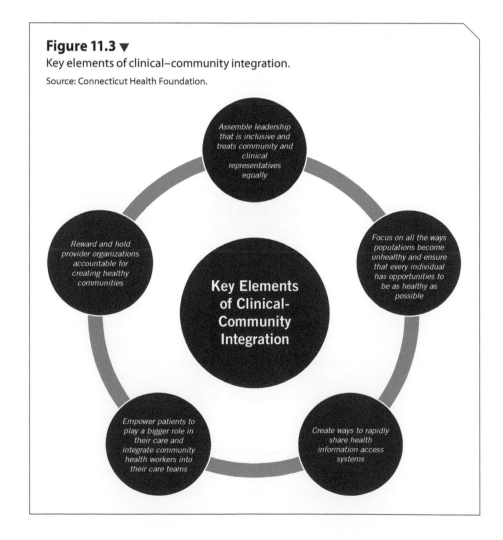

Figure 11.3 ▼
Key elements of clinical–community integration.
Source: Connecticut Health Foundation.

Assemble leadership that is inclusive and treats community and clinical representatives equally

Focus on all the ways populations become unhealthy and ensure that every individual has opportunities to be as healthy as possible

Reward and hold provider organizations accountable for creating healthy communities

Key Elements of Clinical-Community Integration

Empower patients to play a bigger role in their care and integrate community health workers into their care teams

Create ways to rapidly share health information access systems

Assemble Leadership That Is Inclusive and Treats Community and Clinical Representatives Equally

BPN started with HRSA's required partners and added formal partners to expand the reach of client support. After discovering that even more support was needed to provide more equitable healthcare for the mothers in its rural area, BPN added many other informal partners. BPN is expanding its care coordination process via iPad technologies in partner organizations and among obstetric providers to reach out to Bootheel mothers in the most rural areas.

Focus on All the Ways Populations Become Unhealthy and Ensure That Every Individual Has Opportunities to Be as Healthy as Possible

The SCC meets with mothers to gather their unique stories of success, challenges, and gaps in pregnancy care and beyond while giving them a voice for improving maternal care in the Bootheel and utilizing their input to offer culturally appropriate support and resources. Assessment tools include the Edinburgh Postnatal Depression Scale and PRAPARE® (Protocol for Responding to and Assessing Patients' Assets, Risks, and Experiences).

Create Ways to Rapidly Share Health Information across Systems

From the beginning, BPN heard from its partners how vital a referral and resource platform would be for its network. BPN launched the BoRN platform to increase connectivity among resources and to decrease duplication of effort. The platform aims to make partner follow-up easier, to help close gaps, and to prevent mothers from being lost in the system.

Empower Patients to Play a Bigger Role in Their Care and Integrate Community Health Workers/Care Coordinators into Their Care Teams

BPN is unique, in that a maternal fetal medicine (MFM) specialist is available at the lead agency, St. Francis Medical Center, in Cape Girardeau, Missouri. Cape Girardeau is at the eastern edge of the Bootheel, adjacent to the six-county region. Availability of an MFM specialist at the midpoint between the perinatal centers in St. Louis and the southeastern portion of the Bootheel allows for higher levels of care closer to a patient's home. In January 2021, BPN began piloting its care system by embedding an SCC within the local MFM practice, thereby testing the model with patients at the highest medical risk. The primary role of the SCC is to leverage programs already established within the region (communities did not want to add programs). The SCC is responsible for the navigation of agencies working to unite disparate resources to facilitate a clinical–community integrated team that connects prenatal and postpartum women with the support services they need. "You Matter, Your Voice Matters," BPN's care coordination campaign, empowers mothers to use their voices to promote positive changes not only for themselves but for all mothers in the Bootheel and encourages them to use the support services available to them.

Reward and Hold Provider Organizations Accountable for Creating Healthy Communities

Gaps and trends identified through quantitative and qualitative data from the SCC are used to improve processes and make recommendations to local and state representatives. With the introduction of BPN's BoRN platform, partners can more easily track and collect data to assess progress, to make improvements, and to plan for long-term sustainability of services. Aggregating resources on a localized platform decreases time spent searching and connecting clients to resources in a vast area.

Firsthand examples in Box 11.1 and Box 11.2 relate the impact of SCC efforts on telehealth capabilities in a rural clinic and on the health outcomes for a mother and her babies.

Expansion of Resources in the Bootheel

BPN partners participate in standardized simulation training, which is offered at one hospital at a time to help hospital teams build skills relevant to their unit. In April 2021, BPN's perinatal center partner, SSM Health, presented "Response to OB/NICU Emergencies"; 36 individuals ranging from registered nurses, respiratory therapists, and OB-GYNs to pediatricians and a neonatologist attended the training. In addition to in-person simulation trainings, SSM Health's perinatal outreach education team is in the final stages of creating "Response to OB/NICU Emergencies" through a virtual platform. This

---

Box 11.1 | Case Example of SCC Impact on Telehealth Implementation in a Rural Clinic

A s the SCC gained the trust of the medical staff, more complicated situations were referred to the SCC regardless of the type of visit the patient was scheduled for that day. A gap in telehealth services was identified when remote staff reached out for help with transportation of a woman to the main hospital (a three-hour round trip) for same-day access to a medically necessary Level 2 OB ultrasound. This story led to the placement of an ultrasound machine and establishment of telehealth capability in that community, so that emergent ultrasounds can be completed in a timely manner, and mothers can remain in their community to do weekly non-stress testing, thus decreasing time on the road and time away from work and/or family.

> **Box 11.2 | Case Example of How SCC Efforts Improved Pregnancy Outcomes and the Health of Triplets**
>
> An example of early success was the management of a woman pregnant with triplets, who was considered a "no show" for two scheduled appointments already. The patient was on the verge of a third missed visit and not being able to be rescheduled with the provider, per office policy, so staff reached out to the SCC, asking her to contact the mother, which the SCC had already done, to increase the mother's success at making her appointment. At 25 weeks pregnant, this woman was homeless, had limited prenatal care, had admitted to recent drug use, and was at risk of giving birth to her babies at any time. A referral to home visiting services and behavioral health services and the continued follow-up from the SCC provided the mother with the support she needed to make her prenatal visits and to carry her babies until 34 weeks, resulting in a healthier pregnancy outcome and avoidance of a potential nine-week NICU stay for three newborns.

training will be offered to EMS and nondelivering hospital staff, providing continuing education units and increasing the skills and knowledge of frontline medical personnel whom mothers may encounter prior to reaching a facility that is equipped for delivery.

Through its Perinatal LAN, Missouri participated in the Preeclampsia Foundation's cuff kit project. With funding from the Missouri Foundation for Health, the Missouri Hospital Association blanketed the state with cuff kits, making home blood pressure monitoring available to pregnant persons during the COVID-19 pandemic. BPN facilitated the application process for its partners to assist them with obtaining blood pressure cuffs for pregnant mothers. In addition to clinical providers, home visitors and BPN's mental health partners were also provided with cuffs. This gave mothers a tool to monitor and report their blood pressure and helped decrease travel for patients who needed routine blood pressure follow-ups during pregnancy and after delivery. The readings also supported early diagnosis of preeclampsia, giving mothers earlier access to medical treatments to help prevent maternal complications, such as maternal stroke, seizures, preterm delivery, and death.

When focused conversations in BPN's multiple work groups spotlighted a need for improvement of meeting effectiveness, the network established a monthly interactive BPN Connect meeting. BPN Connect is open to any agency that provides services to mothers in the Bootheel to learn about or report updates, opportunities, or suggestions for the communities served and to network with other agencies.

Recognized for its work in rural maternal-child health, BPN has been approached for input and thought partnership by Missouri's Perinatal LAN, by the Maternal Fetal Health work group and subcommittees on substance use and maternal mental health of MO HealthNet (Missouri Medicaid), by Neonatal Abstinence Syndrome (NAS) and Missouri Children's Division, and by the Department of Psychiatry at the University of Missouri.

Eleven BPN partners from eight organizations, including MO HealthNet, had the privilege to attend the 2022 Maternal Health Learning and Innovation (MHLIC) Spring Skills Institute. BPN is proud that a MO HealthNet representative attends the MHLIC opportunities.

After a small number of BPN members completed an Intercultural Development Inventory, the assessment was offered to BPN's equity work group. Members examined their own biases and discussed ways to bring awareness of equity to other partners and community members. This assessment and work group also provided educational opportunities and other equity resources to partners and community members.

DISCUSSION

The BPN offers a range of capabilities for bringing together cross-sector partners to develop programs and services that improve access to quality maternal care in rural communities. The BPN approach has implications for (1) scaling up programs with clinical and community partners that are treated equally, (2) incorporating assessment tools to understand client clinical and social needs, (3) identifying a shared referral system to organize patient activities across providers, (4) leveraging frontline health workers (community health workers and care navigators, for example) to build individual, provider, and community capacity, and (5) utilizing data to make current improvements and future program plans.

1. *Scaling up.* Scaling up, or expanding and replicating, an innovative pilot program to reach more people requires commitment from partners old and new. Health program approaches that are effective and appropriate on a small scale require know-how and capacity to retain effectiveness in different contexts. BPN has learned that scaling up requires partners with historical program knowledge as well as partners with new insights and perspective.

2. *Incorporating assessment tools.* Assessment tools that measure both clinical and social needs assist partnerships in comprehensively addressing client needs. This yields a broad range of partner expertise and services and results in better outcomes for mothers.

3. *Identifying a shared referral system.* A shared and robust referral system allows BPN partners to engage in care coordination that is high quality and high value. Use of the platform results in more efficient workflow processes, saves time for providers, and expands partners' reach.

4. *Leveraging frontline health workers.* Utilizing a trusted workforce that has developed one-on-one relationships with mothers supports patients

in taking a more active role in their care. These frontline staff, such as system care navigators and community health workers, are critical members of the care team and have strong community connections that improve outcomes for mothers and babies.

5. *Utilizing data*. BPN partners actively participate in the collection and use of data. Extensive and varied data are used to monitor progress, make real-time program adjustments, and demonstrate the impact of the program to mothers, organizational leadership, funders, and potential new partners.

SUMMARY

The BPN RMOMS program brings clinical and community partners together to improve maternal health outcomes in rural communities. As an example of rural clinical–community integration, the program unites a broad range of stakeholders that play complementary roles in designing programs and offering services with the goal of reducing maternal morbidity and mortality in rural areas.

REFERENCES

1. The Commonwealth Fund. *The Maternity Care Crisis*. August 15, 2019. https://www.commonwealthfund.org/blog/2019/rural-maternity-care-crisis#:~:text=Pregnant%20women%20living%20in%20rural%20America%20face%20unprecedented%20barriers%20to%20maternity%20care.&text=This%20lack%20of%20prenatal%20care,higher%20rates%20of%20infant%20mortality.

2. Health Resources and Services Administration. Rural counties lose birthing units. *ENews*. 2017. https://www.hrsa.gov/enews/past-issues/2017/march-16/rural-ob.html.

3. Connecticut Health Foundation. Key elements for advancing clinical-community integration. Policy brief. 2018. https://www.cthealth.org/publication/key-elements-advancing-clinical-community-integration/.

4. Krist AH, Shenson D, Woolf SH, et al. Clinial and community delivery systems for preventive care: an integration framework. *Am J Prev Med*. 2013;45(4):508–516.

5. Bascom D. Creating a roadmap to achieving community-integrated health. 2017. https://www.cerner.com/perspectives/roadmap-to-achieving-community-integrated-health.

6. Health Resources and Services Administration. Rural Maternity and Obstetrics Management Strategies (RMOMS) Program. 2022. https://www.hrsa.gov/rural-health/community/rmoms.

7. "Kaizen," Lexico. 2022. https://www.lexico.com/en/definition/kaizen. Accessed February 21, 2022.

8. *Healthy People 2030*. Social determinants of health: what are social determinants of health? Washington, DC: US Department of Health and Human Services; 2020. https://health.gov/healthypeople/objectives-and-data/social-determinants-health. Accessed February 21, 2022.

9. Pathways Community HUB Institute. What is the HUB model? 2019. https://pchi-hub.com/the-institute/. Accessed February 21, 2022.

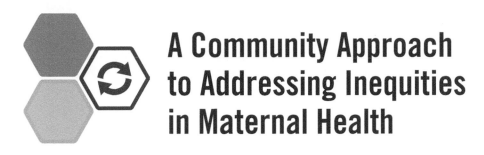

Chapter 12

A Community Approach to Addressing Inequities in Maternal Health

DEIDRE MCDANIEL, VALERIE NEWSOME GARCIA, KAREN CHUSTZ, SAANIE SULLEY, DEBORAH FRAZIER, AND HAYWOOD BROWN

INTRODUCTION

Many interventions designed to address disparities in maternal health target clinical settings. However, many maternal deaths occur outside of a hospital/ birthing facility, anywhere from one week to one year postpartum, and roughly 80% of the deaths are preventable.[1,2] The Alliance for Innovation on Maternal Health Community Care Initiative (AIM CCI) is a community-based, data-driven quality improvement program aimed at decreasing maternal morbidity and preventable maternal mortality, particularly among Black and Indigenous women and birthing persons. The National Healthy Start Association (NHSA) AIM CCI leads the effort to build a clinical–community integration model for addressing maternal morbidity and preventable maternal mortality through the joining of community voices with the voices of both women/birthing persons and partners/fathers.

Activities of the NHSA AIM CCI project include (a) identifying and convening maternal safety workgroups that comprise community-focused public health and clinical experts to guide program activities to ensure integration of community and clinical components, (b) facilitating equity-focused national implementation and adoption of non-hospital-focused maternal safety bundles (MSBs), (c) developing and piloting at least four new non-hospital-focused MSBs for use in outpatient clinical settings and community-based organizations with an emphasis on equity and enhancing capacity to recognize and reduce maternal morbidity and mortality, and (d) collecting and analyzing structure, process, and outcome data to drive continuous improvement in implementation of non-hospital-focused MSBs using a continuous quality improvement framework.

Some unique aspects of the NHSA AIM CCI include:

- Piloting projects in diverse communities in priority areas, such as Georgia and Louisiana, which have the highest rates of maternal mortality in the country. This provides important insight regarding feasibility of bundle implementation in non-hospital-based sites and ensures that bundles, resources, and support strategies resonate in the respective communities.
- Integrating equity practice and solutions that address the social determinants of health, including development of methods, measures, and metrics that enable organizations (using both the non-hospital and hospital-focused bundles) to analyze, track, and devise strategies for advancing health equity.
- Developing an implementation platform with robust opportunities for sharing best practices and lessons learned, and a methodology to promote early adoption and scaling, which includes: invitations for representatives from communities to participate in local non-hospital-focused MSB workgroups and receive capacity-building support for their communities; connections to diverse funding opportunities to address women's health; and promotion of, and connection to, other resources available through new programs in the Health Resources and Services Administration's maternal health portfolio.
- Inculcating equity throughout bundle development. All AIM CCI bundles will contain foundational equity elements that build upon the Self-Assessed Measure of Racial Equity Capacity and the Racial Equity Learning Series (RELS), a seven-module course in racial equity developed by AIM CCI and designed to develop capacity across all levels, from individual to organizational. Modules I through III of RELS are geared to the individual, and Module IV begins the transition to a team focus, promoting external action. Modules V, VI, and VII focus on external equity capacity-building that includes strategies for divisions/departments, institutions/corporations, and regional systems. Each module builds on the previous one to ultimately transform systems. More information on RELS is available from NHSA.

CASE STUDY: NEW ORLEANS

The literature on implementation science is replete with evidence of the difficulties of building collaboratives due to lack of resources, capacity, trust, and stakeholder buy-in. The literature is less clear, however, on what happens when all the players are at the table and the resources are there to support them but there is no defined leadership. Such was the case with the New Orleans AIM CCI collaborative. This case study details the organization's journey to establishing and maintaining a clinical–community stakeholder collaborative to address disparities in maternal morbidity and mortality using a co-leadership model to leverage community resources.

The City of New Orleans was the first community to join the NHSA AIM CCI initiative. The NHSA team traveled to New Orleans in January 2020 to provide an orientation about the program to community leaders and stakeholders, to garner partnership, and to assist the New Orleans community with establishing a local maternal safety workgroup (LMSW), the local collaborative for all AIM CCI pilot sites. NHSA's contact and local convener for this discussion was the City of New Orleans Health Department. While the meeting was well attended and the local stakeholders solidified their commitment to participate, pilot, and implement the AIM CCI MSBs, a local agency needed to be identified to serve as the lead. The lead agency's role is to serve as fiscal agent, to provide program oversight, to coordinate data collection and reporting, and to convene local clinical and community stakeholders that would be charged with using a collaborative equity framework to implement the AIM CCI MSBs locally.

NHSA AIM CCI conducted a survey to identify potential lead agencies, and multiple organizations, including the Louisiana Public Health Institute (LPHI) and the New Orleans Health Department, were identified by community stakeholders as likely choices. Because the local health department was the original convener, the public health entity for the city, and charged with bringing the community stakeholders to the table, it was determined to be the most appropriate to serve as lead agency for the New Orleans pilot. The health department allocated staff and resources to move the initiative forward, obtained buy-in from local hospital systems in New Orleans, and gained support from the Louisiana Perinatal Quality Collaborative, thereby establishing a hierarchical leadership structure for the community collaborative. Local community stakeholders agreed with this decision and were ready to participate in development and piloting of the MSBs. No one, however, foresaw the COVID-19 pandemic and a series of four hurricanes that would abruptly interfere with the local health department's capacity to lead the work.

Although the New Orleans Health Department is well versed in the protocols and management of natural disasters like hurricanes, the demands of the COVID-19 pandemic placed great strain on the department's resources and staffing structures. The effects of COVID-19 were also felt by community partners/stakeholders and local hospital systems. As the end of 2020 approached and the pandemic continued to rage across the globe, it became clear that the health department, community stakeholders, and the local health system needed to realign their priorities to meet the needs of the community during this crisis. The health department quickly realized that, despite its deep desire to do the work, they did not have the capacity to simultaneously lead a new initiative and focus on the staffing and resource demands of pandemic response and the four natural disasters. A new leadership structure would be required to continue momentum for the New Orleans collaborative.

In January 2021, the NHSA team proposed a co-leadership model to the New Orleans Health Department. A co-leadership model allowed the health department to focus on the priorities of COVID-19 while continuing their engagement with AIM CCI. In February 2021, NHSA convened a meeting with the LMSW community stakeholders to propose the co-leadership model and to determine which organization was best suited for the role. Based on its history of cultivating community collaborations, commitment to racial justice and health equity, and long-standing relationship with community stakeholders, the LPHI was identified to serve as co-lead for the New Orleans AIM CCI collaborative. Subsequently, the health department suggested that, because of its fiscal capabilities as a nongovernment agency and its staffing capacity, LPHI serve as the lead agency for the collaborative. LPHI and the health department have a long history of public health collaboration that helped facilitate a smooth leadership transition.

To bring the collaborative one-year-in-the-making to fruition in the midst of a pandemic, LPHI strategized about how best to organize its leadership, to adhere to the scope of work provided by NHSA, and to engage community stakeholders. The solution was to maintain a co-lead infrastructure to manage program requirements. To assist in the transition, NHSA agreed to provide technical assistance to LPHI and to engage and facilitate regular meetings with community partners and stakeholders, reconvene the LMSW, and begin the process of bundle implementation. This gave LPHI time to assess its internal staffing and data capacity, to identify a suitable co-lead, and to develop a suitable model for leadership inclusive of roles and responsibilities as identified in the scope of work. LPHI determined that an agency able to assist with creation and implementation of equity tools, research practices, and capacity-building would be the best fit.

By May 2021, LPHI had identified the Institute of Women's and Ethnic Studies (IWES) as its co-lead to provide data collection and evaluation support, equity resources, and technical assistance. LPHI recruited a dedicated team to coordinate AIM CCI activities, including a lead coordinator and data specialist, and assumed its role as leader of implementation of the New Orleans LMSW.

Under the co-leadership model, the New Orleans collaborative has: facilitated regular meetings of the LMSW, conducted a community needs assessment, created a community-led health equity strategy, created a data infrastructure to adhere to AIM CCI data reporting requirements, created a collaborative strategic work plan, conducted focus groups on the experiences of both mothers and fathers, and begun bundle implementation. Applying the strengths of LPHI and IWES collectively has created a strong backbone for the collaborative's model.

LESSONS LEARNED

Value of a Shared Leadership Model

Shared leadership creates an opportunity to leverage the unique resources and strengths of each organization, resulting in increased bandwidth and expanded expertise. It also provides an example of the collaborative process as a model for development of LMSWs.

Importance of Articulating a Common Goal and Shared Responsibility

Utilize a collective impact model.[3] Collective impact is an intentional method of different entities working together and sharing information for the purpose of solving a complex problem, using a structured form of collaboration.

Establish clear roles and expectations. Having multiple organizations at the table has its benefits ("many hands make light work"), but responsibilities must be clearly defined for each entity to devise a clear strategy for working together and ensure that key elements aren't lost in the flow of synergy.

Ensure leadership buy-in, accessibility of staff, and resources to support the project. Even when unexpected barriers arise, having a team of committed individuals with the time and resources they need to focus on ways to pivot and proceed can make all the difference.

Facilitate Enhanced Data-Sharing

It is important to have data literacy across local partner organizations. Such collaborative data approaches aid all organizations in learning and sharing skills and resources with other members of the LMSW. Moreover, it aids in creating standardized data collection tools and measures across all participating organizations.

There may be a steep learning curve related to collecting, understanding, and sharing data. This can be intimidating and can slow data collection. Taking time early in the partnership to explain what data points are needed, what the numbers mean, why data are important, and how partner organizations can streamline this process (designating a lead data person for each site to manage data and liaise with the lead organization, for example) can reduce some of the hesitancy around engaging with data and enhance communication to avert the common headaches encountered in data-sharing.

CONCLUSION

Feedback from New Orleans, as well as the NHSA's other pilot sites, confirms the importance of a strong collaboration. This has led to the decision by NHSA to design a Clinical Community Integration Roadmap. The roadmap has been developed with the goal of creating the framework for a perinatal system of care in daily processes and organizational and community structure/culture to ensure that no matter where on the continuum women/birthing persons are—from delivery through the first year postpartum—equitable care is a standard of care that addresses their medical, behavioral health, and psychosocial needs. Building on the lessons learned in using a collective impact model for collaborative work, this clinical–community integration model for addressing maternal morbidity and preventable maternal mortality reflects the realities of all birthing experiences by joining the voices of community providers and those with lived experience, thereby increasing its potential for impact and improved outcomes.

REFERENCES

1. Petersen EE, Davis NL, Goodman D, et al. Vital signs: pregnancy-related deaths, United States, 2011–2015, and strategies for prevention, 13 states, 2013–2017. *MMWR*. 2019;68:423–429. http://dx.doi.org/10.15585/mmwr.mm6818e1

2. Trost SL, Beauregard J, Njie F, et al. *Pregnancy-Related Deaths: Data from Maternal Mortality Review Committees in 36 US States, 2017–2019*. Atlanta, GA: Centers for Disease Control and Prevention; 2022.

3. Kania J, Kramer M. Collective impact. *Stanf Soc Innov Rev*. 2011;9(1):36–41. https://doi.org/10.48558/5900-KN19.

Chapter 13

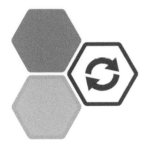

The Broward Healthy Start Program: Cross-Sector Collaboration—Improving Pregnancy Outcomes and Birth Equity Using a Collective-Impact Framework

MARCI RONIK, MONICA FIGUEROA KING, SHARETTA REMIKIE, AND RONEÉ WILSON

INTRODUCTION

We live in a time when women's reproductive freedoms and rights are being questioned and threatened. More than ever, it is important to approach maternal and child health within a reproductive justice framework and through a health equity lens. Maternal and infant mortality, and the factors that contribute to these health indicators, are not experienced in the same way by communities of color, communities of lower socioeconomic status, and communities that encounter different aspects of the social determinants of health, including education, employment, housing, and access to quality healthcare.

This chapter presents a model for examining rates of maternal mortality and maternal characteristics that may lead to adverse birth outcomes at a micro level, and it demonstrates how a small group of community-invested stakeholders used data to develop strategic plans of action that are measurable, meaningful, and sustainable. Ingredients for success, as well as lessons learned, are included at the conclusion of the chapter.

Marci Ronik, Monica Figueroa King, Sharetta Remikie, and Roneé Wilson, *The Broward Healthy Start Program* In: *The Practical Playbook III*. Edited by: Dorothy Cilenti, Alisahah Jackson, Natalie D. Hernandez, Lindsey Yates, Sarah Verbiest, J. Lloyd Michener, and Brian C. Castrucci, Oxford University Press. © de Beaumont Foundation 2024. DOI: 10.1093/oso/9780197662984.003.0013

BROWARD COUNTY'S HEALTHY BABIES ARE WORTH THE WAIT® INITIATIVE

Population health is defined as the "health outcomes of a group of individuals, including the distribution of such outcomes within the group."[1] Understanding complex health and social challenges in the context of the community in which they occur allows stakeholders to identify and implement unique interventions to change the trajectories of these issues. It is necessary to engage a diverse group of community-invested stakeholders across sectors and systems, to use quantitative and qualitative data to drive decision-making, and to maintain continuous monitoring and evaluation of efforts in addressing these challenges. Most importantly, change should be driven by community stakeholders, because they have the most to gain from successful place-based initiatives.

The approach to addressing complications and challenges during pregnancy and birth that may lead to maternal and infant mortality and other adverse birth outcomes in Broward County, Florida, is led by the Broward Healthy Start Coalition (BHSC) in collaboration with its community partners. In November 2018, the March of Dimes launched its Healthy Babies are Worth the Wait® (HBWW) initiative, using a collective-impact (CI) framework[2] and forming an HBWW Committee. The HBWW Committee consisted of community-invested stakeholders, such as funders, healthcare providers, and members of the community, including Zeta Phi Beta sorority sisters. BHSC has used this framework for several years, and the March of Dimes engaged the coalition as the backbone organization. Because this approach is relatively new (although it has roots in community coalition-building, community psychology, and community health), the evolution of the CI approach has been iterative, and lessons have been learned along the way. The HBWW Committee identified criticisms of the CI framework originally presented in 2011 and included methods to address the criticisms in project development, principally the importance of engagement at the community level as a grassroots approach, the need to investigate data using a racial and health equity lens, and the importance of sustained evaluation and involvement. Another criticism of the CI method is that it typically has been used as a top-down approach[3] without engaging those whose lives are affected. The HBWW project therefore emphasized the importance of including women's lived experiences of pregnancy and birthing.

The CI approach does not prescribe a methodology for addressing community-based challenges, so the HBWW Committee chose to guide the project's structure according to strategies associated with results-based accountability (RBA).[4] BHSC used RBA strategies as a road map for change for several years before the HBWW initiative launched, through its partnership with the Children's Services Council of Broward's strategic planning process. RBA strategies are useful in addressing community challenges concretely and systematically in a CI framework. An overview of CI, RBA, and how they relate to one another follows.

THE COLLECTIVE IMPACT FRAMEWORK

The article that introduced the concept of *collective impact* in 2011 defined it as "the commitment of a group of important actors from different sectors to a common agenda for solving a specific social problem."[2] The authors discussed the need to move from "isolated impact"—oriented toward finding and funding solutions embedded in singular organizations or programs—to "collective impact"—a systematic approach that focuses on interorganizational and cross-sector relationships. Five conditions necessary for designing a successful CI initiative were identified:

1. Common agenda: Agree on a shared vision for change.
2. Shared measurement systems: Agree on measurement and reporting of results.
3. Mutually reinforcing activities: Coordinate activities into an overarching plan for success.
4. Continuous communication: Build a culture of trust through ongoing meetings and dialogue.
5. Backbone support: Dedicate a staff, separate from the participating organizations, to plan, manage, and support the initiative.

To its credit, FSG, the consulting firm founded by Mark Kramer and co-led with John Kania that developed CI, took criticisms of its work to heart and addressed several of the criticisms in a 2016 paper, "Collective Impact Principles of Practice."[5] The following eight principles augment the original framework and were designed to help practitioners successfully implement CI initiatives (emphasis in this list come from the 2016 paper).

1. Design and implement the initiative with a priority placed on *equity*.
2. Include *community members* in the collaborative.
3. Recruit and co-create with *cross-sector* partners.
4. Use data to continuously *learn, adapt, and improve*.
5. Cultivate leaders with unique *system leadership* skills.
6. Focus on program and *system strategies*.
7. Build a culture that fosters *relationships, trust, and respect* across participants.
8. Customize for *local context*.

RESULTS BASED ACCOUNTABILITY

Results-based accountability (RBA) is a "disciplined way of thinking and taking action that can be used to improve the quality of life in communities, cities, counties, and nations. RBA can also be used to improve the performance of programs, agencies, and service systems."[4] It starts with "population accountability," the identification of the population of context (Who are we accountable to?), and "performance accountability" (How can we improve the performance of programs, agencies and service systems?). Involving community stakeholders promotes an approach that is engaging, data-driven, and outcomes-focused. It results in "Turn the Curve" reports that are action-oriented, with opportunities for rapid change. The reports include not only trending data but also the "story behind the data," accomplishments, and action steps for implementation.

When using RBA strategies, collaborators identify indicators to use in measuring whether stakeholders are better off. During reviews, they evaluate the strategies for continuous iteration and modification. Data are used to inform the community of the value of the CI initiative and to advocate with decision makers for continued and integrated resource development. Questions that frame the dialogue and take stakeholders from talk to action include:

1. What are the results we want for our community?
2. How will we know when we have achieved these results?
3. What indicators would help us measure whether we have achieved these results? Are they getting better or worse? Are they affecting some subpopulations and geographic locations more than others? What data do we need to have, what data would we like to have, what data would be nice to have?
4. What is the "story behind the curve"? Why are conditions getting better or worse?
5. Who is our "champion"? Who will facilitate the process and sustain our efforts? Who are the likely and unlikely partners who have a potential role to play in improving our conditions? Who else needs to be at our table? How do we "expand our tent"?
6. What works to improve these conditions? What are best practices that have worked in other communities? What are some low-cost, no-cost, and off-the-wall ideas in addition to activities that require funding? What are our next steps?
7. How will we measure how we are doing, and how will we create a continuous communication plan and feedback loop?

INTEGRATION OF CI AND RBA

Table 13.1 compares the five conditions for CI with strategies applied using RBA. Figure 13.1 illustrates the iterative processes for these approaches.

Table 13.1   Comparison of Collective Impact and Results-Based Accountability

Collective Impact	Results-Based Accountability
Backbone organization	Who is our champion organization or individual?
Common agenda	What results are we looking for?
Shared measurement systems	How will we know when we have achieved the results we are looking for? What is our data development agenda?
Continuous communication	How will we know how we are doing? Who else needs to be at the table?
Mutually reinforcing activities	Now what? What works to improve these conditions? What are best practices that have worked in other communities?

OPERATIONALIZING CI AND RBA

Backbone Support/Champion

To support the HBWW initiative, the March of Dimes engaged BHSC as the backbone organization/champion and formed a committee of community stakeholders. Dr. Sharetta Remikie, Florida Maternal Child Health Director of the March of Dimes at the time (and a coauthor of this chapter), and Monica Figueroa King, Chief Executive Officer of BHSC (and also a coauthor of this chapter), co-facilitated the project.

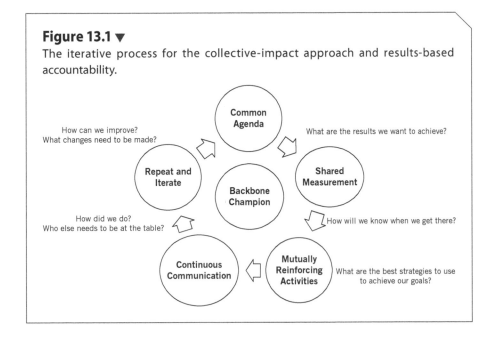

Figure 13.1 ▼
The iterative process for the collective-impact approach and results-based accountability.

Common Agenda: What Is the Result We Are Looking for?

The rate of maternal mortality is defined as the number of maternal deaths per 100,000 live births. The Healthy People 2030 target, established by the US Department of Health and Human Services, is 15.7 per 100,000 live births. In 2007, the rate of maternal mortality in the United States was 12.7.[5] In 2019 (the most recent year for which data are available), the rate was 20.1. This rate was statistically significantly higher than the rate for 2018 (17.4). The rate in 2019 represents a 58.3% increase over 12 years. Recent research suggests that the rates of US maternal mortality may have been higher than previously reported between 2000 and 2014, and place the United States behind other industrialized nations (as is also true for infant mortality rates), spotlighting the need to address this public health crisis.[5] While the number of maternal deaths may seem relatively small (754 women died of maternal causes in the United States in 2019), one maternal death is too many. In Florida, the number of maternal deaths has fluctuated over the past 10 years, from 64 in 2013 to 28 in 2020. The rate has also fluctuated, from a high of 29.7 in 2013 to a low of 13.4 in 2020.

The rates and counts of maternal mortality differ by various characteristics, including race, ethnicity, age of mother, and geographic location. For example, in 2019, the rate for non-Hispanic Black women in the United States was 44.0 deaths per 100,000 live births, which was 2.5 times the rate for non-Hispanic white women (17.9) and 3.5 times the rate for Hispanic women (12.6). Rates also increased with maternal age, with 12.6 deaths per 100,000 live births for women younger than 25 in 2019 and 75.5 for those age 40 and over. The rate for women age 40 and over was six times higher than the rate for women younger than 25.

A report issued in 2021 by www.reviewtoaction.org stated that of the 237 maternal deaths reviewed in nine states, 63.2% were preventable and could be attributed to one of seven leading underlying causes of pregnancy-related death: hemorrhage, cardiovascular and coronary conditions, infection, cardiomyopathy, embolism, preeclampsia and eclampsia, and mental health conditions. A critical intersectionality exists between maternal health, infant health, and the overall health of family and societal units. In the United States, mothers and babies face an urgent crisis. Rates of maternal death and premature birth are on the rise, and prematurity is the leading cause of infant mortality. The United States has the highest maternal death rate among the world's most developed high-income nations. Every 12 hours, a woman dies from pregnancy-related causes.

Because health disparities experienced by subpopulations affect the overall health of a community and where a woman lives can determine her access to care, adequate prenatal care and quality obstetric services are needed to begin to reduce risks for both mothers and babies. The HBWW Committee identified the need to address health at the smallest population level, the census tract. The March of Dimes provided financial support for consultant services for collecting and analyzing data at the census tract level for those areas in Broward County experiencing the highest rates and highest volumes of preterm birth and infant mortality. Persistent underlying racial and ethnic disparities also play a role in birth outcomes. Black women are more likely than white women to experience complications throughout the course of their pregnancies. In the United States, Black women have maternal death rates three times higher than the rates for women of other races or ethnicities. Women of color are up to 50% more likely than white women to experience a preterm birth, and their babies face up to a 130% higher infant death rate.

Shared Measurement: How Will We Know How We Are Doing?

Once the geographic areas experiencing high rates and volumes of preterm birth and infant mortality were identified, the HBWW Committee agreed to focus its efforts on the city of West Park, in south-central Broward County. This community is unique and is distinguished by its assets as well as its barriers, including its own historical and social context, social supports and social capital (faith-based institutions, civic organizations, and neighborhood businesses, for example), and lack of resources (exemplified by food and maternity deserts; lack of access to affordable, safe, and sustainable housing; and neighborhood deprivation).

Quantitative Analysis

The initial tasks of the project included an investigation into the collection and analysis of data at the census tract level. Information included the socioeconomic and maternal and child health characteristics of Broward County, the city of West Park, the ZIP Code in which it is located, and its three associated census tracts. All data were retrieved from the Florida CHARTS Web site or the US Census Bureau's American Community Survey. After reviewing the data, the HBWW Committee determined to focus on one census tract in the area, tract 1007, which is one of 359 census tracts in Broward County. An analysis of the 2017 data revealed that the highest percentage of preterm births in the city and ZIP Code fell in this tract, with 20.5% of all babies born at less than 37 weeks' gestational age. At the time, tract 1007 was 81.8% Black or African American and had the highest rate of poverty in the area, with almost 28% of households living in poverty. Women living in tract 1007 who gave birth in 2017 were more likely to be obese prior to pregnancy, to have their baby's birth covered by Medicaid, and to be less than 20 years old at the time of childbirth. They also were more likely to have a high-risk pregnancy, to deliver by cesarean, and to have no, or late, prenatal care.

Continuous Communication

After presenting the quantitative data, the HBWW Committee made a recommendation to engage stakeholders in the city of West Park. Dr. Remikie of the March of Dimes, Monica Figueroa King of BHSC, and Sheryl Brown of Zeta Phi Beta sorority addressed the West Park city commission, and City Commissioner

Felicia Brunson became a champion of the effort, lending support and facilitating access to local businesses and residents. A town hall meeting took place at Mary Saunders Park Recreation Center, located in the middle of the identified census tract, in November 2018. Marci Ronik, a consultant to BHSC (and coauthor of this chapter), conducted the data analysis and prepared information for a "data walk" for participants.

Approximately 25 attendees representing community members, youth, members of Zeta Phi Beta, researchers, and healthcare providers engaged in the town hall activities. After presenting and explaining the data, Marci Ronik asked participants, "What jumped out at you, and what would you like to know more about?" Facilitators reported small-group responses to the group as a whole, and participants recommended strategies for understanding challenges from the perspective of pregnant and birthing women living in the area. Suggestions included hosting a local baby shower (Shower2Empower) and conducting a focus group with pregnant women from the community.

Mutually Reinforcing Activities

Members of the HBWW Committee continued to engage diverse stakeholders in West Park and planned a Shower2Empower in Mary Saunders Park for December 2019; the city commission sponsored the event. To recruit pregnant women to attend the shower, volunteers from the community, including members of Zeta Phi Beta and public health students, canvassed the neighborhood and distributed flyers. Community-centered settings, including churches, the local recreation center, and the local health clinic, as well as BHSC staff, also distributed information about Shower2Empower. Canvassers asked potential attendees what pregnancy-related topics they would like to learn more about, and these themes were incorporated into the event. Twenty-four pregnant or recently pregnant women and community-invested stakeholders attended the shower. Other stakeholders included family members, partners, and community leaders. In addition to listening to educational presentations, guests were offered healthy snacks and lunch, and 12 community-based pregnancy-related vendors provided information about their services. Each participant received a diaper bag filled with informational materials and baby-related products, and organizers awarded raffle prizes donated by local businesses. Presentations included information about preterm birth, sexually transmitted diseases and infections, and child safety practices. Attendees were invited to take part in a later one-hour focus group to share stories about their pregnancy. Those individuals would receive a Wal-Mart gift card as thanks for their focus-group participation.

Qualitative Analysis

Eight pregnant women attended the focus group. Half indicated that this was their first pregnancy and the other four women reported that their previous pregnancies had been full-term. The mean number of weeks pregnant for participants was 27, with a range of 20 to 38 weeks. All the women were Black or African American. One spoke Creole only, and a BHSC patient navigator provided translation. The mean age of participants was 25, with a range of 19 to 33. Six of the women lived in the neighborhood in which the shower was held, one woman lived in an adjacent community, and one woman lived in the northern part of the county. All the women gave signed consent to participate in the group.

Focus group questions, developed by the HBWW Committee, addressed challenges related to pregnancy, participants' satisfaction with their healthcare providers, methods for accessing information, and ways the women practiced self-care. Dr. Remikie and Marci Ronik co-facilitated. Dr. Remikie, a Black woman who had lived in West Park for many years, has a doctorate in education and focuses her research on understanding health disparities among women of color through their stories. Marci Ronik took notes, which the co-facilitators reviewed and discussed immediately after the group meeting to identify emerging themes.

The group began as participants introduced themselves and shared their name, age, number of weeks pregnant, and whether this was their first pregnancy. Ensuing questions were open-ended, and participants were encouraged to elaborate on their responses. The following is an overview of the conversation's themes.

- *Stress and worry.* Participants described their challenges associated with this pregnancy. Emerging themes included stress related to being tired, managing multiple priorities, transportation, lack of support, and finances. Several women indicated that they were emotional, sad, or depressed and needed respite, self-care, and emotional support.
- *Experiences with healthcare provider.* Participants were satisfied that their healthcare provider gave them information; their dissatisfactions included lack of collaboration with specialty providers, not always being seen by the same provider at their practice, and feeling rushed. Participants also said they did not believe their doctors listened to them or did not speak their language (Creole-speaking participant).
- *Knowledge acquisition and self-care.* Most participants said they used either a mobile application or book to learn about and track their pregnancy. Some said they gained knowledge through family and friends. Methods to engage in self-care were varied and included exercise, meditation, watching television, listening to music, and talking to friends. Some women said they wanted more support, such as groups specific to their culture (Haitian) and support groups in the evenings and on weekends.

Feedback Loop: How Are We Doing?

BHSC shared the information gathered from this project with the HBWW Committee and other committees that focus on maternal and child health in

Figure 13.2 ▼

Overview of maternal and child health committees in Broward County, 2022.

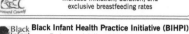

Breastfeeding Coalition of Broward County Increase initiation, duration, and exclusive breastfeeding rates	**Perinatal HIV** Eliminate the rate of perinatal transmission of HIV and reduce rates of STI/STD perinatal infections
Black Infant Health Practice Initiative (BIHPI) Reduce racial disparities in mortality and preterm births	**Safe Sleep** Reduce incidences of infant deaths due to unsafe sleep practices
Infant Health Increase access to programs to address maternal stress and depression; increase access to infant mental health services	
Bringing Babies Home Healthy Reduce rates of substance exposed newborns and families with infants involved in the child welfare system	**Maternal Health/HBWW** Reduce rates of maternal morbidity and mortality; reduce rates of NTSV Cesarean Section deliveries

Broward County. BHSC has a robust structure for reviewing data, sharing information, and developing strategies based on the analysis. Figure 13.2 provides an overview of maternal and child health committees in the county.

Each maternal and child health committee produces an annual Turn the Curve (TTC) report as data from the previous year are released by the Florida Department of Health. BHSC and its partners continue to focus on women's health and social needs. The Maternal Health Committee, a subcommittee of BHSC's Fetal and Infant Mortality Review Community Action Group, is the lead committee for implementing strategies relative to improving maternal health in Broward County. The HBWW Committee has recently merged with the Maternal Health Committee. The 2022 TTC report (2020 data) for the Maternal Health Committee is available at Maternal-Health-TTC-Report-2020-data. docx(live.com).

Recommendations for strategic action are made during the annual review and are incorporated into an action plan that guides the Maternal Health Committee's activities. Some of the recommended actions are:

- Engage the larger community (e.g., businesses, faith-based organizations, civic organizations).
- Continue to implement system mapping. (Who else needs to be at the table? Who are our likely and unlikely partners? Who must be at the table, who should be at the table, who could be at the table?)
- Investigate and study best practices (such as doulas and group education) that may be integrated into services. (Currently, BHSC engages in a curriculum for community-based doulas to provide pregnancy services and to bill Medicaid for such services. BHSC also has started a Facebook Live 10-week curriculum, Parent Connect, that is facilitated by a nurse doula.)

LESSONS LEARNED

The most critical lesson learned from the HBWW project is the need to understand the unique sources of stress faced by Black women throughout their lifetimes and during their pregnancies, as well as the potential role of stress in adverse birth outcomes. Because the HBWW project was community-based and person-centered, it provided an opportunity for pregnant women to have their voices heard and their narratives included. The focus group was facilitated by a Black woman who had lived in the community, which gave participants the opportunity to speak freely with someone whom they considered a trusted partner. The HBWW Committee shared project results with community providers, including healthcare practitioners, local politicians, funding sources, and other diverse stakeholders. It also shared results at the state level at a meeting that included diverse stakeholders representing Black communities throughout Florida, as well as at the annual American Public Health Association conference in San Diego in 2018. Receiving this information has helped others develop a deeper understanding of pregnant women and their personal experiences. Attention has been drawn to the unique needs of pregnant and parenting women in communities of color, which may lead to development of individualized and community-based prevention and early-intervention strategies.

As BHSC continues to collect data on the macro and micro levels, the work has started to focus on other areas of Broward County that experience high rates and volumes of adverse birth outcomes, and a CI initiative will be developed in one of those locations. That community will have its own unique qualities, characteristics, assets, and strengths as well as needs, and BHSC will conduct a comprehensive needs assessment using a similar approach to the one described here, and the approach will be iterated as needed during implementation.

INGREDIENTS FOR SUCCESS

Get Proximate

Getting to know the community and the stakeholders in the community, hearing the lived experiences of pregnant and birthing women, and engaging them in decision-making allowed us to get close and understand the unique needs of individuals; the community context in which they live, work, and raise their families; and the community's resources and assets as well as its barriers and stressors.

Use Disaggregated Data to Understand Unique Circumstances and to Inform Decision-Making

Had we looked only at the infant mortality rates and preterm birth rates for Broward County as a whole, we might not have focused on West Park and census tract 1007. While we knew there were disparities in birth outcomes, we had not looked in depth to understand the unique needs of communities. We learned by being curious and asking questions. This work needs to be investigated through a racial equity lens and include data from other sectors that may affect people of reproductive age and their families. BHSC works with the educational system, child welfare, early childhood education, criminal justice, behavioral health, and housing. Navigating between systems is challenging and requires continual effort to break down silos and integrate services.

Engage Community-Invested Stakeholders

Ask who else needs to be at the table. Think outside the box. Our choice of West Park as an area to investigate was serendipitous: The parks and recreation manager for West Park attended a leadership course taught by Marci Ronik, consultant to BHSC, and in the course of conversation, the manager mentioned that the city was seeking opportunities to bring in community providers. After Marci Ronik later looked at the data for West Park, the process began.

Encourage and Promote Collaboration

System and community-invested stakeholders often do not understand the challenges, or the strengths, within their communities and systems. When we presented the data to City Commissioner Brunson and then to doctors and nurses at the birthing hospital, they were surprised to learn the statistics for their community. If we don't share information and engage others in the improvement process, we will continue to work in silos. Healthcare providers were interested in the map of maternity deserts[6] and the lack of geographically accessible OB-GYN offices in the most vulnerable areas. Because Broward County is so large and has eight birthing hospitals, it is commonly believed that OB-GYN offices are easy to access and easy to use. After the data were shared with the hospital system that serves the area, efforts were undertaken to potentially locate a mobile clinic in the community. Clearly, the data provided a significant moment of awareness for West Park healthcare providers.

Develop a Tolerance for Frustration

This work is challenging and can be disappointing and frustrating. It also can be rewarding, as when we look at the data for West Park and see a decrease in preterm births since the HBWW project was implemented. Change takes time, and long-term outcomes are not recognized in months or even years.

Celebrate Small (and Large) Successes

Small wins lead to larger wins, and the reason to have a champion or backbone organization is to provide the push to keep up momentum. It is easy to lose sight of the importance of the work, so applaud even small successes.

Remember Why You Do This Work

Listening to the lived experiences of pregnant and birthing individuals and engaging them in the work is critical to successful outcomes. Listening is hard work; it takes time and effort and is often the most rewarding aspect of what we do. Remember the result you are looking for—in our case, it is for Broward mothers to have healthy pregnancies and positive birth outcomes. We are only as healthy as the least healthy among us, and we need to lift each other up to improve our population's health.

REFERENCES

1. Kindig D, Stoddart G. What is population health? *Am J Public Health*. 2003;93(3): 380–383.

2. Kania J, Kramer M. Collective impact. *Stanf Soc Innov Rev*. 2011;9(1):36–41.

3. Wolff T. Ten places where collective impact gets it wrong. *Glob J Community Psychol Pract*. 2016;7(1):1–11.

4. Friedman M. *Trying Hard is Not Good Enough*. 3rd ed. Santa Fe: Parse Publishing; 2018.

5. Collective Impact Forum. Collective Impact Principles of Practice. April 20, 2016, https://collectiveimpactforum.org/wp-content/uploads/2021/12/Collective-Imp act-Principles-of-Practice.pdf. Accessed September 9, 2023.

6. March of Dimes. *Nowhere To Go: Maternity Care Deserts Across the U.S.* 2018. https://www.marchofdimes.org/sites/default/files/2022-10/2018_Maternity_Care_ Report.pdf. Accessed January 19, 2020.

Chapter 14

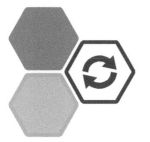

Impacting Maternal and Prenatal Care Together: A Harris County/Houston Collaborative

JUNE HANKE, JAMIE FREENY, AND RUTH S. BUZI

INTRODUCTION

Harris County is the largest county in Texas and the third most populous county in the nation, with 4.7 million residents.[1] The county has a minority population of 3 million, comprising 63.5% of its total. Harris County residents are diverse: 44.6% are Hispanic and almost 20% are African American. The county has a large disadvantaged and uninsured population: 22.4% of the population are uninsured, 15.9% live in poverty, and 21.7% of children live below poverty level. Houston is the major city in Harris County and is regarded as the most diverse city in the nation.

Harris County's maternal health outcomes in 2010 alarmed public health leaders and led to discussions about possible solutions. A review of the latest available birth outcomes data at that time indicated rates of adverse outcomes had not improved and had instead worsened.[2] The data indicated that between 2000 and 2007, preterm birth rates increased from 9.4% to 13.5% and infant mortality rates increased from 5.4 to 6.8 per 1,000 live births. Pregnancy-related mortality ratios, based on aggregated data, doubled from 11.2 to 23.5 per 100,000 births, and only 52.4% of births received prenatal care in the first trimester of pregnancy. These outcomes were worse in low-income communities. Figure 14.1 shows first-trimester entry into prenatal care in 2007 in Harris County.

The leadership at the community services division of the local public healthcare system led the efforts to address the Harris County's maternal health disparities. Their goals became increasing awareness of the health status of mothers and infants and elevating these issues to a public health priority at the county

June Hanke, Jamie Freeny, and Ruth S. Buzi, *Impacting Maternal and Prenatal Care Together* In: *The Practical Playbook III.* Edited by: Dorothy Cilenti, Alisahah Jackson, Natalie D. Hernandez, Lindsey Yates, Sarah Verbiest, J. Lloyd Michener, and Brian C. Castrucci, Oxford University Press. © de Beaumont Foundation 2024.
DOI: 10.1093/oso/9780197662984.003.0014

Figure 14.1 ▼
2007 Harris County births with prenatal care beginning in the 1st trimester.

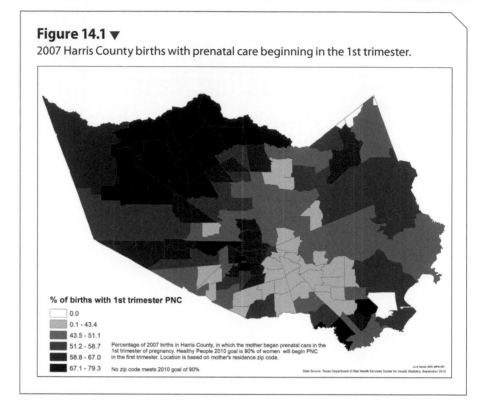

% of births with 1st trimester PNC

☐	0.0
	0.1 - 43.4
	43.5 - 51.1
	51.2 - 58.7
	58.8 - 67.0
	67.1 - 79.3

Percentage of 2007 births in Harris County, in which the mother began prenatal care in the 1st trimester of pregnancy. Healthy People 2010 goal is 90% of women will begin PNC in the first trimester. Location is based on mother's residence zip code.

No zip code meets 2010 goal of 90%

June Hardie MSH, MPH, RN

Data Source: Texas Department of Stat Health Services Center for Health Statistics, September 2010

level. Executive-level leaders of organizations that serve the population held a series of conversations, citing statistics that were staggering. But graphs that tracked only state and city data did not garner enough attention. To generate more responsiveness, geographic information system (GIS) mapping was used by the public health system leadership.[3] The GIS maps showed how infant mortality rates and preterm birth rates varied among Harris County communities at the ZIP Code level. Using the ZIP Code maps, presentations were made by the public health system leadership to community-based resource groups, including local health coalitions, local health systems, and local nurses' associations, to increase awareness of the prevalence of adverse birth outcomes at the community level.

WORKING ACROSS SECTORS TO ADDRESS HEALTH DISPARITIES: THE IMPACT COLLABORATIVE

Initial Planning Meetings

In May 2010, the public health system leadership called a stakeholder meeting. Attendees brainstormed the barriers, system challenges, and other underlying issues that were leading to poor birth outcomes. The first task was to analyze the complex factors that lead to poor birth outcomes and the burdensome costs of those outcomes to families and the community. That complexity suggested that one agency or organization alone could not address all aspects of the problem.

During the stakeholder meeting, four priority areas were identified as critical to creating sustainable solutions: quality of care/service delivery, public awareness, resource enrollment, and legislative advocacy. A SWOT analysis (strengths, weaknesses, opportunities, and threats) was completed for each priority area.[4] Experts in each area gathered evidence supporting the identified problems and potential solutions to present at a collaborative stakeholder meeting and additional stakeholders were identified and invited to that gathering. These discussions led to formation of the Impacting Maternal and Prenatal Care Together (IMPACT) Collaborative.

Collaborative Structure

Designing the structure of the collaborative followed the steps outlined in the Prevention Institute's guide for successful collaboration.[5] Strategic planning tools and the SMART (specific, measurable, attainable, realistic, timely) framework were used by the public health system leadership to determine and assess objectives and need. IMPACT members were recruited deliberately to ensure that there were representatives from the community, healthcare providers, governmental and nongovernmental organizations, health departments, and local universities. The collaborative used an iterative formation process, created work groups, and employed community-based activities to ensure that the work and outcomes met the needs and utilized the strengths and diversity of the members. Organizers held regularly scheduled meetings for consistent engagement and to discuss funding opportunities among members. IMPACT's structure was devised to include members in decision-making and to ensure sustainability.

Convening the Collaborative

The first IMPACT Collaborative meeting was held in June 2010.[6] It began with an overview of the prevalence of infant mortality, preterm births, prenatal care, and maternal mortality in Harris County. Presentations highlighted problems and concerns in each of the four priority areas identified during the initial planning meeting. Attendees completed action cards that compiled their contact information, interest in serving on the steering committee, priority area of interest, and their feedback.

Steering Committee

The steering committee was formed at the initial planning meeting and became the governing body of the IMPACT Collaborative. The purpose of the committee is to discuss research and issues related to maternal and child health disparities, to identify best-practice interventions and measures, to explore funding opportunities, to share resources, to promote ongoing communication among members, to plan full IMPACT Collaborative meetings, to continue to generate interest, and to obtain stakeholder commitment. This structure has allowed for continued involvement and participation of multiple organizations and individuals, from executives to students. Action groups have continued their efforts and the collaborative was able to obtain grant funding for implementation of community-based interventions.

Action Groups
Quality of Care/Service Delivery

IMPACT worked with advocacy groups to increase and improve care for high-risk pregnant women. This action group partnered with the March of Dimes on its Healthy Babies are Worth the Wait and Go Before You Show campaigns to target pregnant women in high-risk communities through patient and provider education and facilitating their access to services.

Public Awareness

The public awareness action group's goal was raising awareness about the maternal and child health issues that affect select communities by working with community members to develop sustainable solutions specific to those communities. The goal was accomplished through a series of education forums in targeted ZIP Code areas. Education forums engaged leaders and residents in a dialogue on the most effective methods for eliminating health disparities and solicited input regarding creation of a public awareness and education campaign targeting women in select communities. The series of education forums also raised awareness of the IMPACT Collaborative and helped members share resources. The first part of each forum was dedicated to sharing birth outcome data for the targeted community. The second part was a facilitated discussion with community members about their perspectives and their suggested solutions for increasing utilization of early prenatal, interconception, and postpartum care.

Resource Enrollment

IMPACT provided application assistance, health education, screenings, and referral for obstetric prenatal care visits to pregnant women in need of a medical home. The goal was to identify and overcome barriers women face when applying for various health insurance policies—such as Medicaid and Texas Children's Health Insurance Program (CHIP) Perinatal—to receive prenatal care. The action group partnered with local organizations to bring resources to women in communities at risk for adverse birth outcomes.

Legislative Advocacy

The legislative advocacy action group successfully lobbied Texas's 83rd legislature for creation of a maternal mortality and morbidity task force. The task force studied and recommended how to reduce pregnancy-related deaths and maternal morbidity in the state. The legislative advocacy group earlier partnered with Amnesty International and the Motherhood Center in Houston to host a Mother's Day discussion and poetry reading in support of the federal Maternal Health Accountability Act of 2011.

Community Programs
Women With IMPACT

The Healthy Texas Baby Coalition of the Department of State Health Services (DSHS) awarded the IMPACT Collaborative a grant to implement the Women With IMPACT (WWI) program. The program's goal is to reduce pre-term birth and infant mortality rates by improving the physical and psychological health of women ages 18 to 35 in high-risk communities in Harris County through preconception and interconception health education and referrals to care. Objectives of the WWI program are to increase behavioral intent and self-efficacy for healthy behaviors related to physical activity, adequate diet, maintaining a smoke-free home, alcohol use, multivitamin use, and stress reduction. The program also focuses on increasing knowledge and utilization of local resources and primary care services. Care Connections is an enhanced referral process for educational workshop participants as well as other women participating in recruitment activities who may have psychosocial or medical needs. The goal of enhancing the referral process is to build sustained linkages between women in the community, service providers, and IMPACT.

IMPACT For Families

The goals of IMPACT For Families include connecting pregnant women to a medical home and access to prenatal care; offering information on available community resources, case management, and health education; and providing application assistance for Medicaid, CHIP Perinatal, Harris Health System Financial Assistance, and the Texas Women's Health Program. The program hosts events at residential complexes in target communities; during the events, resource information, application assistance, health education, screenings, referrals for prenatal care visits, refreshments, and door prizes valued at less than $10 are provided to all participants.

Community Engagement

IMPACT uses a variety of strategies to recruit participants to community programs. Interactive methods include direct communication between recruiters and potential participants and direct referral by IMPACT Collaborative partners located in target communities. Passive methods include outreach events, posters, and flyers. Posters and flyers are distributed to potential participants at churches, apartment complexes, work sources, salons, corner stores, community centers, and beauty supply stores in targeted communities.

THE EVOLUTION OF IMPACT

Through the years, IMPACT has been supported by several initiatives that helped increase skills and competencies for addressing maternal health disparities in the community. In 2014, IMPACT underwent some administrative and leadership expansions. The IMPACT Collaborative applied for funding through DSHS to support coalitions focused on improving maternal health.[7] The goal of the funding opportunity was to expand the network of active, effective perinatal coalitions in Texas and to address geographic and racial disparities in birth outcomes through community-informed, participatory programming. The funding also aimed to support projects that address priority factors in poor maternal and infant health and to collect data on the impact of those projects on health outcomes.

With the support of multiple organizations, IMPACT successfully secured the DSHS funding. The department's requirements were to establish formal memorandums of understanding (MOUs) with all coalition members, to finalize the leadership structure of the IMPACT Collaborative, and to develop a plan for recruitment and orientation strategy for new members. Another requirement was to track data on key outcomes. The state also required meetings with communitywide stakeholders to educate the broader community on the plan and to conduct IMPACT Collaborative satisfaction surveys.

With the addition of DSHS funding, new members from various sectors in the community joined the collaborative. MOUs helped cement the support of member organizations, and community outreach helped increase awareness of maternal health challenges in the community. Satisfaction surveys were effective in identifying strengths and weaknesses of the collaborative and helped in creating improvement plans. DSHS assisted with the evaluation process, which enhanced the effectiveness of the collaboration to address community needs.

In 2017, IMPACT was accepted to the Collective Impact Learning Collaborative (CILC) by maternal and child health national advocate CityMatCH.[8] CILC was designed to increase the capacity of communities to implement collective-impact strategies to address maternal and child health priorities at the community level. IMPACT members completed the Best Change Process Assessment, which covers domains like identified problems or goals to be addressed, community engagement in analyzing information about an issue, and assessment of organizational or community resources that can be used to help address goals. Members of the collaborative's backbone leadership participated in two-day training and received continuous technical assistance to improve the capacity of IMPACT to reach its identified goals. The technical assistance supported establishment of a common agenda. After reviewing local data, members decided to focus on early entry to prenatal care and planned community activities to achieve the goal. Adapting shared measurement systems to track changes was an important goal, and members with expertise in evaluation were instrumental in leading discussions about appropriate measures. Engaging additional members to facilitate a dialogue about the needs of the community was also a priority. Members completed the Top 100 Partners Exercise to brainstorm and prioritize influential leaders who could be engaged in the collective impact effort. After identifying the organizations, members developed a recruitment script that reflected the spirit of collective impact for inviting potential new members.

The collaborative also received funding from the March of Dimes. Funding provided support for outreach activities to educate the community about the importance of preconception care and to encourage enrollment in Healthy Texas Women, a funding source for family planning services. IMPACT conducted outreach activities at housing projects and community centers to encourage pregnant women to obtain early prenatal care. Funding also supported development of an educational campaign and conferences to give health professionals the latest information on early entry to prenatal care and improving preconception health.

As part of its response to community needs, the IMPACT Collaborative addressed natural disasters (e.g., floods) by developing an emergency preparedness card to be used by pregnant women to access their prenatal information in the event of being unable to reach their regular health provider. The card captures pertinent health information and is available in English and Spanish. IMPACT organized a conference on emergency preparedness and made the card available to health professionals who attended.

IMPACT SUCCESSES

Work accomplished by the collaborative through its action groups and community programs implemented interventions, mobilized the Harris County community, and created public interest in improving maternal health outcomes. IMPACT meets monthly, includes program participants, and maintains a common vision among members. From the beginning, the collaborative has shared ideas, built consensus, and achieved a unified commitment to sustainable solutions. Over the years, IMPACT has reached a significant number of community members through its initiatives. Some of those activities include the following:

- Conducted outreach events at various community venues to inform women and men on the importance of preconception health, early prenatal care, and interconceptional health.

- Informed and enrolled women in the Healthy Texas Women program at community events.
- Organized events at residential settings and community centers to encourage pregnant women to access early prenatal care and to fill out an emergency preparedness card.
- Organized presentations at community multiservice centers in communities with the highest disparities.
- Coordinated conferences with stakeholders/providers of prenatal, gynecologic, pediatric, and postpartum care to educate health professionals about the latest evidence-based strategies to improve interconceptional health and prenatal care.
- Coordinated educational conferences to engage and educate healthcare professionals in distributing the emergency preparedness card at their facilities.

Surveys completed by participants in the various outreach programs demonstrated success in connecting nonpregnant women to family planning and primary care and pregnant women to prenatal care; improved access to social resources; and improvement in knowledge and behaviors that promote health and well-being.

COLLABORATIVE SUSTAINABILITY/LESSONS LEARNED

The IMPACT Collaborative has been active since 2010. Several factors contribute to its longevity and sustainability:

- *Building relationships among stakeholders.* Building and sustaining relationships with coalition members is an essential element of successful partnerships. IMPACT accomplishes this by showing general interest in every stakeholder who comes to the table, emphasizing respect and inclusiveness, allocating time for networking and sharing, and providing refreshments or ice breakers to create a welcoming, relaxing, friendly atmosphere.
- *Securing backbone leadership.* Creating a collaborative of individuals committed to the cause was essential. Engaging organizations that already were committed to the work and whose mission was aligned with the collaborative increased the likelihood of having ongoing support.
- *Engaging member organizations in continuous communication.* It is essential to communicate authentically with member organizations to garner support for the IMPACT agenda.
- *Engaging individuals with lived experiences.* It was crucial to obtain input from members of the community who were directly affected by the identified health disparities and who represent the communities served. Engaging them in initial conversations helped set the collaborative structure and guide the programmatic work, including goal-setting,

use of funding, and solution-building. Although such things as meeting times and travel to meeting locations can be barriers, overcoming them for all members is crucial. Obtaining members' input and finding ways to compensate them for their time facilitate meaningful and consistent participation.

- *Specifying goals and creating measurement tools to evaluate progress.* It is essential to identify goals that respond to the needs of the community, and input can come from community members and community stakeholders at the state and local levels. Once specific goals are identified, it is important to define measures to track changes.
- *Staying current with local data and continuing to inform members.* Collecting data about maternal health trends is helpful in keeping members engaged and interested. Data should highlight inequities and the burden of health disparities in the community.
- *Conducting satisfaction surveys.* Obtaining input from members about the effectiveness of the collaborative and ways to improve it is essential. Surveying members about the needs of the collaborative in a changing environment helps ensure that the work is perceived as meaningful and relevant.
- *Engaging in advocacy.* Connecting with political representatives helps support a legislative agenda that addresses community needs. Identifying lawmakers from the community who care about maternal health and inviting them and their staff to meetings is an effective way to create connections.
- *Developing relationships with university institutions.* Partnerships with universities on supporting data collection as well as outreach in the community have enhanced the work of the collaborative.
- *Securing funding to support the work of the collaborative.* Applying for funding from organizations whose priorities line up with the collaborative's strengthens IMPACT and enhances competencies for addressing the maternal health needs of the community.

CONCLUSION

Despite the success of the IMPACT Collaborative and work done in the community for more than a decade, maternal health outcomes in Harris County remain challenging. Some maternal health outcomes have improved: Data suggest that between 2014 and 2019, preterm births decreased from 12.1% to 11.9%. Between 2010 and 2019, infant mortality rates decreased from 6.3 to 5.9 per 1,000 live births.[2] However, in 2010, 55.6% of births entered first-trimester prenatal care, but the percentage declined to 54.5% in 2015 and 48.9% in 2019. Inequities in birth outcomes persist in the county, with 16.7% of Black infants born preterm, compared with 10.1% of white infants. Inequity also persists for

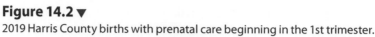

Figure 14.2 ▼
2019 Harris County births with prenatal care beginning in the 1st trimester.

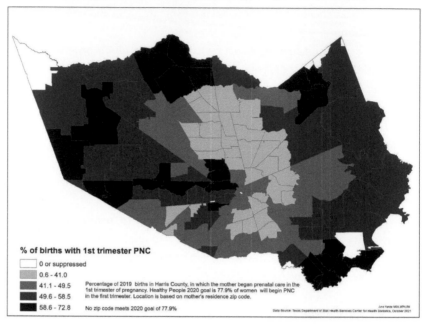

% of births with 1st trimester PNC

- 0 or suppressed
- 0.6 - 41.0
- 41.1 - 49.5
- 49.6 - 58.5
- 58.6 - 72.8

Percentage of 2019 births in Harris County, in which the mother began prenatal care in the 1st trimester of pregnancy. Healthy People 2020 goal is 77.9% of women will begin PNC in the first trimester. Location is based on mother's residence zip code.

No zip code meets 2020 goal of 77.9%

Jone Hande MIS,MPH,RN

Data Source: Texas Department of Stat Health Services Center for Health Statistics, October 2021

infant mortality rates: the rate is 12.3 per 1,000 live births for Black infants and 4.7 for white infants. Entry into first-trimester prenatal care follows the same pattern: 42.5% for Black mothers and 63% for white. Figure 14.2 shows first-trimester entry into prenatal care in 2019.

Maternal mortality and morbidity data trends for Harris County are limited, but some data are available from a study conducted in 2017.[9] The data suggest that between 2008 and 2015, severe maternal morbidity (SMM) in Harris County increased by 53%, compared with 15% statewide. In 2015, the SMM rate was 2.38 per 10,000 deliveries or 2.4%, which is 20% higher than the state average. The data also suggest that 3.1% of Black women experience SMM, compared with 2% of white and Asian women and 2.5% of Hispanic and other groups.

Continued work on maternal health outcomes will require engaging in broader collaborations with community organizations, engaging individuals with lived experiences as active participants, obtaining additional funding to enhance the capacity to reach the community, and ensuring consistent leadership. Securing 501(c)(3) nonprofit status for IMPACT could help the collaborative attain financial independence and eliminate the need to rely on community organizations as fiscal agents. Continuation of IMPACT will depend on its ability to garner support from individuals and organizations that will engage in authentic collaborations.

REFERENCES

1. United States Census Bureau. QuickFacts, Harris County, Texas. 2020. https://www.census.gov/quickfacts/harriscountytexas. Accessed February 1, 2022.

2. Health disparity and health inequity: trends and data reports. 2019. https://www.houstontx.gov/health/chs/documents/Health-Disparities-Data-Report-II-2019-Morbidity-and-Mortality.pdf. Accessed February 1, 2022.

3. What is GIS? https://www.esri.com/en-us/what-is-gis/overview. Accessed February 1, 2022.

4. SWOT analysis: Strengths, weaknesses, opportunities, and threats. Community Toolbox. https://ctb.ku.edu/en/table-of-contents/assessment/assessing-community-needs-and-resources/swot-analysis/main. Accessed February 1, 2022.

5. Cohen L, Baer N, Satterwhite P. Developing effective coalitions: an eight-step guide. In: Wurzbach ME, ed. *Community Health Education and Promotion: A Guide to Program Design and Evaluation*. 2nd ed. Gaithersburg, MD: Aspen; 2002:144–161. http://thrive.preventioninstitute.org/pdf/eightstep.pdf. Accessed February 1, 2022.

6. Freeny J, Cummings A, Hillard Alford M, Hanke J, Lloyd L, Boswell D. Impacting maternal and prenatal care together: a collaborative effort to improve birth outcomes. *J Appl Res Child*. 2014;5(1):18. https://digitalcommons.library.tmc.edu/childrenatrisk/vol5/iss1/18.

7. Healthy Texas Mothers and Babies. https://www.dshs.texas.gov/HealthyTexasBabies/home.aspx. Accessed February 1, 2022.

8. Using Collective Impact to Address MCH Priorities. 2017. https://www.citymatch.org/test1/. Accessed February 1, 2022.

9. Severe Maternal Morbidity in Harris County. 2017. University of Houston School of Public Health Center for Health Care Research.

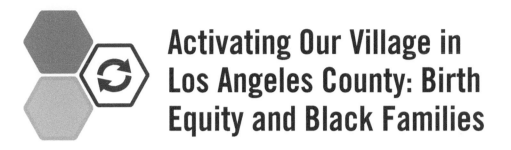

Chapter 15

Activating Our Village in Los Angeles County: Birth Equity and Black Families

BRANDI SIMS DESJOLAIS, MELISSA FRANKLIN, HELEN O'CONNOR, KACI PATTERSON, SONYA YOUNG AADAM, DEBORAH ALLEN, ADJOA JONES, AND SYLVIA SWILLEY

INTRODUCTION

This is a story of two mothers and two babies. Each mother has a graduate degree, a good job, and a stable relationship, is at a healthy weight, and was consistent with prenatal appointments throughout pregnancy. Yet, at birth, their stories diverge. One mother left the hospital two days postpartum with her chubby daughter, born at 39 weeks, in her arms. The other mother left her baby behind in the hospital and was herself lucky to leave the hospital alive. She returned for days and nights to watch, weep over, and pump breast milk for her 27-week-old daughter, who fought for her life until finally she could be sent home. The only difference between the two mothers is that one is white and one is Black. How can race, which we know has no biological meaning, make such a difference? The answer is that while race has no biological meaning, it has overwhelming social meaning. Black women and birthing people, in the aggregate, experience a lifetime of racism, from microaggressions to overt and systemic discrimination. These experiences translate into the unjust inequality in premature births, infant mortality and morbidity, and maternal mortality. Race is not biologically real, but it has a very real biological impact.

The story of the two mothers ultimately became one of joy and abundance, of resilience and strength, of coming together. In the story there is hurt, hope, help, and healing. There is locking of arms and facing off for hard conversations. There are activists, funders, and allies. There are clinicians, birth workers, epidemiologists, academics, parents, and people who simply care about at last achieving change for Black people. We call this the Village.

Brandi Sims Desjolais, Melissa Franklin, Helen O'Connor, Kaci Patterson, Sonya Young Aadam, Deborah Allen, Adjoa Jones, and Sylvia Swilley, *Activating Our Village in Los Angeles County* In: *The Practical Playbook III*. Edited by: Dorothy Cilenti, Alisahah Jackson, Natalie D. Hernandez, Lindsey Yates, Sarah Verbiest, J. Lloyd Michener, and Brian C. Castrucci, Oxford University Press. © de Beaumont Foundation 2024. DOI: 10.1093/oso/9780197662984.003.0015

It is important to reflect on where every story begins for each Black woman/birthing person and child. I want to ensure that other mothers like me have options—support, love, equity in care, and resources at their reach to create healthy and loving environments for themselves and their children.

—Adjoa Jones

THE AAIMM PUBLIC-PRIVATE-COMMUNITY PARTNERSHIP

The Los Angeles County African American Infant and Maternal Mortality (AAIMM) Prevention Initiative is a coalition of the Los Angeles County departments of public health, health services, and mental health; First 5 LA; community- and faith-based organizations; and healthcare providers, birth workers, funders, universities, and community members. AAIMM is united with one purpose: to address the unacceptably high rates of Black infant and maternal death and to ensure healthy and joyous births for Black families in Los Angeles County.

Black babies in Los Angeles County die before their first birthday at two to three times the rate of babies of any other race, and Black women die from complications of pregnancy and childbirth at four times the rate of women of other races (see Figures 15.1 and 15.2). These statistics for Los Angeles mirror figures for the entire country.

Figure 15.1 ▼

Infant mortality rate is defined as the number of deaths to infants within the first year of life per 1,000 live births. Data not shown for Native Americans, Pacific Islander, Other, and Unknown races. Three-year averages used to account for random and annual rate fluctuations.

Data Source: 2004-2017 California Department of Public Health, Birth and Death Statistical Master Files. 2018-2021 data downloaded from the Vital Record Business Intelligence System (VRBIS).

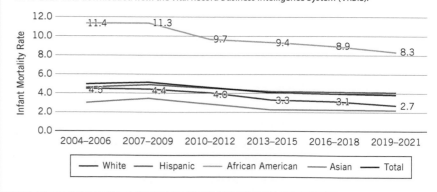

Figure 15.2 ▼

"Maternal Mortality Rate" is defined as the number of female deaths due to obstetric causes (ICD-10 codes A34, O00-O95, O98-O99) within 42 days of a pregnancy per 100,000 live births.

Sources: California Integrated Vital Records System, 2018-2020, California Department of Public Health, Birth and Death Statistical Files, 2011-2017. Perinatal Indicators Report 2020.

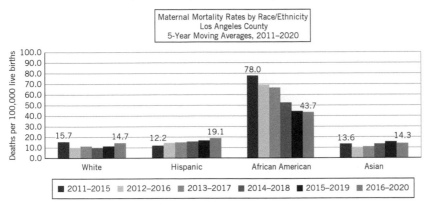

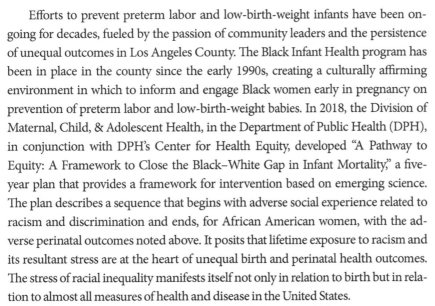

Maternal Mortality Rates by Race/Ethnicity
Los Angeles County
5-Year Moving Averages, 2011–2020

Legend: ■ 2011–2015 ■ 2012–2016 ■ 2013–2017 ■ 2014–2018 ■ 2015–2019 ■ 2016–2020

Efforts to prevent preterm labor and low-birth-weight infants have been ongoing for decades, fueled by the passion of community leaders and the persistence of unequal outcomes in Los Angeles County. The Black Infant Health program has been in place in the county since the early 1990s, creating a culturally affirming environment in which to inform and engage Black women early in pregnancy on prevention of preterm labor and low-birth-weight babies. In 2018, the Division of Maternal, Child, & Adolescent Health, in the Department of Public Health (DPH), in conjunction with DPH's Center for Health Equity, developed "A Pathway to Equity: A Framework to Close the Black–White Gap in Infant Mortality," a five-year plan that provides a framework for intervention based on emerging science. The plan describes a sequence that begins with adverse social experience related to racism and discrimination and ends, for African American women, with the adverse perinatal outcomes noted above. It posits that lifetime exposure to racism and its resultant stress are at the heart of unequal birth and perinatal health outcomes. The stress of racial inequality manifests itself not only in relation to birth but in relation to almost all measures of health and disease in the United States.

The five-year plan, with a goal to reduce the Black–White infant mortality gap by 30%, focuses on four strategies grounded in evidence that exposure to the stress of racism is a root cause of the disparity in birth outcomes:

- Strategy 1: Create collaborative structures to support progress at local and county levels.
- Strategy 2: Reduce women's exposure to stressors in the social environment.
- Strategy 3: Block the pathway from social stress to physiological stress.

- Strategy 4: Intervene as early as possible when stress has taken a toll on health.

After release of the framework, DPH partnered with First 5 LA, an independent public agency that promotes the safe and healthy development of young children, to launch the AAIMM Prevention Initiative. Simultaneously, the LA County Department of Health Services (DHS) was preparing to launch an AAIMM community action team (CAT) in one of the most affected communities, laying the foundation for AAIMM as a government–community partnership. A fellowship funded by the Pritzker Foundation's National Collaborative for Infants and Toddlers also seeded the effort, informed by emergent research and by focus groups of over 100 Black women. Together with many partners, AAIMM now operates as a countywide steering committee and four regional CATs.

Eighteen entities make up the LA County AAIMM Steering Committee (see Figure 15.3), which guides implementation of the five-year plan and is responsible for developing and implementing complementary strategies. Committee members advance advocacy, awareness, and policy change.

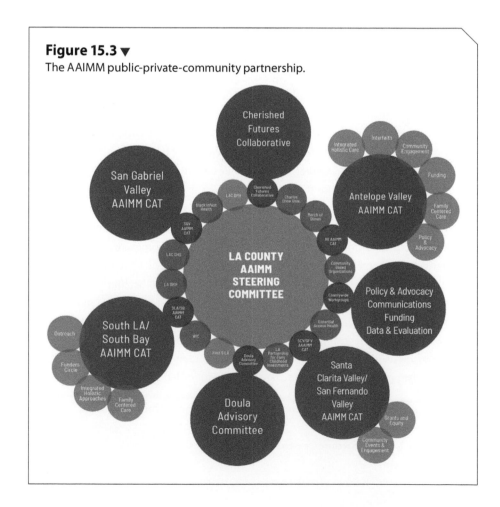

Figure 15.3 ▼
The AAIMM public-private-community partnership.

Figure 15.4 ▼
The AAIMM theory of causality.

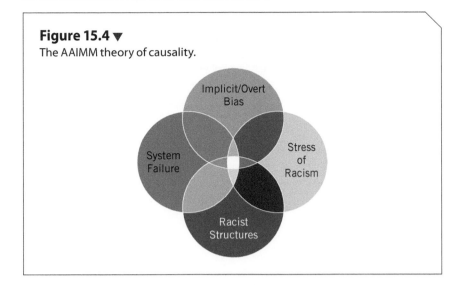

Although members work on different priorities, the countywide steering committee serves as a hub for collective efforts, a place of solidarity versus hierarchy, to strategize and to hold each other—especially governmental and healthcare entities—accountable.

Shaping the collective work is a theory of causality that lands at the intersection of implicit and overt bias against Black women and birthing people that they experience in clinical settings; the failures of support systems to effectively strengthen the well-being of Black families in a way that centers the Black person and not the system; racist structures within society that work together to thwart opportunity and well-being of Black individuals; and the stress of racism (see Figure 15.4).

INTENTIONAL VALUES OF THE AAIMM PREVENTION INITIATIVE

Los Angeles County is huge, and finding solidarity in an area with so many people and so much spread is not easy. Creating the conditions for solidarity and authentic collaboration on behalf of a group of people rarely centered in policy or funding priorities is daunting, especially when one considers the storied history of public health and Black communities. What has always been needed is intention, and values to guide that intention, a place of shared vision that extends beyond "closing the gap," to joyous and healthy births and lives. AAIMM decided upon its shared intentional values, described in detail later, and out of those were born the following activities:

- *Collaborative backbone support.* DPH and First 5 LA, in an innovative bidirectional backbone structure, provide infrastructure support and

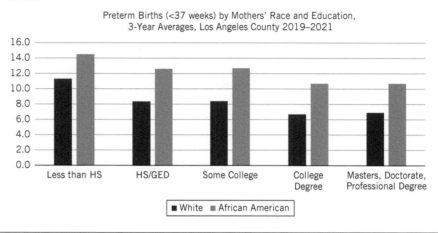

Figure 15.5 ▼

Preterm births are defined as gestational age less than 37 weeks at birth. Educational attainment is based on mother's highest level of education at the time of delivery. Gestational age based on obstetrical estimation. Thee-year averages used to account for random annual rate fluctuations. Data for unknown education level not shown. Data not shown for Hispanic, Asian, Native American, Pacific Islander, Other, and Unknown races.

Data Source: 2019-2021 birth records downloaded from the Vital Record Business Intelligence System (VRBIS).

Preterm Births (<37 weeks) by Mothers' Race and Education,
3-Year Averages, Los Angeles County 2019–2021

■ White ■ African American

management oversight while fostering stakeholder autonomy within and between the AAIMM steering committee, CATs, and their own agencies.

- *Community partnership that drives engagement.* Four CATs serve six service planning areas, four of which have high rates of African American infant births and deaths and much higher rates of Black maternal and infant deaths than for any other race (see Figure 15.5). CATs are regionally based collaborative partnerships between the LA County Health Agency, community-based organizations, healthcare providers, community residents, faith-based organizations, birth workers, allies, and community businesses. CATs inform and raise awareness through community engagement; increase support from providers, clinics, and hospitals currently providing perinatal health services; and train communities and clinicians in strategies to revise harmful practices and build resources, with a goal of shifting power by uplifting the voices of community in decision-making and advocacy regarding public health crises and persistent inequities in health and social services. With such large geographic boundaries, CATs ensure that the work has the regional specificity the community desires.

- *Funding.* AAIMM began with one Pritzker Fellow and a small but mighty team at DPH, DHS, and First 5 LA. Today, there are multiple state and local grants, a pooled fund for philanthropic investors as well as private programmatic investments, and pending federal funds. There is a central AAIMM funding work group that oversees equitable and transparent proposals and use of funds.

- *Communications.* Serving as both an internal and external landing place for sharing information, building solidarity, and fostering action that centers values, communications efforts have included development of a website (www.blackinfantsandfamilies.org), social media channels, core messaging, and broad-reaching campaigns. AAIMM does not do "promotions" for promotions' sake, nor does AAIMM "craft" messages.
- *Black Maternal Health Center of Excellence.* Charles Drew University of Medicine and Science in Los Angeles developed a Center of Excellence that focuses on research, pipeline and workforce development and sustainability, and cultivation of community-based health infrastructure to support wraparound, interdisciplinary, holistic, culturally and racially concordant services for Black birthing people.
- *Father engagement.* The AAIMM Fatherhood Program promotes the importance of having fathers/partners engaged in and navigating pregnancy alongside their partner, which bolsters mental, emotional, and physical health throughout the perinatal period. The program includes culturally congruent social support in a group atmosphere and technical assistance to service and medical providers to best serve African American fathers from pregnancy through the postpartum period.
- *Cherished Futures for Black Moms & Babies.* Cherished Futures is a multisector collaborative effort aligned with the comprehensive AAIMM initiative to reduce infant mortality and to improve maternal patient experiences and safety for Black mothers and babies. Cherished Futures unites key decision makers from local birthing hospitals, public health, community-based organizations, and advocates to implement systems-change interventions at the clinical, institutional, and community levels.
- *Doula program.* The AAIMM Doula Program provides free, culturally congruent doula support to Black/African American pregnant people countywide. Clients receive educational, emotional, and physical support to reduce medical interventions (including cesareans), to improve mental health, to increase satisfaction with the birth experience, and to increase breastfeeding success. The program commits to providing doulas a living wage and a range of workforce development opportunities.
- *Village Fund.* The Village Fund seeks to reinforce the broad goals of the AAIMM initiative by funding community-led efforts that support the physical and mental well-being of Black families before, during, and after birth. Organizations, networks, coalitions, individual service providers, micro-enterprises, and small businesses are eligible to apply for grants of up to $30,000, with priority consideration given to Black-led entities. The Village Fund was developed by a team of Black women and allies. It

is managed by the LA Partnership for Early Childhood Investment and is capitalized by a combination of public and private philanthropic dollars.

None of the above would have been possible without our values. What started as a strategic planning best practice became the DNA of our steps forward and informed program design, communications and outreach, training, challenges to long-held notions, and even rubrics for grant-making and hiring practices. The intentional values are:

1. Racism as a root cause
2. Black women/people up front and leading
3. Fighting inequity while fostering equity
4. No blame game
5. We are all pieces of the puzzle

Value 1: Racism as a Root Cause

Los Angeles's reputation as a beacon of progressive values can conceal the racist history it shares with the rest of the country and the experiences of racism that continue to happen in the city. Doing antiracist work in Los Angeles is by no means a breeze. Prior to 2017, public health officials in the county had not declared racism a leading cause of Black infant mortality. Interventions were focused on a mother's activities and behavior until today's leadership began presenting public health data to demonstrate the societal ills at play: Black women across socioeconomic statuses and education levels were faring worse around pregnancy than white women who had not completed high school (see Figure 15.6). This problem was not a result of personal behavior but system behavior, whose reality was increasingly highlighted in national news headlines. National media outlets were highlighting the same disparity.

If you ask the average person why babies born to Black mothers are so much more likely to die in their first year of life or why Black mothers themselves are so much more likely to die from complications related to pregnancy and childbirth, you will probably get one of the four answers listed in Table 15.1.

Centering race as a social determinant of health was a breakthrough moment that opened doors to many more breakthroughs: DPH and First 5 LA appointed dedicated staff to AAIMM; state and private investment came to the county; program development centered Black women's experiences, leading to a myriad of interventions that demand systemic change and explore individual need instead of individual behavior change; a commitment to ongoing anti-racism education enabled new and varied sectors to find their role in this work.

Value 2: Black Women/People Up Front and Leading

"Why does AAIMM center Black women/people? Don't all moms and babies need more support?" This is a question we commonly heard in the early stages of the AAIMM Prevention Initiative as we educated stakeholders about the Los

Figure 15.6 ▼

The Equity-System Readiness Tool.

Source: Melissa R. Franklin, 2019.

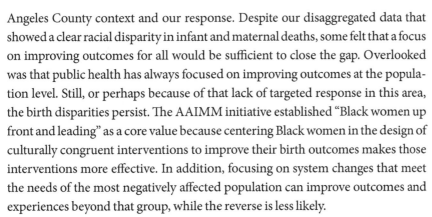

Equity-System Readiness Check

☐ Are your people and your leadership ready to have difficult conversations (about race and racism) and slow down/end projects in order to get the work done with respect and cultural humility?

☐ Do you have the right staff (representative of the community, advocates, authentic allies)?

☐ Do you have members of the impacted group (in this case African Americans) up front and leading (representation) as staff, grantees, contractors, organizational leaders?

☐ Do you have hiring and promotion practices in place that support equity and equitable advancement?

☐ Are you willing to identify/adjust practices in order to foster equity?

☐ Do you have the right data? Is it disaggregated by race/ethnicity/class? Do you require your partners/grantees to do the same?

☐ Have you established a culture of self-reflection and cultural humility?

☐ Is everyone, including leadership, speaking about root causes and approach to solutions from an equity frame?

☐ Are you willing to invest in addressing disparity among a few (versus focusing on the big numbers)?

☐ Are your contracting practices aligned in such a way that organizations that represent the community you endeavor to impact can participate in strategic planning and grantmaking, as well as receive grants?

☐ Do you understand the community's history and the trauma contained within?

☐ Have you embraced knowledge sharing, continuous learning, collaboration, and solidarity as a frame for stakeholder engagement?

☐ Has your leadership and staff undergone implicit bias, cultural humility, and anti-racism (with a focus on the impacted race) education?

Angeles County context and our response. Despite our disaggregated data that showed a clear racial disparity in infant and maternal deaths, some felt that a focus on improving outcomes for all would be sufficient to close the gap. Overlooked was that public health has always focused on improving outcomes at the population level. Still, or perhaps because of that lack of targeted response in this area, the birth disparities persist. The AAIMM initiative established "Black women up front and leading" as a core value because centering Black women in the design of culturally congruent interventions to improve their birth outcomes makes those interventions more effective. In addition, focusing on system changes that meet the needs of the most negatively affected population can improve outcomes and experiences beyond that group, while the reverse is less likely.

Beyond centering Black women in the design of interventions, AAIMM also ensures representation of Black women as leaders and decision makers across stakeholder groups. Their lived experience enhances their expertise in their respective fields, and elevating their voices within the initiative helps correct for the effects of structural racism on organizational leadership pipelines. We see this as a form of restorative practice, with county systems making lasting changes to how they approach the design, implementation, evaluation, and funding of public health interventions for populations that experience disparities. This type of power-sharing can also have a healing effect, rebuilding trust between institutions and communities.

Table 15.1	Perception vs Facts about Black Infant Mortality and Maternal Mortality	
The Perception	**The Facts**	
Socioeconomic Status Does a higher level of poverty among Black women explain the difference?	We know that a secure job, a safe home, and healthy food all contribute to health. And when you look at white mothers alone or Black mothers alone, better-off mothers have healthier babies. Los Angeles County data tell us that Black women who have private insurance, which means they are employed, have worse outcomes than white women who receive public insurance.	
Mother's Education Could the gap in LA be due to a lower average education level among Black women?	All over the world, women's education is associated with healthier births. White and Black women who are well educated do have an advantage over those of the same race with less education. But county data show that better-educated Black mothers have worse birth outcomes than white women who did not complete high school!	
Mother's Behavior Could it be that Black women engage in riskier behavior than white women?	That's not what the data tell us. While Black and white women tend to engage in different kinds of risky behavior, risk-taking seems to be evenly divided. For example, white women drink alcohol more than Black women, while Black women in LA County smoke more than whites during pregnancy. But the more fundamental point is that risk-taking doesn't explain the gap. Black mothers in LA County who do not smoke have worse outcomes than white women who do.	
Access to Healthcare Perhaps the fact that Black women are less likely to have private insurance, or a car, means they are less able to get to prenatal care than white women?	Once again, this is a real concern, but it doesn't explain the inequality we see in birth outcomes. Data show that Black women who had adequate care had worse outcomes than white women who did not.	

AAIMM has been deliberate in operationalizing this value. Like all AAIMM values, the commitment to Black women up front and leading is publicly articulated on the initiative's website and in all overview presentations and materials. Making this commitment explicit establishes an expectation and supports accountability within the collaborative.

Perhaps the most effective place this is codified is in the AAIMM steering committee itself. The steering committee's charter states that the committee will endeavor to maintain a membership that is at least 51% African American and 51% non-county entities. It also stipulates that the committee will have representation from each of the regional CATs, Black-led community-based organizations, reproductive justice organizations, midwifery practices, faith-based leaders, and parents unaffiliated with organizations. This ensures that those guiding the initiative not only represent the affected community (Black women) but also represent their inherent diversity of experience, environment, and perspective. As the birth-disparities data remind us, educational and economic status are not protective factors for Black women. Black women are not a monolith, and interventions that seek to improve their birth outcomes and the representatives shaping them must account for that. The Black women on the steering committee are nonprofit leaders, program participants, decision makers in philanthropy and health plans, mothers, scholars, birth workers, and county agency representatives. They combine lived experience with topical expertise and community wisdom to shift the systems within which they operate, to enhance the efficacy of interventions, and to improve the county's ability to meet the needs of Black women and their families.

The value of Black women up front and leading is shared and affirmed across the AAIMM network, including through strategies implemented by partners. For example, the Cherished Futures for Black Moms & Babies multisector hospital quality improvement effort created a Community Advisor Collective to inform improvement strategies and ensure that Black women are part of the decision-making process. The advisers are a group of respected Black community leaders, researchers, philanthropists, and clinicians with lived experience in Cherished Futures' priority communities. These advisers are embedded as experts within each hospital team and participate in monthly coaching calls with their hospital teams, attend site visits, present at collaborative convenings, and provide additional technical assistance and strategic thought partnership as needed.

As expected, shifting the paradigm to elevate the experience and leadership of Black women across a network of private, public, and community-based institutions has presented challenges. First, we continue to contend with historic and contemporary structural racism that has impeded the pipeline of Black female leadership in institutions. While Black women may be well represented in frontline staff as community health workers, home visitors, and case workers, far fewer have been elevated to leadership, have decision-making power, or are given the flexibility within their workday to attend collaborative meetings.

Simultaneously, while the pipeline of Black leadership has thrived within community-based organizations, Black-led nonprofits in Los Angeles County continuously face funding scarcity that limits their capacity to participate in collaborative meetings or to redirect resources to collaborative efforts when compared with county agencies and private organizations.

These two issues combined can often result in a core group of Black women stretched thin across many meetings and projects and taking on additional work to help move the needle. While their lived experience has a positive effect on the quality and effectiveness of the work, many leaders have reported that their personal connections to this issue create a sense of urgency and that the tendency to overextend themselves to shift systems and to improve outcomes can lead to burnout.

It is essential that collaborative efforts to elevate the leadership of Black women employ strategies to make the work sustainable for them. This has become a recent focus for the AAIMM initiative as we enter our fourth year, and the COVID-19 pandemic has created both complexities and new opportunities to improve the experience of the work. The steering committee and CATs have deliberately cultivated a "safe space" for Black women from which all participants benefit. This allows for authentic discussion and the ability to raise and address concerns as needed, ranging from collective response to police brutality to the pace of the work and frequency of meetings. From the beginning, AAIMM has also prioritized reducing barriers to participation by paying for the time of community members and community-based representatives. Payments align with the federal consulting rate and signal that the presence and input of these stakeholders are valued.

> There are days in this work when the problem seems so big, so unchangeable when I worry that my own children will not be preserved from the traumatic birth experience we had, if they decide to have children. What gives me great hope is the village of leaders who both pour into this work and pour into each other. I think that is the secret sauce of change—solidarity of purpose and unwavering commitment to our shared values. These are the things that signal that change is not only possible, it is imminent.
>
> —*Melissa Franklin*

Box 15.1 | Power-Sharing with Black Women: Principles of Engagement

1. *Center Black Voices.* Generate meaningful and relevant results and outcomes for Black women, birthing persons, and mothers in accordance with their specific needs, priorities, and preferences.
2. *Respect Their Rights.* Work in ways to protect, facilitate, and enable Black women, birthing persons, and mothers to exercise their right to high-quality care and equitable access to services and resources, and respect their right to share their views and opinions about services, policies, and/or decisions that affect them.
3. *Build Trust.* Build relationships of trust based on mutual respect, transparency, power-sharing, and two-way communication.
4. *End-to-End Participation.* End-to-end participation requires both integrating Black perspectives into the content of policies, services, and programs, and representation of Black people in the decision-making process.

Source: Davies-Balch, S. Operational Guidance for Power-Sharing with Black Girls, Women, Birthing Persons, and Mothers. Black Wellness & Prosperity Center. 2021.

Value 3: Fighting Inequity While Fostering Equity

Closely related to the first two values, the third value demands that we walk the talk. Before we can expect lasting change, all individuals and institutions involved in AAIMM must be prepared to assess their own biases, name their institution's harmful histories and practices, and bring reflections and solutions. Self-reflection must become a habit, and prospective partnerships and collaborations must align. The Equity-System Readiness tool (see Figure 15.7) is useful in such self-reflection.

Naming racism and working toward equity means looking and listening internally and committing to structural change. DPH and First 5 LA model this for large bureaucracies by recognizing that the workplace is not separate from the social conditions and experiences of its employees and is made stronger by enabling that context to shape workplace equity. Actionable steps for fostering equity in the workplace include alerting all staff to identified inequities (hiring practices, policy revisions, or microaggressions, for example), identifying tools for further assessment and the goals of change, hosting and facilitating conversations, soliciting leadership on and review of potential changes, and regularly sharing progress toward goals.

Walking the talk also means racism is not met with Band-Aids or figureheads. When Black people are leading, there must be genuine allyship. Allyship does not look or feel like oversight; it is support. The ones experiencing should be the voices being heard, receiving acknowledgment of the inequities in their lives and what change would look like.

AAIMM offers implicit bias and antiracism training toward personal growth and regularly provides grounding exercises during meetings. We align our activities and language with a reproductive justice frame (https://www.sistersong.net/reproductive-justice),[2] recognizing that Black women's health sits at the intersection of racism and sexism. We use inclusive language to welcome all who may experience pregnancy and anyone who is affected by anti-Black racism. This includes using the terms *Black* and *African American* together or interchangeably, as we do for *birthing people* and *women*.

This value also pertains to the focus of our efforts—that they go further than "closing a gap" and "surviving." We celebrate and advocate for healthy and joyous births and beyond for Black families, acknowledging that a family can emerge from a birth experience alive yet still have been harmed by the experience.

Whether referencing equity in our systems, our partners, or our interactions with each other, we seek healing and reconciliation while not recreating harm with each other. It is important that our interventions, our conversations, and our partnerships reflect that. Often that means slowing down and being intentional. If the voices of those most affected are not represented, if our values are not reflected in practice, we slow down or stop altogether to ensure that forward movement is just.

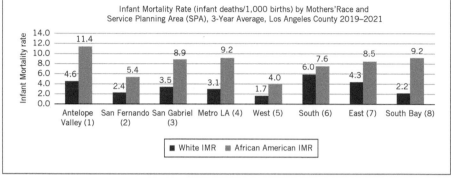

Figure 15.7 ▼
Infant mortality rate is defined as the number of deaths to infants within the first year of life per 1,000 live births. Data not shown for Hispanic, Asian, Native American, Pacific Islander, Other, and Unknown race. Three-year averages used to account for random annual rate fluctuations. Birth data for 485 White and 157 Black births, and data for 2 White deaths where SPA designation was missing are excluded. SPA designations based on 2010 census data.

Data Source: 2019 -2021 data downloaded from the Vital Record Business Intelligence System (VRBIS).

Infant Mortality Rate (infant deaths/1,000 births) by Mothers' Race and Service Planning Area (SPA), 3-Year Average, Los Angeles County 2019–2021

Value 4: No Blame Game

Be it smoking, sex, or nutrition, the American public health field historically has utilized a strategy of scaring people into healthy behavior. While fear-based messaging and programs abound, recent years have brought greater recognition that this tactic is harmful in two connected ways: it removes any responsibility from the discriminatory institutions and capitalist interests that make health practically unattainable for many and instead puts the onus of making healthy choices—and the guilt and stress of not achieving them—on individuals.

Remember the Black mother at the beginning of this chapter? Imagine caring for a premature infant while carrying the burden of thinking the circumstance was your fault. The AAIMM initiative seeks to undo the harm this strategic redirection of responsibility causes Black women and families during the perinatal period.

The central message of the initiative is, "Healthy and joyous births take a village." It is purposefully positive, strengths-based instead of fear-based, and does not imply that Black pregnant women and families need to modify their behaviors. AAIMM staff educate, refer to resources, and provide culturally congruent services that do not place blame on Black families. In alignment with the messaging campaign, the direct services for Black families offered through AAIMM prepare them for encountering systems that are not set up for them and assure families that they are deserving of, and entitled to, respectful, optimal care.

The AAIMM fatherhood and doula programs are designed for empowerment and stress reduction. Instead of a strictly didactic or formulaic set of

> ## Box 15.2 | Questions That Do Not Place Blame on the Client
>
> - Is your employer respecting your legal right to time off?
> - Do you need help finding stable housing or food programs?
> - If you are not feeling respected and supported by your current provider, may we find a different provider in your network?
> - Did your hospital schedule your follow-up lactation visit to set you up for success with breastfeeding?
> - Who do you call when you're feeling down?

interactions, staff build relationships and individualized support. Black pregnant women should, in a sense, always be considered high-risk because of the burden they have borne since before the pregnancy began.

Concurrent with direct services, AAIMM seeks to transform systems and how they respond to Black families. A critical first step in the work with hospitals, health plans, housing authorities, policymakers, and government agencies is to ask them to disaggregate their patient/member/resident data by race to see what disparities exist within their own walls. Data are a needed tool to demonstrate that the problem is right here, not "over there," and to hold institutions accountable for change.

Next, we ask what policies and practices can be modified to eliminate disparities and that all staff receive training on the modifications. For housing, this has meant developing explicit policies that prioritize pregnant people for family housing (and not single housing). For health plans and hospitals, this has included implicit bias training for all staff, seeking feedback and guidance from Black patients, hiring staff who reflect the community served, partnering with midwives and doulas, and implementing protocols for clinical interventions that reduce preterm birth. We have engaged philanthropic agencies about the need to move toward and fund such systems-level change, to prioritize funding policy and service interventions led by Black women, and to change the nature of their relationship with grant-making from one of top-down decision-making to one of inclusive facilitation. We ask all stakeholders to speak openly about the disparity they are addressing and to name racism as its root cause.

To that end, trainings are a starting point for hard conversations. AAIMM is a constant reminder that we are here not to fix a problem in the Black community but to fix the systems that enable the problem to exist. That kind of antiracist work takes personal and institutional perseverance. We accept the challenge so that when an expectant Black family activates its village of support, we, the village, will be ready to act, in joy.

As a white woman, I could say that this work doesn't impact me or my family, that it's too complicated to effect change, so why bother. But how does one turn her back on injustice? Moreover, how does one bear witness to the joys of Black parenthood and feel the high of solidarity and then choose to walk away?

—Helen O'Connor

Value 5: We Are All Pieces of the Puzzle (Everyone Has a Role)

The two mothers described earlier could have absorbed their birth experiences—one mother traumatized, one unaware—not knowing that their voices could make a difference. Instead, each is a coauthor of this chapter.

Our initiative is a collective of collectives by design, one that centers Black women and birthing persons, communities, and community leaders and is supported by allies and collaborators. The organizations that form the AAIMM Prevention Initiative have come together in a collaboration that characterizes what the collective-impact framework dictates: shared vision with complementary activities—different organizations with different strengths that benefit the overall objective.[3]

To counter the adverse physiological effects of chronic stress on the body and the social determinants of health, solutions require a multifaceted approach. Stakeholders endeavor to affect Black maternal mortality by contributing their own expertise with programs geared to their specific areas of focus.

- Having two managing organizations share responsibilities for the AAIMM initiative promotes cross-talk and understanding that enable an enriching range of expertise and perspectives. Just as the management agencies are committed to the initiative, the managers are committed to working with each other. Communication at all levels and devotion to the vision encourages a willingness to work out differences, to develop relationships among stakeholders, and to cultivate trust.
- The prominent position of the CATs that represent diverse communities is the heartbeat of the initiative in communities, bridges gaps, fosters awareness, and drives innovative incubators.
- Community-based organizations bring historical wisdom, courageous conversations, and deep understanding of what will best center and honor Black families in their respective communities.
- Our funding and policy advocacy partners bring unique stakeholders to the table, translating public health language and community needs for funders and policymakers, and vice versa.
- Our hospital and clinical partners, including Cherished Futures and the Association of Black Women Physicians, add expertise, strengthening the AAIMM workforce with accurate information, and serve as clinical ambassadors, modeling for other providers and institutions what it looks like to reimagine maternal health.

> **Box 15.3 | AAIMM Collaborators**
>
> Association of Black Women Physicians, March of Dimes, LA County DPH, and First 5 LA teamed up to present a series of physician trainings on eliminating birth disparities. One notable training was "Doulas and Doctors and Mamas, Oh My!" This training addressed the sensationalized and strained relationships between doulas and doctors and other misconceptions while promoting improved collaboration between the two as part of a village of support for expectant families.

Trust and respect are fundamental to our collective. Communication among the stakeholders in AAIMM promotes interorganizational referral to ensure maximal benefit to the mothers. It is necessary for the collaborating organizations to align with the values of AAIMM while building authentic relationships with fellow partners. Collaborators are simultaneously transformed by their participation, leading to transformation within their organizations, networks, and spheres of influence.

Little did we know that our values would become both strategy and intervention. They weave us together in a fabric that we hope will not be easily unraveled as it grows stronger, and that will usher in change. This is the story of us, and who we are can be found in our values. The story never will be perfect, but it is our love story, our becoming one with impact and not a separate entity from it. We organize our love story by the values that joined us together, flawed and clunky as that story is. Such is love.

CONCLUSION

Ultimately, this is a story about the lessons of intentionality. In language. In design. In shared purpose and action. Our collective work is to manifest joyous and healthy births for Black women and birthing people and their families through the method of intentionality.

Intentional Language

American culture long has insisted that the path to equality is best pursued through race-neutral and colorblind policies. However, eliminating race from the discussion eradicated racism from neither policy nor practice in any faction of society. DPH's decision to name racism as a root cause and to target interventions toward the population most disproportionately affected by that harm was a bold one, even when the department's conclusion was backed by rigorous data. Amid some pushback, DPH remained committed to focusing on who the data represented: Black women. The department's courage gave others courage as well: namely, funders. In philanthropy, the conversations around equity had almost exclusively adopted sanitized language that was intentionally non-race-specific. "Communities of color," "marginalized communities," "underrepresented," "underserved," and now "BIPOC" are all terms used to avoid the tough but necessary conversations around race and racism. Thankfully, that's changing.

Similarly, in seeking strategic partners, philanthropy often looks toward counterparts in the public sector to animate "public–private partnerships" and signal collaboration among the sectors as it pursues bold ideas. For AAIMM, it was critical to insert the community as an equal partner and stakeholder in the design and execution of our bold idea. We intentionally adopted the phrase "public-private-community partnership." We understood that we cannot and will not center community if we don't even name it as a core pillar of the work. Language always will matter.

Intentional Design

"Nothing about us without us," says the adage. Throughout this chapter, we detail the importance of intentional design. From the steering committee and CATs to outreach and engagement, the Village Fund and community grant-making to clinical interventions and hospital quality improvement, each element of the AAIMM Prevention Initiative was intentionally designed to center the voices, experiences, and leadership of Black women. It is essential that collaborative efforts seeking to elevate the leadership of Black women employ strategies to make the work sustainable for them. This includes actively removing financial and emotional barriers to participation, fostering urgency while not contributing to burnout, and listening—to Black women and for one's own biases.

Intentional Purpose and Action

For the work to work, it is essential to know and understand the change you seek and the conditions required for change to happen and be sustained. We constantly reiterate the goal: joyous and healthy births for Black women and birthing people and their families. We understand that to both achieve and sustain that goal, we must change conditions so that systems perpetuating harm, and actors within those systems, change behaviors. We need systems that prioritize family needs at a structural level. We need shared values grounded both in what Black women and birthing people and their families need to thrive and how they experience it, as a village. We need solidarity and authentic collaboration grounded in the same values that brought us together. We need to act in a way that focuses our energy on changing conditions. We need accountability to the Black women who have led this work for decades without fame or fortune and who continue to serve and heal their communities every day. And we need humility in understanding that the more we learn, the more we need to learn. As we implement our work and drive toward outcomes that deliver joyous and healthy births for Black families, we evaluate our efforts to amplify what works and to move away from what doesn't, so that good practice can become good public policy. We offer these lessons as part of our own continuous improvement and invite others to join with us in this intentional space.

Equity

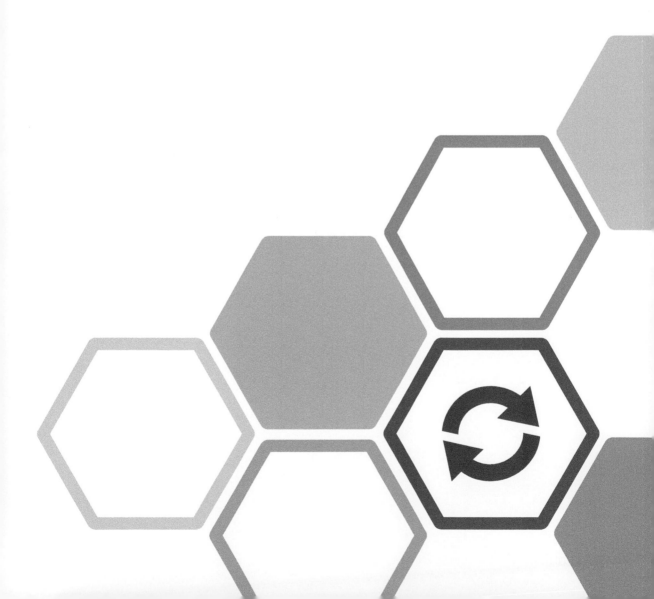

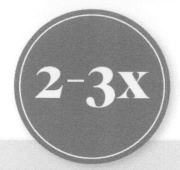

Black, American Indian, and Alaska Native women are 2-3x more likely to die from pregnancy-related causes than white women

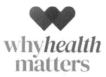

Sources: Hoyert DL. Maternal mortality rates in the United States, 2021. *NCHS Health E-Stats*. 2023. https://dx.doi.org/10.15620/cdc:124678; and Petersen EE, Davis NL, Goodman D, et al. Racial/ethnic disparities in pregnancy-related deaths—United States, 2007–2016. *MMWR*. 2019;68:762–765. http://dx.doi.org/10.15585/mmwr.mm6835a3

Infographic Created By: Why Health Matters and Imaginari

Chapter 16

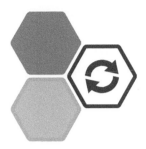

Centering Equity: Systemic Racism and Social Determinants of Maternal Health

NATALIE D. HERNANDEZ AND TAMARON A. JOHNSON

Persistent racial inequities in maternal health have existed for decades despite investments and advancements in the US healthcare system. There have been considerable efforts to improve maternal healthcare, but measures that only focus on clinical causes of maternal mortality and morbidity are insufficient. As a result, many racial and minoritized communities do not have access to quality care, do not receive the respect they deserve, and continue to suffer disproportionately from dismal maternal health outcomes. Embedded within the persistent inequities are the ongoing effects of racism, bias, sexism, and other forms of oppression that intersect to adversely affect maternal health outcomes.[1] To advance maternal health equity, we need to address the social, structural, and political determinants of health.[2] By understanding the root causes, when they started, and the impact of power structures that create an imbalance of opportunities and resources, we will be better equipped to develop actionable solutions to address the maternal health crisis.

The first few chapters of this section provide a framing and foundation for the rest of the chapters, which discuss the root causes of poor maternal health outcomes. The chapters dig deep and discuss how systemic racism and social and structural determinants contribute to maternal health inequities. The chapters detail various equity-based solutions to maternal health disparities. They discuss the historical context of maternal health, environmental impacts on maternal health, and laws and institutions that influence it. Furthermore, the chapters promote a reproductive justice framework that illuminates the past and present atrocities seen in maternal health while offering solutions to address reproductive health disparities.

Natalie D. Hernandez and Tamaron A. Johnson, *Centering Equity* In: *The Practical Playbook III*. Edited by: Dorothy Cilenti, Alisahah Jackson, Natalie D. Hernandez, Lindsey Yates, Sarah Verbiest, J. Lloyd Michener, and Brian C. Castrucci, Oxford University Press. © de Beaumont Foundation 2024. DOI: 10.1093/oso/9780197662984.003.0016

The racial disparities in maternal health find their roots deep in American history. In Chapter 17, Velez and Avila provide the historical context to assist us in our understanding of the impact of structural racism on maternal health outcomes in the United States. They detail how the context of colonialism, slavery, and oppression relates to present-day maternal health outcomes. The authors illuminate the utility of reproductive justice as an equity-focused framework to combat structural racism in maternal health outcomes by providing some examples of how reproductive justice can, and should, be used in public health.

In Chapter 18, Webb introduces the current state of maternal health in the United States and describes a brief history of structural racism and how its role has given rise to such bleak conditions for birthing individuals. The chapter also provides a path forward by recommending equity-centered and justice-centered frameworks for informing research, training, and practices and for centering communities in solutions.

Unlike health equity, which has been defined, maternal health equity lacks a clear definition, but a definition is needed to reach a consensus and to align stakeholders for action. In Chapter 19, Mosley identifies a definition for maternal health equity along with research priorities to improve health equity in Georgia using the Delphi method. (Georgia tops the list of states with the highest maternal mortality rate.[3]) This chapter provides a basis for discussion, ensuring a standard definition for, and an understanding of, what constitutes maternal health equity.

An example of centering Black women and using community-based approaches is highlighted in Chapter 20, "Redesigning Systems with Black Women to Improve Maternal Health in Atlanta." The chapter features the Institute for Healthcare Improvement (IHI) and the Redesigning Systems with Black Women project. The project aimed to improve equity, dignity, and safety while reducing racial inequities in maternal outcomes for Black birthing people. The chapter authors describe their work, conducted in Atlanta, GA, and detail their experience. Throughout the careful exploration of their processes, they share the lessons their team has learned when communicating and developing solutions with those affected most by the maternal health crisis. The chapter promotes a crucial step in addressing the maternal health crisis: centering the solution around the voices of those most afflicted.

In Chapter 21, Hayes and Pizii focus on reproductive justice and antiracism in carceral institutions. The chapter is written as an autoethnographic discussion and interview between the two authors about their experiences. The discussion centers the experiences of Black women in an account of the complexities and nuances of partnering with carceral institutions to provide doulas for incarcerated pregnant people. The authors define reproductive justice and highlight its importance as an analytical tool to examine the cultures and systems that have become the status quo and shape bodily autonomy. The chapter illuminates the additional struggles incarcerated women face regarding their reproductive rights and provides recommendations on utilizing reproductive justice to advance incarcerated pregnant people's health and quality of life.

In Chapter 22, "Environmental Impacts on Maternal Health," Okoh introduces readers to the foundations of environmental justice and how socioeconomic, physiological, and environmental factors collectively affect health. The chapter also provides strategies for addressing environmental factors to combat their effects on maternal health while affirming the pregnant person's agency in their health.

In the last chapter of this section, Warren-Clem and McGee focus on designing a justice-conscious approach to reproductive health. They discuss the role of health-related legal doctrines and their impact on the delivery of healthcare and health outcomes. Through the analysis of two case studies, they argue that medical-legal partnerships and viewing care through a health justice lens can create and increase equity in maternal health.

This section aims to give readers a better understanding of the historical context, structures, policies, and environmental factors that contribute to maternal health inequities. The lessons, tools, equity-and-justice frameworks, and practices described in the chapters will assist readers with developing and implementing promising approaches to advance maternal health equity. The chapters also emphasize the importance of working in partnership with communities, healthcare systems, and stakeholders that address the structural determinants of health to be more effective in reducing maternal morbidity and mortality and improving outcomes for pregnant people. Ideally, the lessons and tools imparted by the chapters will reinvigorate readers' desire to create equity in maternal health.

REFERENCES

1. Clark A, Wescott P, Mitchell N, Mahdi I, Crear-Perry J. Centering equity: addressing structural and social determinants of health to improve maternal and infant health outcomes. *Semin Perinatol*. 2022;46(8):151661. doi:10.1016/j.semperi.2022.151661.

2. Dawes DE. *The Political Determinants of Health*. Baltimore, MD: Johns Hopkins University Press; 2020.

3. America's Health Rankings. *Health of Women and Children Report*. 2022. https://www.americashealthrankings.org/health-topics/58/heat-map?topics=6. Accessed January 15, 2023.

Chapter 17

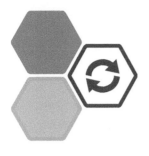

Historical Context Matters: Structural Racism, Maternal Health, and Reproductive Justice

CHRISTINE M. VELEZ AND MARIA MERCEDES ÁVILA

INTRODUCTION

The United States is beset by some of the highest maternal mortality rates compared to other economically advanced countries.[1-5] The World Health Organization defines maternal health as women's health during pregnancy, labor, and postpartum.[5] According to the Centers for Disease Control and Prevention (CDC), 700 women die yearly due to pregnancy-related complications. This statistic is alarming for all American women.[4] Black women, in particular, are dying more than any racial or ethnic group in the United States, as Black women are two to three times more likely than white women to die of pregnancy-related causes.[2,6-10] The social determinants of health, such as poverty and educational attainment, alone are not responsible for the disproportionately high rates of maternal mortality rates in the United States, particularly among Black women.[3,8] Racially and ethnically diverse women disproportionately face higher incidences of STIs, reproductive cancers, maternal and infant mortality rates, challenges with breastfeeding, and delayed identification of services for children with dis/abilities and mental health challenges.[4,5] Racially and ethnically diverse women and women of low socioeconomic status also face barriers to accessing behavioral healthcare.[7] This is extremely important because maternal depression has been associated with child abuse, neglect, and foster care placement.[7] If racially and ethnically diverse women and poor women are met with discrimination and racism when accessing mental health support, we can assume they are at higher risk of losing their children to the child welfare system, among

Christine M. Velez and Maria Mercedes Ávila, *Historical Context Matters* In: *The Practical Playbook III*. Edited by: Dorothy Cilenti, Alisahah Jackson, Natalie D. Hernandez, Lindsey Yates, Sarah Verbiest, J. Lloyd Michener, and Brian C. Castrucci, Oxford University Press. © de Beaumont Foundation 2024. DOI: 10.1093/oso/9780197662984.003.0017

other consequences of structural racism in maternal health. The United States has the highest maternal mortality rate of any high-income country.[1-5] However, one of the most troubling statistics is that approximately 63.280% of all maternal deaths in the United States are preventable.[4]

The American Public Health Association has identified racism as a public health emergency.[11] This chapter argues that structural racism significantly contributes to maternal health disparities for women of color in the United States. The chapter offers definitions of structural racism and the social determinants of health, and it presents a preliminary historical overview of reproductive health abuses against women of color in the United States. Finally, reproductive justice (RJ) is discussed as an equity-focused framework useful for challenging and combating structural racism in maternal health.

STRUCTURAL RACISM AND SOCIAL DETERMINANTS OF HEALTH

Although intertwined, structural racism and the social determinants of health are two distinct concepts. In this chapter, structural racism is understood as a social determinant of health, and structural racism is defined as a system in which public policies, institutional practices, cultural representations, and other norms work in various, often reinforcing, ways to perpetuate racial group inequity. The chapter identifies dimensions of history and culture that have allowed privileges associated with "whiteness" and disadvantages associated with "color" to endure and to adapt over time. Structural racism is not something that a few people or institutions choose to practice. Instead, it has been a feature of the social, economic, and political systems in which we all exist.[12]

In contrast, the social determinants of health are "conditions that affect the health and quality of life of people in a given environment, including where a person works, lives, or plays." According to the CDC, this definition includes the following five components: economic stability, education access and quality, healthcare access and quality, neighborhood and built environment, and social and community context.[4,6] Thus, health disparities are understood as "preventable differences in the burden of disease, injury, violence, or opportunities to achieve optimal health that are experienced by socially disadvantaged people."[7] Health inequities are avoidable inequalities between groups of people. Racism in all its forms, but particularly structural racism, is a preventable component of the US healthcare system. Racism is not an inherent trait one is born with; it is a learned behavior. Learned racist beliefs and actions have always been central to US policy and legislation. They have life-or-death consequences for racially and ethnically diverse communities, especially those of lower socioeconomic backgrounds.

HISTORICAL CONTEXT

To understand the disproportionately high maternal mortality rates in the United States today, especially among racially and ethnically diverse women, it is essential to understand the historical context that contributes to ongoing health disparities. The history of colonization of the Americas, including the trans-Atlantic slave trade, is critical to understanding the current reproductive reality facing racially and ethnically diverse women. The Americas were colonized under systems of imperialism and colonialism, and sexual violence was a tool frequently used by early European colonists against Indigenous women and communities during the Spanish and Portuguese "conquest" of the Americas.[13]

This was followed by close to 400 years of the trans-Atlantic slave trade, which set the conditions for unequal treatment of Blacks and other marginalized groups. What we now call the social determinants of health, such as education, income, neighborhood characteristics, access to care, safety, and food stability, "have all been dictated by the very structure of American society from the time of slavery."[14] In the US antebellum South, the slave economy determined the reproductive destinies of Black reproducing bodies as "slave owners sought the assistance of physicians in the management of Black women's fertility."[6,13,14] After 1808, when the United States formally stopped the importation of enslaved people from Africa, slave owners routinely turned to new practices and surgical procedures around women's health to enhance reproduction and ensure a steady supply of slave labor.[6] Unfortunately, the ban on the importation of slaves exacerbated slave owner control and vigilance over the reproduction of slave women, and thus increased the value of the reproduction of slave labor and encouraged slave owners to "take extreme measures to ensure that these women could not only conceive, but also could bring a fetus to full term."[6] The use of a 'scientific approach' to reproductive management of enslaved people "ushered in a new era of slave breeding, coercion, medical experimentation, and the neglect for reproductive freedom."[6] The treatment of infertility among slave women became a topic of concern for slave owners, and "infertile enslaved women were treated like damaged goods; slave owners wreaked havoc on these women with physical abuse and torment in times where they perceived the failure to bear children as a loss to profit."[6] The treatment of infertility in slave women was mainly experimental. The only concern was the successful breeding of more enslaved people; there was a complete lack of care or concern about the health of enslaved women. Pregnant enslaved women were often provided little to no reprieve from work responsibilities and were expected to carry on without rest or proper care.

Ultimately, the distrust of medical systems and providers by racially and ethnically diverse women is due to historical abuses by medical professionals and systems.[6,13] There is a history of medical and surgical experimentation on enslaved women and racially and ethnically diverse women. Forced and coerced sterilization, eugenics, and social control came after the formal end of slavery. The American South became the first region to perform forced sterilizations on women of color, specifically Black women, although forced sterilizations were also conducted with regularity in other geographic locations, such as in Boston and in New York State: "physicians, social workers, and members of state eugenics boards worked together in the sterilization of low-income Black women with the intention of reducing the number of Black women eligible for public assistance."[6]

Other groups of women, such as women with dis/abilities, Indigenous women, and Latina women (specifically Puerto Rican women), have faced the indignity of coerced and forced sterilizations and coerced medical experimentation.[15,16] Indigenous women were targeted by the eugenics movement and the state's forced removal of their children from their homes.[17] Puerto Rican women, in particular, were targets of medical experimentation in birth control trials where they were unknowingly given extremely high doses of estrogen, which resulted in health problems and death for many of the women in those studies.[18] The lists of egregious and even subtle forms of reproductive abuses can go on and on. The eugenics movement was justified by labeling Black women (as well as other racial and ethnically diverse groups of women) as bad mothers and as hypersexual.[19] Other groups, such as Indigenous and Latina women, were also labeled as bad mothers, hypersexual, and essentially "deserving" of abuse and violence.[19]

REPRODUCTIVE JUSTICE AS AN EQUITY- AND JUSTICE-CENTERED FRAMEWORK

Reproductive justice (RJ) is a multipronged framework developed by women of color activists to address aspects of reproductive health that they felt were absent from the white mainstream feminist movement of the 1960s and 1970s, which mainly focused on abortion access.[15,16,20] Although access to abortion is a crucial part of the RJ agenda, women of color felt that as racialized women, their reproductive health concerns reached beyond abortion access and that the issues affecting them were not reflected in second-wave feminist movements.[15,16,20] Thus, the RJ movement, which has since developed into a framework, was initiated by Black, Asian, Latinx, and Indigenous women who acknowledged that identities at the intersection of race, ethnicity, and gender had unique needs that differed from those of white women. The right to bodily autonomy and self-determination undergirds RJ frameworks and approaches. An RJ framework contests rationales that blame women for poor health outcomes by focusing on the structural context, instead of individual behavior, as "no matter how empowered, knowledgeable or willing someone is to change their behavior, they may not be able to because of structural determinants of health"[14]

RJ demands a decidedly antiracist approach to addressing health inequities and disparities. RJ strongly focuses on race/ethnicity and acknowledges the negative effects of racism and discrimination on health.[20] Resistance and resilience of Black women are "a notable component of the historical foundations of reproductive oppression."[6] RJ acknowledges that despite the legacies of oppression, marginalized communities also have histories of resistance and resilience, community-building, and self-advocacy. An RJ approach highlights these strengths and underscores how women of color have resisted oppression and organized informal community care and support systems.[15,16]

At its core, RJ recognizes the right of every person to have children, not to have children, and to parent in safe and healthy environments.[15,16,20] RJ includes reproductive health (which focuses on service provision) as a component, but RJ is focused on human rights as part of equitable service provision for all people. RJ is informed by intersectionality and emphasizes the "interconnectivity of reproductive rights, human rights, and economic justice."[6,21,22] Intersectionality underscores power and access to resources by highlighting the marginalization of multiply minoritized people and communities.[21,22] RJ frameworks can help highlight social determinants of health and structural inequities that perpetuate maternal and child health disparities for racially and ethnically diverse birthing people.[14] Frameworks that connect structural racism to health outcomes can "further elucidate the web of causation between the structural and social determinants of health for Black women and other disenfranchised groups" and have "the potential to facilitate the identification of interventions and policies that can remediate and eliminate inequalities in health across the population."[14] Along with structural racism in systems and policy, racism experienced at the micro/individual level in the process of accessing healthcare also contributes to disproportionately high rates of maternal mortality, especially for Black women, as "it is racist attitudes toward Black women that are the dispositive factor in whether these mothers live or die."[2]

USING RJ TO ADDRESS STRUCTURAL CHANGE

RJ has the potential to identify and remove barriers to healthcare access as well as racism's role in perpetuating these barriers. An RJ-focused approach is also focused on visibility and representation. It acknowledges that a more racially/ethnically diverse and culturally/linguistically responsive healthcare workforce trained in structural racism and the social determinants of health can promote a system of care that centers on the reproductive needs of all people but especially those of racially/ethnically diverse birthing people. People of color remain underrepresented in the health workforce, despite research establishing that a racially and ethnically diverse workforce can help facilitate and expand access to healthcare for vulnerable people and meet the needs of an increasingly diverse population.[23] Pipeline program interventions that focus on the barriers faced by those seeking to enter the health workforce have the potential to recruit and retain racially and ethnically diverse professionals.[23] Although much work remains, many areas, such as psychiatry, nursing, oncology, and surgery, are actively trying to find ways to diversify, noting that diversity can improve patient care and reduce health disparities. [24-27]

An RJ-focused approach centers on access to healthcare and health insurance. It supports the full expansion of Medicaid in all states, because "disparities in health not only emerge from how healthcare systems operate, but also from the legal, regulatory, and policy climate within which healthcare is delivered."[6] Although the Affordable Care Act of 2010 brought about many significant changes in Medicaid and health insurance coverage, it still allowed states to opt out of expanding Medicaid coverage to underinsured and uninsured populations, which many states chose to do. States that decided not to expand Medicaid had the highest numbers of underinsured and uninsured residents. Since almost half of US births are covered by Medicaid, when individual states decided not to expand it, they made access to prenatal, birthing, and postnatal care even more challenging for poor women, especially impoverished women of color. Medicaid is also the largest payer of family planning and maternal healthcare services, including prenatal care, labor and delivery care, contraception, and screenings for reproductive cancers. The hardships created by limiting access to healthcare are preventable and a clear example of structural racism that can be addressed through policy initiatives that expand and sustain healthcare access for all populations, particularly racial and ethnic minorities and people of color.

There are helpful examples of researchers and policymakers who have used an RJ-focused approach to address health disparities broadly and maternal health specifically. One example is a research study conducted with a state-recognized Gulf Coast tribe that utilized an RJ-informed approach to explore the effect of environmental degradation on tribal members' health by conducting interviews with Indigenous women. Findings showed that participants communicated high rates of chronic illness, significant issues with infertility, and hindrance of their ability to parent in safe and healthy environments.[28] A recently introduced policy (HR 959), called the Black Maternal Health Momnibus Act of 2021, is an example of an RJ-informed policy that directs multiagency efforts to improve maternal health, in particular, for racial and ethnic minorities and demands that the Department of Health and Human Services (HHS) address the social determinants of health.[29] These two examples demonstrate the innovative ways in which RJ can be applied to improve maternal health outcomes in the United States.

CONCLUSION

Racially and ethnically diverse communities are disproportionately affected by health disparities and inequities. Although this chapter identifies some research on this topic, specifically the impact of structural racism on Black women's health, more research is needed. Future research also needs to consider the health implications of structural racism on other racial and ethnically diverse groups. All birthing people, regardless of gender, should be included in future research, as RJ demonstrates that the intersection of multiply minoritized identities can negatively affect reproductive health. People in the United States, particularly racially and ethnically diverse communities, have a long history of distrusting the healthcare system. Meaningfully addressing health disparities and inequities can potentially dismantle systemic and structural racism. Exposure to systemic racism, discrimination, and incarceration falls under the social and community context of the social determinants of health as one of the five key areas representing the majority of a person's life in our society. We must focus on improving the five key areas disproportionately affecting racially and ethnically diverse communities. Equity and justice mean everyone has a fair opportunity to be as healthy as possible and to thrive. They mean living in a society where providers can identify their biases and prejudices and not expose communities to substandard levels of care. In a society where every provider is concerned about having migrant children in internment camps, Black children murdered in our streets, or Native Indigenous children buried in cemeteries across our country, many around or near what are now hospitals or universities, workforce diversity and development are key aspects of addressing and eliminating health disparities and inequities. Workforce development needs to happen in meaningful ways to ensure providers receive education and training on systemic racism and the history of systemic racism in healthcare in the United States.[4,6,12]

An RJ-informed approach to care provision, healthcare practice, and health-related research can help expose and break down structural oppression faced by communities of color seeking reproductive care. Researchers can apply and use an RJ-informed framework in their work to address maternal health disparities, especially through participatory action research methodologies, and they should keep in mind the foundational tenets of RJ from design through dissemination.[30] In practice, educational programs across all health-related disciplines should teach RJ, replete with a focus on the historical context affecting current outcomes.[30,31] An awareness of the social determinants of health, combined with centering on vulnerable populations, is one way for professionals to adopt culturally appropriate care practices that can benefit racially and ethnically diverse patients. From a policy standpoint, RJ's emphasis on rights and social justice can be leveraged to address maternal health disparities, at the local, state, and federal levels.[30,31] Black women and women of color should be treated equitably and with dignity and respect. RJ focuses on these women and all birthing people in its mission to achieve safe and equitable systems for all communities. Due to the multilevel and complex influence of racism in health inequities, transdisciplinary approaches are "necessary to disrupt both [racism's] legacies and [its] contemporary manifestations."[8] RJ as a movement and a framework emerged from the transdisciplinary efforts of women of color, including professionals, activists, and community members alike. Hence, the emphasis on a multilevel approach aligns well with RJ.

REFERENCES

1. Hardeman RR, Kheyfets A, Mantha AB, et al. Developing tools to report racism in maternal health for the CDC Maternal Mortality Review Information Application (MMRIA): findings from the MMRIA Racism & Discrimination Working Group. *Matern Child Health J*. 2022 26(4): 661–669.

2. Wynn GT. The impact of racism on maternal health outcomes for black women. *U Miami Race Soc Just L Rev*. 2019;10:85.

3. Baiden D, Parry M, Nerenburg K, et al. Connecting the dots: structural racism, intersectionality, and cardiovascular health outcomes for African, Caribbean, and Black mothers. *Health Equity*. 2022;6(1):402–405.

4. Trost S, Beauregard J, Chandra G, et al. Pregnancy-related deaths: *data from Maternal Mortality Review Committees in 36 states, 2017–2019*. Education (Chula Vista). 2022;45(10):1. https://www.cdc.gov/reproductivehealth/maternal-mortality/docs/pdf/Pregnancy-Related-Deaths-Data-MMRCs-2017-2019-H.pdf. Accessed January 28, 2023..

5. World Health Organization. *Maternal Health*. https://www.who.int/health-topics/maternal-health#tab=tab_1. Accessed June 9, 2022.

6. Taylor JK. Structural racism and maternal health among Black women. *J Law Med Ethics*. 2020;48(3):506–517.

7. Klawetter S, Frankel K. Infant mental health: a lens for maternal and child mental health disparities. *J Hum Behav Soc Environ*. 2018;28(5):557–569.

8. Neely AN, Ivey AS, Duarte C, et al. Building the transdisciplinary resistance collective for research and policy: implications for dismantling structural racism as a determinant of health inequity. *Ethn Dis*. 2020;30(3):381.

9. Williams DR, Lawrence J, Davis B. Racism and health: evidence and needed research. *Annu Rev Public Health*. 2019;40:105.

10. Chambers BD, Taylor B, Nelson T, et al. Clinicians' perspectives on racism and Black women's maternal health. *Womens Health Rep*. 2022;3(1):476–482.

11. American Public Health Association. *Racism Is a Public Health Crisis*. https://www.apha.org/topics-and-issues/health-equity/racism-and-health/racism-declarations. Accessed June 9, 2022.

12. The Aspen Institute. *11 Terms You Should Know to Better Understand Structural Racism*. https://www.aspeninstitute.org/blog-posts/structural-racism-definition/ Published July 11, 2016. Accessed June 9, 2022.

13. Washington HA. *Medical Apartheid: The Dark History of Medical Experimentation on Black Americans from Colonial Times to the Present*. New York: Doubleday Books; 2006.

14. Crear-Perry J, Correa-de-Araujo R, Lewis Johnson T, et al. Social and structural determinants of health inequities in maternal health. *J Womens Health*. 2021;30(2):230–235.

15. Ross LJ. Reproductive justice as intersectional feminist activism. *Souls*. 20173;19(3):286–314.

16. Ross LJ, Solinger, R. *Reproductive Justice: An Introduction*. Oakland: University of California Press; 2018.

17. Ralstin-Lewis DM. The continuing struggle against genocide: Indigenous women's reproductive rights. *Wicazo Sa Rev*. 2005;20(1):71–95.

18. Womack ML. US colonialism in Puerto Rico: why intersectionality must be addressed in reproductive rights. *St Antonys Int Rev*. 2020;16(1):74–85.

19. Scott KA, Britton L, McLemore MR. The ethics of perinatal care for Black women: dismantling the structural racism in "mother blame" narratives. *J Perinat Neonatal Nurs*. 2019;33(2):108–115.

20. SisterSong. *Reproductive Justice*. https://www.sistersong.net/reproductive-justice Accessed on June 9, 2022.

21. Crenshaw K. Mapping the margins: intersectionality, identity politics, and violence against women of color. *Stanf L Rev*. 1990;43:1241.

22. Cho S, Crenshaw KW, McCall L. Toward a field of intersectionality studies: theory, applications, and praxis. *Signs*. 2013;38(4):785–810.

23. Snyder CR, Frogner BK, Skillman SM. Facilitating racial and ethnic diversity in the health workforce. *J Allied Health*. 2018;47(1):58–69.

24. Lokko HN, Chen JA, Parekh RI, Stern TA. Racial and ethnic diversity in the US psychiatric workforce: a perspective and recommendations. *Acad Psychiatry*. 2016;40(6):898–904.

25. Kozhimannil KB, Almanza J, Hardeman R, Karbeah JM. Racial and ethnic diversity in the nursing workforce: a focus on maternity care. *Policy Polit Nurs Pract*. 2021;22(3):170–179.

26. Winkfield KM, Flowers CR, Patel JD, et al. American Society of Clinical Oncology strategic plan for increasing racial and ethnic diversity in the oncology workforce. *J Clin Oncol*. 2017;35(22):2576–2579.

27. Burks CA, Russell TI, Goss D, et al. Strategies to increase racial and ethnic diversity in the surgical workforce: a state of the art review. *Otolaryngol Head Neck Surg*. 2022;166(6):1182–1191.

28. Liddell JL, Kington SG. "Something was attacking them and their reproductive organs": environmental reproductive justice in an Indigenous tribe in the United States Gulf Coast. *Int J Environ Res Public Health*. 2021;18(2):666.

29. The Black Maternal Momnibus Act of 2021. HR 959. https://www.congress.gov/bill/117th-congress/house-bill/959. Accessed July 21, 2022.

30. Luna Z, Luker K. Reproductive justice. In: Carole Joffe and Jennifer Reich, eds. *Reproduction and Society*. Abingdon, UK: Routledge; 2014:244–249.

31. Gilliam ML, Neustadt A, Gordon R. A call to incorporate a reproductive justice agenda into reproductive health clinical practice and policy. *Contraception*. 2009;79(4):243–246.

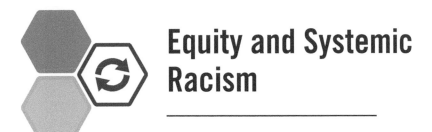

Chapter 18

Equity and Systemic Racism

JONATHAN WEBB

INTRODUCTION

The United States has the highest maternal death rate among developed high-income countries despite some recent success in addressing this problem. Most maternal deaths are preventable.[1] According to a 2020 Commonwealth Fund study, the United States is among the worst of developed countries for overall maternal health due to its high maternal mortality rate, overrepresentation of obstetrician-gynecologists relative to midwives, and shortage of maternity care providers. In addition, the United States is the only country not to guarantee access to provider home visits or paid parental leave.[2,3] Within the grim maternal mortality issue, a more nuanced challenge exists: the Black maternal mortality crisis.

THE PROBLEM AND THE COVID-19 PANDEMIC

In the United States, significant attention has been given to addressing the maternal mortality problem and the Black maternal mortality crisis; a 2020 report released by the National Center for Health Statistics indicated that the maternal mortality rate for non-Hispanic Black women was three times the rate for non-Hispanic white women. The report noted that the rate for non-Hispanic Black women was significantly higher than those for non-Hispanic white and Hispanic women. The increases in the maternal mortality rates from 2019 to 2020 among non-Hispanic Black and Hispanic women were significant, while the increase among non-Hispanic white women during the same period was not.[4] The unprecedented COVID-19 pandemic contributed to the widening disparity and compounded many foundational systemic equity and health equity concerns. Lower-wage employees were classified as essential workers during the

Jonathan Webb, *Equity and Systemic Racism* In: *The Practical Playbook III*. Edited by: Dorothy Cilenti, Alisahah Jackson, Natalie D. Hernandez, Lindsey Yates, Sarah Verbiest, J. Lloyd Michener, and Brian C. Castrucci, Oxford University Press.

pandemic, requiring them to place themselves in harm's way to keep the country financially afloat and able to access basic needs, like food, public safety, utilities, and so on. Most of their jobs couldn't be performed remotely. These "essential workers" are the employees who have the most difficulty receiving adequate healthcare, due to an overburdened and already biased system and a societal infrastructure that has created a class of working poor, wherein people sometimes must decide between working for an hourly wage on a particular day and taking time off for a healthcare appointment. Additionally, these individuals are more likely to experience the challenges associated with chronic stress, which was increased during the pandemic. These inequitable situations were exacerbated by COVID-19 and contributed to the rising disparity in maternal mortality rates.

In his book *We Still Here*, Dr. Marc Lamont Hill wrote, "COVID-19 didn't merely spotlight the profound inequalities within our social arrangement. In many ways, it made them worse."[5] Dr. Hill highlighted the disparity by challenging us to consider why "African Americans accounted for 60% of the COVID-related deaths, but only account for 13% of the population."[5] He concluded that racist systems don't merely deny certain groups access to social good and fair treatment but also render them vulnerable to premature death. Likewise, he suggested that COVID-19 infection and survival are linked to the disproportionate economic vulnerability experienced by Blacks. "Black people remain near the top of every index of social misery and hover close to the bottom of every measure of social prosperity. Black families have a net worth ten times less than their white counterparts. We are consistently denied access to housing, healthcare, education, food security, and living-wage jobs. These realities create the conditions for Black vulnerability."[5] These conditions placed Black mothers at risk for poorer health outcomes during the pandemic because they consistently endured tremendous personal sacrifice to earn a living.

Given the complexity of the maternal mortality problem and growing Black maternal mortality in the United States, we must act with urgency, innovate in our approach to problem-solving, and intentionally focus on the root cause, which will require an honest interrogation of our systems and infrastructures and their role in affecting outcomes. Each maternal death statistic is a lost life—a mother, sister, wife, daughter—and affects a family and community. We must acknowledge that, despite our best efforts, the unacceptably high US maternal mortality rate persists. Those interested in working to address the problem must be willing to "think outside the box" and to take different approaches to developing solutions or thoughtfully identifying ways to scale up current strategies that have seen incremental success. It is important to adjust our efforts to focus on the systems that create the environments of inequity within which our target populations function.

Figure 18.1 ▼

Equality/Equity/Liberation.

Source: The Equality/Equity/Liberation image is a collaboration between the Center for Story-based Strategy (https://www.storybasedstrategy.org/the4thbox) and the Interaction Institute for Social Change (http://interactioninstitute.org/). released and licensed under a Creative Commons Noncommercial Sharealike 4.0 license.

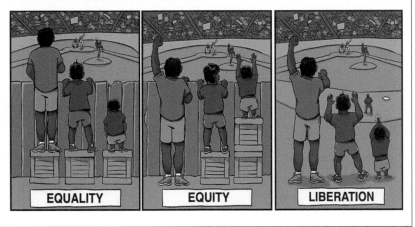

SEEING THE PROBLEM FROM A DIFFERENT VANTAGE POINT

Addressing maternal health inequities through a different lens requires exploring two essential areas: (1) a standard definition of health and health equity and (2) the historical context for how the United States, as a developed nation, ranks so poorly as a safe place to birth for all people. These two elements are critical to our collective understanding of the issue. Likewise, their context allows us to move urgently to implement solutions commensurate to the challenge.

Figure 18.1 is a popular visual for illustrating the distinction between equality and equity. It challenges the viewer to embrace the notion that every individual presents with a specific and unique set of circumstances. To identify a singular solution to satisfy the needs for all persons ignores the situational nuance that comes from a deeper understanding of the individual or community. In this context, equity provides a customized solution that removes the barriers that prevent people from accessing the services, tools, and systems that would allow them to thrive. Another element of this visual is the concept that partnering in developing the customized solution requires an understanding of an individual's reality. The historical context surrounding the inequities related to marginalized populations becomes extremely relevant.

The preamble of the Constitution of the World Health Organization outlines a few key principles related to health. It sets out that health is a state of complete physical, mental, and social well-being and not merely the absence of disease or infirmity; that enjoyment of the highest attainable standard of health is a fundamental right of every human being regardless of race, religion, political belief, and economic or social condition; and that the health of all people is essential to attaining peace and security and is dependent on the fullest cooperation of individuals and states.[6,7] This framing offers additional insight that health extends beyond simply managing disease states and lays the groundwork for a holistic view of what it means to be healthy. It acknowledges the direct link between physical health and social and emotional well-being. The public health community offers a more correlative perspective and explanation that expands the understanding of this symbiotic relationship through the social determinants of health (SDOH) and life-course theory (LCT).

The SDOH are conditions in the places where people live, learn, work, and play that affect a wide range of health and quality-of-life risks and outcomes.[8] Through this lens, physical, mental, and social health not only are linked, but also are influenced by the environment in which people live, their access to quality healthcare, the availability of educational opportunities, economic health and stability, and the developmental circumstances that surround them. The distribution and disparity of power and resources shape these circumstances at the global, national, and local levels. SDOH are directly responsible for the health inequities our nation faces.

Building on this relationship between resource distribution, social infrastructure influence, and health outcomes, LCT, an emerging interdisciplinary theory, draws a connection to SDOH and the health outcomes of the patient and future generations. Conversely, the generational link outlined by LCT illuminates the influence that ancestors have had on a patient's health. LCT "is an integration of advances in multiple disciplines over the past century in understanding the interconnectedness, interdependence, and dynamic interactions across time and space of persons and their environments; a way of understanding human development and adaptation across the life span."[9] LCT provides a framework "to explore the intergenerational transmission of health, expressed biologically (epigenetically) or by nature of shared family/ community exposures."[9] LCT has evolved from identifying four domains— timeline, timing, environment, and equity—as foundational components and focuses on two core constructs—early programming and cumulative pathways. Early programming draws attention to developmental biology's influence on long-term health outcomes. Cumulative pathways suggest that "chronic stress (both biological and psychological) can cause wear and tear on the body's regulatory system, which can lead to a decline in health and function. LCT posits that the impact of biological, behavioral, and social risk factors builds up over time, resulting in 'weathering' or the gradual degradation of health."[9] The health trajectory for individuals and communities alike, therefore, can be influenced early on by factors that can either introduce risk or offer a protective benefit.

SDOH and LCT show that the factors in people's immediate social surroundings and the circumstances they inhabit affect their health. We also have a frame for (1) how SDOH and associated situational stress influence the health and well-being of generations and (2) how distribution of resources can affect SDOH and create inequity in our systems. Recently, increased attention has been given to understanding the underlying causes of these inequities, and those efforts have focused on racism. When we align to the thinking that overall health (including physical, mental, and social well-being) is affected by the circumstances in which people live, learn, work, and play (SDOH) and that these influences have generational health outcomes, our efforts should lead us to seek clarity about how power has been distributed and how individuals find themselves in their current circumstances. From this vantage point, we must acknowledge the role that racism plays in allocating resources and therefore determine that racism is the root cause of health inequity in our nation. Racism has influenced our policies, systems, and structures in a manner that benefits some while disadvantaging others. The disadvantages affect the current generation's maternal health, their health outcomes, and the health of future generations.

A BRIEF HISTORY OF STRUCTURAL RACISM

The systems that underpin our nation are built on a foundation of racism and inequity. They were established during a time when people of color were seen as property, were devalued, and were considered to be "less than." The lack of diversity (of any kind, but primarily race/ethnicity and gender) among the Founders ensured that a necessary perspective for equity was missing during the birth of our nation. The systems the Founders established define our societal infrastructure and are intentionally skewed. Dr. M. Gabriela Alcade said:

> The United States intentionally structured its systems to (repeatedly) exclude certain groups of people from full participation and representation based on their race and ethnicity. Even so-called race-neutral policies enacted recently (and today) have harmful effects on communities of color because of ingrained biases and hierarchies built to favor those who are seen as white. The system is not broken—it works as it was intended. The current visible and invisible hierarchies were erected to benefit whiteness, to the detriment of those seen as "other."[10]

To bring about genuine change that supports equitable outcomes, the current system must be analyzed through a different lens and then dismantled.

The people indigenous to this country had their lands taken from them and efforts were made for them to be assimilated into the cultures of those who colonized them. For most Black Americans, the introduction to American soil was by way of slavery. "Between 1525 and 1866, according to the Trans-Atlantic Slave Trade database, 12.5 million Africans were shipped to the New World; 10.7 million survived Middle Passage, disembarking in North America, the Caribbean and South America."[11] Scholars estimate that 450,000 Africans arrived in the United States over the course of the slave trade and most of the 42 million members of the African American community descend from this group of less than half a million Africans.[11]

The enslaved people were brought to the New World as part of an estimated $5.9 trillion to $14.2 trillion business (according to 2009 estimates) to support the domestic and agricultural needs of the New World. The forced removal of people from their homeland and native culture resulted in a loss of cultural identity and objectification of a group of people for profit. Enslaved people were seen as property and were treated as such. Families were torn apart. Enslaved people were dehumanized and devalued in every sense. Enslaved people had no voting rights, and prior to the Civil War, the US Constitution included the Three-Fifths Compromise, which indicated that for purposes of representation in Congress, a Black person counted as three-fifths of a white inhabitant of a state.[12] In the medical environment, Blacks were experimented on. Most famously in Black maternal health history, Anarcha, Betsy, and Lucy, three enslaved women who lived and worked on plantations near Alabama, were subjected to experimentation. Dr. J. Marion Sims, the 19th-century physician considered the father of modern gynecology, practiced medical procedures on enslaved women, often without anesthesia, to perfect his fistula technique. Medical professionals, then and now, believed that Blacks had different levels of pain tolerance, had genetic differences that affected their intelligence, had thicker skin, were more fertile than their white counterparts, and had stronger immune systems.[13] This foundational medical myth and others like it allowed for dehumanization and provided justification for the mistreatment of enslaved people. Even in today's system, these myths and a history of systemic dehumanizing have contributed to Black patient and physician interactions where patient concerns are discounted, individuals struggle to be heard and to have their health concerns taken seriously, and treatment protocols may differ based upon the physician's perception of the patient's situation, believability, and credibility.

At the abolishment of slavery, it was understood that the financial impact on states that were losing a key component of their workforce and industrial infrastructure was significant, so Black Codes ("vagrancy laws") were imposed to try to re-enslave the "free" labor force. The laws required formerly enslaved people to have written evidence of employment to avoid being forced to work again on plantations for no compensation. Black Codes restricted land ownership for Blacks and prevented them from gaining full citizenship rights, which manifested in conditions ranging from unequal employment opportunities to involuntary labor through debt. Many Blacks fled the South for more welcoming conditions in the North or enlisted in the US military, hoping for opportunities to better their families or to take advantage of the benefits afforded to veterans. The reality of their new situations, however, didn't live up to their vision of the new American dream. In a system that historically and consistently placed minimal value on their existence, it was hard (and in some cases, impossible) for Blacks to obtain GI Bill benefits, even as veterans who had earned them. For example, the GI Bill allowed veterans to obtain home loans and to purchase property, thus laying a foundation on which to build family and generational wealth, but in the North, Black veterans encountered redlining, a practice that made it nearly impossible for Black families to purchase homes in desirable areas. Redlining is "the illegal practice of refusing to offer credit or insurance in a particular community on a discriminatory basis (as because of the race or ethnicity of its residents)."[14] Banks wouldn't lend to Black families moving into predominantly white areas; the neighborhoods and homes that Black families were relegated to were consequently deemed uninsurable, were perceived as less valuable, and had a paucity of resources, such as schools, clean environments, and accessible healthcare. Black people and their communities also received more attention from law enforcement, resulting in criminal violations at disparate rates. Even today,

the United States has the highest incarceration rate in the world. The overwhelming burden of contact with the system has fallen on communities of color, especially African Americans. African American adults are five times more likely to be imprisoned than white Americans. African Americans are twice as likely as their white counterparts to have a family member imprisoned at some point during their childhood.[15]

While these statistics may lead one to surmise that Blacks commit crimes at a higher rate than their white counterparts, data do not support that conjecture.

Understanding this historical context is essential if the public health community and its partners intend to bring about meaningful change and equitable health outcomes. Through this historical lens, the role that structural racism plays in health becomes more evident. According to the Center for American Progress, "structural racism is defined as the system of public policies, institutional practices, cultural representations, and other norms that work in reinforcing ways to perpetuate racial inequality."

A thorough history analysis provides insight into the systemic inequities created by structural racism and the resulting stress experienced by communities of color due to policies and infrastructure that have devalued their existence, denied them access to home ownership, experimented on them, and criminalized their activity. For people of color, the policies that influence their interaction with educational, criminal justice, medical, and housing systems, for example, have been problematic and traumatic. This pervasive and chronic stress directly affects the health of mothers, children, and communities. As indicated in LCT, consistent exposure to stressors results in chronic stress and can cause wear and tear on the body, which over time may result in "weathering," the gradual degradation of health. The stressors directly affect the health of the individual; for a pregnant person, they may influence the health of a budding young life during a critical period of development. For instance, "maternal stress during pregnancy could program the fetal brain in a way that influences the way the infant's system regulates stress over the life course, elevating risk for ADHD, future chronic health conditions, infectious diseases and preterm birth in the infant's future offspring."[9]

The nation's dark history of racism has created inequitable structures and biased systems that directly contribute to the adverse health and maternal health outcomes of communities of color. Given what we know to be true, we must become comfortable with this fact. Identifying the root cause of the problem is the only way to address it appropriately. Acknowledging structural racism and its impact on health generally and maternal health specifically reframes the narrative around the population we're supporting and the problem we're solving. The blame for current outcomes shifts from the individual to the system and allows us to focus efforts on improving the societal and foundational factors that will bring measurable change. This new understanding also challenges us to identify holistic approaches to improving health that don't solely focus on clinical experiences (although these efforts are impactful and important), but to also address the many contributing factors that exist around the whole person. It allows solutions to be built in partnership with a population, and not despite them.

A PATH FORWARD

Improving the US maternal health reality will require a focus on systemic change, not simply new programs. The efforts must center on affected communities in a way we are unaccustomed to. Our approach to maternal health equity must abandon the paternalistic, "we know best" philosophy that views those whose health we are trying to improve as victims of or, worse, part of the problem. We must begin to partner with the marginalized in development and implementation of a shared solution. Likewise, the historical understanding we have reached should challenge us to interrogate the systems that affect a community's health instead of seeing that community as a problem that must be solved.

Solutions that promote equitable maternal health outcomes must contain a few key elements. They must center the community or the affected population, set up shared power and decision-making authority with the marginalized entities, establish genuine partnerships, define those they intend to serve as assets and not as problems, and facilitate interrogating the current situation/system (and not people) for historical context through a racial justice lens. Several frameworks strive to center the community and approach solutions with a partnership mindset. They include human-centered design, community-based participatory research, barrier analysis, and community asset mapping.

Human-Centered Design

Human-centered design is a problem-solving technique that puts real people at the center of the development process, enabling creation of products and services that resonate with, and are tailored to, the end user or target audience.[16] It includes three phases: inspiration, ideation, and implementation. Inspiration requires empathy and a connection to the end-user group. Ideation encourages innovative solution development that ideally is based on a firm understanding of the issue. Innovation should expand across multiple areas, including programming, system, and legislation. Implementation is critical because ideas without action and an execution plan are not helpful and may even be harmful if stakeholders have engaged and invested their time and trust in a process to bring forth solutions but that process lacks a thoughtful rollout strategy. As author and scholar Lee Bolman said, "Vision without a strategy remains an illusion."[17]

Community-Based Participatory Research

Community-based participatory research supports collaborative interventions that involve scientific researchers and community members in addressing diseases and conditions that disproportionately affect health-disparity populations.[18] It encourages and recognizes the strength of each partner across the multiple disciplines required to bring forth quality solutions. The definition of a partner is extended to include the community, the power of residents' lived experience, and knowledge of the situations in which they currently exist. This approach supports community capacity-building by developing solutions that will directly benefit residents. It likewise ensures sustainability of solutions because interventions are built on understanding the barriers and the assets in a community. Last, this approach supports translating research findings into culturally congruent and appropriate interventions.

Barrier Analysis

Barrier analysis assesses behavioral determinants associated with a particular behavior by analyzing the people who engage in the desired behavior (doers) and those who don't (non-doers).[19] This approach is often seen in global health settings but can be applied effectively in domestic environments. The assessment requires learning from affected community members how they achieve the desired behavior given their current resources and identifying barriers as well as the organic community solutions that can circumvent them. Barrier analysis leans into the thinking that the solution to a community's problem exists in that community. Lessons learned from the analysis are then built into a sustainable community strategy or educational curriculum.

Community Asset Mapping

Community asset mapping is an approach that identifies current community capacity and ability and maps strengths and resources to uncover solutions. Building on existing assets to address community needs is a solid approach to promoting community involvement and ownership of sustainable solutions.[20]

CONCLUSION

The US maternal health outlook is bleak. Reversing the negative trend in maternal health and birth outcomes is possible but will require intentional strategic focus. The adverse maternal health outcomes experienced today result from historical, institutionalized racism. Racism has created a limited set of circumstances, a disadvantaged group, and the resulting Black maternal mortality crisis. The problem wasn't created overnight and is not one that any single group can solve. To achieve the collective goal of equitable maternal and birth outcomes for all, we must be willing to partner with traditional and nontraditional stakeholders and be innovative in developing solutions. Given the multifaceted nature of the disparities in maternal outcomes created by an inequitable system, our focus cannot simply be on program development. The essential components of a thoughtful strategy include system change firmly rooted in historical understanding, cultural humility, and a willingness to reframe the narrative from a problem we're solving for the target population, to valuing the target population as a partner in the work.

Affected communities must be considered an asset and must be thoughtfully engaged in problem-solving. The solutions to improving maternal health outcomes exist in the communities we serve. We must be willing to work meaningfully alongside impacted individuals and the community-based organizations that serve them. A brighter future for maternal health in the United States is within reach. To realize it, however, we must acknowledge our country's past, build equitable systems and solutions that are on scale with the problem, and be ready to boldly engage with those affected by the problem we're solving. We are stronger together.

REFERENCES

1. Robeznieks A. U.S. has highest maternal death rate among developed countries. *Modern Healthcare*. 2015. https://www.modernhealthcare.com/article/20150506/NEWS/150509 941/u-s-has-highest-maternal-death-rate-among-developed-countries.
2. The Commonwealth Fund. *Maternal Mortality and Maternity Care in the United States Compared to 10 Other Developed Countries*. 2020. https://www.commonwea

lthfund.org/publications/issue-briefs/2020/nov/maternal-mortality-maternity-care-us-compared-10-countries.

3. U.S. ranks worst developed country for maternal health. *Time*. 2015. https://time.com/3847755/mothers-children-health-save-the-children-report/.

4. Centers for Disease Control and Prevention, National Center for Health Statistics. Maternal mortality rates in the United States, 2020. https://www.cdc.gov/nchs/data/hestat/maternal-mortality/2020/maternal-mortality-rates-2020.htm. Accessed February 23, 2022.

5. Hill ML, Barat F, Taylor K. *We Still Here: Pandemic, Policing, Protest, and Possibility*. Chicago: Haymarket Books; 2020.

6. World Health Organization. Constitution. In: *World Health Organization: Basic Documents*. 45th ed. Geneva, Switzerland: World Health Organization; 2005.

7. World Health Organization. Constitution. 2022. https://www.who.int/about/governance/constitution.

8. Centers for Disease Control and Prevention. About social determinants of health (SDOH). https://www.cdc.gov/socialdeterminants/about.html. Published March 1, 2012.

9. Verbiest S. *Moving Life Course Theory Into Action: Making Change Happen*. Washington, DC: American Public Health Association; 2018.

10. Alcalde MG. Zip codes don't kill people—racism does. Health Affairs Blog. 2018.

11. Gates HL Jr. How many Africans were really taken to the U.S. during the slave trade? America's Black Holocaust Museum. https://www.abhmuseum.org/how-many-africans-were-really-taken-to-the-u-s-during-the-slave-trade/. Published January 6, 2014.

12. Simba M. The three-fifths clause of the United States Constitution (1787). Blackpast. September 18, 2019. https://www.blackpast.org/african-american-history/events-african-american-history/three-fifths-clause-united-states-constitution-1787/.

13. Trawalter S, Hoffman KM, Jordan R. Racial bias in pain assessment. *Proc Natl Acad Sci*. 2016;113(16):4296–4301. https://doi.org/10.1073/pnas.1516047113.

14. redlining. The Merriam-Webster.Com Dictionary. 2022. https://www.merriam-webster.com/legal/redlining.

15. Center for American Progress. Mass incarceration, stress, and Black infant mortality: a case study in structural racism. https://www.americanprogress.org/article/mass-incarceration-stress-black-infant-mortality/. Published June 5, 2018.

16. Landry L. What is human-centered design? Business Insights Blog. https://online.hbs.edu/blog/post/what-is-human-centered-design. Published December 15, 2020.

17. Lee's home page. Lee Bolman. 2022. http://www.bolman.com/index.html.

18. National Institute on Minority Health and Health Disparities (NIMHD). Community-based participatory research program (CBPR). 2022. https://www.nimhd.nih.gov/programs/extramural/community-based-participatory.html.

19. Kittle B. *A Practical Guide to Conducting a Barrier Analysis*. New York, NY: Helen Keller International; 2013. https://pdf.usaid.gov/pdf_docs/PA00JMZW.pdf.

20. UCLA Center for Health Policy Research. Asset mapping. http://healthpolicy.ucla.edu/programs/health-data/trainings/documents/tw_cba20.pdf

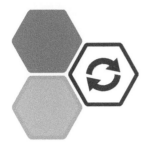

Introduction to Maternal Health Equity: A Consensus-Driven Definition and Research Priorities

BACKGROUND ON MATERNAL HEALTH EQUITY

In the United States, maternal morbidity and mortality rates are greater than in other high-income countries. The rates have been increasing over the past four decades despite decreasing trends globally.[1-3] Maternal morbidity and mortality refer to disability and deaths attributed to pregnancy-related causes before, during, and up to 6 weeks after childbirth.[1] An estimated 17 people in the United States die per 100,000 live births, compared to 6.5 deaths in the United Kingdom and 1.7 in New Zealand.[1] And for every maternal death, another 70 people experience severe complications or a so-called near miss.[4]

Moreover, inequities in US maternal health—particularly by race/ethnicity—are stark and persistent. The risk of death from pregnancy is over three times greater for Black women and two times greater for Alaska Native/Native American people than for white Americans.[1,2,5,6] Greater risk of poor maternal health outcomes and negative perinatal healthcare experiences have also been documented for marginalized groups, including some immigrants and refugees,[7,8] LGBTQ people,[9] rural communities,[10] and people with disabilities.[11] Despite these long-standing inequities and substantial community-based advocacy,[12-14] there has been little consensus among researchers on the definition of maternal health equity or priority areas for research and action.

An estimated 80% of all maternal deaths in the United States are preventable.[1,2,5] Today, the leading causes of maternal death include mental health conditions, cardiovascular conditions, infections, and hemorrhage. However, the causes and their

Elizabeth A. Mosley, *Introduction to Maternal Health Equity* In: *The Practical Playbook III*. Edited by: Dorothy Cilenti, Alisahah Jackson, Natalie D. Hernandez, Lindsey Yates, Sarah Verbiest, J. Lloyd Michener, and Brian C. Castrucci, Oxford University Press. © de Beaumont Foundation 2024. DOI: 10.1093/oso/9780197662984.003.0019

rankings vary by timing (during pregnancy, delivery, and postpartum) and race/ethnicity. For example, the leading cause of maternal mortality for white people is mental health conditions (14.9%), while the leading causes for Black people are cardiovascular conditions (13.9%) and cardiomyopathy (13.9%). Among the maternal deaths deemed preventable, Maternal Mortality Review Commissions have identified common contributing factors: patient/family factors (e.g., lack of knowledge about warning signs), provider factors (e.g., misdiagnosis and ineffective treatment), health facilities (e.g., lack of guiding protocols, poor coordination of care), and community factors (e.g., poor access to clinical care, unstable housing). Notably, reproductive justice organizations led by women of Color—such as Black Mamas Matter Alliance and the National Birth Equity Collaborative—have consistently emphasized the need for solutions beyond proximal causes that address the structural and social determinants (or "root causes") of maternal health inequities, including the healthcare system (e.g., a shortage of primary care providers, financial barriers to care, racism), educational system, built environment (e.g., housing segregation), and federal/state policies, such as paid family leave and health insurance coverage.[12,14]

CASE STUDY: MOREHOUSE SCHOOL OF MEDICINE CENTER FOR MATERNAL HEALTH EQUITY

Across the United States, Georgia consistently has one of the highest maternal mortality rates: an estimated 26 deaths for every 100,000 live births, or nearly double the national average.[15] As is true for national data, the Georgia data reflect severe racial/ethnic disparities: Black women in Georgia are 3.3 times more likely to die from pregnancy-related complications than white women. Approximately 66% of maternal deaths in Georgia have been deemed preventable. One potential contributing factor has been the declining maternity care workforce across the state, particularly in rural areas. Today, 93 of the state's 159 counties have no hospital with a labor and delivery unit.[16] And there are only two birthing centers: one in metro Atlanta and one in Savannah. Moreover, the state legislature passed HB 481, outlawing abortion as early as six weeks.

To address the maternal health crisis in Georgia, particularly issues of racial/ethnic inequality for Black women, the Center for Maternal Health Equity at the Morehouse School of Medicine (hereafter, Center for Maternal Health Equity) and the Johnson & Johnson Health of Women Team in the Office of the Chief Medical Officer partnered to establish the Georgia Maternal Health Research for Action Steering Committee (hereafter, Research Steering Committee). The Research Steering Committee brings together researchers, clinicians, policy experts, and community leaders to align inclusive, actionable, sustainable, and scalable evidence-based approaches for improving maternal health outcomes among Black mothers in Georgia. This chapter presents the Center for Maternal Health Equity and its work as a case study, which can be replicated across the country.

The partnership of the Center for Maternal Health Equity and Johnson & Johnson Women's Health Team was established to provide strategic and technical input regarding current and upcoming research supported by Johnson & Johnson and the Center for Maternal Health Equity to understand and ultimately improve maternal health for Black women in Georgia. The work is guided by two stakeholder groups: the Georgia Community for Action Group and the Research Steering Committee (of which the author is a member). The Community Action Group is tasked with identifying priorities for community advocacy and mobilization and is led by Healthy Mothers Healthy Babies Coalition of Georgia along with other community and public health practice leaders, including the Center for Black Women's Wellness, doulas, March of Dimes, SisterLove, SisterSong, and the Department of Public Health.

Working closely with the Community Action Group, the Research Steering Committee was tasked with defining maternal health equity and setting research priority areas for the state. The Research Steering Committee's 13 members (see Table 19.1) include representatives from Black Mamas Matter Alliance, local health systems, public health researchers, midwives, physicians, Georgia Perinatal Quality Collaborative, and the Centers for Disease Control and Prevention Division of Reproductive Health.

Delphi Consensus Process

Given the need to establish a clear consensus on a definition of maternal health equity and to set clear priorities for actionable research, a three-round Delphi approach was used, with the 13 Research Steering Committee members serving as a panel of experts (see Figure 19.1). The Delphi method is a widely used analytic approach for obtaining consensus from experts, particularly for improving decision-making on health and social issues.[17] It begins with problem identification (i.e., defining maternal health equity), then proceeds with open-ended questions and qualitative analysis to determine the scope of opinions on an issue, followed by structured questionnaires and quantitative analysis to rank the order of the possibilities. This can be repeated as often as needed until consensus (ideally set a priori—70% in this case) is reached. Summary results are reported to participants during or after the surveys.

First, Research Steering Committee members responded to an online survey with the following open-ended questions: (1) "How do you define maternal health equity?" (2) "What are the most important research priorities to address maternal health equity in Georgia?" Responses were analyzed using inductive content analysis to develop a list of potential definition components for rank-ordering.[18] For Round 2, participants were given a structured questionnaire to rank the potential definition components (1–9) by relevance, importance, and feasibility and the potential research priorities (1–7) by importance and urgency. Next, Research Steering Committee members reviewed the survey results and had large- and small-group discussions of necessary additions and

Table 19.1	Demographic Characteristics of the 13 Experts on the Georgia Maternal Health Research for Action Steering Committee (GMHRA-SC)
Parameter	**Experts [n (%)]**
Female sex	12 (92%)
Race/ethnicity	
Black/African American	9 (69%)
White	3 (23%)
Hispanic	1 (8%)
Degree	
PhD	7 (54%)
MD	4 (31%)
MPH	2 (15%)
Setting	
Academic	7 (54%)
Clinical	3 (23%)
Health advocacy	2 (15%)
Industry	1 (8%)
Focus	
Public health	4 (31%)
Obstetrician/gynecologist	3 (23%)
Nurse/midwife/doula	3 (23%)
Research/technology	3 (23%)

Source: Hernandez ND, Aina AD, Baker LJ, et al. Maternal Health Equity in Georgia: A Delphi Consensus Approach to Definition and Research Priorities. *BMC Public Health* 2023;23:596.

revisions. For Round 3, participants were given a revised list of definitions and research priorities, then were asked to re-rank them using the same criteria.

Maternal Health Equity Defined

The group's open-ended answers defining maternal health equity emphasized health disparities; structural and social determinants of health; gender, racial, socioeconomic, and sexual equity; life-course perspectives; and bias-free and safe healthcare (see Figure 19.2). Qualitative analysis of all open-ended answers resulted in nine potential components of a maternal health equity definition (see Table 19.2). The group was asked to rank the nine potential components using an anonymized survey; then, the group had an open discussion of the results. The group decided maternal health equity must include

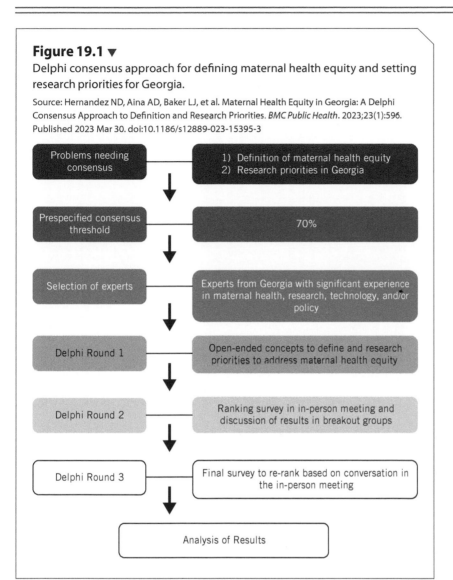

Figure 19.1 ▼

Delphi consensus approach for defining maternal health equity and setting research priorities for Georgia.

Source: Hernandez ND, Aina AD, Baker LJ, et al. Maternal Health Equity in Georgia: A Delphi Consensus Approach to Definition and Research Priorities. *BMC Public Health*. 2023;23(1):596. Published 2023 Mar 30. doi:10.1186/s12889-023-15395-3

Problems needing consensus	1) Definition of maternal health equity 2) Research priorities in Georgia
Prespecified consensus threshold	70%
Selection of experts	Experts from Georgia with significant experience in maternal health, research, technology, and/or policy
Delphi Round 1	Open-ended concepts to define and research priorities to address maternal health equity
Delphi Round 2	Ranking survey in in-person meeting and discussion of results in breakout groups
Delphi Round 3	Final survey to re-rank based on conversation in the in-person meeting
Analysis of Results	

pregnant people of all genders and life-course perspectives. However, these components were ranked low, so they were combined into more significant concepts on the ranking list (i.e., through gender-inclusive language and adding "across the life course").

After another final round of ranking, the Research Steering Committee reached a consensus on the definition. Maternal health equity was defined as:

> the ultimate goal and ongoing process of ensuring optimal perinatal experiences and outcomes for everyone as the result of practices and policies free of interpersonal or structural bias that tackle current and historical injustices, including social, structural, and political determinants of health impacting the perinatal period and life course.

Figure 19.2 ▼

Open-ended concepts of maternal health equity from 12 experts.

Source: Hernandez ND, Aina AD, Baker LJ, et al. Maternal Health Equity in Georgia: A Delphi Consensus Approach to Definition and Research Priorities. Under Review.

How do you define maternal health equity?

...both a social justice and a practical issue. It is achieved when the its root causes are addressed. It requires addressing the immediate health needs of individuals, communities, and populations, and most importantly, tackling current and historical injustices manifested [in] social, structural, and political structures.

Elimination of underlying advantages and disadvantages which contribute to gaps in maternal health outcomes between groups

Racial and sociodemographic equity in maternal health. Maternal health status cannot be predicted by race, SES, geography/zip code

Accessible maternal care for all women regardless of their race, socioeconomic background, education level, or cultural background

All mothers should have equal access to safe, affordable, and unbiased maternal healthcare

The process by which social determinants and health risk factors are addressed on an individual level so that each woman achieves optimal health outcomes during pregnancy

When all pregnant people experience the best pregnancy-related health outcomes possible, free of systematic disadvantage for certain groups due to power imbalances created by social oppression, including racism, sexism, ableism, poverty, ethnocentrism, and heterosexism

...all pregnant women and mothers have fair opportunities to achieve a state of well-being, live healthy lives, fulfill the goals for their lives, and carry out the various roles that they inhabit (mother, wife, sister, friend, employee, etc.). To achieve health equity, we must ensure that all women, regardless of socioeconomic status, where they live, their racial/ethnic identity, disability status, sexual orientation, religion, or other social category, have equal and fair opportunities to achieve positive physical, emotional, psychological, and social well-being.

Equal opportunity to thrive in the perinatal space

When outcomes for pregnant and birthing persons are not defined by their socioeconomic and educational status, access to service, geography, race, or ethnicity, and where these factors are not a predictor for morbidity or mortality

The right environment and right care at the right time for each woman. Health equity spans the life course and goes well beyond access to health-care, including economic and social life chances.

...the destination for optimizing maternal and birth outcomes through practices and policies that ensure that every expectant and birthing mother gets [what] she needs that is fair and just in order to achieve health and wellness

#	Definition of Maternal Health Equity[a]	Mean Ranking Score	
		Round 2, ranked 1–9[b] (n = 14)[c]	Round 3, ranked 1–7[b] (n = 12)[d]
1	Eliminating underlying drivers (advantages and disadvantages between groups) of disparities *across the life course*[e]	4.00	2.92
2	Tackling current and historical injustices manifested in the social determinants of health and the structural and political structures that impact the perinatal experience	3.64	2.00
3	All mothers *and birthing people of all genders*[f] have equal opportunity to have a positive perinatal experience and achieve well-being	2.36	4.00
4	Appropriate and high-quality clinical care services for each mother's *and birthing person's*[g] individual needs	5.00	3.75
5	Care is free from interpersonal or structural bias	3.93	4.33
6	Include pregnant people of all genders	8.57	N/A
7	Access to safe services	5.79	5.33
8	Access to affordable care	5.00	5.67
9	Approaches health from a life-course perspective	6.71	N/A

Table 19.2 Ranking of Maternal Health Equity Definition (Delphi Rounds 2 and 3)

Source: Hernandez ND, Aina AD, Baker LJ, et al. Maternal Health Equity in Georgia: A Delphi Consensus Approach to Definition and Research Priorities. *BMC Public Health* 2023;23:596.
Abbreviation: N/A, not applicable (the question was not included in Round 3).
[a] Question to experts: Noting that all of these are important to improve maternal health, what needs to be included in a definition of maternal health equity for Georgia?
[b] 1 represented the highest priority.
[c] Includes one anonymous respondent during a live meeting who responded likely not knowing that they were not requested to provide feedback.
[d] One expert was unavailable.
[e] The phrase "across the life course" was added for Round 3 after removal of concept #9.
[f] The phrase "and birthing people of all genders" was added for Round 3 after removal of concept #6.
[g] The phrase "and birthing person's" was included only in Round 3.

Research Priorities

The Research Steering Committee members identified 14 potential research priorities, which were then rank-ordered by importance and urgency (see Table 19.3). The group reviewed the results and decided that "causes of, and solutions to, racial inequity in maternal health outcomes and services"—unanimously ranked as essential and urgent—needed to be integrated into all research priorities. Ultimately, the four highest-ranked priorities (with over 75% agreement they are critical) were:

- Evaluating what's worked in reducing disparities and how to translate results to Georgia
- Policy-related factors that impede access to high-quality maternal health services
- Understand and measure the causes of, and solutions to, social, structural, and political drivers of maternal health disparities
- Effects of stress and sleep health on maternal morbidity

At the same time, in the surveys and during the open discussion, the Research Steering Committee members emphasized the importance of studying maternal mental health; patient-centered care; life course factors, particularly for Black and low-income pregnant people; full-spectrum care, including midwifery and abortion services; and radical care models for care coordination and social support.

CALLS TO ACTION

Ultimately, the Research Steering Committee—a diverse panel of 13 experts in maternal health—reached a clear consensus on the definition of maternal health equity and priorities for actionable research. The group emphasized upstream and root influences on maternal health equity,[14] including structural, social, and political factors, while de-emphasizing individual-level and clinical factors. They also utilized a life-course perspective[19] that addresses current injustices and historical oppressions contributing to observed differences in maternal health between groups. Furthermore, Research Steering Committee members broadly defined maternal health equity to include equity across all social axes of race/ethnicity, socioeconomic status, gender, sexuality, and more. At the same time, they named the specific and urgent needs of Black women, who bear the burden of maternal mortality in our state and country.

The group established a clear research agenda:

1. Determine what's been proven to work and implement it in Georgia
2. Identify policy priorities to expand access to high-quality care
3. Understand and measure the social, structural, and political determinants
4. Address stress-related factors and, relatedly, sleep

These research goals align with advocacy efforts in Georgia communities and at the state legislature, including Medicaid expansion. The state recently expanded Medicaid coverage from six weeks to six months postpartum. However, clinicians, advocates, and researchers agree that what is needed is at least one

#	Research Priorities to Address Maternal Health Equity in Georgia[a]	Round 2 (N = 14)[b]			Round 3 (N = 12)[c]		
		UI	I not U [n (%)]	I and U [n (%)]	UI	I not U [n (%)]	I and U [n (%)]
1	Evaluating what's worked in reducing disparities and how to translate results to Georgia	0	3 (21%)	11 (79%)	0	0	12 (100%)
2	Policy-related factors that impede access to high-quality maternal health services[d]	0	1 (8%)	12 (92%)	0	2 (17%)	10 (83%)
3	Understand and measure the *causes of, and solutions to*[e] social, structural, and political drivers of maternal health disparities	0	3 (21%)	11 (79%)	0	3 (25%)	9 (75%)
4	Effects of stress *and sleep health*[f] on maternal morbidity	0	10 (71%)	4 (29%)	0	3 (25%)	9 (75%)
5	Understanding maternal mental health[d]	0	5 (38%)	8 (62%)	0	4 (33%)	8 (67%)
6	Patient-centered maternal care, including provider-level factors that impede that care	0	3 (21%)	11 (79%)	1 (8%)	4 (33%)	7 (58%)
7	Life-course factors that contribute to higher risk of poor maternal health outcomes, particularly for Black and low-income mothers	0	5 (36%)	9 (64%)	0	5 (42%)	7 (58%)
8	Evaluating barriers to *and benefits of*[g] full-spectrum care, including midwives, doulas, postpartum care, and abortion services	0	4 (29%)	10 (71%)	0	6 (50%)	6 (50%)

(continued)

	Table 19.3 Continued						
9	Protective effects of *safe, affordable, and accessible*[h] radical care models/intensive care coordination and social supports	0	7 (50%)	7 (50%)	0	6 (50%)	6 (50%)
10	Uncovering the interactions of challenges and assets within Black communities and families and how they produce risks and resilience for maternal and birth outcomes[i]	0	7 (50%)	7 (50%)	0	6 (55%)	5 (45%)
11	Understanding patients' *clinical and nonclinical*[j] expectations of their care	0	7 (50%)	7 (50%)	1 (8%)	6 (50%)	5 (42%)
12	Evaluating Black women's *and birthing people's nonclinical*[k] experience of maternal care services	0	4 (29%)	10 (71%)	1 (8%)	6 (50%)	5 (42%)
13	Factors that contribute to patient distrust of providers	0	8 (57%)	6 (43%)	0	9 (75%)	3 (25%)
14	Causes of, and solutions to, racial inequity in maternal health outcomes and services[e]	0	1 (8%)	12 (92%)	N/A		

Abbreviations: I, important; N/A, not applicable (the priority was incorporated into other choices for Round 3); NR, no response; U, urgent; UI, unimportant.

[a] Question to experts: What are the most important research priorities to address maternal health equity in Georgia?

[b] Includes one anonymous respondent during a live meeting who responded likely not knowing that they were not requested to provide feedback.

[c] One expert was unavailable.

[d] N = 13 in Round 2.

[e] The phrase "causes of, and solutions to," was included only in Round 3.

[f] The phrase "and sleep health" was included only in Round 2.

[g] The phrase "and benefits of" was included only in Round 3.

[h] The phrase "safe, affordable, and accessible" was included only in Round 3.

[i] N = 11 in Round 3.

[j] The phrase "clinical and nonclinical" was included only in Round 3.

[k] The phrase "and birthing people's nonclinical" was included only in Round 3.

year of postpartum Medicaid or, ideally, Medicaid expansion to all people who fall below 138% of the federal poverty level.[12,20,21]

Moreover, the 2018 Black Mamas Matter Toolkit for Advancing the Human Right to Safe and Respectful Maternal Health Care was created to help implement evidence-based solutions at the state level. These include:

- Increasing affordability of reproductive health services (e.g., Medicaid expansion)
- Improving access to comprehensive sexual health education
- Ensuring access to safe and legal abortion services
- Improving the quality of maternal healthcare
- Ensuring acceptability of maternal healthcare for high-risk groups (e.g., cultural humility of providers, culture of respect for bodily autonomy)
- Ensuring availability of maternal health services
- Ensuring nondiscrimination (e.g., addressing social determinants, rights of incarcerated people)
- Ensuring accountability (e.g., improving monitoring systems and maternal health review process)

The process of convening the Research Steering Committee, gathering consensus on a definition of maternal health equity, and setting research priorities can easily be replicated in other settings. In the coming years, the Center for Maternal Health Equity and other stakeholders will implement this research agenda alongside community-driven advocacy efforts to reduce maternal morbidity, mortality, and disparities. Time will tell if this multisector, community-clinical-academic coalition can shift the tide in Georgia, where the stakes are so high and the challenges so numerous.

REFERENCES

1. Tikkanen R, Gunja MZ, FitzGerald M, Zephyrin L. *Maternal Mortality and Maternity Care in the United States Compared to 10 Other Developed Countries.* The Commonwealth Fund; 2020. https://www.commonwealthfund.org/publications/issue-briefs/2020/nov/maternal-mortality-maternity-care-us-compared-10-countries. Accessed May 3, 2021.

2. MacDorman MF, Declercq E, Cabral H, Morton C. Recent increases in the U.S. maternal mortality rate: disentangling trends from measurement issues. *Obstet Gynecol.* 2016;128(3):447–455. doi:10.1097/AOG.0000000000001556.

3. Creanga AA, Berg CJ, Syverson C, Seed K, Bruce FC, Callaghan WM. Pregnancy-related mortality in the United States, 2006–2010. *Obstet Gynecol.* 2015;125(1):5–12. doi:10.1097/AOG.0000000000000564.

4. Simpson KR. Severe maternal morbidity and maternal mortality: what can be learned from reviewing near miss and adverse events? *Am J Matern Child Nurs.* 2018;43(4):240. doi:10.1097/NMC.0000000000000446.

5. Trost S, Beauregard J, Chandra G, et al. Pregnancy-related deaths: data from Maternal Mortality *Review Committees in 36 states*, 2017–2019. Education (Chula Vista). 2022;45(10):1. https://www.cdc.gov/reproductivehealth/maternal-mortality/docs/pdf/Pregnancy-Related-Deaths-Data-MMRCs-2017-2019-H.pdf. Accessed January 28, 2023.

6. Building U.S. Capacity to Review and Prevent Maternal Deaths. Report from Nine Maternal Mortality Review Committees. *Review to Action*; 2018. https://www.cdcfoundation.org/sites/default/files/files/ReportfromNineMMRCs.pdf. Accessed January 3, 2022.

7. Kentoffio K, Berkowitz SA, Atlas SJ, Oo SA, Percac-Lima S. Use of maternal health services: comparing refugee, immigrant and US-born populations. *Matern Child Health J*. 2016;20(12):2494–2501. doi:10.1007/s10995-016-2072-3.

8. Gagnon AJ, Merry L, Robinson C. A systematic review of refugee women's reproductive health. *Refuge*. 2002;21(1):6–17. doi:10.25071/1920-7336.21279.

9. McManus AJ, Hunter LP, Renn H. Lesbian experiences and needs during childbirth: guidance for health care providers. *J Obstet Gynecol Neonatal Nurs*. 2006;35(1):13–23. doi:10.1111/j.1552-6909.2006.00008.x.

10. Shah NT. Eroding access and quality of childbirth care in rural US counties. *JAMA*. 2018;319(12):1203–1204. doi:10.1001/jama.2018.1646.

11. Signore C, Davis M, Tingen CM, Cernich AN. The intersection of disability and pregnancy: risks for maternal morbidity and mortality. *J Womens Health*. 2021;30(2):147–153. doi:10.1089/jwh.2020.8864.

12. Center for Reproductive Rights. *Black Mamas Matter: Advancing the Human Right to Safe and Respectful Maternal Health Care*. Center for Reproductive Rights; 2018. http://blackmamasmatter.org/wp-content/uploads/2018/05/USPA_BMMA_Toolkit_Booklet-Final-Update_Web-Pages-1.pdf. Accessed August 5, 2019.

13. SisterSong, National Latina Institute for Reproductive Justice, Center for Reproductive Rights. *Reproductive Injustice: Racial and Gender Discrimination in U.S. Health Care*. Center for Reproductive Rights; 2014. https://reproductiverights.org/reproductive-injustice-racial-and-gender-discrimination-in-u-s-health-care/.

14. Crear-Perry J, Correa-de-Araujo R, Lewis Johnson T, McLemore MR, Neilson E, Wallace M. Social and structural determinants of health inequities in maternal health. *J Womens Health*. 2021;30(2):230–235. doi:10.1089/jwh.2020.8882.

15. Department of Public Health Maternal Mortality Review Committee. *Maternal Mortality Report 2014*. Department of Public Health; 2019. https://dph.georgia.gov/document/publication/maternal-mortality-2014-case-review/download. Accessed May 3, 2021.

16. Miller A. The ripple effect when rural hospitals drop birthing services. *Georgia Health News*. http://www.georgiahealthnews.com/2021/12/rural-hospitals-drop-birthing-services/. Published December 20, 2021. Accessed January 3, 2022.

17. Hasson F, Keeney S, McKenna H. Research guidelines for the Delphi survey technique. *J Adv Nurs*. 2000;32(4):1008–1015.

18. Miles MB, Huberman AM, Saldaña J. *Qualitative Data Analysis: A Methods Sourcebook*. 3rd ed. Thousand Oaks: SAGE Publications; 2014.

19. Braveman P. What is health equity: and how does a life-course approach take us further toward it? *Matern Child Health J.* 2014;18(2):366–372. doi:10.1007/s10995-013-1226-9.

20. American Academy of Family Physicians, American Academy of Pediatrics, American College of Obstetricians and Gynecologists, American College of Physicians, American Osteopathic Association, American Psychiatric Association. Helping ensure healthy mothers and healthy babies: eliminating preventable maternal mortality and morbidity. 2019. http://www.groupof6.org/dam/AAFP/documents/advocacy/prevention/women/ST-G6-MaternalMortality-091619.pdf. Accessed January 3, 2022.

21. Eliason EL. Adoption of Medicaid expansion is associated with lower maternal mortality. *Womens Health Issues.* 2020;30(3):147–152. doi:10.1016/j.whi.2020.01.005.

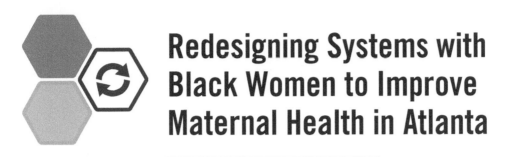

Chapter 20

Redesigning Systems with Black Women to Improve Maternal Health in Atlanta

JEMEA DORSEY AND KAPRICE WELSH

A PERVASIVE HEALTH CRISIS

In 2010, Amnesty International published a groundbreaking 154-page report, "Deadly Delivery: The Maternal Health Care Crisis in the USA." The report highlighted the human cost of systemic failures and the steps that were "urgently needed to move toward a healthcare system that respects, protects, and fulfills the human right to health without discrimination."[1]

Over 12 years later, we continue to grapple with this issue. The pregnancy-related mortality rate in the United States exceeds that of other developed nations and is marked by significant disparities in outcomes by race. Despite recent medical advances in obstetric care, the risks associated with pregnancy have not declined—and for Black women the risks have worsened. Black women continue to die at two to four times the rate of white women, experience health inequities, and face discrimination and disrespectful care in birthing facilities across the nation. Evidence from maternal mortality review committees suggests that delays in diagnosis, delays in initiation of treatment, and use of ineffective treatments contribute to preventable cases of maternal death.

In 2019, in the Giving Voice to Mothers Study, researchers concluded that mistreatment was experienced more frequently by women of color, when birth occurred in a hospital, and among those with social, economic, or health challenges. Mistreatment was exacerbated by unexpected obstetric interventions as well as by patient–provider disagreements.[2] Since 2013, the Council on Patient Safety in Women's Health Care and the Alliance for Innovation on Maternal Health (AIM) have developed patient safety bundles that target maternal health (including maternal venous thromboembolism, obstetric hemorrhage, and

Jemea Dorsey and Kaprice Welsh, *Redesigning Systems with Black Women to Improve Maternal Health in Atlanta* In: *The Practical Playbook III*. Edited by: Dorothy Cilenti, Alisahah Jackson, Natalie D. Hernandez, Lindsey Yates, Sarah Verbiest, J. Lloyd Michener, and Brian C. Castrucci, Oxford University Press. © de Beaumont Foundation 2024. DOI: 10.1093/oso/9780197662984.003.0020

severe hypertension in pregnancy), postpartum care basics for maternal safety, and safe reduction of primary cesarean delivery.[3] These care bundles, collections of best practices based on robust evidence when properly implemented across all care settings, have been shown to improve outcomes overall and to reduce racial and ethnic disparities.[4]

In recent years, many local and national organizations have dedicated time and money to reducing the rates of maternal mortality and morbidity. What we now understand from their efforts is that there is no single solution to the problem, and it will require multiple interventions at all levels if we want to achieve better outcomes.

A COMMUNITY APPROACH

While there have been many approaches to addressing the maternal health crisis in the United States, few of them have incorporated, or been designed with, communities, nor have they centered the unique needs and voices of Black women. In 2019, Joia Crear-Perry, founder and president of the National Birth Equity Collaborative and a member of the board of the Black Mamas Matter Alliance, made an introduction between the Institute for Healthcare Improvement (IHI) and the Center for Black Women's Wellness (CBWW). IHI had begun a three-year, multicity quality-improvement project, Better Maternal Outcomes: Redesigning Systems with Black Women, supported by a grant from Merck for Mothers. The Better Maternal Outcomes project was created to facilitate locally driven, codesigned, rapid improvements in four cities—Atlanta, Detroit, New Orleans, and Washington, DC. The initiative aimed to improve equity, dignity, and safety while reducing racial inequities in outcomes for Black birthing people. Specifically, the project was tasked with engaging and supporting a strengthened collaboration between the healthcare delivery system, community organizations, and workers, and centering the experience of Black birthing people in redesigning the system of care during the prenatal, birth, and postpartum periods. IHI was seeking a lead agency to anchor the work in Atlanta.

While much of IHI's work focuses on driving change within healthcare systems, CBWW offered a unique voice as a Black-led, community-based organization with a long history in maternal and child health programming. Housed in a busy multipurpose community center southwest of downtown Atlanta, CBWW was adept at working with predominantly Black, low-to-moderate-income communities to design, implement, and evaluate interventions for their diverse needs. Throughout its more than 30-year history, CBWW has placed community engagement at the center of its programming: A highly visible and engaged outreach department uses mechanisms like focus groups and surveys to collect community feedback, and the center builds community leadership groups to ensure that those most affected by a community problem are at the table to help identify solutions.

CBWW is a long-time grantee of Healthy Start, the signature federal program focused on improving birth outcomes in communities with infant mortality rates that are at least one and a half times the US national average. Through this program, CBWW's Atlanta Healthy Start Initiative provides home-based case management services to pregnant and postpartum women until infants reach 18 months, and it executes activities focused on improving family and community wellness (among them, promoting women's health, mental health linkages, and a fatherhood program). The initiative serves approximately 700 mothers, fathers, and infants each year. In addition, Healthy Start projects form and sustain a Community Action Network, a cross-section of agencies and community residents who work collaboratively to strengthen the system of care for women and families and to enact community-level change. Partners are diverse, with individuals and agencies representing local and state government entities, early childhood centers, hospitals, community-based agencies, universities, healthcare centers, workforce development agencies, and health systems. CBWW relied on these existing partnerships for the Better Maternal Outcomes project, inviting several of the partners, along with others, to participate.

The Process

Atlanta's Better Maternal Outcomes project ran from 2019 to 2021 and used an Equity Action Lab model to guide the work. An Equity Action Lab is a flexible model that uses the Community of Solutions Framework to guide participants through a structured set of activities in an equitable codesign process to set a health equity goal that is important to the participants.[5] Over 30 individuals took part in the one-and-a-half-day action lab; one-quarter of the participants were women with lived experience (current or former pregnant and postpartum Healthy Start participants with recent interaction with the healthcare system). Other participants represented healthcare systems, direct-service community-based organizations, advocacy groups, universities, healthcare insurance payers, local foundations, and birth workers (doulas and family support specialists, for example).

The Equity Action Lab agenda was developed by IHI, CBWW, and a small group of partners comprising a leadership team. The action lab included presentations and panel discussions with subject matter experts to ground the work, provided historical context, centered themes of racism and its impact on maternal health outcomes, and defined terminology. Women with lived experience shared stories of interfacing with the healthcare system, perceived lack of respectful care, challenges navigating the system, and resources and services they felt had been supportive. Attendees did journey mapping and were guided through a set of activities to identify and prioritize work for the group to do collectively to address improved maternal health. Participants praised the action lab and commented about the best aspects of the process: "seeing that medical professionals care about the work as well," "highlighting real women's stories," and "connecting with others."

The action lab resulted in the formation of three design teams to focus on key areas of maternal health: respectful care, shared leadership, and supporting women across silos. Attendees selected their group of interest, helped draft an aim statement for their team, identified change ideas, wrote a charter, and selected team leadership. Dr. Nikkia Worrell, a quality specialist in a major safety-net hospital system, served as design team co-lead for the Supporting Women Across Silos team and led development of the driver diagram that centered the entire group's work and collaboration around a common aim (see Figure 20.1).

CBWW relied on its strength as a partner convener and as a conduit for amplifying the voices of Black women. However, recognizing that quality-improvement work involved rapid tests of change, frequent touchpoints, and strong communications mechanisms, CBWW chose to hire a consultant to provide project management support, facilitate communications with the three design teams, and oversee reporting to IHI. Design team leaders convened meetings with their teams, led tests of change ideas, and reported on progress during routine meetings with IHI. Importantly, IHI provided substantial coaching and support throughout the process. Two "momentum" labs were

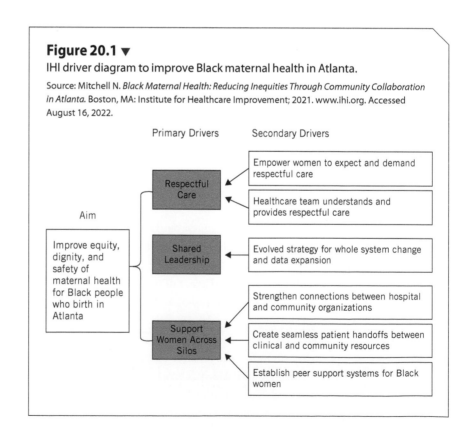

Figure 20.1 ▼

IHI driver diagram to improve Black maternal health in Atlanta.

Source: Mitchell N. *Black Maternal Health: Reducing Inequities Through Community Collaboration in Atlanta.* Boston, MA: Institute for Healthcare Improvement; 2021. www.ihi.org. Accessed August 16, 2022.

held, one at the six-month and one at the 12-month mark of the project, to share work of the design teams and plans for further action. A culminating lab served as a final debriefing and celebration.

Codesigning and Testing Ideas

Over the first year, the three design teams convened to test strategies using the Plan-Do-Study-Act (PDSA) cycle. This rapid process of testing change ideas— planning an idea, trying it, observing the results, and acting on it—helped move the work along, as teams were able to implement what they learned to make improvements. Each design team completed between three and five PDSA cycles over the 18-month project. Below are descriptions of how each team approached the process.

Respectful Care

The Respectful Care team sought to identify a definition of respectful care that encompassed all ideas they considered important. They reviewed various definitions, including definitions from the White Ribbon Alliance, the New York City Department of Health, and other national organizations, and concluded that development of their definition needed to be centered on the experiences of Black women and birthing people in Georgia. The team created and tested a survey, ultimately learning from over 40 pregnant and postpartum women about their birthing experience over the course of several months and gathering comments (two of which are below), as survey respondents defined what made care respectful or not.

> I think I should have been asked if my water could be broken instead of told that it was going to happen. Yes, that was the plan, but I felt like we should have talked about it. I would have liked to have had a conversation after the [cesarean] section about what all happened before, during, and after, because I don't remember why some things happened and it's not in my medical record.
>
> *— Survey respondent*

> My doctor made me feel empowered by letting me know that certain procedures were my choice. She did a great job of going into detail and explaining things when I didn't necessarily understand. She did all of this from the very beginning, so it made it easier to speak with her and express my concerns from that point.
>
> *— Survey respondent*

Feedback from respondents about experiences with their doctors and midwives became the backdrop not only for the Respectful Care team's definition but also the testing of other ideas, such as a respectful care simulation experience, modeled after the poverty simulation[6] experience and designed to increase providers' awareness about racism and bias and their impact on patients' experience and outcomes. The team shared its surveys with the other two design teams to inform their PDSA cycles.

Supporting Women across Silos

This team focused on improving connections among community-based organizations, social-support opportunities, and clinical services, as well as the connections between these services and patients. The unique makeup of its leadership helped drive Supporting Women Across Silos to begin testing ideas early on. The group leaders were a physician who directs quality improvement in a key hospital system in Atlanta and a woman with lived experience as a mother of eight and a strong advocate in her community and the school system. The physician's deep experience with quality-improvement work and PDSA cycles helped the team focus on key strategies, test them, and use lessons learned to formulate their work. The other leader's familiarity with community resources and experience with the hospital system made the team dynamic. Ideas tested included a referral system between community-based programs and Grady Health System (a safety-net hospital system) and working with a payer to increase patients' knowledge of available resources. As a result of these cycles, Grady Health System and CBWW re-established a formal agreement to facilitate referrals and information-sharing.

Shared Leadership

The Shared Leadership team focused its efforts on engaging healthcare delivery system leaders in deeper conversation, education, and action regarding the effects of racism on Black maternal health. They conducted two test cycles to determine the best messaging for a communication piece for hospital leadership. The team drafted a cover letter and one-page infographic and obtained feedback from approximately 10 leaders, including physicians, hospital leaders, and Medicaid payers, to learn which information, data, and messaging was most compelling, as well as potential calls for action. Based on that feedback, Shared Leadership redesigned and retested the infographic. This team relied on additional sources to develop their materials, including public health graduate students. Consensus was developed that the call to action for hospital leadership was to implement AIM's Reduction of Peripartum Racial/Ethnic Disparities bundle with fidelity. The team concluded that a future action for leaders was to support their staff to participate in the respectful care simulator experience being tested by the Respectful Care team.

The Shared Leadership team included several local funders, which generated ongoing discussions about how to sustain the committee's work. Ideas included identifying potential anchor organizations, such as Morehouse School of Medicine's Center for Maternal Health Equity, to support the work of the design team after the duration of the project.

Rapid Cycles Amid a Rapidly Changing World

While some partners involved in this highly collaborative effort had experience with quality improvement and rapid tests of change using PDSA cycles, most did not. IHI committed staff and resources to support the effort in a commitment to build quality-improvement capability for each of the cities involved in this Merck for Mothers initiative. Not all partners were intensively engaged in the design team work, whose rapid cycles necessitated frequent touchpoints. Design teams initially met every two weeks, then reduced meetings to once per month. Partners unable to participate in the design teams were invited to the momentum labs—convenings held approximately every six months—to keep abreast of the teams' progress and key lessons.

Some design teams modified leadership or membership because of job changes, changes in individuals' capacity, and differences among the group about how the work should be executed. This resulted in some teams' identifying new leadership or individuals stepping up to take on unofficial co-leads to help keep the work moving forward. Navigating stakeholder relationships was a critical dynamic of this process, delicately facilitated by the project management consultant who worked with each design team and staff at CBWW.

COVID-19 affected the speed at which cycles occurred, brought disruptions and delays in the way some ideas were tested, and suspended all in-person labs and design team meetings. In recognition of the stress the pandemic was causing to individuals, organizations, and systems, the IHI team gave space for the groups to process emotions, slow the pace, and recalibrate; the project's timeline was adjusted and moved out a few months. Celebration was an important component of this project, including a final lab to share what had been learned and to acknowledge representatives from the other three peer cities. These appreciations were critical, and likely more impactful given the unique circumstances of an unprecedented pandemic.

LESSONS LEARNED

Lessons from this quality-improvement project have implications for people committed to advancing health equity in maternal health.

Redesign Systems with Those Most Affected by the System

For the quality-improvement project directed at Black maternal health outcomes, it was crucial to amplify the voices of Black women. CBWW spent time during the planning phase communicating about the initiative to women served by the organization, encouraging participation in the Equity Action Lab and design team work, and alleviating barriers to participation (transportation and child care among them). Women with lived experiences were encouraged to take on leadership roles with the design teams, and one volunteered to serve as a team co-lead. Creating space for all to share their experiences and perspectives was important. This included Black women representing agencies and health-care systems who shared their own experiences as college-educated women experiencing disrespectful care. Seeing these commonalities, including among Black female physicians who were negatively affected by the system they are part of, was illuminating and built connection.

Build and Strengthen Collaborations

The project started with a base of strong partners and expanded from there. Inviting established partners who already were involved with CBWW's Atlanta Healthy Start Community Action Network ensured an established trust and commitment to driving change and achieving collective impact to improve health outcomes. The partner group grew to include other necessary voices, such as advocates, policymakers, health systems, and funders. The necessity of valuing and creating opportunities for shared leadership and of embracing varied degrees of engagement in the process became clear.

Create a Shared Impactful Experience

The Equity Action Lab was an essential first step to ground the work, create a shared experience, center the voices of Black women with lived experience, and build buy-in and commitment from a large group of partners. This day-and-a-half intensive gathering was a necessary starting point and introduction to quality-improvement work.

Sustain the Work

Support from Merck for Mothers and resources and technical assistance support from IHI built quality-improvement capacity among organizations. From the beginning, CBWW knew it was important to include local funders in the effort to increase awareness of Black maternal health in Atlanta and to codesign strategies for improvement. CBWW invited a handful of local funders to kick off the Equity Action Lab, and all invited funders remained involved in the work, some of them serving on a design team and even providing leadership.

THE FUTURE

Improving Black maternal health continues to be a priority for CBWW and the partners involved in Better Maternal Outcomes: Redesigning Systems with Black Women. Because CBWW's quality-improvement capacity increased through this process, in 2020 the group was invited to work with the National Healthy Start Association as part of its five-year cooperative agreement with the US Department of Health and Human Services for AIM's Community

Care Initiative (AIM CCI). As the lead agency in Atlanta, CBWW is focused on convening partners to pilot postpartum safety bundles in community-based and outpatient clinical settings using an equity framework. CBWW uses evidence-based patient-safety and quality-improvement resources and data collection to track outcomes. Examples of bundle elements include providing education on postpartum warning signs that are culturally responsive and utilize core principles of holistic and respectful maternity care, and screening for, and responding to, common medical and behavioral health morbidities and social determinants of health, such as exposure to violence, unstable housing, and food insecurity. Several of the partners involved in the Better Maternal Outcomes project continued to pilot postpartum safety bundles through AIM CCI, solidifying a strong base of partners committed to a coordinated, collaborative, and equitable approach to fully meeting the postpartum needs of Black women.

Several local foundations that were a part of the Better Maternal Outcomes project now have funding initiatives focused on maternal and child health, including Healthcare Georgia Foundation and United Way of Greater Atlanta. Their participation in this quality-improvement process illuminated the barriers systems imposed on Black women and forged unique relationships with an array of providers, payors, community workers, and women with lived experience, providing important context and resulting in a deepened commitment to centering equity and the voices of Black women in future funding initiatives.

The Respectful Care team's big idea of a simulation experience gained significant traction, and a small group of partners continues to implement and fine-tune this hands-on education, which has reached providers as well as public health, nursing, and medical students in Georgia and other states.

Since the project concluded, multiple other maternal health initiatives have begun as increased attention to the Black maternal health crisis continues. The capacity of partner organizations and the trust built through this intensive collaborative process have accelerated momentum and motivated participation. Overall, Atlanta partners are in a unique position to coordinate efforts and embed an equity framework in all they do to eradicate inequities in Black maternal health.

REFERENCES

1. Amnesty International. Deadly delivery: the maternal health care crisis in the USA. https://www.amnesty.org/en/documents/amr51/007/2010/en/. Published August 10, 2021.

2. Vedam S, Stoll K, Taiwo TK, et al. The Giving Voice to Mothers study: inequity and mistreatment during pregnancy and childbirth in the United States. *Reprod Health*. 2019;16:77. https://doi.org/10.1186/s12978-019-0729-2.

3. Eppes CS, Han SB, Haddock AJ, Buckler AG, Davidson CM, Hollier LM. Enhancing obstetric safety through best practices. *J Womens Health*. 2021;30(2):265–269. Published online February 2, 2021. doi:10.1089/jwh.2020.8878.

4. Main EK, Chang S-C, Dhurjati R, Cape V, Profit J, Gould JB. Reduction in racial disparities in severe maternal morbidity from hemorrhage in a large-scale quality improvement collaborative. *Am J Obstet Gynecol.* 2020;223:123.e1–123.e14.

5. Mitchell N. *Black Maternal Health: Reducing Inequities Through Community Collaboration in Atlanta.* Boston, MA: Institute for Healthcare Improvement; 2021. www.ihi.org. Accessed August 16, 2022.

6. Why a Simulation? The Poverty Simulation. Missouri Community Action Network, Jefferson City. https://www.povertysimulation.net/about/. Accessed August 23, 2022.

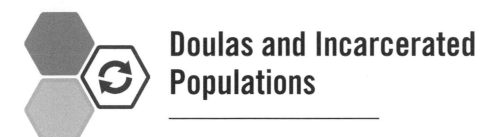

Chapter 21

Doulas and Incarcerated Populations

CRYSTAL HAYES AND MARISA PIZII

INTRODUCTION

Shortly after Prison Birth Project member Larissa (not her real name) gave birth to her son, a white woman said to her, "Your baby is so cute, I just want to take him and hide him under my coat and sneak him out. And my husband is Black so the baby will fit right in." She meant this as a compliment, but Larissa was incarcerated, and her baby was about to be taken away from her while she went back to prison. What is most disturbing about this comment is that there was so much unconscious racism both in the comment that the baby would "fit right in" and in the reality that Black[†] mothers are far more likely to lose babies to the state, and those babies are often given to white families to raise. Larissa's doula was there and heard the comment. She supported Larissa, validating Larissa's feelings about the hurtful comment.[1]

The authors of this chapter are two prison-based doulas and childbirth educators. We are Black women affected by the carceral system whose lived experiences provide a unique context for analyzing and addressing conscious and unconscious racism in correctional institutions and the broader carceral system. One author's father was in prison for 45 years and her mother was incarcerated when she was a toddler. The other author has a close family member who was incarcerated on and off for several years as they struggled with substance and alcohol

---

† In the tradition of the Black press and scholars like W.E.B. Du Bois, who argued that Black always be capitalized as a form of respect when talking about the Black experience,[27] we choose to also capitalize Women of Color. We do so as a sign of respect and to center their humanity in a world dominated by racism and gender-based violence. In this chapter we also capitalize Indigenous, Women of Color, and People of Color (and not white when referring to white people or white communities) to not only pay People of Color respect, but also to politically call attention to the use of power that is embedded in language. Capitalizing Black and not white helps to signal the ongoing need to demarginalize Blackness and decenter whiteness in the face of enduring white supremacy and racial inequality.

Crystal Hayes and Marisa Pizii, *Doulas and Incarcerated Populations* In: *The Practical Playbook III*. Edited by: Dorothy Cilenti, Alisahah Jackson, Natalie D. Hernandez, Lindsey Yates, Sarah Verbiest, J. Lloyd Michener, and Brian C. Castrucci, Oxford University Press. © de Beaumont Foundation 2024. DOI: 10.1093/oso/9780197662984.003.0021

use disorder while battling poor access to mental health services. We write this chapter to add our voices to the work being done to promote reproductive justice as a strategy to help dismantle white supremacy and mass incarceration and their impact on racial inequities in maternal health. The chapter is written to share some of the challenges, complexities, and inherent liberatory possibilities that doula providers can offer when they hold a reproductive justice framework at the center of their work. This is particularly true for doula providers in carceral environments (e.g., prisons, jails, detention centers, and the child welfare and foster care system).

This chapter also aims to highlight reproductive justice as a powerful analytical and organizing tool. This framework is an alternative to prison reform work that does not sufficiently address issues of systemic oppression. Ultimately, the chapter is an opportunity to talk about how to use the reproductive justice framework as a strategy to move the dialogue away from debates about prison reform. As reproductive justice advocates and doulas, we believe that this framework forces us to examine the culture (white supremacy) and systems (e.g., police brutality, tough-on-crime laws, family surveillance and separation policies, etc.) that allow mass incarceration to exist where reproductive oppression is the norm, and not the exception.

HISTORY OF THE CREATION OF REPRODUCTIVE JUSTICE

Reproductive justice is a human rights, feminist, and intersectional theoretical paradigm that compels us to dismantle all forms of abuse and abuses of power that violate our human right to control our own families and sexual bodies.[2] Reproductive justice is a radical analysis of institutionalized inequality and oppression. The term was first coined and defined in July 1994 by a group of 12 Black women who called themselves the Women of African Descent for Reproductive Justice (WADRJ).[3] In 1994, WADRJ gathered in a hotel room in Chicago, Illinois, after attending the Clinton Administration's presentation of their proposed healthcare plan. The Clinton healthcare plan excluded any mention of the need for reproductive and sexual health. For example, the plan de-emphasized the need for screenings for sexually transmitted infections or diseases, treatment of fibroids, or even pregnancy care. Immediately realizing that the Clinton healthcare plan was racist and set to severely restrict bodily autonomy, violate a woman's reproductive rights and choices, and endanger women's sexual health, WADRJ took out a full-page ad in the *Washington Post* denouncing it. In their ad, WADRJ also demanded that there be a new plan put in place that would provide access to all needed sexual and reproductive care, no matter the region of the country or the ability to pay, including abortion healthcare, comprehensive pregnancy and postpartum services and care, comprehensive sexual education, and screenings for sexually transmitted infections and diseases, among others.

The WADRJ also offered a racial and gender analysis and critique of white supremacy that is the basis of the reproductive justice framework and the root cause of reproductive oppression. This framework centers the lives of Black and Brown women, underscoring that the history of anti-Black racism and white supremacy are embedded in reproductive decision-making and bodily autonomy.[4] This history is reflected in the three core tenets of reproductive justice, which include: "(1) the right to have a child under the conditions of one's choosing; (2) the right not to have a child using birth control, abortion, or abstinence; and (3) the right to parent children in safe and healthy environments free from violence by individuals or the state."[2]

The 12 Black women who pioneered reproductive justice organized the three core principles of reproductive justice to counter the untrue assumption that all women, no matter their race and socioeconomic status, have access to the resources that they need to make healthy reproductive choices for themselves and their families. Reproductive justice not only decenters whiteness but also separates reproductive rights from being solely focused on fertility and termination of pregnancy. The framework sheds light on the racial and social justice contexts that shape bodily autonomy and the options to determine our own destinies. As reproductive justice continued to evolve, a fourth principle was added in recognition of the needs of queer and nonbinary people. This principle specifically sought to include bodily autonomy, sexuality, and sexual health to be free from all forms of reproduction and reproductive oppression.

As reproductive justice scholars and advocates whose work focuses on addressing carceral systems, the incarceration of pregnant and parenting people and anyone assigned female at birth (AFABS) who can become pregnant creates alarming concerns for their reproductive health. This is particularly important because, once arrested and incarcerated, people have limited autonomy and independence to make health decisions for themselves. As a result, some scholars are beginning to recognize that mass incarceration is a major driver of reproductive oppression, with major health implications for Black women and other Women of Color (WOC), who are disproportionately incarcerated when compared to their white counterparts.[5,6]

REPRODUCTIVE JUSTICE AND PRISON MATERNAL HEALTHCARE FOR INCARCERATED PREGNANT WOMEN

Although it is not always realized, incarcerated people are the only group who have a constitutionally protected right to healthcare. The two landmark cases that protect their right to healthcare are *Estelle v Gamble* and *Brown v. Plata*. Despite the *Estelle v Gamble* decision that guarantees healthcare for incarcerated people,[7] prisons are not mandated to follow basic healthcare standards. Consequently, healthcare, including reproductive healthcare, is inconsistent and often inadequate to meet the needs of incarcerated pregnant women.[8] The lack of accountability in prison healthcare not only violates incarcerated pregnant women's constitutionally protected right to healthcare but also leaves them particularly vulnerable to decisions that are not always in the best interests of their health.[9,10]

Incarcerated pregnant women are often dangerously shackled to beds, are forced to labor alone, and have their newborn infants stripped from them less than 24 hours after birth.[8,10,11] As women's incarceration rates continue to climb,[12] so should the concern for women's reproductive health. This is especially true given that 4% of women are pregnant at the time of their arrest.[13] This is crucial for Black women, who not only have higher rates of incarceration than white women[14,15] but are also more vulnerable, given their high rates of maternal and infant mortality[16] and the history of racialized reproductive oppression.[17]

Pregnant women in the US carceral system and their reproductive healthcare needs remain largely invisible to the world,[18] while Black women's over-incarceration is treated mainly as an afterthought, usually deemed relevant only in discussions of incarcerated Black men.[19] However, given Black women's historic experience of systemic brutality and exploitation, few institutional protections and supports, and their vulnerability to reproductive oppression, it is urgent that research illuminate their unique stories in the carceral system. This is critical when most incarcerated women are imprisoned during critical reproductive health years; moreover, many have high-risk pregnancies due to poor health and poverty prior to incarceration.[8,10,20,21] Thus, barriers to basic reproductive care can have major implications for incarcerated women's health and open them up to practices with long-term health implications (such as forced sterilization).[8,22–25]

The ability to freely make decisions about their own lives and pregnant bodies, and the lives of their children—as core reproductive values—has been stolen by the carceral system. As Black women, doulas, and childbirth educators who work in carceral spaces, the authors are committed to telling the stories of incarcerated women and shifting the discourse around reproductive politics to center questions about power and privilege at the intersections of race and pregnancy. The following is an excerpt from an autoethnographic discussion and interview between the two authors about their experiences, and some of the challenges that they faced as Black doulas working toward reproductive justice within a women's facility.

Crystal: You worked for a long time with the Prison Birth Project (PBP), but I am curious—how was PBP born?

Marissa: That's a really interesting story. The three co-founders met at the conference that's hosted by my current organization, formerly known as the Civil Liberties and Public Policy Collective Power for Reproductive Justice. They were really inspired by the electric energy of Tina Reynolds, who is a formerly incarcerated Black woman doing organizing work in New York. She came to the conference to speak, and they were energized and felt like we needed to do something here in Massachusetts because they had all just been or some of them had been somehow involved with the protest against the building of the women's jail in Chicopee, Massachusetts. It was clear that that protest was not going to disrupt the plans and the building was moving forward and actually opened. It then became very clear to the three people who had just witnessed Tina Reynolds that something had to be done to ensure that pregnant women would be provided with the care that they needed.

Crystal: Okay, so when I came along during my PhD program, we met a lot about how to advance the organization's reproductive justice lens. Can you talk about how it came to be that you all wanted to include an RJ lens in PBP?

Marissa: Communication was clear very early that there needed to be something to support people with a more reproductive justice–based liberatory lens.

Crystal: Why is that—because was the term [reproductive justice] even popularized during that time the way it is now?

Marissa: Yes, true. Now it's really funny to say reproductive justice–based in the sense that RJ was something that was still moving into the lexicon. The awareness of RJ and the understanding for many people at that point where RJ was picking up a lot of steam [are] not really clear to me. The conflict around not being able to stop the jail from being built pushed people to come up with something that could be used to reduce as much harm as possible, and we all believed RJ was it. Also, all three of the founders were either formerly incarcerated themselves or had immediate family members who had been incarcerated and were continuing to have struggles with the carceral system. So they knew and they felt the impact on themselves, and they also saw the impact that the system had on human bodies and that it doesn't actually create rehabilitation and readjustment and course correcting, it just creates further harm and trauma. And so they made the decision to reach out to the jail and suggested that that the jail provide some kind of programming for pregnant folk, and the jail was like, "What do you all want to offer to us? It's just a program." And so that's where the Prison Birth Project began.

Crystal: Does it surprise you that the jail was open to suggestions about what kind of programming to offer women?

Marissa: To be honest, we fit right into their plan. They were operating from this idea that they were building a gender-specific jail to solve the problem of what incarcerated women face when they are locked up in jails designed for men. They saw the idea of building a gender-specific jail as a liberatory step in prison reform work, so they were okay with inviting us to think about next steps. You know, their ideas were rooted in carceral feminism, right? It was a liberatory step to somehow make women more liberated in a cage. [Pause] I'm not quite sure how they arrived at that.

Crystal: So, they believed that [in] building this jail for women they were protecting and supporting women?

Marissa: [Sigh] Yup. That's exactly what they believed. And in some ways, they were right. Before this women's jail, they housed women in the same jail as men. They just had a gender-specific floor for women. So they saw this work to open up this new jail as a way to enhance services for women but also just to get them out of a facility where men were being incarcerated. We need to hold that thought for one second.

Crystal: *Yeah, that's a lot to hold right now. Yeah. I have lots of thoughts right now. Okay, so what was it like for you? What did you do?*

Marissa: *My work always centered around being the codirector of programs for the PBP. Directing means a lot of things, right? I was codirector, meaning it was really just me and two other folk that were responsible for moving things forward in the organization from every aspect that an organization needs in order to be successful and thrive. So I did fundraising. Any kind of internal affairs, HR work, as well as all of the public and external programming. I was responsible for a multitude of those things throughout the years. But the most important pieces of my work that were externally based were around the programs that we ran within the jail. We ran programs for about 10 years, but we started out there running the doula-based program where we came in and we supported pregnant women with doulas.*

Crystal: *When I arrived at PBP, you all had several programs by that time.*

Marissa: *Yes. The jail hadn't really thought about any of this stuff before we engaged them, so we were happy to get a doula program up and running. We then asked the people behind the wall what was in their best interest for us to continue. What are ways we could grow programming and grow impact of support behind the wall for them? And they said, well, we're moms and we would like a group for moms, and so that's where "Mothers Among Us" came from. We eventually, as you know, also started a breastfeeding program in the jail, too. So, we had the doula program, childbirth educator class, and Mothers Among Us.*

Crystal: *Did you feel like RJ was rooted in the programs, and, if so, how?*

Marissa: *It was hard. I'd say yes and no. We didn't have any control, right? Like the Mothers Among Us program was completely controlled by the jail. They decided who could attend and for how long. They only allowed women to attend who had elementary school-age children. If you were a grandmother, mother of older children, or mothered children in your family that you did not give birth to, you could not be involved. It was frustrating to us, because we wanted all of them, but [the jail's] rationale was that only people with younger children needed the parenting support. It's ridiculous. You don't stop being a parent, even if your role changes. The jail had complete control over who they would even identify as a mother. It definitely caused some trauma for all of us.*

Crystal: *This reminds me that prison-based doula work is all about timing, too. You all appeared at the right time, with the right administration in place, and the right agenda. Would you agree?*

Marissa: *Oh, absolutely. We slid in right on time. We had the right administrator, who I believe had a doula work with their own family at one point, so they knew the benefits of it. We were lucky in that way.*

Crystal: *Which leads me the next question about how you operate from within a reproductive justice lens in a women's jail. It seems to me that your philosophies would be in constant conflict. How did you reconcile it? Did it matter? Were you okay with the cognitive dissonance? We used to talk about this, actually, when we were together at PBP.*

Marissa: *I never did. I mean, I never felt like it was reconciled or resolved. I knew that we were there only by their grace. We had an administration at the jail that was brand new. They didn't have anything, so we pioneered the reproductive health stuff at the jail, and it was huge to bear witness to women in that position knowing life would be even harder at the jail without our programs. For a long time, that helped me not feel like I was in complete conflict with my own values by being in the jail.*

Crystal: *Right, because I am often feeling like I am even betraying my own father and mother, who were both incarcerated—my dad for 45 years. I really think there's a fine line between intervening on behalf of incarcerated people and upholding the system's unjust policies and practices.*

Marissa: *Right, because now, because of the work we did, that jail is the "model" facility for the state! Now they look to that jail when building new jails, etc. So, how do we sit with that?*

Crystal: *Whew, what an RJ agenda. I mean, it's the fear that I have, too, with my work—designing RJ programs for prisons that will be used to help build more prisons, with the argument that they are better, when no one is better off simply locked up. Tell me how RJ was put to practice in the work.*

Marissa: *Hmmm. Well, our childbirth education program was a peer-to-peer program. We were not interested in certificates and professionalized programs. We felt like those programs were white-centered and rooted in racist ideas and beliefs. So, we didn't require people to have those certificates. We built our own curriculum in some ways with the women behind the wall. Sometimes it was hard trying to explain some of the language, etc. I think what was complicated by our work is the fact that in doing so, we were acting like peers, but we weren't peers. We got to leave the facility. We were not incarcerated, even though some of us were formerly incarcerated. It was a struggle to deal with that positioning piece.*

Crystal: *Yes, I struggle with that currently in my work with the local women's prison now. I still very much identify as that poor working-class Black girl from NYC with an incarcerated father. I have a lot of privilege now. I have my PhD. I am at a university. I have a lot of privileges. And I am also a Black woman, so I still very much feel targeted.*

FINAL THOUGHTS

The criminal legal system presents unique challenges for pregnant women once they become entangled in it. Larissa's experience that was narrated at the beginning of this chapter is not an uncommon experience or story for incarcerated Black women. There are lots of cases like hers where well-intentioned (and not so well-intentioned) people say and do harmful things aimed at incarcerated pregnant people. For Black women, these issues are linked to a long history of reproductive injustices and other forms of structural violence.[26] Incarcerated pregnant Black women deal with people's internalized anti-Black racist and classist sentiments about who is deserving of motherhood, and who is not, and all the general assumptions that people make about "prisoners."

Carceral institutions (e.g., prisons and jails) and policies are intrinsically dehumanizing and violent and undermine the core tenet of reproductive justice that says that every human being has the right to parent their own children. This basic core tenet of reproductive justice is violated every time a parent of dependent children is incarcerated. Nearly 80% of incarcerated women are mothers and the sole providers for dependent children. In other words, reproductive justice requires fresh new thinking and a willingness to dismantle a system that relies heavily on incarcerating people for crimes associated with having a history of abuse, addiction, and poverty. For instance, the majority of incarcerated women are survivors of untreated trauma and abuse during their prime reproductive years. Given this trauma history, many incarcerated women are at risk for adverse pregnancy-related outcomes. Therefore, applying a reproductive justice lens can help advocates push for a full range of comprehensive pregnancy and postpartum care and supports for incarcerated pregnant women that include opportunities for new mothers and infants to stay together. Reproductive justice provides the foundation for improving the overall quality of life for incarcerated pregnant people. Incarcerated pregnant people are frequently subject to daily indignities, such as being denied access to basic hygiene products (e.g., feminine napkins, breastfeeding pumps, maternity clothes, etc.), to the cruel and inhuman policy of having their newborns taken away from them within hours after delivery. Adhering to reproductive justice principles requires that we design a system that is both just and humane.[6]

REFERENCES

1. *The Prison Birth Project Legacy Report, 2008–2017*. Five College Compass—Digital Collections. 2018. https://compass.fivecolleges.edu/object/smith:85906. Accessed October 18, 2022.

2. Ross L, Solinger R. Reproductive justice. Oakland, CA: UC Press; 2017. https://www.ucpress.edu/book/9780520288201/reproductive-justice. Published online December 31, 2019.

3. Ross LJ. The Black scholar: a personal journey from women's rights to civil rights to human rights. doi:10.1080/00064246.2006.11413347. Published online 2017.

4. Ross LJ. The color of choice: white supremacy and reproductive justice In: INCITE! Women of Color against Violence, ed. *Color of Violence: The INCITE! Anthology*. Duke University Press; 2016:53–65.

5. Hayes C, Sufrin C, Perritt J. Where choice ends. *Inquest*. https://inquest.org/where-choice-ends/. Published October 5, 2021. Accessed October 14, 2021.

6. Hayes CM, Sufrin C, Perritt JB. Reproductive justice disrupted: mass incarceration as a driver of reproductive oppression. *Am J Public Health*. 2020;110(Suppl 1): S21–S24. doi:10.2105/AJPH.2019.305407.

7. *Estelle v Gamble*, 429 US 97 (1976). https://supreme.justia.com/cases/federal/us/429/97/. Accessed April 3, 2022.

8. Sufrin C. *Jailcare: Finding the Safety Net for Women Behind Bars*. Oakland, CA: University of California Press; 2017.

9. Ferszt GG, Clarke JG. Health care of pregnant women in U.S. state prisons. *J Health Care Poor Underserved*. 2012;23(2):557–569. doi:10.1353/hpu.2012.0048.

10. Hotelling BA. Perinatal needs of pregnant, incarcerated women. *J Perinat Educ*. 2008;17(2):37–44. doi:10.1624/105812408X298372.

11. Braithwaite RL, Treadwell HM, Arriola KRJ. Health disparities and incarcerated women: a population ignored. *Am J Public Health*. 2005;95(10):1679–1681. doi:10.2105/AJPH.2005.065375.

12. Equal Justice Initiative. Shackling of pregnant women in jails and prisons continues. 2020. https://eji.org/news/shackling-of-pregnant-women-in-jails-and-prisons-continues/. Accessed January 11, 2022.

13. Sufrin C, Beal L, Clarke J, Jones R, Mosher WD. Pregnancy outcomes in US prisons, 2016–2017. *Am J Public Health*. 2019;109(5):799–805. doi:10.2105/AJPH.2019.305006.

14. Crenshaw K. Black girls matter: pushed out, overpoliced and undeprotected. *Afr Am Policy Forum*. https://scholarship.law.columbia.edu/cgi/viewcontent.cgi?article=4236&context=faculty_scholarship. Published online 2014.

15. Maurer B. The Anthropology of Money. *Annual Review of Anthropology* 2014;35(2006):15–36. doi:10.1146/annurev.anthro.35.081705.123127

16. Centers for Disease Control and Prevention. Pregnancy Mortality Surveillance System. https://www.cdc.gov/reproductivehealth/maternal-mortality/pregnancy-mortality-surveillance-system.htm. Published 2015. Accessed May 3, 2017.

17. Silliman J, Fried MG, Ross L, Gutierrez E, Bader EJ. Undivided Rights: Women of Color organize for reproductive justice. 2016. http://www.jstor.org.ezproxy.lib.uconn.edu/stable/pdf/20838731.pdf. Accessed April 28, 2017.

18. Sawyer W. Visualizing the racial disparities in mass incarceration. *Prison Policy Initiative*. https://www.prisonpolicy.org/blog/2020/07/27/disparities/ Published online 2020. Accessed October 27, 2021.

19. Gross KN. African American women, mass incarceration, and the politics of protection. *J Am Hist*. 2015;102(1):25–33. doi:10.1093/JAHIST/JAV226.

20. Fogel CI. Pregnant inmates: risk factors and pregnancy outcomes. *J Obstet Gynecol Neonatal Nurs*. 1993;23(1):33–39. doi:10.1111/j.1552-6909.1993.tb01780.x. Published online 1993.

21. Kyei-Aboagye K, Vragnovic O, Chong D. Birth outcome in incarcerated, high-risk pregnant women. *J Reprod Med*. 2000;45(3):190–194. http://journals.lww.com/obgynsurvey/Abstract/2000/11000/Birth_Outcome_in_Incarcerated,_High_Risk_Pregnant.11.aspx. Published 2000. Accessed December 7, 2017.

22. Roth R, Ainsworth S. "If they hand you a paper, you sign it": a call to end the sterilization of women in prison. *Hastings Womens Law J*. 2015;26(1):5–45.

23. Roth R. No new babies—gender inequality and reproductive control in the criminal justice and prison systems. *Am U J Gender & Soc Pol'y & L*. 2004;12:391.

24. Roth R. Obstructing justice: prisons as barriers to medical care for pregnant women. *UCLA Womens Law J.* 2010;18(1):79–105. http://search.ebscohost.com/login.aspx?direct=true&db=a9h&AN=63698304&site=ehost-live&scope=site.

25. Roth R. Searching for the state: who governs prisoners' reproductive rights? *Soc Polit.* 2004;11(3):411–438. doi:10.1093/sp/jxh043.

26. Dyer L, Hardeman R, Vilda D, Theall K, Wallace M. Mass incarceration and public health: the association between Black jail incarceration and adverse birth outcomes among Black women in Louisiana. *BMC Pregnancy Childbirth.* 2019;19(1):1–10. doi:10.1186/S12884-019-2690-Z/TABLES/5.

27. Tharps LL. The Case for Black With a Capital B: Commentary. *New York Times.* Nov 19, 2014. https://www.nytimes.com/2014/11/19/opinion/the-case-for-black-with-a-capital-b.html. Accessed September 12, 2023.

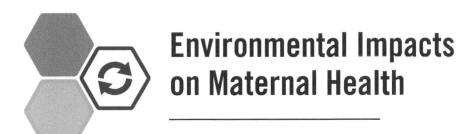

Chapter 22

Environmental Impacts on Maternal Health

MICHELE OKOH

This is America. We're not supposed to have these kinds of problems—at least, that's what we tell ourselves. But we do.
—Catherine Coleman Flowers

In recognition of growing scientific evidence demonstrating that environmental health exposures, both before and during pregnancy, can affect maternal health and the health of offspring throughout life, the American College of Obstetricians and Gynecologists (ACOG) has issued *Committee Opinion Number 832* (Opinion), which replaced *Committee Opinion Number 575* issued in October 2013. The American College of Nurse-Midwives has endorsed the Opinion. The Opinion acknowledges the significant role gynecologists and other obstetric healthcare clinicians play in addressing environmental impacts on maternal health.[1] According to ACOG, these practitioners "are uniquely positioned to educate patients about the effects of environmental exposure before and during pregnancy."[1] Therefore, maternal healthcare providers should be "knowledgeable about toxic environmental agents in relation to environmental health risk assessment, exposure reduction, and clinical counseling."[1] ACOG recommends that providers assess for, counsel about, and advocate regarding environmental impacts on maternal health.

This chapter aims to prepare providers to achieve this mission. First, the chapter introduces basic concepts related to understanding environmental impacts on maternal health. This coverage includes a foundational presentation of environmental health and environmental justice. Second, the chapter offers specific examples of environmental justice issues related to maternal health. This section discusses potential risk factors as though they are separate and distinct, but the examples do not promote the misconception that one risk

Michele Okoh, *Environmental Impacts on Maternal Health* In: *The Practical Playbook III*. Edited by: Dorothy Cilenti, Alisahah Jackson, Natalie D. Hernandez, Lindsey Yates, Sarah Verbiest, J. Lloyd Michener, and Brian C. Castrucci, Oxford University Press. © de Beaumont Foundation 2024. DOI: 10.1093/oso/9780197662984.003.0022

factor overshadows another. The purpose of the select population-based risk factors is the opposite. It underscores that pregnant women belong to different populations, and each carries the risk factors associated with all the populations combined. Providers need to understand the intersectionality underlying maternal health. Providers must not view pregnant women[†] on a single dimension. Physiological, socioeconomic, and environmental factors interact to produce synergistic effects that impact overall health. With that relationship comes an environment fraught with inequity. Pregnant women come from a diversity of races, cultures, and backgrounds, aspects that do not disappear simply because they are pregnant. Similarly, their womanhood does not erase their race, culture, and other aspects of their background. They are whole people, and providers must view them from this perspective. Third, this chapter suggests strategies for improving maternal environmental health. The strategies are mainly based on recommendations from ACOG, but they are meant to be more practical. The strategies primarily address assessment and counseling, but the knowledge gained from the previous sections should assist providers in advocating for policies that promote maternal environmental health. While it is impossible to educate providers on all aspects of the relationship between the environment and maternal health in a single chapter, this chapter should give providers a basic understanding of environmental impacts on maternal health and tools they can use to further maternal environmental health.

OVERVIEW OF ENVIRONMENTAL IMPACTS ON MATERNAL HEALTH

Understanding Environmental Health

The term *environment* means the world in which one lives. However, seeing the environment as separate from oneself creates a false dichotomy. People affect their environments, and their environments affect their health. *Environmental health* refers to a person's relationship to this environment. One's environment can both positively and negatively affect one's health. In other words, the environment can benefit and burden an individual's health. For example, greenness (exposure to vegetation) positively affects physical and mental health.[2] However, the environment also includes adverse exposures. The environment includes "exposure to pollution and chemicals (e.g., air, water, soil, products), physical exposures (e.g., noise, radiation), the built environment (e.g., housing,

---

[†] Throughout this chapter, the terms *mother* and *woman* are used. The usage of these terms should be understood to include pregnant persons and people who have given birth who do not identify as women. For further discussion on sexed language, *see* Gribble KD, Bewley S, Bartick MC, et al. Effective communication about pregnancy, birth, lactation, breastfeeding and newborn care: The importance of sexed language. *Front Global Womens Health.* 2022;3. doi:10.3389/fgwh.2022.818856.

land-use, infrastructure), other anthropogenic changes (e.g., climate change, vector breeding places), related behaviors, and the work environment."[3]

According to the World Health Organization (WHO), environmental factors account for approximately one-quarter of the global burden of disease: 23% of global deaths and 22% of global disability-adjusted life years (DALYs) were attributable to environmental risks.[3] However, this estimate underestimates the actual disease burden from environmental factors because it does not capture the full impact of lead and air pollution.[4] It also does not account for the effects of neurotoxicants, endocrine-disrupting chemicals, and climate change.[4] Factors in one's environment also interact with each other. Greenness can reduce exposure to air, noise, and heat pollution.[2] Due to the significant impact that environmental health has on overall health, environmental health should also be considered in addressing maternal health.

Getting to the Root of the Problem

Environmental exposures, both chemical and nonchemical, are not evenly distributed.[5] Social inequity drives disparities in maternal health. Black women especially have a higher rate of maternal morbidity and mortality. Nationally, the Black infant mortality rate is more than twice that of white infants (10.8 per 1,000 Black babies, compared with 4.6 per 1,000 white babies).[6]

The structural determinants of health are the underlying causes of these disparities. They include the policies, institutions, and cultural norms that create the conditions for the social determinants of health. The structural determinants of health are rooted in how power and resources are distributed across society. These structures stem from the racial, gender, and class systems originating with the creation of the United States and its economy.[7] Due to structural determinants, people of color live in vastly different social and physical environments than their white counterparts do.[5]

The same structures that bore social inequity also cause disparities in environmental health. Environmental health cannot be understood devoid of its social and institutional context. The environments people live in are inextricably linked to this context, and there is an interplay between environmental risk factors and the social determinants of health. The physiological and socioeconomic approaches, the two dominant approaches to understanding maternal health morbidity, mortality, and disparities, ignore the underlying cause.[7] Attempts to understand this inequity by focusing on individual behaviors and socioeconomics lead to a narrative of blaming the individual. In contrast, a focus on biological susceptibility leads to the misconception that race is a risk factor.[7] Neither of these is true. Providers consider how a pregnant woman's environment impacts maternal health. Therefore, addressing environmental health requires providers to understand how environmental justice affects maternal health.

Environmental Justice

At its core, environmental justice is about people and how their environments affect their health. However, environmental benefits and burdens are not equitably distributed in society. The effort to address these inequities is known as environmental justice. Dr. Robert D. Bullard, also known as the father of environmental justice, has described environmental justice as "nothing more than this whole principle: people have the right to a clean, healthy, sustainable environment without regard to race, color, or national origin. It's just that simple."[8] Whereas environmental health focuses on the environment's effect on people's health; environmental justice addresses the underlying societal structures leading to environmental inequity. Environmental justice seeks to remedy the underlying structural determinants of health that lead to health disparities.

Environmental Justice and Maternal Health

The physiological changes mediating fetal development, childbirth, and breastfeeding make pregnant people especially vulnerable to environmental exposures.[9] Most environmental chemicals on the market have not been evaluated for their effects on maternal health.[1] The body burden, concentrations of chemicals in the body, is higher in women of color due to differences in environmental exposures from housing, occupations, and consumer products.[5] Eurocentric beauty standards lead to the use and marketing to women of color of chemical products like hair relaxers and skin lighteners.[5] Discriminatory housing policies contribute to food apartheid and poor housing conditions.[5] People of color are more likely to live near sources of air and water pollution and are less likely to benefit from remediation of environmental contaminants.[5]

EXAMPLES OF MATERNAL ENVIRONMENTAL HEALTH CONCERNS

Both place-based and product-based exposures affect maternal health, before and during pregnancy. ACOG has emphasized, "Chemicals can be found in a wide range of consumer products, personal care products, food packaging, and household materials, as well as in air and water."[1] Providers should assess pregnant women for environmental exposures stemming from where they work, live, and engage in recreation.[1] However, a place-based approach, while imperative, is not sufficient to address environmental factors affecting maternal health. People can move from place to place. Furthermore, even excluding factors related to migration, an individual can expose themselves to products independent of their location. Therefore, providers should consider both place-based and product-based exposures. This section provides examples of place-based and product-based exposures. Specifically, this section discusses chemical exposures from endocrine-disrupting personal care products and the lack of access to safe drinking water.

Personal Care Products

Personal care product use has been associated with multiple health effects. The effects are believed to be related to the chemicals contained in these products, such as phthalates, parabens, and per- and polyfluoroalkyl substances (PFAS). In laboratory and animal studies, personal care product use has been associated with an increased risk of breast cancer.[9] In these studies, endocrine-disrupting chemicals in personal care products were observed to interfere with hormonal signaling and reproductive development.[9]

Personal care product use is a complex source of exposure. Each product is a mixture of multiple chemicals, and products are often used simultaneously or in immediate succession.[9,10] This type of exposure may lead to additive and interacting effects.[9] When considering risks associated with personal care product usage, it is crucial to consider cumulative risks.[11]

Endocrine Disruption

Although there is a scientific consensus that developing fetuses are vulnerable to environmental exposures from endocrine-disrupting chemicals, pregnant women still do not perceive the severity of this risk.[12] Pregnancy is considered a time when women are highly motivated to make behavioral changes to protect the health of their expected child.[12] However, this does not seem to be the case concerning endocrine-disrupting chemicals. Although there is increased knowledge of the presence of endocrine-disrupting chemicals in products, many pregnant may not receive enough information about the risks of using products containing endocrine-disrupting chemicals.[13] Most pregnant women attempt to make safe product use choices, yet because they may not always be aware of environmental chemicals in personal care products, they may not change their personal care product use patterns.[14]

Personal Care Products as Factors in Maternal Health Disparities

Women are disproportionality exposed to chemicals through their usage of personal care products.[9] On average, American women use 12 personal care products daily, exposing them to approximately 126 different chemicals.[9] A quarter of American women use more than 15 personal care products daily.[9] A large prospective study mainly involving non-Hispanic white women found a 10% to 15% increase in the risk of breast cancer among non-Hispanic white women who were moderate and frequent users of personal care products.[9] An increased risk is even more concerning in relation to Black women, who have higher breast cancer mortality rates than their white counterparts despite similar or slightly higher rates of mammography screening among Black women.[9]

Racial discrimination based on European beauty norms may also lead to the disproportionate use of personal care products among Black women. Personal care product use may be a physical manifestation of societal racism.[15] Products that straighten hair, lighten skin, and mask odors reinforce European beauty norms.[15] Historically, imagined odor was used to control sexual behavior, and Black women who deodorized and used vaginal douches were identified as more sexually virtuous.[15] Odor discrimination led to the targeted marketing of these products to Black women.[15] Black women are more likely than white women to use fragranced feminine products and vaginal douches.[15] Vaginal douching alone may contribute to phthalate exposure disparities.[15] Women who frequently douche have 150% higher exposures to phthalates than nonusers.[15] These ideas eventually became cultural norms and persisted beyond current marketing.[15]

Racial differences in personal care product use may factor in health disparities among Black women.[11] Black consumers spend nine times more than other groups on hair and beauty products.[15] Black women spend more on personal care products associated with increased urinary phthalate metabolite levels, including deodorizing, feminine hygiene, and fragrance products.[11] Hair products frequently used by Black women are more likely to contain endocrine-disrupting chemicals, including phthalates.[16] Because of societal pressures cultural norms favoring long, straight hair, Black women are more likely to use hair dyes and products marketed for hair growth, straightening, and moisturizing.[16] In addition to the products' differences in chemical composition, Black women use more of the products and with greater frequency.[16] This exposure may factor in differences in health outcomes, such as increased incidences of fibroids and early menarche.[16]

Cultural norms associated with race further complicate the issue. For example, socioeconomic status cannot explain the difference in phthalate levels among Black women.[15] Black women of higher socioeconomic status are more likely to use multiple personal care products.[16] This behavior is counterintuitive, because one would expect individuals with more education to be more knowledgeable and to act to reduce exposure.[16] Black women continue to use hair products, knowing they harm their self-worth, identity, and societal acceptance.[16] This suggests that, while costs may be a barrier, economic factors do not seem to drive these behaviors.

Furthermore, Black women are more susceptible to these exposures due to the cumulative impact of other co-occurring environmental and social risk factors.[15] Due to coexisting place-based environmental stressors, the health impacts on Black women related to phthalate exposure through personal care products may be more significant.[15]

Access to Safe Drinking Water

The United States is known internationally for providing access to safe drinking water to its population. However, this is not universally true. Americans facing water insecurity are generally low-income people of color. The Latino and Black populations are twice as likely not to have indoor plumbing as their white counterparts. This disparity is even greater among Native Americans, who are 19 times more likely not to have indoor plumbing.[17]

Over 43 million people, or approximately 15% of the population in the United States, are dependent on well water because they do not have access to public water.[18] They must rely on private water wells that are unregulated by the Safe Drinking Water Act (SDWA). These individuals are instead subject to widely differing state regulations. Most of the states do not have any standards related to drinking water quality.[19] The owners are responsible for the safety of their well water. However, many private well owners believe they can detect contamination by the water's taste, appearance, or smell and believe well testing is unnecessary.[18]

Well contamination remains prevalent. After sampling wells in 48 states, the United States Geological Survey (USGS) found that over one-fifth of the wells had contaminants that exceeded SDWA standards. One-fourth of the wells in primarily agricultural areas exceeded safe drinking water standards.[20] Most emergency department visits for acute gastrointestinal illness are associated with private well contamination.[21]

Lead-based paint, soil, and water from lead pipes and plumbing fixtures are the most common sources of lead exposure in the United States.[22] Although often overlooked as a population, children who consume water from private wells are at an increased risk of lead exposure in comparison to their counterparts who drink water from community water systems (CWS).[23] Whereas CWS must implement corrosion-control measures to reduce lead exposure, individual well owners maintain private wells.[24] A study found that children who depend on private wells average blood lead levels (BLLs) that are 20% higher than the levels in children with access to CWS.[23] Few private well owners know the risk of lead exposure from private wells and fail to manage corrosion control to reduce lead. [23]

A lack of infrastructure translates to a lack of standards. The SDWA covers public water systems that provide water to at least 25 people. Most Americans consume drinking water protected by the SDWA, but the statute does not cover private wells.

Colonias

Colonias are unincorporated areas along the United States–Mexico border,[25] and communities like colonias are typically not included in international reporting statistics related to access to water.[17] Colonias are home to 5.5 million Americans, most of whom are in low-income families. The communities are typically peri-urban, which means that, despite being outside city limits, they are within commuting distance of an incorporated municipality. The communities developed out of poverty and broken promises. Much of the land in colonias was sold to migrant workers with the understanding that they would soon receive basic amenities.[26] However, the amenities ultimately never came, leaving the communities responsible for providing essential services like safe drinking water and sewage. Socioeconomic factors exacerbate the severity of the lack of access to basic infrastructure and further reduce residents' access to safe drinking water.[25] Because the communities typically do not have access to public water systems, they must construct private wells. The wells are built by residents to meet their immediate needs, independent of standards, and thus the wells are often shallow.[25] In addition to being vulnerable to contamination, these unprotected wells can also serve as sources of groundwater contamination.[27] Shallow, unprotected wells like those in colonias are susceptible to contamination from flood waters.[28] Additionally, the lack of infrastructure leads to exposure to waste from septic systems. And, of course, standing water from flooding is a mosquito breeding medium, increasing the risk for mosquito-borne diseases.

Underbound Black Communities

Throughout the South, the lack of access to essential services is bound in institutional racism. Many communities are excluded from municipal water, sewer, and trash services through "municipal underbounding."[24] Municipal underbounding is similar to redlining, an exclusionary practice exercised by a governmental entity. Whereas redlining restricted where Black residents could live, municipal underbounding involves drawing municipal boundaries to exclude existing Black communities.[24] The communities are neighboring, and sometimes fully enclosed within, municipal boundaries, but they are excluded from municipal services.[23] Children living in these areas have much higher BLLs‡ than children living within municipal boundaries as well as children in rural areas that are well dependent. [24] One study found a 29% increase in BLLs for every 10% increase in the non-Hispanic Black population in a census block.[23] Research indicates that extending public services like access to CWS may be associated with race.[29] Black peri-urban communities relying on private wells are exposed to more microbial contamination than communities in neighboring areas receiving water from public water systems.

---

‡ Recently, the Centers for Disease Control and Prevention (CDC) reduced the BLL reference value from 5 µg/dL to 3.5 µg/dL and updated its guidance on case management for BLLs. The new value is not a health-based standard but instead represents the top 2.5% among US children 1 to 5 years old with the highest BLLs based on the 2015–2016 and 2017–2018 NHANES.

STRATEGIES FOR IMPROVING MATERNAL ENVIRONMENTAL HEALTH

Environmental threats to maternal health are ubiquitous and numerous. This is an area of public health needing additional research and development, but providers do not need to be environmental health experts to address environmental factors in maternal health.[1] Indeed, ACOG recommends not delaying addressing environmental impacts on maternal health due to scientific uncertainty, because the threat is "severe and irreversible."[1] Providers can help improve environmental implications for maternal health through assessment, counseling, and advocacy.[1]

For providers working on an individual level, the Health Belief Model may provide a helpful approach to addressing maternal environmental health. The Health Belief Model is useful for understanding how target populations perceive and respond to risks. In the context of this chapter, it is essential to educate the target population on risks associated with phthalate exposure because of the absence of counseling provided by healthcare providers. The Health Belief Model has been previously used in education about endocrine-disrupting chemicals, such as phthalates. The Health Belief Model is especially significant because the risk associated with these chemicals is unclear. Therefore, it is essential to understand whether target populations perceive associated risks as enough to justify a behavior change.[12] The Health Belief Model has six constructs: (1) perceived susceptibility, (2) perceived severity, (3) perceived barriers, (4) perceived benefit, (5) cue to action, and (6) perceived self-efficacy. All six constructs apply in the phthalate risk program. Perceived susceptibility is an individual's perception that she will personally experience an adverse health outcome associated with phthalate exposure. Perceived severity is an individual's perception of the significance of the adverse health outcome associated with phthalate exposure. Barriers are obstacles to engaging in behavioral changes to reduce phthalate exposure, and benefits relate to the rewards of engaging in healthy behavioral changes.[12] Cue to action refers to internal and external stimuli that lead a person to take action to reduce phthalate exposure. Self-efficacy relates to an individual's belief that they can engage in and maintain the behaviors.[30] This model is a basis for providers to use in thinking through approaches as they address assessment, counseling, and advocacy concerning maternal health.

Providers should incorporate questions regarding environmental exposures into patients' health histories before and during pregnancy. This assessment should consider the occupational, home, and recreational environment. The Director of the Alliance of Nurses for Healthy Environments, Katie Huffling, has created the "Environmental Exposure Assessment" for use during prenatal care.*

---

* For additional screening tools evaluated by Bonnie Hamilton Bogart for the National Collaborating Centre for Environmental Health and BC Centre for Disease Control, see Bogart BH. Environmental health risks in children: screening tools for community health nurses and paraprofessional home visitors and their integration within public health practice. Environmental Health Resources for Health Professionals. https://nben.ca/en/ceh-resources-for-health-professionals. Published 2014. Accessed March 24, 2022.

A focus group of nurses favored this assessment.[31] However, an assessment alone is not enough. The provider must also address how the pregnant person perceives their susceptibility, severity, benefits, and burdens concerning environmental risk factors.[12] These areas can be addressed through provider counseling.

Many environmental risk factors, such as endocrine disruptors, are not obvious. Therefore, providers must be clear about the links between maternal health and birth outcomes associated with environmental exposures. The counseling should be patient-centered and include advice specific to that pregnant person's exposure risks.[12] Overall, pregnant women have expressed an interest in learning more about environmental exposures during pregnancy, but physicians typically do not counsel pregnant women on such issues.[32] A provider does not have to limit counseling to the clinical setting. Classes and written materials can be used to supplement information.[1]

Self-efficacy should be affirmed with guidance about how the pregnant person can reduce their risk of environmental exposures. Pregnant persons can use an app like Detox Me, Healthy Living App, or Think Dirty to address perceived barriers, self-efficacy, and cues to action to identify toxins in personal care products. These apps include barcode scanners that allow participants to scan items of interest to determine whether toxins are present, including phthalates. This removes the barrier of having to review multiple labels and having extensive knowledge of listed chemicals. The apps will do that for participants. These apps also suggest alternative products if they do contain toxic chemicals. The app will increase self-efficacy by empowering women to take meaningful action to reduce phthalate exposure through personal care products. The ubiquitous nature of phthalates can make engaging in behavioral changes to reduce exposure overwhelming. Using an app will make this process seem more manageable and achievable. The app also provides a cue to action through in-app reminders.

REFERENCES

1. American College of Obstetricians and Gynecologists. Reducing prenatal exposure to toxic environmental agents. ACOG Committee Opinion No. 832. *Obstet Gynecol.* 2021;138:e40–e54.

2. Lee KJ, Moon H, Yun HR, et al. Greenness, civil environment, and pregnancy outcomes: perspectives with a systematic review and meta-analysis. *Environ Health.* 2020;19:91. https://doi.org/10.1186/s12940-020-00649-z.

3. Prüss-Ustün A, Wolf J, Corvalán C, Neville T, Bos R, Neira M. Diseases due to unhealthy environments: an updated estimate of the global burden of disease attributable to environmental determinants of health. *J Public Health.* 2016;39(3):464–475. doi:10.1093/pubmed/fdw085.

4. Shaffer RM, Sellers SP, Baker MG, et al. Improving and expanding estimates of the global burden of disease due to environmental health risk factors. *Environ Health Perspect.* 2019;127(10):105001. doi:10.1289/ehp5496.

5. Boyles AL, Beverly BE, Fenton SE, et al. Environmental factors involved in maternal morbidity and mortality. *J Womens Health.* 2021;30(2):245–252. doi:10.1089/jwh.2020.8855.

6. Office of Minority Health. Infant mortality and African Americans. https://minorit yhealth.hhs.gov/omh/browse.aspx?lvl=4&lvlid=23. Published July 8, 2021. Accessed February 1, 2022.

7. Crear-Perry J, Correa-de-Araujo R, Lewis Johnson T, McLemore MR, Neilson E, Wallace M. Social and structural determinants of health inequities in maternal health. *J Womens Health*. 2021;30(2):230-235. doi:10.1089/jwh.2020.8882.

8. Smith J. The father of environmental justice, on whether we're all doomed. *Vox*. https://www.vox.com/2021/12/10/22826247/robert-bullard-environmental-just ice-vox-conversations-interview. Published December 10, 2021. Accessed January 28, 2022.

9. Taylor KW, Troester MA, Herring AH, et al. Associations between personal care product use patterns and breast cancer risk among white and Black women in the Sister Study. *Environ Health Perspect*. 2018;126(2):027011. doi:10.1289/ehp1480.

10. Parlett LE, Calafat AM, Swan SH. Women's exposure to phthalates in relation to use of personal care products. *J Expo Sci Environ Epidemiol*. 2012;23(2):197–206. doi:10.1038/jes.2012.105.

11. Helm JS, Nishioka M, Brody JG, Rudel RA, Dodson RE. Measurement of endocrine disrupting and asthma-associated chemicals in hair products used by black women. *Environ Res*. 2018;165:448–458. doi:10.1016/j.envres.2018.03.030.

12. Che S-R, Barrett ES, Velez M, Conn K, Heinert S, Qiu X. Using the health belief model to illustrate factors that influence risk assessment during pregnancy and implications for prenatal education about endocrine disruptors. *Policy Futures Educ*. 2014;12(7):961-974. doi:10.2304/pfie.2014.12.7.961.

13. Rouillon S, El Ouazzani H, Hardouin J-B, et al. How to educate pregnant women about endocrine disruptors? *Int J Environ Res Public Health*. 2020;17(6):2156. doi:10.3390/ijerph17062156.

14. Barrett ES, Sathyanarayana S, Janssen S, et al. Environmental health attitudes and behaviors: findings from a large pregnancy cohort study. *Eur J Obstet Gynecol Reprod Biol*. 2014;176:119–125. doi:10.1016/j.ejogrb.2014.02.029.

15. Zota AR, Shamasunder B. The environmental injustice of beauty: framing chemical exposures from beauty products as a health disparities concern. *Am J Obstet Gynecol*. 2017;217(4):418e1–418e6. doi:10.1016/j.ajog.2017.07.020.

16. Gaston SA, James-Todd T, Harmon Q, Taylor KW, Baird D, Jackson CL. Chemical/ straightening and other hair product usage during childhood, adolescence, and adulthood among African-American women: potential implications for health. *J Expo Sci Environ Epidemiol*. 2019;30(1):86–96. doi:10.1038/s41370-019-0186-6.

17. Tippin C. The household water insecurity nexus: portraits of hardship and resilience in U.S.–Mexico border colonias. *Geoforum*. 2021;124:65–74. doi:10.1016/ j.geoforum.2021.05.019.

18. Water Resources. Domestic (private) supply wells. https://www.usgs.gov/miss ion-areas/water-resources/science/domestic-private-supply-wells?qt-science_cen ter_objects=0#qt-science_center_objects. Published March 1, 2019. Accessed April 28, 2022.

19. Bowen K, Krishna T, Backer L, Hodgins K, Waller LA, Gribble MO. State-level policies concerning private wells in the United States. *Water Policy*. 2019;21(2):428–435. doi:10.2166/wp.2019.205.

20. DeSimone LA. Quality of water from domestic wells in principal aquifers of the United States, 1991–2004. USGS sir 2008–5227. https://pubs.usgs.gov/sir/2008/5227/. Published 2009. Accessed April 28, 2022.

21. DeFelice NB, Johnston JE, Gibson JMD. Reducing emergency department visits for acute gastrointestinal illnesses in North Carolina (USA) by extending community water service. *Environ Health Perspect*. 2016;124(10):1583–1591. doi:10.1289/ehp160.

22. Ruckart PZ, Jones RL, Courtney JG, et al. Update of the blood lead reference value—United States, 2021. *MMWR*. 2021;70(43):1509–1512. doi:10.15585/mmwr.mm7043a4.

23. Gibson JMD, Fisher M, Clonch A, MacDonald JM, Cook PJ. Children drinking private well water have higher blood lead than those with city water. *Proc Natl Acad Sci*. 2020;117(29):16898–16907. doi:10.1073/pnas.2002729117.

24. Stillo F, Gibson JM. Racial disparities in access to municipal water supplies in the American South: impacts on children's health. *Int Public Health J*. 2018;10(3):309–323.

25. Rowles LS III, Hossain AI, Ramirez I, et al. Seasonal contamination of well-water in flood-prone colonias and other unincorporated U.S. communities. *Sci Total Environ*. 2020;740:140111. doi:10.1016/j.scitotenv.2020.140111.

26. Cuellar C. Colonias bear the heaviest burden when rain falls in the Rio Grande Valley. Texas Public Radio. September 2, 2021. https://www.tpr.org/border-immigration/2021-07-22/colonias-bear-the-heaviest-burden-when-rain-falls-in-the-rio-grande-valley. Accessed April 28, 2022.

27. Martínez-Santos P, Martín-Loeches M, García-Castro N, et al. A survey of domestic wells and pit latrines in rural settlements of Mali: implications of on-site sanitation on the quality of water supplies. *Int J Hyg Environ Health*. 2017;220(7):1179–1189. doi:10.1016/j.ijheh.2017.08.001.

28. Aladejana JA, Kalin RM, Sentenac P, Hassan I. Assessing the impact of climate change on groundwater quality of the shallow coastal aquifer of Eastern Dahomey Basin, southwestern Nigeria. *Water*. 2020;12(1):224. doi:10.3390/w12010224.

29. Leker HG, MacDonald Gibson J. Relationship between race and community water and sewer service in North Carolina, USA. *PLOS One*. 2018;13(3):e0193225. doi:10.1371/journal.pone.0193225.

30. Tola HH, Shojaeizadeh D, Tol A, et al. Psychological and educational intervention to improve tuberculosis treatment adherence in Ethiopia based on Health Belief Model: a cluster randomized control trial. *PLOS One*. 2016;11(5):e0155147. doi:10.1371/journal.pone.0155147

31. Huffling K. Prenatal preconception assessment. https://envirn.org/wp-content/uploads/2017/03/prenatal-preconception-assessment.pdf. Published 2011. Accessed March 24, 2022.

32. Sharma S, Ashley JM, Hodgson A, Nisker J. Views of pregnant women and clinicians regarding discussion of exposure to phthalate plasticizers. *Reprod Health*. 2014;11(47). https://reproductive-health-journal.biomedcentral.com/articles/10.1186/1742-4755-11-47#citeas.

Chapter 23

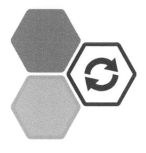

Reimagining Prenatal Care: Designing a Justice-Conscious Approach to Reproductive Health, Pregnancy, and Early Parenthood

KEEGAN D. WARREN AND DAPHNE MCGEE

HEALTH EQUITY AND SOCIAL DETERMINANTS

The World Health Organization (WHO) defines social determinants of health as "the conditions in which people are born, grow, work, live, and age, and the wider set of forces and systems shaping the conditions of daily life." Frequently, though, the second half of the definition is left out of the on-the-ground delivery of healthcare, despite movement toward value-based care and alternative payment methodologies. That is, too few healthcare entities actively integrate the forces and systems—in the WHO's words: "the economic policies, development agendas, social norms, social policies, and politics"—into individual patient care, clinical decision-making, and community-based advocacy. This chapter explores both through two case studies. In so doing, it adopts a definition of health that aligns with the WHO charter preamble, incorporating notions of not just the absence of illness but also the presence of wellness—and that may simply be summarized as how well and how long people live.

As attorneys with expertise at the intersection of health and law, the authors feel compelled to begin by acknowledging and emphasizing that how the courts and legislatures understand and approach legal analysis and law shapes health even when "health law" is not the apparent subject. That is, health and law intersect in ways beyond regulation of entities, professionals, products, and services,

Keegan D. Warren and Daphne McGee, *Reimagining Prenatal Care* In: *The Practical Playbook III*. Edited by: Dorothy Cilenti, Alisahah Jackson, Natalie D. Hernandez, Lindsey Yates, Sarah Verbiest, J. Lloyd Michener, and Brian C. Castrucci, Oxford University Press. © de Beaumont Foundation 2024. DOI: 10.1093/oso/9780197662984.003.0023

and the civil justice structure in particular informs health and well-being long before a person becomes a patient.

Consider how civil law shapes access to care. For example, Tyler and Teitelbaum described how the tort law concept of "duty"—the question of whether one individual owes a legal obligation to act for the benefit of another individual—means in the context of the delivery of healthcare that a physician has no requirement to treat any given would-be patient.[1] From the patient perspective, this means there is no right to access healthcare—including pregnancy care. Indeed, insofar as there is a right to pregnancy care, it is due to legislative action that is explicit about some aspect of health. The Emergency Medical Treatment and Active Labor Act (EMTALA) is an apt example here because it has been traditionally understood to require treatment and stabilization or transfer of, inter alia, pregnant persons who present in the emergency department and may be about to deliver. Not coincidentally, EMTALA grew from grassroots outrage about physician rejection of low-income pregnant persons, demonstrating the power of advocating for law that is structured to create better health outcomes.

A second salient example is the much broader approach to access to prenatal care, which is critical to good outcomes for parent and baby. Title 19 of the Social Security Act—that is, Medicaid—creates a limited right to coverage of healthcare for pregnancy-related conditions during and immediately after pregnancy, in the process covering nearly half of all births in the United States. The efficacy is clear: in comparison to uninsured women, women with Medicaid are significantly more likely to receive adequate prenatal care.[2]

While there are countless such examples, the takeaway is that health-related legal doctrines exist—and that they offer a unique opportunity to integrate what occurs outside the walls of clinics and hospitals into the delivery of healthcare in a way that improves health outcomes. But we cannot achieve equitable health outcomes without grounding doctrines and laws in the context in which they were created.

An excellent example is that lack of transportation—and transportation is a commonly cited health-related social need—may be the legacy of residential segregation laws in the first half of the 20th century, which in turn shaped our modern cities and suburbs. Those laws deliberately achieved segregation by using race to restrict freedom to contract and to inform access to utilities and schools. That same expressly race-based approach to neighborhoods also informed the federal law that founded our national hospital system. Thus, programs that offer travel vouchers in response to an acute need may help a patient get to the next prenatal visit, but they do not help the person get to specialty care, school, or work because they do not operate at the level of the fundamentally inequitable system in which the need arises. We and others advocate for health equity not to be reduced to a response to individual crises, and that healthcare delivery systems employ a more holistic and longitudinal model. By thinking about the why, how, and who of health inequities, we can deploy a justice-conscious approach to health equity that creates structural change as identified and driven by those most affected.[3]

UNMET LEGAL NEEDS

That law is a key social determinant of health is embodied by the concept of "health-harming legal needs." Programs that respond to immediate health-related social needs without incorporating law risk exacerbating the inequities because they do not undo the harm that is the root cause of the need. For this reason, legal care must be understood as healthcare.

At the individual level, health-harming legal needs can be understood through the national IHELP™ model, which describes concrete interventions that can remediate some unmet needs as part of the delivery of healthcare[4] (see Figure 23.1).

Given that law broadly affects health, it should be of little surprise that the professionals who study and practice law also affect health. Notably, Teufel and Mace have demonstrated that access to lawyers is as predictive of community health as income inequality,[5] and the National Academy of Medicine has recommended that lawyers further be studied in terms of their contributions to health.[6]

The national medical-legal partnership (MLP) model embeds law into the delivery of healthcare by making attorneys and paralegals an onsite, collaborating part of the care team. MLPs integrate legal expertise into healthcare settings to help clinicians, case managers, and social workers address structural problems at the root of so many health inequities. The National Center for Medical-Legal Partnership is an excellent resource. Based at George Washington University, it leads education, research, and technical assistance efforts to help every health organization in the United States leverage legal services as a standard part of the way they respond to social needs. Visit their virtual home at https://medical-legalpartnership.org/.

MLP also means that the notion of structural competency—the idea that clinicians should appreciate the forces that influence health outcomes at levels above individual interactions—is complemented and surpassed because legal professionals are necessarily structural experts. Thus, MLP attorneys are able to bring structural expertise to bear on individual patient needs as well as on clinical transformation, and to do so in a way that studies show helps medical professionals practice at the top of their licenses.

In addition to bolstering the workforce, the MLP approach has had demonstrable health impact, including reduced admissions and improved health for patient populations as diverse as asthmatic children[7,8] and adults,[9]

Figure 23.1 ▼
The IHELP™ model.

Source: Marple K. Framing legal care as health care. National Center for Medical-Legal Partnership. 2015. medical-legalpartnership.org/mlp-resources/messaging-guide/.

Common Social Determinant of Health	How Legal Services Can Help	Impact of Legal Services on Health/Healthcare
INCOME Resources to meet daily basic needs	• Appeal denials of food stamps, health insurance, cash benefits, and disability benefits	1. Increasing someone's income means s/he makes fewer trade-offs between affording food and healthcare, including medications 2. Being able to afford enough healthy food helps people manage chronic diseases and helps children grow and develop.
HOUSING & UTILITIES A healthy physical environment	• Secure housing subsidies • Improve substandard conditions • Prevent evictions • Protect against utility shut-off	1. A stable, decent, affordable home helps a person avoid costly emergency room visits related to homelessness. 2. Consistent housing, heat and electricity helps people follow their medical treatment plans.
EDUCATION & EMPLOYMENT Quality educational and job opportunities	• Secure specialized education services • Prevent and remedy employment discrimination • Enforce workplace rights	1. A quality education is the single greatest predictor of a person's adult health. 2. Consistent employment helps provide money for food and safe housing, which also helps avoid costly emergency health care services. 3. Access to health insurance is often linked to employment.
LEGAL STATUS Access to jobs	• Resolve veteran discharge status • Clear criminal/credit histories • Assist with asylum applications and other immigration issues • Provide assistance with name and gender marker changes.	1. Clearing a person's criminal history or helping a veteran change their discharge status helps make consistent employment and access to public benefits possible. 2. Consistent employment provides money for food and safe housing, which helps people avoid costly emergency healthcare services. 3. Helping a transgender person change their name and gender on their forms of ID to match their identity can help remove barriers to employment.
PERSONAL & FAMILY STABILITY Safe homes and social support	• Secure restraining orders for domestic violence • Secure adoption, custody and guardianship for children	1. Less violence at home means less need for costly emergency healthcare services. 2. Stable family relationships significantly reduce stress and allow for better decision-making, including decisions related to healthcare.

diabetic youth,[10] sickle-cell patients,[11] high-utilizing patients,[12] and even healthy newborns.[13]

The MLP model also provides a closed-loop system that works at the individual, population, and community levels. Not only are MLP lawyers onsite in a way that facilitates timely interventions, but they also routinely use case-management systems with well-defined and structured data fields. Information-sharing in MLPs is an opportunity to move seamlessly from patients to policy in the clinical redress of social determinants of health.[14]

Finally, as value-based care increasingly becomes the expectation, evidence-driven approaches like MLP are critical to achieving evaluable improvements in health equity.

CASE STUDY 1: RESPONDING TO A CRISIS

MLP can remediate specific structural barriers to health equity for pregnant and parenting persons and reduce frustrations among the workforce. For example, in a model financed through local public health dollars and then supplemented by a Medicaid §1115 waiver, California Rural Legal Assistance, Inc., and the Monterey County Health Department partnered to address the health-harming legal needs of patients at a local federally qualified health center.[15] Physicians and families there had struggled for decades with the effects of fetal pesticide exposure, which research links with ADHD, autism, asthma, and low IQ. Once on site, the MLP attorney was able to demonstrate how various laws led to pesticide exposure during pregnancy, and then to solve the problem through collaborative, practical efforts with physicians at the individual, population, and community levels. For example, individual patients received direct and referral representation by the MLP attorney, a concrete and measurable intervention of an acute need. Second, the MLP attorney trained clinicians to write letters for pregnant patients in a way that better aligned with pertinent law and thus triggered legal protections, a population-focused tactic that also increased provider willingness and ability to advocate. Third, the patient experiences informed successful advocacy to change a state law so that pesticide exposure decreased for all pregnant Californians. By employing a justice-conscious lens, the interprofessional team redressed an inequity born of laws that were not written with a critical approach to health impact on pregnant persons and their children, and that disproportionately affected the Latinx population.

The example also demonstrates that the MLP approach occurs along a continuum (see Figure 23.2): legal representation for affected individuals complemented by training of clinicians as well as evolution of clinical policy to reflect the structural realities that patients are experiencing. In moving from patients to policy, MLP is a powerful tool in the population health management toolkit, and it presents a pragmatic approach to increasing health equity.

CASE STUDY 2: INTEGRATING STRUCTURAL EXPERTISE INTO PRENATAL CARE

People's Community Clinic (PCC) is a federally qualified health center in Austin, Texas. It runs the Center for Women's Health (CWH), which provides prenatal care, family planning, and other reproductive health services.

In 2017, CWH began incorporating group visits into its prenatal care model. The basic group care curriculum included discussions of health-related needs, such as insurance and employment, but the curriculum did not have legal expertise or information built in to rectify the newly identified issues affecting the pregnancies of the participating patients. CWH had access to an MLP attorney through PCC's existing MLP, which was funded as enabling services through

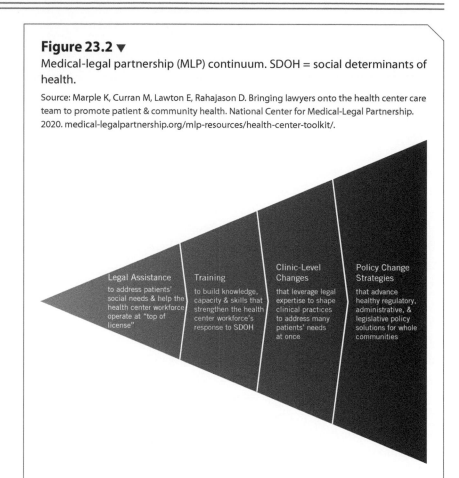

Figure 23.2 ▼

Medical-legal partnership (MLP) continuum. SDOH = social determinants of health.

Source: Marple K, Curran M, Lawton E, Rahajason D. Bringing lawyers onto the health center care team to promote patient & community health. National Center for Medical-Legal Partnership. 2020. medical-legalpartnership.org/mlp-resources/health-center-toolkit/.

Legal Assistance
to address patients' social needs & help the health center workforce operate at "top of license"

Training
to build knowledge, capacity & skills that strengthen the health center workforce's response to SDOH

Clinic-Level Changes
that leverage legal expertise to shape clinical practices to address many patients' needs at once

Policy Change Strategies
that advance healthy regulatory, administrative, & legislative policy solutions for whole communities

the Health Resources and Services Administration (HRSA), and the MLP champions team identified the transition to group prenatal care as an opportunity to move the legal services more upstream. By embedding an additional attorney as co-facilitator of the group visits, CWH would be able to equip patients with legal information to address issues affecting parenting—and to do so as preventive care along the MLP continuum, not focusing solely on acute crises.

The project was strategically designed to integrate into the CWH's medical model of group care by giving shape to the legal checkup concept as a means for upstream legal practice. For each group visit, the attorney, health educator, and nurse-midwife would meet to plan the topics to be discussed. Then, each of the three practitioners would facilitate discussions during the group meetings, allowing expectant parents and their families to voice concerns and both share and receive support. Importantly, these questions were already arising for clinicians; the difference is that the MLP approach meant the care team had onsite, integrated expertise to mitigate the health-related needs. Group participants generally reported that not only did they improve legal literacy skills, but also that legal knowledge reduced stress during pregnancy.

Participating providers also reported increased self-efficacy in understanding the effects of health-harming legal needs and helping patients navigate them.

To ensure sustainability, the co-facilitators observed patients and interviewed providers over the course of several group cohorts. Their findings became the basis for the Prenatal Legal Checkup, an open-source curriculum hosted at https://texaslawhelp.org/article/prenatal-legal-checkup and https://www.austinpcc.org/pregnancy-resources/prenatal-legal-checkup-videos/. The care team believe that some of the more salient topics around familial and personal stability represent a unique health-affirming opportunity if embedded into routine family-planning healthcare.

REIMAGINING CARE FOR PREGNANT PERSONS

Here are two primary suggestions that every healthcare facility should follow.

Recommendation 1: MLP Should Be a Funded, Standard Approach to Care

If inequity occurs at the structural level—that is, as a matter of social priorities written proscribed into law—then MLP represents the translational approach to addressing health equity. At its simplest, MLP embeds legal professionals in the delivery of healthcare to remediate health-harming legal needs at the point of service. But a truly integrated model means that the collaborative legal interventions occur along a continuum, ranging from addressing the needs of individuals in acute crisis, to solving problems for whole populations, to incorporating structural realities into clinical practices and, ultimately, to moving from patient to policy to achieve broader policy gains across communities.

But getting started is not necessarily easy. Legal services, like healthcare services, are regulated at the federal, state, and even local level. Effectively and efficiently navigating the regulatory schema in tandem may be aided by an expert, such as via the services of one of the authors (KW). Additionally, respectful screening for needs, appropriate financing of interventions, compliant sharing of data, and maximized metrics and evaluation of the services are best facilitated by someone well versed in the law, policy, and history of both the healthcare and legal services industries. Because MLP is most effective as a fully integrated model, a third party can also be helpful for strategically planning continuum activities, or those that embed the MLP legal team's structural expertise in administrative and clinical activity in a way that multiplies frontline capacity. Whether it is practicable to engage a professional in the tailored design, strategy, and implementation of a new MLP (or in the analytical revamping of an established program), the authors recommend that medical and legal entities alike become familiar with the toolkit offered by the National Center for Medical-Legal Partnership (see Figure 23.3.) The toolkit delves into options instrumental for success of an integrated care-delivery model, ranging from assessing health-harming legal needs to establishing organizational relationships, and from financing legal care to forming service-delivery workflows.

But successful deployment of best practices necessitates that managed care organizations and states who seek to catalyze and sustain equitable approaches to the delivery of healthcare recognize and incentivize providers to collaborate with the legal sector. Moreover, financial incentives must flow to the professionals providing the collaborative legal services, on whatever basis works for the parties (e.g., fixed rate, shared savings, or per-member/per-month). Importantly, MLP represents a practicable opportunity within the greater shift from volume to value to align with alternative payment methodologies, consistent with, for instance, the Center for Medicare and Medicaid Services' Health Care Payment Learning and Action Network Categories 3 and 4.[16] Finally, public health departments can be important partners in evaluation and advocacy, bringing critical legal epidemiological expertise to bear.

Recommendation 2: Employ a Health Justice Lens to Increase Equity

There is abundant opportunity to move further upstream in imagining law as a tool to improve health. Because the practice of medicine is regulated at federal, state, and institutional levels, law can bridge the gap to create a mechanism to

Figure 23.3 ▼

The National Center for Medical-Legal Partnership's planning, implementation, and practice guide for building and sustaining a health center-based medical-legal partnership.

Source: Based on Marple K, Curran M, Lawton E, Rahajason D. Bringing lawyers onto the health center care team to promote patient & community health. 2020. https://medical-legalpartnership.org/mlp-resources/health-center-toolkit/.

In October 2020, the National Center for Medical-Legal Partnership promulgated a toolkit outlining nine conversations that a health center team should have with its legal partners to plan for an MLP's long-term success and to integrate it into the health center's operations.

- ☐ Conversation 1: What SDOH problems do we want to address?
- ☐ Conversation 2: How many lawyers do we need to meet the need(s) we identified and accomplish our goals?
- ☐ Conversation 3: Build it as a direct service or contract it: How will we staff our integrated legal services?
- ☐ Conversation 4: How are we going to pay for it?
- ☐ Conversation 5: What are our goals and expectations for the program, ourselves, and our legal partners?
- ☐ Conversation 6: What other partners in our community can be helpful?
- ☐ Conversation 7: How will we address patient consent and information-sharing?
- ☐ Conversation 8: How will we integrate legal services into our workflows and systems?
- ☐ Conversation 9: How will we make sure the program is effective and that it lasts?

require providers-in-training to receive inclusive education that mitigates the negative health impacts of bias, particularly in reproductive care.

Similarly, institutional rules can act like law in furthering equity in pregnancy outcomes. For example, in December 2021, an illustration of a cross-section of a pregnant person, drawn by Chidiebere Ibe, a Nigerian medical illustrator and student, went viral.[17] It's not often that a medical illustration reaches a wide Internet audience, but this one did for one particular reason: the skin of the person and the fetus was more melanated than typical illustrations found in textbooks. At a time when the maternal mortality rates for Black persons have become a more prevalent concern, the image catalyzed discussion about the importance of representation from medical and nonmedical professions alike. After all, representation—or the lack thereof—in medical education can have significant consequences in terms of clinicians' recognition of conditions as well as patients' sense of inclusion in their own medical care. It is critical that institutional policy, procedures, and pathways are understood as law-adjacent opportunities to improve health equity, and that such efforts are recognized in value-based purchasing frameworks.

Law can bridge the gap in a concrete, upstream way to facilitate inclusive medical education, which can positively affect the health of expectant parents in minoritized groups. Competencies regarding social determinants of health, implicit bias, and health justice can, and should, be developed by accrediting bodies across health professions.

Additionally, healthcare law for pregnant and parenting persons must not be limited, as a field, to just medical care during and immediately after pregnancy. A whole-person approach is necessary and appropriate to redress health inequities. That requires evolution of healthcare financing laws to create payment incentives and structures that fund justice services as the health services that they are. It also requires collection and co-location of intersectoral data related to health disparities, which legal services can, and should, contribute to. Integrating data from community-based and integrated legal services, court data, and other medical, public health, and social services data would also help identify opportunities and set concrete goals for improving health equity. Furthermore, it requires recognition in laws like Medicaid legislation that pregnancy care is not a single episode that ends 45 days after delivery; rather, health outcomes for parenting persons start with access to adequate care long before conception.

But we must also understand that not all law that affects healthcare is readily apparent as law that affects health. Similarly, not all law that affects pregnancy and parenting is crafted through a health justice lens. Rather, as suggested by the examples of the tort concept of duty and a disability law indirectly catalyzing increased exposure to pesticides, health-harming legal doctrines can take many forms because health disparities for pregnant persons do not begin or end solely in a medical office. With innumerable ways in which the law and systems affect health, there are innumerable opportunities to advocate for changes in law and policy to facilitate holistic reproductive care. Research and advocacy for policies like paid parental leave and comprehensive universal medical coverage that includes mental healthcare can help to shift the focus from mitigating disparities to creating laws that explicitly seek to improve health and quality of life.

Ultimately, a health justice lens means acknowledging the context in which people seek reproductive care and addressing systemic barriers to reproductive health, however they manifest. It means addressing health equity not only as a matter of meeting an acute need, but also at the structural level that enables, creates, and sustains inequities. It means inquiring who wrote a given law and for whom it was written as well as who is affected by it. And it means including the excluded in designing a solution. Medicine alone cannot solve problems fundamentally ingrained in social structure through law and policy.

REFERENCES

1. Tyler TE, Teitelbaum JB. In: *Essentials of Health Justice: A Primer*. Burlington, MA: Jones & Bartlett; 2019:4–6.

2. Medicaid and CHIP Payment and Access Commission. Medicaid's role in financing maternity care. https://www.macpac.gov/wp-content/uploads/2020/01/Medicaid%E2%80%99s-Role-in-Financing-Maternity-Care.pdf. Published January 2020. Accessed August 21, 2022.

3. Tyler TE, Teitelbaum JB. In: *Essentials of Health Justice: Law, Policy, and Structural Change*. Burlington, MA: Jones & Bartlett Learning; 2022.

4. Marple K. National Center for Medical-Legal Partnership; 2015. Framing Legal Care as Health Care Messaging Guide. https://medical-legalpartnership.org/wp-content/uploads/2015/01/Framing-Legal-Care-as-Health-Care-Messaging-Guide.pdf. Accessed August 21, 2022.

5. Teufel J, Mace S. Legal Aid inequities predict health disparities. *Hamline L Rev*. 2015;38(2):329–360. https://digitalcommons.hamline.edu/hlr/vol38/iss2/7. Accessed August 21, 2022.

6. National Academies of Sciences, Engineering, and Medicine. 2019. *Integrating Social Care into the Delivery of Health Care: Moving Upstream to Improve the Nation's Health*. Washington, DC: The National Academies Press; 2019:171. See Recommendation 5C. https://doi.org/10.17226/25467.

7. Klein MD, Beck AF, Henize AW, Parrish DS, Fink EE, Kahn RS. Doctors and lawyers collaborating to help children: outcomes from a successful partnership between professions. *J Health Care Poor Underserved*. 2013;24(3):1063–1073. doi:10.1353/hpu.2013.0147.

8. Pettignano R, Bliss LR, Caley SB, McLaren S. Can access to a medical-legal partnership benefit patients with asthma who live in an urban community? *J Health Care Poor Underserved*. 2013;24(2):706–717. doi:10.1353/hpu.2013.0055.

9. O'Sullivan MM, Brandfield J, Hoskote SS, et al. Environmental improvements brought by the legal interventions in the homes of poorly controlled inner-city adult asthmatic patients: a proof-of-concept study. *J Asthma*. 2012;49(9):911–917. doi:10.3109/02770903.2012.724131.

10. Malik FS, Yi-Frazier JP, Taplin CE, et al. Improving the care of youth with type 1 diabetes with a novel medical-legal community intervention: the Diabetes Community Care Ambassador Program. *Diabetes Educator*. 2018;44(2):168–177. doi:10.1177/0145721717750346.

11. Pettignano R, Caley SB, Bliss LR. Medical-legal partnership: impact on patients with sickle cell disease. *Pediatrics*. 2011;128(6):e1482–e1488. doi:10.1542/peds.2011-0082.

12. Martin J, Martin A, Schultz C, Sandel M. Embedding civil Legal Aid services in care for high-utilizing patients using medical-legal partnership: health affairs forefront. *Health Affairs*. https://www.healthaffairs.org/do/10.1377/forefront.20150422.047 143/full/. Published April 22, 201520150422.047143/full/.

13. Sege R, Preer G, Morton SJ, et al. Medical-legal strategies to improve infant health care: a randomized trial. *Pediatrics*. 2015;136(1):97–106. doi:10.1542/peds.2014-2955.

14. National Center for Medical-Legal Partnership. Information-sharing in medical-legal partnerships. 2017. https://medical-legalpartnership.org/wp-content/uploads/2017/07/Information-Sharing-in-MLPs.pdf.

15. California Rural Legal Assistance, Inc., Monterey County Health Department. Rural health equity—Monterey County, California. https://www.co.monterey.ca.us/home/showdocument?id=78913. Accessed August 21, 2022.

16. The Mitre Corporation. Alternative Payment Model Framework. 2017. https://hcp-lan.org/workproducts/apm-refresh-whitepaper-final.pdf.

17. Orie A. The creator of the viral black fetus image will have his illustrations published in a book. CNN. https://www.cnn.com/2022/01/13/health/chidiebere-ibe-medical-illustrations-published-nigeria-spc-intl/index.html. Published January 19, 2022. Accessed August 21, 2022.

Data

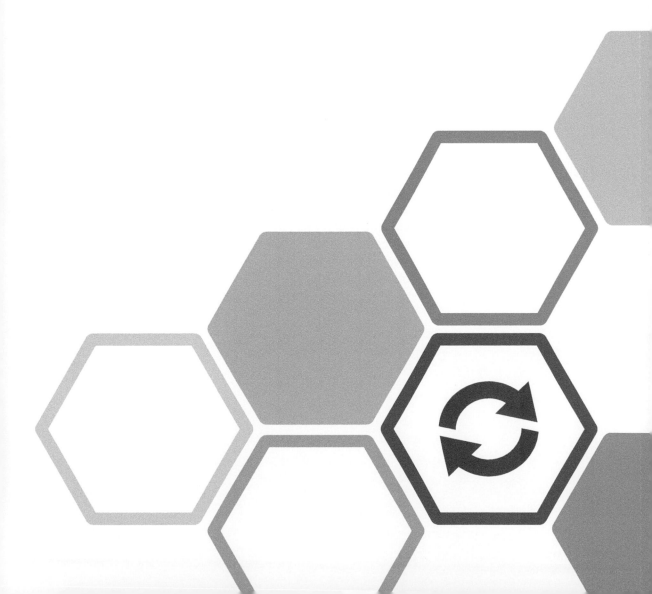

Carrita's Story

"You need to stop coming in here every time your belly hurts. There's nothing wrong with you. We can't help you."

It was the third time in a week that I had been in the emergency department. I was 25 weeks pregnant and something was wrong, but nobody was listening. "Please, I can't risk losing another child," I begged.

The nurse knew my pregnancy was high risk. Four weeks earlier, at a routine appointment, my doctor said, "You've got an incompetent cervix." *Incompetent*—as if I had done something wrong—but what it meant was my cervix had shortened significantly and I needed an emergency cervical cerclage. For the fourth time that week, I was back. At 26 weeks, I was having contractions.

They triaged me and put baby monitors on my belly. I gripped the bed rails in pain while my pregnant nurse told me all about her pregnancy and once again that nothing was wrong with me.

Why won't anyone believe me? Help me?

Finally, my doctor came in and said she'd check my cervix. Finally! For a week, I've been begging someone to just check. The color drained from her face. "You're already six centimeters dilated, and I can feel his feet." Her voice sounded urgent. I was in labor, but the cerclage was still there, and I was terrified.

"Will he survive? Will I survive?" were some of my last thoughts before heading back for an emergency C-section. Fourteen weeks early, this wasn't supposed to happen.

Immediately after my delivery, my son was rushed to the NICU, but not before letting me hear him cry. Something doctors said he wouldn't do because of his underdeveloped lungs. Everything in my high-risk pregnancy had been a fight. I had to be my own advocate. I fought for my son, and now he was fighting for me, I told myself when I heard him cry. My fight didn't end after I gave birth or when we left the NICU. Yeah, I'd given birth to a fighter, two of them.

Source: Illinois Maternal Health Digital Storytelling Project. Carrita's Story. September 8, 2022. https://www.youtube.com/watch?v=jGKjPWgkQQU

Chapter 24

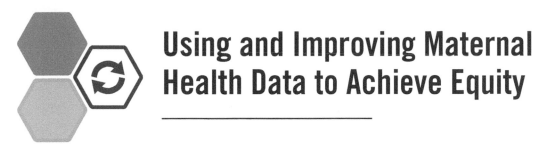

Using and Improving Maternal Health Data to Achieve Equity

LINDSEY YATES

R eaders may have noticed all the statistics in this book. In addition to the infographics spaced throughout, many of the chapters include data. Data are more than percentages, rates, or a series of numbers. Data are systematically collected to help us understand what is happening to us or around us. Data are collected and used for making key decisions. Data help us determine what we will prioritize, whom to include in our efforts, and how much time or money to invest to solve a problem.

In this section of the *Practical Playbook,* data are central. Data are foundational to any playbook: Imagine a coach, their staff, and their team facing a critical moment in a game. To determine what to do, they will consult a playbook that lists data they can use to optimize their chances to win. We are facing a critical moment for maternal health, and in this playbook we also provide data. The statistics we cite, however, are not just numbers for succeeding at a game. These numbers represent people. They represent lived experiences, including children and families who are navigating life without a parent, partner, or family member. They represent affected communities that unjustly and disproportionately experience poor outcomes. They represent community groups, organizations, and neighborhoods that have lost contributing members.

We know that maternal health data are important and have significant meaning, but other questions need to be answered. For example: What data are available? How should we collect maternal health data? Which data-collection methods can we use? The purpose of this section of the playbook is not to list statistics but to answer some of these questions by describing and evaluating current US maternal health data, including data metrics and data-collection methods.

Lindsey Yates, *Using and Improving Maternal Health Data to Achieve Equity* In: *The Practical Playbook III.* Edited by: Dorothy Cilenti, Alisahah Jackson, Natalie D. Hernandez, Lindsey Yates, Sarah Verbiest, J. Lloyd Michener, and Brian C. Castrucci, Oxford University Press. © de Beaumont Foundation 2024. DOI: 10.1093/oso/9780197662984.003.0024

The chapters in this section aim:

- To highlight the strengths and challenges of collecting, analyzing, and using current data sources to address inequities in maternal health
- To identify opportunities and novel designs to better address data inequities
- To describe how to partner with communities to collect and disseminate data for research and program evaluation

Like all data, maternal health data have many features and present some challenges. Each chapter in this section describes a feature of maternal health data or a challenge to collecting and using it. Contributing authors provide practical strategies, tools, and methods that stakeholders can leverage in the collection and use of maternal health information.

The United States collects a lot of data about maternal health. People and organizations invested in improving maternal health outcomes want to use that data to inform their work. This section begins by summarizing the available maternal morbidity and mortality data at the federal and state levels. In "Democratizing Data: Understanding the Challenges and Opportunities for Community-Based Utilization of Maternal Mortality Data and In Maternal Health Interventions," Athena Cross and Pam Silberman describe US maternal morbidity and mortality data and outline opportunities for making that information more accessible to communities.

Data should be collected ethically and address questions that are meaningful to the people about whom research is undertaken. Researchers also must acknowledge the harmful ways research has been used to exploit and traumatize marginalized people. Alayah Jennings-Johnson, author of the chapter "Decolonizing Maternal Health Research: An Introduction to Indigenous Research Methods and a Decolonial Framework for Indigenous Maternal Health Research," describes Indigenous research methods and how we can be better data users and partners to Indigenous communities.

Many of the data cited in this playbook are quantitative—numbers. Maternal health data also can be qualitative. It can, and should, include stories from those who experience poor maternal health outcomes: women and birthing people. In one of the chapters dedicated to qualitative data, "Maternal Health and Gathering Evidence of Structural Racism," Lauri Andress addresses the importance of using qualitative data to understand the impact of racism on maternal health outcomes. In the chapter, "Using Narrative Medicine and Longitudinal Qualitative Research to Examine Maternal Health Outcomes," which follows the chapter by Andress, Burcu Bozkurt outlines how to use two novel research methods to better understand women and birthing people's experiences.

In addition to yielding aggregated data, or data that summarize population-level outcomes, data measures can be applied to understanding individual-level health status. A variety of data measures—each with strengths and limitations—are used to inform clinical decisions about childbirth and pregnancy. "Garbage In, Garbage Out: Examining How Maternal Health Data Tools Misuse Race," the chapter by Marie V. Plaisime, examines the origins of two data measures—body mass index and the algorithm for vaginal birth after caesarean—and their implications for racial disparities in maternal health outcomes.

In addition to using data to try to understand what is happening, we use data to evaluate what we have done. Program evaluation is an essential function of health programs and interventions, especially if we want to replicate or scale them. To successfully evaluate a program or intervention we need local data, and we need strong community engagement. The chapter "Culturally Responsive Evaluation," written by Kimberley Broomfield-Massey, Rakiah Anderson, Calondra Tibbs, and Christine Tucker, describes a framework that centers community and supports use of local data.

Some data issues not covered in these chapters are important to highlight. First, although the United States has a robust maternal health data system, some data are missing. For example, there are limited data about childbirth and pregnancy complications among transgender and nonbinary populations. Missing data are a multifaceted issue. When we do not have data about certain groups, it means that their outcomes are often invisible, which limits our use of evidence-based strategies to improve outcomes. While data often are absent because we can't or won't prioritize their value, exclusion from data systems may offer protection from harmful surveillance or the politicized efforts to hurt certain populations.[1] Next, not all researchers who regularly analyze data are adept at making their results easy for others to understand. We create and share charts and graphs, but we do not always do a good job of explaining what the information means—we make data literacy the responsibility of the reader and the audience. Instead, we should endeavor to make data easier to understand as well as useful to everyone. Finally, there is a long history of racial disparities in maternal health outcomes. We know that those outcomes are rooted in racism, sexism, poverty, and other systems of oppression, yet our data systems do not typically include measures that account for that reality. There is ongoing work to develop standard measures for structural racism and structural sexism.[2-6] Including those measures in data sets will better inform our approach to addressing racial disparities in maternal health.

The chapters in this section are written for anyone who needs or wants to use maternal health data, including students, community organizers, researchers, and evaluators. No data set or system is perfect, and it is imperative to understand what information we have, how we can use it, and how we can improve it.

REFERENCES

1. Onuoha M, Sampath S, Braithwaite M, Faife C. On missing data sets. https://github.com/MimiOnuoha/missing-datasets?msclkid=6158c200a93011ec8b2abd718ffa00c1. Published January 24, 2018. Accessed January 18, 2023.

2. Homan P. Structural sexism and health in the United States: a new perspective on health inequality and the gender system. *Am Sociol Rev*. 2019;84(3):486–516. doi:10.1177/0003122419848723.

3. Brown TH, Homan PA. Frontiers in measuring structural racism and its health effects. *Health Serv Res*. 2022;57(3):443–447. https://doi.org/10.1111/1475-6773.13978.

4. Hardeman RR, Homan PA, Chantarat T, Davis BA, Brown TH. Improving the measurement of structural racism to achieve antiracist health policy. *Health Aff*. 2022;41(2):179–186. doi:10.1377/hlthaff.2021.01489.

5. Chantarat T, van Riper DC, Hardeman RR. Multidimensional structural racism predicts birth outcomes for Black and white Minnesotans. *Health Serv Res*. 2022;57(3):448–457. https://doi.org/10.1111/1475-6773.13976.

6. Adkins-Jackson PB, Chantarat T, Bailey ZD, Ponce NA. Measuring structural racism: a guide for epidemiologists and other health researchers. *Am J Epidemiol*. 2022;191(4):539–547. doi:10.1093/aje/kwab239.

Chapter 25

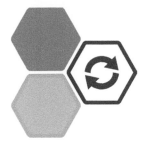

Democratizing Data: Understanding the Challenges and Opportunities for Community-Based Utilization of Maternal Mortality Data and Maternal Health Interventions

ATHENA CROSS AND PAM SILBERMAN

INTRODUCTION

Historically, egregious inequities in maternal mortality and morbidity, exacerbated by policies and strategies grounded in white supremacy, have perpetuated inequities in maternal health. Today, policymakers and advocates agree that for any strategy that addresses maternal mortality and morbidity to be successful, it must include investments in community-based resources. This realization is reflected in the Biden administration's White House Blueprint for Addressing the Maternal Health Crisis[1] and in policies like the 2021 Build Back Better Act's Kira Johnson Act (S 1042/HR 1212),[2,3] Social Determinants for Moms Act (S 851/HR 943),[4,5] and the Perinatal Workforce Act of 2021 (S 287/HR 945).[6-8] These policies and the maternal health crisis blueprint recognize that improvements in maternal health cannot happen without resources for community-based and community-driven interventions.

Despite research supporting the need for community-based resources, existing policies and practices make it difficult for community groups to engage meaningfully in efforts to address maternal mortality and morbidity.[9] This is in part related to a lack of access to maternal health data.

Athena Cross and Pam Silberman, *Democratizing Data* In: *The Practical Playbook III*. Edited by: Dorothy Cilenti, Alisahah Jackson, Natalie D. Hernandez, Lindsey Yates, Sarah Verbiest, J. Lloyd Michener, and Brian C. Castrucci, Oxford University Press. © de Beaumont Foundation 2024. DOI: 10.1093/oso/9780197662984.003.0025

Maternal health data provide communities with necessary information on maternal mortality rates, trends in maternal death, leading causes of death, racial inequities in maternal death, and, often, preventability. A recent national review found that, despite momentum and increased attention in the nation to racial disparities in maternal mortality, our ability to truly understand the scope of the problem and leverage data is limited.[10]

This chapter explores publicly available data and data sources, shortcomings of the data, and opportunities to improve data availability for community-based use. The chapter discusses state and federal sources of maternal health data and the advantages and disadvantages of the data for community utilization. It also highlights promising state and federal interventions that may affect community-based organizations that focus on improving maternal health outcomes.

STATE DATA

Maternal Mortality Review Information Application

In 2019, the Centers for Disease Control and Prevention (CDC) created the Enhancing Reviews and Surveillance to Eliminate Maternal Mortality (ERASE MM) program to work with Maternal Mortality Review Committee (MMRC) review processes that inform recommendations for preventing deaths.[11,12] Through the ERASE MM program, a standardized data-collection framework called the Maternal Mortality Review Information Application (MMRIA, commonly referred to as "Maria") was developed; it was designed to facilitate MMRC functions through a common data language.[11] MMRIA was created as a data standardization tool and a first step toward fully understanding the causes of maternal mortality and eliminating preventable maternal deaths.[11] Currently, 30 MMRCs covering 31 states are funded by the CDC and participate in MMRIA data collection.[11]

MMRIA collects qualitative data in the form of narrative reports from MMRCs, hospitals, physicians, transportation/ambulance services, and coroners.[13] Additionally, MMRIA collects maternal death data, including whether a death was pregnancy-related, pregnancy-associated, or pregnancy-related but not pregnancy-associated, cause of death, preventability, demographics, prenatal/labor and delivery/postpartum data, hospitalizations, and social and environmental considerations.[13] MMRIA also recommends that states review any other sources of medical care and conduct informant interviews with families, friends, personal support, and medical staff.[13] The breadth of information collected in the MMRIA database is robust, and because race/ethnicity data are collected, MMRIA allows for the evaluation of maternal death with racial/ethnic consideration. A CDC working group has developed definitions for racism and interventions aimed at addressing racism that MMRCs can use as part of the MMRIA tool.[14]

While the MMRIA database is the most comprehensive resource for state-level maternal mortality data, this information has important limitations. First, not all states participate and use these data-collection standards. Further, MMRIA data are not publicly available and are only accessible to the CDC and the state MMRC. Finally, despite adoption of MMRIA's standardized data collection, there are no standardized data publication requirements, resulting in inconsistency in the way MMRCs present mortality data.

The MMRIA data set contains standardized information across states that could help community groups identify the states that appear over time to do the best job addressing maternal mortality. It is imperative that the CDC democratize MMRIA data and make it publicly available. Furthermore, it is important not only to create standardization in data collection but also to develop public reporting standards that will help advocates and community members better understand and interpret maternal mortality in their states.

MMRCs

The most pertinent place to get publicly available state data on maternal deaths is the state MMRC report. In 2018, Congress enacted the Preventing Maternal Deaths Act (HR 1318), which established the creation of MMRCs. MMRCs are multidisciplinary bodies convened at the state and/or jurisdictional level to comprehensively review maternal deaths during, or within one year of, pregnancy.[11] MMRCs have access to both clinical and nonclinical information, including vital records, medical records, police reports, and social service records. The MMRCs use these data to better understand the circumstances surrounding each maternal death.[11] They also develop recommendations for preventing similar deaths.[11] MMRCs collect a broad range of statewide maternal mortality data, and this information is shared with the public through published reporting. As of 2022, 49 states and three cities have an MMRC; 33 states formed an MMRC between 2011 and 2022.[10]

Categorization of Maternal Deaths

The definitions of maternal deaths and maternal mortality rates vary by MMRC. Such deaths are categorized in two primary ways:

- Pregnancy-related deaths are deaths that occur as a result of a pregnancy complication during pregnancy or within one year of the end of pregnancy.[15] For instance, a pregnancy-related death may be related to cardiac conditions, hemorrhage, or infection (to name a few causes). Identification of pregnancy-related deaths has improved with changes in how coroners code causes of death and because a pregnancy checkbox has been added to death records, which aids in identifying such deaths. Nonetheless, errors in reported pregnancy status on death records still occur and can lead to over- or underestimation of the number of pregnancy-related deaths.[16]

- Pregnancy-associated deaths are deaths due to any cause during pregnancy or within one year of the end of pregnancy.[15] Causes of pregnancy-associated deaths include suicide, homicide, accidental drug overdose, and unrelated cancer.

Other Maternal Health Data Available Through MMRC Reports

In addition to mortality data, states have the option to present data on preventability, leading cause of death, race/ethnicity, and maternal morbidity. Like maternal mortality data, data on these outcomes vary by MMRC.

Preventability

Thirty-two states and the city of Philadelphia publish preventability data, which usually are expressed as a percentage.[10] In a recent review of state MMRCs, the preventability percentage ranged from 100% in Idaho to 19% in Wisconsin.[10] Generally, in the states that report pregnancy-related deaths (24 of 32 states), 60% to 100% of deaths were preventable.[10] Eleven states also publish a pregnancy-associated preventability percentage, which may include drug overdose, car accidents, and suicide. In eight states that provided these data, preventability percentages range from 60% to 100%.[10,15] Mortality rates and preventability percentages combine to tell a story of not only how pregnant and birthing people die but also whether the deaths were preventable. This information is critical to community-based efforts and can inform and shape the types of resources and interventions created. The dimension of preventability indicates that, with "reasonable" intervention, the deaths may have been prevented, providing the opportunity to develop targeted interventions to address the preventable causes.

Leading Cause of Death

In reporting the leading cause of death (LCD), states may publish pregnancy-related LCD, pregnancy-associated LCD, or both. Forty-two states plus New York City and Philadelphia publish the leading causes of maternal death.[10] Understanding the LCD can help community-based organizations to develop interventions that address one or several specific causes.

Race/Ethnicity

Some states also publish race- and ethnicity-based mortality data, which are particularly helpful in tracking efforts to reduce disparities in maternal mortality or morbidity. Thirty-four states, plus the cities of New York and Philadelphia, publish race data for pregnancy-related deaths, and 26 states and

Philadelphia publish race data for pregnancy-associated deaths.[10] Twenty-two states plus Philadelphia publish race data for both pregnancy-related and pregnancy-associated deaths.[10] However, 15 states plus Washington, DC, have not published any maternal race data.[10] Even among states that report the data, the information varies from state to state and even within states over time. States may report on different races/ethnicities or publish the data in one report but not a subsequent one. This hinders external stakeholders from developing effective interventions aimed at addressing racial/ethnic disparities.[10]

Maternal Morbidity

Six states plus Washington, DC, and New York City also focus on maternal morbidity. Tracking morbidity cases or trends allows states to investigate and develop recommendations for interventions that may potentially reduce maternal death and better target state-based efforts. The fact that so few states track morbidity data demonstrates a gap in state-based efforts.[10]

Other Data

Some MMRC reports provide additional maternal demographic data, including maternal age, education, and insurance status. Although not often reported, the timing of death from pregnancy is provided by some states, which offers more insight into when people are dying and helps to target interventions. Some states provide the timing of prenatal care initiation, demonstrating whether maternal mortality is influenced by when a person initiates prenatal care. Additionally, some states provide data on mental health and substance use, suicide, obesity, and hypertension. Finally, some states provide county-level data.

Challenges of Using MMRC Data

MMRC published reports are not without flaws, and meaningful interpretation of state data is challenging. Because states present data inconsistently, state-to-state comparison and even state-based analysis from one report to the next can be impossible. States have different reporting frequencies, different definitions of maternal death (death within one year, death within 42 days postpartum), and different ways of reporting racial and ethnic differences in mortality (if this information is provided at all). Even basic components, such as the state-established MMRC report frequency, ranges from every six months (in Hawaii and Philadelphia, for example) to every five years (in Massachusetts, for example).[10] Within states, one report may cover one year while another may cover multiple years. This means that individuals and community-based organizations cannot rely on consistent availability of MMRC data. Further, after a state publishes its MMRC report, it may not consistently present the same information in its next one, adding to the challenge for community-based organizations to understand state maternal mortality trends.

FEDERAL DATA

Federal data sets are aggregates of state-level data that are provided to the federal government. Federal data may come from several sources, including state departments of health, Medicaid claims data, and mortality data provided by the state, city, or county coroner's office. Standardization in data collection is guided by the CDC Model Surveillance Protocols, which provide guidance on surveillance methods to foster consistency in practice and to result in data that are more accurate and comparable.[17] The CDC protocols provide standardization of case definitions (uniform criteria for reporting cases), indicator development (environmental and public health indicators and indicators for chronic disease), and classifications of disease (classification of disease for morbidity coding). These standards help to ensure that jurisdictions are using a common language with common definitions so that state data can be compared.[17]

In the case of the Pregnancy Risk Assessment Monitoring System (PRAMS), the protocols ensure the standardization of data-collection methodologies that allows single-jurisdiction or multijurisdictional analysis.

PRAMS Data

PRAMS was developed in 1987 to collect site-specific, population-based data on maternal attitudes and experiences before, during, and shortly after pregnancy.[18] PRAMS provides data unavailable from other sources, and its surveillance currently covers about 81% of all US births.[18] The data are used to investigate emerging issues in the field of reproductive health and to plan and review programs and policies aimed at reducing health problems among mothers and infants.[18]

PRAMS collects de-identified data through a two-part survey tool given to a sample of people who recently have given birth.[18] The first part of the survey includes core questions focused on the participant's most recent birth, preconception and prenatal care, cigarette and alcohol use, breastfeeding, and physical abuse.[18] Questions in the second portion of the survey are chosen from a list developed by the CDC or state.[18]

The assessment provides overarching race and ethnicity data for survey participants; however, there is no way to determine racial and ethnic differences in survey responses. For instance, while some questions ask about the experience of "discrimination," without the overlay of race/ethnicity, it is impossible to determine who is experiencing discrimination and whether race or ethnicity factors into this experience.

The CDC publishes state-level maternal and child health indicators on the PRAMS website. States also may publish a more comprehensive state-based report. Community-based organizations or individuals researching or working on maternal health can use PRAMS data to understand a broad range of information related to pregnancy. However, they may be challenged when attempting to understand racial/ethnic considerations in these data. While PRAMS does not provide mortality statistics, it is a good example of democratized state- and territory-level data that are publicly available for broad utilization.

Pregnancy Mortality Surveillance System

The Pregnancy Mortality Surveillance System (PMSS), developed in 1986, is another federal data set about maternal health, specifically maternal mortality. PMSS uses epidemiologists to review and analyze death records, birth records, and fetal death records, if applicable, from all 50 states, New York City, and Washington, DC.[16] PMSS uses the National Vital Statistics System (NVSS) via the Wide-ranging Online Data for Epidemiologic Research (CDC WONDER) database to calculate the national pregnancy-related mortality rate. This rate is an estimate of the number of pregnancy-related deaths for every 100,000 live births.[16] This data set counts births for US residents and nonresidents that occur within the United States.[16] Counts can be obtained by state, county, urbanization, child's gender and weight, mother's race, age, education, gestation period, prenatal care, birth plurality, and medical and tobacco-use risk factors.[16]

The main difference between PMSS mortality data and NVSS data is that while NVSS reviews deaths up to 42 days postpartum, PMSS defines a pregnancy-related death as the death of a woman while pregnant or within one year of the end of pregnancy from any cause related to or aggravated by the pregnancy.[16] PMSS data are limited by a significant time lag, and available reporting covers maternal deaths only from 1987 through 2018 (the most recent data available).[16] Other sources, such as MMRC reports, potentially can provide more granular and up-to-date mortality data.

STATE INTERVENTIONS TO ADDRESS MATERNAL HEALTH

MMRC and Perinatal Quality Collaborative Interventions

MMRCs may create interventions, and these efforts may include development of policies or targeted interventions for healthcare providers or families. Only two states (Arizona and Colorado), however, publicly state that they develop interventions around maternal health equity.[10] While MMRCs may occasionally take a role in developing interventions, the majority of state-based interventions are formed through a state Perinatal Quality Collaborative (PQC).

Forty-seven states have a PQC, most of which were formed between 2010 and 2020 and build systems-level interventions centered on hospitals (primarily labor and delivery). In 2022, 36 of 47 states with a PQC focused on implementing Alliance for Innovation in Maternal Health (AIM) interventions, or patient safety bundles. Of the 11 states with a PQC that have not implemented an AIM bundle, six are not enrolled in AIM interventions and five are in development. Most states that have implemented AIM bundles focus on reducing severe hypertension in pregnancy, helping pregnant or postpartum people with substance-use disorder, or reducing cesarean births or obstetric hemorrhage.[10] Community-based organizations can learn from the PQC which interventions are being implemented in the state and then seek information about whether the efforts have led to changes in maternal mortality.

State Interventions to Address Racial Disparities in Maternal Health Outcomes

If we look holistically at both MMRC and PQC approaches to maternal mortality, efforts to address racial inequities can be found in 23 states and two jurisdictions (New York City and Washington, DC).[10] States may implement one or multiple interventions to address racial inequities. Ten states have implemented the AIM Reduction in Peripartum Racial and Ethnic Disparities (RED) safety bundle, 12 states investigate or consider racial disparities in their scope of work, two states have PQC committees focused on racial inequities, and seven states developed recommendations to address racial disparities in maternal mortality.[10]

The RED bundle is intended to provide health systems with insight into racial and ethnic disparities in maternal outcomes, the factors that are modifiable in a healthcare system, and resources that can be used to address these factors to achieve safe and equitable health.[19] The interventions focus on data, training, and communication to improve the quality of care offered by healthcare providers to people of color,[19] and although the RED bundle builds the framework for beginning to recognize racial inequities, it focuses on the modifiable factors in a hospital system.

The biggest shortcoming in the reliance on AIM bundles as a primary statewide collaborative effort to address maternal mortality is that these interventions are directed at the hospital level. Research shows that only 17% of US maternal deaths occur during labor and delivery.[20] Approximately 31% of deaths occur during pregnancy and 52% of deaths occur between one and 365 days postpartum. Despite the fact that nearly 83% of maternal deaths occur outside of labor and delivery settings, no coordinated statewide efforts exist to address this problem.[20]

FEDERAL INTERVENTIONS TO ADDRESS MATERNAL HEALTH

Numerous federal policies, such as the state option for expanded postpartum Medicaid coverage, support expansion of federal resources to address maternal mortality and morbidity. Medicaid coverage provides needed access to birthing services—it covers 42% of US births and approximately 65% of births to Black birthing people. Research suggests that expanded postpartum Medicaid coverage plays an important role in improving maternal and perinatal health outcomes. Timely postpartum visits provide the opportunity to assess a woman's physical recovery from pregnancy and childbirth.[21,22] Such policies and medical strategies focused on increasing access to services and quality of care can help address maternal deaths.

Yet, while there is a focus on increasing access to some services, there are competing policy changes that threaten any potential progress. For example, the US Supreme Court's decision in *Dobbs v Jackson Women's Health Organization*, overturning *Roe v Wade,* will force people to bring to term unintended or mistimed pregnancies. The duality of our national approaches, the push and pull between supporting birthing people and concurrently enacting policies likely to cause harm, is indicative of the challenges of creating national efforts to address maternal mortality and morbidity.

OPPORTUNITIES FOR COMMUNITY-BASED ORGANIZATIONS TO USE DATA AND LEVERAGE INTERVENTIONS

Despite the shortcomings of MMRC reports, MMRCs still are the most relevant source of maternal mortality data. Although community-based organizations looking to leverage state data in developing interventions may be challenged in determining trends or racial inequities, the wealth of information contained in these reports is the most reliable source of state-based data. Community-based organizations and other advocates should compel their MMRCs to commit to providing consistent data in all published reports to enhance the usability of these resources.

Policies and interventions aimed at increasing access to medical providers need to be coupled with community-based strategies. Community-based resources, such as doulas and perinatal health workers, have been shown to reduce preterm and low-birth-weight babies, increase initiation of breastfeeding, facilitate culturally specific birthing practices, and successfully serve as advocates, coaches, and support throughout the prenatal, labor and delivery, and postpartum periods.[23,24] But Medicaid reimbursement for doulas, perinatal health workers, midwifery, and lactation support may be insufficiently covered or not covered at all and may include costly licensure or certification requirements that exclude community-based providers. Without a focus on implementation practices, policy changes by themselves may not be effective in improving health outcomes for underserved populations. Expansion of Medicaid coverage should also encompass increases in reimbursements and reasonable contracting language to allow community-based providers to fully participate in delivery of care.[25]

If we are to address maternal mortality and severe maternal morbidity in this nation, it is imperative that multilevel, multidisciplinary, coordinated interventions be implemented across the entire perinatal continuum. Community-based organizations can help develop strategies that are grounded in actual need, as opposed to strategies that may be influenced by misconceptions rooted in white supremacy when community involvement is absent.[25] To do this, community-based organizations need not only private and public resources and fair insurance reimbursements but also access to reliable, meaningful data.[25] For this, data must be democratized and made available to all parties interested in developing interventions, not just federal and state agencies.

REFERENCES

1. White House. White House blueprint for addressing the maternal health crisis. 2022. https://www.whitehouse.gov/wp-content/uploads/2022/06/Maternal-Health-Blueprint.pdf.

2. Kira Johnson Act. S 1042, 117th Cong, 2021.

3. Kira Johnson Act. HR 1212, 117th Cong, 2021. https://www.congress.gov/bill/117th-congress/house-bill/1212.

4. Social Determinants for Moms Act. S 851, 117th Cong, 2021.

5. Social Determinants for Moms Act. HR 943, 117th Cong, 2021.

6. A Bill to Direct the Secretary of Health and Human Services to Issue Guidance to States to Educate Providers, Managed Care Entities, and Other Insurers about the Value and Process of Delivering Respectful Maternal Health Care through Diverse and Multidisciplinary Care Provider Models, and for Other Processes. S 287, 117th Cong, 2022.

7. To Direct the Secretary of Health and Human Services to Issue Guidance to States to Educate Providers, Managed Care Entities, and Other Insurers about the Value and Process of Delivering Respectful Maternal Health Care through Diverse and Multidisciplinary Care Provider Models, and for Other Processes. HR 945, 117th Cong, 2022. https://www.congress.gov/bill/117th-congress/house-bill/945.

8. Taylor J, Bernstein A. Tracking progress of the Black Maternal Health Momnibus. https://tcf.org/content/data/black-maternal-health-momnibus-tracker/?agreed=1. Published online January 24, 2022. Accessed November 11, 2022.

9. Chinn JJ, Eisenberg E, Artis Dickerson S, et al. Maternal mortality in the United States: research gaps, opportunities, and priorities. *Am J Obstet Gynecol.* 2020;223(4):486–492. doi:10.1016/j.ajog.2020.07.021.

10. Cross A. Killing Black mothers: A review of maternal mortality and severe maternal morbidity of black women in the united states. Published online 2022.

11. Centers for Disease Control and Prevention. Enhancing reviews and surveillance to eliminate maternal mortality (ERASE MM). https://www.cdc.gov/reproductivehealth/maternal-mortality/erase-mm/index.html. Published 2022. Accessed November 11, 2022.

12. Callahan T, Zaharatos J, St Pierre A, Merkt PT, Goodman D. Enhancing reviews and surveillance to eliminate maternal mortality. *J Womens Health.* 2021;30(8):1068–1073. doi:10.1089/jwh.2021.0357.

13. Review to Action. *Maternal Mortality Review Committee Abstractor Manual*. 2020. https://www.reviewtoaction.org/national-resource/maternal-mortality-review-committee-abstractor-manual. Accessed November 11, 2022.

14. Hardeman RR, Kheyfets A, Mantha AB, et al. Developing tools to report racism in maternal health for the CDC Maternal Mortality Review Information Application (MMRIA): findings from the MMRIA Racism & Discrimination Working Group. *Matern Child Health J*. 2022;26(4):661–669. doi:10.1007/s10995-021-03284-3.

15. Review to Action. Definitions. https://reviewtoaction.org/learn/definitions. Accessed November 11, 2022.

16. Centers for Disease Control and Prevention. Pregnancy Mortality Surveillance System. https://www.cdc.gov/reproductivehealth/maternal-mortality/pregnancy-mortality-surveillance-system.htm. Published 2022. Accessed November 11, 2022.

17. Centers for Disease Control and Prevention Surveillance Resource Center. Methods. https://www.cdc.gov/surveillancepractice/guide.html. Published 2022. Accessed November 11, 2022.

18. Centers for Disease Control and Prevention. PRAMS. https://www.cdc.gov/prams/index.htm. Published 2022.

19. Howell EA, Brown H, Brumley J, et al. Reduction of peripartum racial and ethnic disparities: a conceptual framework and maternal safety consensus bundle. *Obstet Gynecol*. 2018;131(5):770–782. doi:10.1097/AOG.0000000000002475.

20. Tikkanen R, Gunja M, FitzGerald M, et al. Maternal Mortality Maternity Care US Compared to 10 Other Countries| Commonwealth Fund. https://www.commonwealthfund.org/publications/issue-briefs/2020/nov/maternal-mortality-maternity-care-us-compared-10-countries. Published online November 2020.

21. The Kaiser Family Foundation. Births financed by Medicaid. https://www.kff.org/medicaid/state-indicator/births-financed-by-medicaid/?currentTimeframe=0&sortModel=%7B%22colId%22:%22Location%22,%22sort%22:%22asc%22%7D. Published 2020. Accessed November 11, 2022.

22. Centers for Medicare & Medicaid Services. Prenatal and postpartum care: postpartum care. https://www.medicaid.gov/state-overviews/scorecard/postpartum-care/index.html. Accessed November 11, 2022.

23. Kett PM, van Eijk MS, Guenther GA, Skillman SM. "This work that we're doing is bigger than ourselves": A qualitative study with community-based birth doulas in the United States. *Perspect Sex Reprod Health*. 2022;54(3):99–108. doi:10.1363/psrh.12203.

24. Thomas M-P, Ammann G, Brazier E, Noyes P, Maybank A. Doula services within a Healthy Start program: increasing access for an underserved population. *Matern Child Health J*. 2017;21(suppl 1):59–64. doi:10.1007/s10995-017-2402-0.

25. HealthConnect One Issue Brief: Creating policy for equitable doula access. https://healthconnectone.org/wp-content/uploads/bsk-pdf-manager/2019/10/HCO_Issue_Brief-final_102419.pdf. Published online October 24, 2019.

Chapter 26

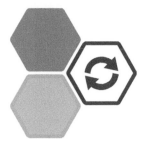

Decolonizing Maternal Health Research: An Introduction to Indigenous Research Methods and a Decolonial Framework for Indigenous Maternal Health Research

ALAYAH JOHNSON-JENNINGS

INTRODUCTION

The idea of "decolonizing" research is becoming more prevalent, especially among, and in recognition of, Indigenous women, who continue to experience large-scale oppression and marginalization. Using the term *decolonize* represents a commitment to rewriting and re-righting history. Decolonization must be an action, rather than a buzzword for the public.[1] When conducting Indigenous health research, individuals must decolonize their work because of the legacy of harm, mistrust, and historical trauma that many Indigenous women and children continue to face. Recognizing the inequities among Indigenous populations, maternal and child health stakeholders should seek to decolonize their work. This goes beyond talking about decolonization and includes considering if decolonization of a research study or program will transcend traditional boundaries and create actionable change.

As an Indigenous woman from the Choctaw, Quapaw, Sauk and Fox, and Miami nations, I seek to advance the various methods and approaches that go into collecting data and performing research with a decolonial lens. My approach to centering decolonial research and data stems from the need to give voice and power of an investigation to the participants. This includes the

Alayah Johnson-Jennings, *Decolonizing Maternal Health Research* In: *The Practical Playbook III*. Edited by: Dorothy Cilenti, Alisahah Jackson, Natalie D. Hernandez, Lindsey Yates, Sarah Verbiest, J. Lloyd Michener, and Brian C. Castrucci, Oxford University Press. © de Beaumont Foundation 2024. DOI: 10.1093/oso/9780197662984.003.0026

decolonial responsibility of deeming traditional practices, culture, and knowledge as acceptable and on par with Western practices, culture, and knowledge. When working with Indigenous women and children (and, arguably, all people), investigators must understand that their role is simply to facilitate the relationship between the tools they have access to and the desires of the population they are engaging. The community should always be the leader of the research. With this, it is important to keep in mind that the data one collects or chooses to use do not belong to the researcher but to the community, given Indigenous tribal data sovereignty over their citizens' data.[2]

This chapter provides background on Indigenous research methods, a discussion of the ethics involved when conducting research with Indigenous communities, and a description of a decolonial framework to utilize with Indigenous maternal and child health stakeholders. It summarizes how stakeholders can participate in the movement to decolonize research and data and go beyond using the term *decolonization* merely as a placeholder.

It is important to note that American Indian/Alaska Native persons and Indigenous populations are not a monolith. As of 2022, there were 574 federally recognized tribes in 35 states[3] and 63 state-recognized tribes in 11 states[4], and other tribes are seeking federal or state recognition. These communities have individual languages, cultures, and histories that should be respected. Furthermore, many Indigenous people do not live on reservations, but in urban communities.[3] Indigenous research methods and strategies for decolonizing data can be applied when interacting with any Indigenous populations.

INDIGENOUS RESEARCH METHODS

A plethora of information describes Indigenous research methods (IRM) and how they may be applied to Indigenous maternal and child health studies. In addition to exploring the literature about IRM, I have had the privilege of learning from Indigenous researchers who shared their understanding and use of IRM.[5] Most notable among them is Māori professor and activist Linda Tuhiwai Smith, who published her book *Decolonizing Methodologies: Research and Indigenous Peoples* in 1999, with subsequent editions in 2012 and 2021. This hallmark work is a guide for decolonizing Indigenous research, and her framework directs and affects research worldwide.[1] Shawn Wilson's *Research Is Ceremony*, published in 2008, further defined Indigenous research methods by emphasizing the role of relationships along the Indigenous research continuum.[6]

To properly conduct Indigenous research, a critical lens of decolonization and a recognition of relationships are crucial. Any research method needs to be reciprocal between the investigator and the community, with the understanding that the community and researcher have equal footing throughout the journey.

As Cameron et al wrote, "In Indigenous methodology, the process of research is more than the production of new knowledge."[7] A study of IRM's facilitators and barriers found that IRM requires more time than typical Western research. Hence, investigators who wish to pursue Indigenous maternal and child health issues need first to consider the ethics of doing so and how to appropriately undertake a study.

The Ethics of Doing Research in Indigenous Communities

Today, many Indigenous communities strongly advocate against researchers who are not connected to, or do not recognize their responsibility to, the community. A tragic history of unethical research on Indigenous women and children has been brought to light, demonstrating the impact of researchers who viewed Indigenous women and children as mere objects without recognizing them as humans deserving of the utmost respect. Brief descriptions of unethical treatment of Indigenous people during the 20th century, some of which took place under the auspices of the Indian Health Service, appear in Box 26.1. Investigators have been known to disappear after completing a study, never witnessing the lasting effects of their inquiry. The legacy of "helicopter research"—the idea that a researcher comes into the community to extract and exploit data for personal gain[8]—lives on in Indigenous communities, and Indigenous researchers have actively taken a position against the method by conducting their own studies in their own communities.[1] Sovereign nations within the United States also have established protocols to reduce the risk of helicopter research and harm being perpetuated in a particular Tribal community.

Tribal Approval

In addition to meeting the usual requirements of an institutional review board, a researcher must receive the approval of a Tribal ethics review board before beginning to collect data among Indigenous peoples or gaining access to data that a Tribe possesses. Tribal research permits have an array of styles and requirements and may require descriptions of all potential harms a study may incur, how the data could aid the Tribe in its development, how the data will be stored, who will have access to the found data, or how to connect to a Tribal community member who can vouch for the investigator and the need for the proposed study.

Whoever designs research tools and interprets data has great power. By designing our own tools, Indigenous peoples can highlight Indigenous theory and our traditional beliefs, histories, and related scientific research to appropriately answer our own questions. By requiring research permits, Tribal nations are taking a hand in redesigning research tools and ensuring their citizens' safety. All such requirements are established to reaffirm the investigator's responsibility and relationship to the community.

Box 26.1 | Historical Abuses of Indigenous Communities

Indigenous communities have a grim history when it comes to all things colonial, including research, especially among those most vulnerable, such as Indigenous women and children. Notoriously, in *Decolonizing Methodologies*, Linda Tuhiwai Smith wrote, "The word itself, 'research,' is probably one of the dirtiest words in the Indigenous world's vocabulary."[i] She went on to describe the reactions that we, as Indigenous peoples, feel upon hearing the word: bad memories, distrust, damage, exploitation. In documented reports filed by the US government, Indigenous women and children often experienced unethical medical abuses and were the subject of unethical research. Some examples are:

- 1900s–1930s: Before widespread use of sulfa, Indigenous women and children's eyelids were radically removed (in a procedure known as a tarsectomy) to prevent trachoma, an infectious bacterial eye disease. These are typically referred to as the "trachoma experiments."
- 1967–1973: The Indian Health Service (IHS) conducted trachoma experiments at three boarding schools in Utah, Arizona, and Nevada.[i] Indigenous children were typically sent against their family's will, treated inhumanely, and subject to rampant abuse in addition to unethical research. In these experiments, Indigenous children 6 to 12 years old—without parental consent and no documented child assent—were forced to take medications and undergo experimental treatment for preventing the eye disease.[ii]
- 1968–1982: It is estimated that 42% of American Indian/Alaska Native (AI/AN) women of childbearing age were forcibly sterilized.[i] Often, the sterilizations were completed by physicians working for the IHS. It was thought that AI/AN women were not sufficiently responsible to manage birth control effectively and that fewer AI/AN births would diminish the amount of taxpayer dollars directed toward welfare for this population.[i] Women who went into the hospital to deliver a child often left sterilized. If not forcibly sterilized, AI/AN patients were given birth control by the IHS that had not yet been approved for use by the Food and Drug Administration.[i-iv]
- 1972: The IHS used 300 children at three different boarding schools on the Navajo reservation as subjects to determine maximum dosing for iron.
- 1973–1974: The IHS and the University of Pittsburgh tested over 1,500 Indigenous children for a vitamin C study, again without obtaining parental consent or child assent.
- 1975: The IHS conducted experiments on 94 Apache children to study respiratory illnesses. Without fully informed parental consent, experimenters subjected the children to invasive laryngoscopy, aspirated their stomachs, and performed invasive blood draws.[i,ii]

Given past and present abuses and unethical research in Indigenous communities, decolonizing data requires learning from the past and following new protocols to protect the communities investigators work with.

REFERENCES

i. Smith LT. *Decolonizing Methodologies: Research and Indigenous Peoples.* Bloomsbury Academic & Professional; 2012. http://ebookcentral.proquest.com/lib/unc/detail.action?docID=1426837

ii. US Government Accountability Office. Investigation of allegations concerning Indian Health Service HRD-77-3. https://www.gao.gov/assets/hrd-77-3.pdf. Published 1976.

iii. Hodge FS. No meaningful apology for American Indian unethical research abuses. *Ethics Behav.* 2012;22(6):431–444.

iv. Lawrence J. The Indian Health Service and the sterilization of Native American women. *Am Indian Q.* 2000;24(3):400–419. http://www.jstor.org.libproxy.lib.unc.edu/stable/1185911.

Engaging with the Community through Partnerships

Relationships are necessary and critical when working to decolonize research and data. Many investigators wait to propose a project until after they have established ties and connection to a community. This can be as simple as attending community events to get involved. Some Tribes require researchers to first visit the community—the Cherokee Nation, for example, requires a two-week visit in the Tribal health clinic prior to initiating a study.[9] Working with a familiar face helps reduce power dynamics that may be introduced through the Western academy. In addition, the introductory interactions reinforce the researcher's obligations to the community.

Community ties must be maintained throughout the process, and consistent discussions with community stakeholders will ensure that the research continues to be appropriate for all stakeholders. Research is an evolving process, and the question one set out to answer may change. Being open to this change is key to creating meaningful work. However, the decision about changes should be led by the community rather than instituted by the investigator.

Finally, the relationship researchers develop with a community should be nurtured well after the project ends. The legacy of helicopter research created the need to continue bonds and trust between communities and individuals. Thinking of research as "kincentric" recognizes the relationships among everything in our world. Once ties are created, there is an expectation they will be maintained for years and decades beyond. If investigators cannot commit the time to properly engage with the community, they should reconsider conducting the study.

Community Involvement with Data

Indigenous communities maintain ownership of all data, and dissemination of the data is based on Indigenous data sovereignty—the inherent right of

Indigenous nations to govern the collection, analysis, and dissemination of their data—as well as ongoing ownership.[10] Since all data are owned by the community and not the researcher or university/entity, although the latter may steward the data, communities must be in control and voice their need for the data prior to collection.[2] "Specific data needs vary across Indigenous peoples and geographies, but there is broad agreement on the need for data [that] meet Indigenous data needs and aspirations."[11] Community direction and ownership do not cease with data collection but continue through data analysis—communities must also oversee and approve how data will be disseminated and used.

Although most Indigenous nations have an ethics review board to oversee research through dissemination, additional steps, such as creating a community advisory board (CAB) that includes key representatives from the Indigenous community, often are expected or required. Consistent meetings with the CAB provide a community the opportunity to influence a project each step of the way and to ensure that research is being done ethically to protect the population involved. Community engagement promotes the efficiency of a study and creates stronger results, and transparent research allows communities to suggest appropriate research techniques. Further, lessons will be learned on both sides to carry forward throughout the study and the researcher's career. Many times, these relationships have resulted in a community's seeking a researcher to conduct a project (rather than the opposite—a researcher approaching the community). These relationships also situate the researcher as a facilitator and an asset for participants to access for addressing their questions on their own terms. This is different from a situation in which an investigator engages in a project to further their career or to gain a grant, with the potential for exploiting Indigenous peoples in service to a funding mechanism or a manuscript.

When conducting a study or publishing data, stakeholders must develop agreements with the community about how data will be used and shared. For instance, Tribes sometimes prefer to keep data for their own use, without broader dissemination, an approach that may not align with the researcher's goals but must be respected nonetheless. Many times, researchers find themselves making two reports, one for the Tribal community and one for the academy. Prioritizing a report that has the information the Tribe seeks will emphasize the Tribe's control of the research and data.

IMPLEMENTING A DECOLONIAL FRAMEWORK FOR INDIGENOUS MATERNAL AND CHILD HEALTH RESEARCH

Tuhiwai Smith argued that decolonizing research is a risky but necessary endeavor when working with Indigenous communities.[1] She discussed the challenges of going against dominant Western paradigms and working to create space within dominant Western narratives, which may ostracize researchers from other colleagues. Her proposed decolonial framework includes the following actions: recovering subjugated knowledge, such as Indigenous traditional practices that were outlawed, and documenting social injustices, such as the research atrocities against Indigenous communities and forced sterilizations of Indigenous people. At the same time, she argued for Indigenous researchers and allies to give voice to those silenced and to challenge both colonialism and racism.[1] This can be done with both qualitative and quantitative data. For example, Indigenous quantitative data can be used to reaffirm Indigenous worldviews, well-being, and appropriate risk and protective factors, and many communities are using data this way today.[1] Using a decolonial framework requires that researchers engage with the community in which the study takes place and that they appreciate the community's history. Following are some factors to consider when gathering data using a decolonial lens.

Determine Whether the Research Is Wanted

Addressing the question of whether a study is desired by the community is the first step in creating decolonial research among Indigenous women and children. This action will shift the power dynamic and help to create meaningful change. The question is intertwined with involving the community with the data: The community should take the lead in data collection and must want the data in their own hands, perhaps even storing the data until an appropriate need arises.

Recognize Biased Perceptions of Indigenous People's Health

Western research has created a legacy of inherent bias, utilizing a paradigm of the individual that does not take into account the holistic nature of Indigenous thought and societies. In the Indigenous worldview, every piece of data and representation of such has a story to tell. Cunningham et al, for instance, debunked a common myth that Indigenous people suffer from alcoholism at higher rates than other groups; when the data are contextualized, Indigenous people's rates are lower than or equal to the rates of whites who live nearby.[12] Data from Indigenous communities can be examined for the purpose of reifying inherent biases or it can be contextualized and operationalized to demonstrate the health and well-being that exist in the community.

Within Indigenous communities, many investigators have focused on health disparities, including high rates of diabetes, obesity, and substance abuse, instead of examining why the disparities exist and what has contributed to these outcomes. These issues stem from the history of colonization that encouraged researchers to view Indigenous peoples as inferior and having deficits; colonialism and contextual factors that have affected the collective have not been thoroughly addressed. Without applying the lens of historical trauma and on-going oppression, we risk placing blame on the community for health disparities instead of on the systemic structures that have influenced them.

The social determinants of health (SDOH), or everyday lived and environmental factors that influence health and well-being, often go unnoticed in data that represent health disparities. Indigenous-specific SDOH include colonialism and related historical trauma.[13-15] For example, during the COVID-19 pandemic, data showed that American Indians and Alaska Natives were at increased risk of being infected with, and dying from, COVID,[16,17] but it is important to contextualize the data. These outcomes are related to SDOH and historical traumas, like long-standing poorly funded infrastructure, limited access to running water, and discrimination.[16,17] By contextualizing the findings, we can challenge colonialism in research, as Tuhiwai Smith advocates; we can begin to provide space for the voice of the silenced. Indigenous researchers and allies are working to include and address SDOH in their work: Instead of focusing on deficits, Indigenous researchers identify health through Indigenous worldviews, especially for Indigenous youth and women/mothers.[18-20] Indigenous communities and investigators are entering a time of thriving for our peoples in which we direct our research and our data on our own terms.

Acknowledge the Indigenous History That Impacts Women and Children

Indigenous communities strive to disrupt narratives that describe individual deficits and aim instead to contextualize the role of historical trauma in a colonial history of genocide. Indigenous peoples have endured hundreds of years of sexual violence being used as a tool for colonization and genocide. Particularly after European arrival, Indigenous women who were leaders, chiefs, and honored in Indigenous communities in the New World were attacked with sexual violence and the refusal to recognize their rightful roles as diplomats.[21,22] Today, the violence initiated at first contact lives on, with Indigenous women, girls, and two-spirit peoples going missing and being murdered at alarmingly high rates. Only recently has there been a surge in data and willingness to collect this information to address the epidemic of missing and murdered Indigenous women, girls, and two-spirit peoples.[23] From the mid-1800s through the 1960s, thousands of children as young as four years old were forcibly removed from their mothers and subjected to rampant sexual and physical abuse in Indian boarding schools far from home.[24] Traditional medicine, which many Indigenous women and mothers performed, was made illegal from the late 1800s until 1978 and was punishable by imprisonment.[25] Therefore, Indigenous mothers and children were unable to openly utilize traditional birthing practices and caretaking. Indigenous women were further subjected to shame and potentially losing their children to the federal government for utilizing traditional practices to raise babies, such as co-sleeping and breastfeeding for longer than 12 months. Not only were they subjected to unethical research, but also Indigenous females, both adults and children, were forcibly sterilized.[26] All of these traumatic events have an impact today in Indigenous communities and are frequently discussed among families.

These atrocities have resulted in ongoing disparities in maternal and child health. Indigenous peoples, and more particularly American Indian and Alaska Native (AI/AN) communities, face high rates of maternal and infant mortality in comparison to their white counterparts, and research suggests that AI/AN people also experience many maternal and infant health disparities that parallel the experiences of African American mothers and children.[27] The Urban Indian Health Institute released a report in 2016 that assessed the state of AI/AN health between 2010 and 2012 and found that the AI/AN maternal mortality rate was 4.5 times higher than the rate for non-Hispanic white women.[28] In the same study, only 60% of AI/AN pregnant people initiated prenatal care, compared with 81.6% of non-Hispanic white women. In the first year of life, AI/AN infants were 2.5 times more likely to die than their non-Hispanic white counterparts.[28]

It is important to recognize the ongoing impact the history of colonization and medical malpractice has on Indigenous peoples and their perceptions of research. Reasons for Indigenous people to mistrust the medical system are found across the history of abuse the population has experienced. There is considerable pan-Indigenous and Tribal-specific history to be acknowledged when working with Indigenous communities; researcher stakeholders must understand the specific history of the Indigenous population with which they intend to engage.

Celebrate Indigenous People's Strengths

Recognizing the strength of the Indigenous community and culture in data and research is vital. Often, data fixate on the negatives of a marginalized population. Indigenous mothers and children are strong and resilient—we have survived centuries of attempted genocide and brutal attempted colonization, yet we are still here, practicing our traditional ways. As Indigenous peoples, we take pride in who we are and the resiliency and willingness of our ancestors to survive as we move toward a renewed period of thriving.

Many Indigenous mothers and families rely on Indigenous cultural teachings and knowledge to raise resilient and healthy children, and many communities are seeking to identify how these practices best support maternal and child health. Therefore, in data collection for qualitative, quantitative, and mixed-method inquiries, researchers must also recognize and support how Indigenous peoples utilize their traditions and traditional knowledge. Studies have shown that maternal and child health can improve with the recognition of Indigenous knowledge about maternal and child health and by increasing cultural continuity and identity.[29-31] Commonly, ceremony is a significant part of bringing mind, body, and spirit together to develop a whole being and community.

Indigenous thought and worldview rely heavily on community ties. We understand that our ancestors survived on behalf of future generations, just as we are committed to creating a world where we are good ancestors for those who come after us. We use traditional knowledge to learn about the Earth, and many times, we have held traditional ecological knowledge in advance of its being deemed "scientifically acceptable" by the Western academy. Our stories are passed from generation to generation to promote our values and culture. We are a strengthened, full community that is learning to attain the thriving health we had before colonization.

Clearly Articulate the Potential Impact of Research

Research has long-standing implications for the community in which data are gathered. By not considering the impact of a study, stakeholders risk further stigmatizing communities. The study should be beneficial for the Tribal participant. To undertake an investigation or use Indigenous data, researchers must ask: Is the research beneficial for the community? Will the research open doors for future projects to benefit the community? What are the possible implications of the research? How will this study influence the relationships among the researcher, the researcher's institution, and the community?

Thinking about impact and doing effective work are vital in collecting decolonial data. Western thinking often promotes focusing on the moment rather than looking at long-term impact, and although this is changing with community-based participatory research and long-term research interventions that prioritize sustainability, it is always an important consideration.

CONCLUSION

Applying a decolonial lens requires relationships and a willingness to rethink the ways we collect and use data. Working in partnership creates the biggest difference. Researchers must interrogate the ways we gather evidence, our own biases, and the history of abuse against Indigenous communities. Although I write this from my positionality as an Indigenous woman, I believe that this information and epistemology can be applied among many historically marginalized populations, including non-Indigenous, racialized communities.

ACKNOWLEDGMENT

Thank you to Ronny Bell, PhD, MS (enrolled member of the Lumbee tribe) for reading a draft of this chapter and providing feedback.

REFERENCES

1. Smith LT. *Decolonizing Methodologies: Research and Indigenous Peoples*. New York: Bloomsbury Academic & Professional; 2012.

2. Tsosie R. Tribal data governance and informational privacy: constructing Indigenous data sovereignty. *Mont L Rev*. 2019;80:229.

3. US Department of Health and Human Services Office of Minority Health. American Indian/Alaska Native. https://www.minorityhealth.hhs.gov/omh/browse.aspx?lvl=3&lvlid=62#:~:text=Approximately%2070%20percent%20of%20American%20Indians%20and%20Alaska,areas%2C%20and%20are%20eligible%20to%20utilize%20this%20program. Published February 24, 2023. Accessed April 13, 2023.

4. National Conference of State Legislatures. State recognition of American Indian Tribes. https://www.ncsl.org/quad-caucus/state-recognition-of-american-indian-tribes. Published October 10, 2016. Accessed April 13, 2023.

5. Johnson-Jennings AC. Coming full circle: the facilitators and barriers of Indigenous research methods in the academy. Published online 2021.

6. Wilson, S. *Research Is Ceremony: Indigenous Research Methods*. Black Point, Nova Scotia: Fernwood; 2008.

7. Cameron BL, Carmargo Plazas MDP, Salas AS, Bourque Bearskin RL. Understanding inequalities in access to health care services for Aboriginal people: a call for nursing action. *Adv Nurs Sci*. 2014;37(3):E1–E16. doi:10.1097/ANS.0000000000000039.

8. Davis JD, Keemer K. A brief history of and future considerations for research in American Indian and Alaska Native communities. https://eric.ed.gov/?id=ED473270. Published online 2002.

9. Manson SM, Garroutte E, Goins RT, Henderson PN. Access, relevance, and control in the research process. *J Aging Health*. 2004;16(5 suppl):58S–77S.

10. Carroll SR, Rodriguez-Lonebear D, Martinez A. Indigenous data governance: strategies from United States Native Nations. *Data Sci J*. 2019;18:31. doi:10.5334/dsj-2019-031.

11. Walter M, Suina M. Indigenous data, Indigenous methodologies and Indigenous data sovereignty. *Int J Soc Res Methodol*. 2018;22(3):233–243. https://www.researchgate.net/publication/328148405_Indigenous_data_indigenous_methodologies_and_indigenous_data_sovereignty.

12. Cunningham JK, Solomon TA, Muramoto ML. Alcohol use among Native Americans compared to whites: examining the veracity of the 'Native American elevated alcohol consumption' belief. *Drug Alcohol Dependence*. 2016;160:65–75. https://doi.org/10.1016/j.drugalcdep.2015.12.015.

13. Czyzewski K. Colonialism as a broader social determinant of health. *Int Indigenous Policy J*. 2011;2(1):5. https://doi.org/10.18584/iipj.2011.2.1.5.

14. Weaver HN, Brave Heart MYH. Examining two facets of American Indian identity: exposure to other cultures and the influence of historical trauma. *J Hum Behav Soc Environ*. 1999;2(1-2):19–33.

15. Warne D, Lajimodiere D. American Indian health disparities: psychosocial influences. *Soc Pers Psychol Compass*. 2015;9(10):567–579. doi:10.1111/spc3.12198.

16. Hatcher SM, Agnew-Brune C, Anderson M, et al. COVID-19 among American Indian and Alaska Native persons—23 states, January 31–July 3, 2020. http://dx.doi.org/10.15585/mmwr.mm6934e1. Published 2020. Accessed April 13, 2023.

17. Arrazola J, Masiello MM, Joshi S, et al. COVID-19 mortality among American Indian and Alaska native persons—14 states, January–June 2020. *MMWR*. 2020;69(49):1853.

18. Jennings D, Lowe J. Photovoice: giving voice to Indigenous youth. *Pimatisiwin*. 2013;11(3):521–537.

19. Johnson-Jennings M, Billiot S, Walters K. Returning to our roots: Tribal health and wellness through land-based healing. *Genealogy*. 2020;4(3):91.

20. Minthorn RZ tah hol ah. Indigenous motherhood in the academy: building our children to be good relatives. *Wicazo Sa Rev*. 2018;33(2):62–75. doi:10.5749/wicazosareview.33.2.0062.

21. Deer S, Clairmont B, Martell CA, White Eagle ML. *Sharing Our Stories of Survival: Native Women Surviving Violence*. Walnut Creek, CA: AltaMira Press; 2007.

22. Guerrero MAJ. "Patriarchal colonialism" and indigenism: implications for Native feminist spirituality and Native womanism. *Hypatia*. 2003;18(2):58–69.

23. Urban Indian Health Institute. Missing and murdered Indigenous women and girls. https://www.uihi.org/resources/missing-and-murdered-indigenous-women-girls/. Published 2018. Accessed September 18, 2022.

24. Curcio AA. Civil claims for uncivilized acts: filing suit against the government for American Indian boarding school abuses. *Hastings Race Poverty L J*. 2006;4:45.

25. Suagee DB. American Indian religious freedom and cultural resources management: protecting Mother Earth's caretakers. *Am Indian L Rev*. 1982;10(1):1–58.

26. Lawrence J. The Indian Health Service and the sterilization of Native American women. *Am Indian Q*. 2000;24(3):400–419.

27. Truschel L, Novoa C. American Indian and Alaska Native maternal and infant mortality: challenges and opportunities. https://www.americanprogress.org/article/american-indian-alaska-native-maternal-infant-mortality-challenges-opportunities/. Published July 9, 2018. Accessed September 18, 2022.

28. Urban Indian Health Institute. Community health profile: national aggregate of Urban Indian Health Program service areas. Seattle, WA. Published online October 2016.

29. Johnson-Jennings M, Koushik P, Olson D, LaBeau M, Jennings D. Ode'imin Giizis: proposing and piloting gardening as an Indigenous childhood health intervention. *J Health Care Poor Underserved*. 2020;31(2):871–888. https://doi.org/10.1353/hpu.2020.0066.

30. Hallett D, Chandler MJ, Lalonde CE. Aboriginal language knowledge and youth suicide. *Cogn Dev*. 2007;22(3):392–399. https://doi.org/10.1016/j.cogdev.2007.02.001.

31. Weibel-Orlando J. Worlds of difference: inequality in the aging experience. doi:10.4135/9781483328539. Published online 2000.

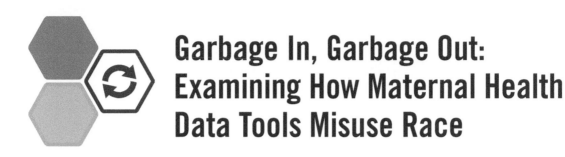

Chapter 27

Garbage In, Garbage Out: Examining How Maternal Health Data Tools Misuse Race

MARIE V. PLAISIME

INTRODUCTION

"Garbage in, garbage out" is a phrase often used in computer science to describe the quality and use of data points. Data, the information we use to make decisions, can be characterized as "good" or "bad." In general, good data are accurate, complete, and collected ethically. Bad data are insufficient and structurally flawed in some way. The type of data one uses affects the results one gets. As scientists, researchers, and health providers, our analysis and findings are only as good as our data. We rely on data to inform knowledge and best practices. When medical devices, tools, calculators, and even algorithms use bad data, the repercussions have unintended consequences, with extensive effects on patient populations.

This chapter describes how flawed data tools affect racial disparities in maternal health outcomes. First, the chapter addresses the concept of race and its relationship to maternal health. Next, the chapter offers two examples of medical tools that have historically used flawed data and discusses the effect on maternal health outcomes of using those tools. For example, the vaginal birth after cesarean (VBAC) algorithm and body mass index (BMI) are widely used to assess health conditions, yet they rely on biased, racialized data. The chapter concludes with critical questions to consider when selecting data points for practice, research, and evaluation.

Marie V. Plaisime, *Garbage In, Garbage Out* In: *The Practical Playbook III*. Edited by: Dorothy Cilenti, Alisahah Jackson, Natalie D. Hernandez, Lindsey Yates, Sarah Verbiest, J. Lloyd Michener, and Brian C. Castrucci, Oxford University Press.
© de Beaumont Foundation 2024. DOI: 10.1093/oso/9780197662984.003.0027

UNDERSTANDING RACE AND ITS IMPACT ON MATERNAL HEALTH

Race is a social construct, meaning that individuals are not born with an intrinsic sense of what it means to be a racialized identity (Black, American Indian/Alaska Native, white, as examples). Individuals learn the rules of racial identities through interactions with other people, the policies and practices of various institutions, and the environments in which they live. Race-associated differences in health outcomes, including maternal health, are routinely quantitatively and qualitatively documented in the United States.[1] These differences are rooted in access to, and interactions with, systems that were intentionally designed to provide benefits to certain racialized groups (white people) while simultaneously harming other racialized groups (Black people, for example). This is structural racism. (Further descriptions of structural racism and its impact on maternal health are found in Chapters 17 and 18.)

Race-based medicine uses a patient's race as the basis for clinical diagnosis or treatment. Here, race is considered an essential biological factor, even though we know that race is not biological. Using race to make medical decisions may harm patient care by providing separate care to different patient groups. For example, several clinical algorithms (formulas or mathematical equations that help doctors assess treatment plans for patients) and clinical tools have been adjusted to include race as an essential component for diagnosis and treatment. Some examples are the estimated glomerular filtration rate (eGFR), pulmonary function tests (PFTs), and the VBAC calculator.[2]

Every year in the United States, nearly 700 women die from preventable pregnancy-related or labor complications. An additional 60,000 women experience a highly preventable birth injury. When we further examine these outcomes by race, we see that Black women are three times more likely than white women to die from those complications or to experience a birth injury.[3] The rates can be even higher depending on where a Black woman lives.

For centuries, scientists and researchers believed that Black women had worse health outcomes because of their behaviors or because their bodies were naturally predisposed to bad health. The ideas that Black women were bad people and had bad health were part of the foundation of the field of obstetrics and gynecology and many data tools in use today. We now know that the poor outcomes Black women experience are the result of social and structural factors that disproportionately harm them. Two of the tools most used in maternal health, in fact, are based on bad data about Black women.

THE VBAC ALGORITHM

Birthing people have the option to give birth vaginally or through a surgical procedure known as a cesarean delivery, or C-section. Cesarean deliveries are essential procedures, but they have many potential complications, including infection, blood loss, damage to organs, extended recovery periods, and increased complications in future pregnancies. Cesarean deliveries also are associated with higher rates of maternal mortality and morbidity.[4] Furthermore, recent evidence shows that they may be overused, particularly for Black birthing people. Black women have higher rates of cesarean deliveries than white women.[5] For women who choose to have more than one child, having a cesarean for their first delivery may have implications for each of their future pregnancies. Every year, 20% of women who had a cesarean delivery with their first child face the decision of how to deliver their second child—they can opt to go through labor and attempt a vaginal delivery (VBAC) or they can choose a cesarean delivery.[6] Evidence demonstrates that birthing people can safely deliver a baby vaginally even if they had a cesarean in the past, but many hospitals and healthcare providers do not strongly support or offer VBAC.[7]

In 2007, the Eunice Kennedy Shriver National Institute of Child Health and Human Development (NICHD) created the VBAC calculator, which was designed to predict the success of VBAC. Various characteristics that had been shown to be associated with delivery were included in the VBAC calculator (Figure 27.1), including race, and when doctors entered race in the calculator, the algorithm predicted lower levels of VBAC success for women of color. This led to doctors' not offering VBAC to women of color.[2] The calculator inadvertently furthered racial disparities in cesarean delivery rates for Black women, thereby creating implications for maternal mortality and morbidity outcomes for Black women.

Citing these implications, health providers and researchers noted that including race in the calculator yielded flawed results, and they called for removing race from the algorithm. In 2021, the American College of Obstetricians and Gynecologists (ACOG) updated the VBAC calculator to no longer include race. Although this change in the calculator represents an important shift in how we use data to help patients make decisions about giving birth, it does not eliminate racism in obstetrics.[8] Removal of race from the VBAC algorithm alone does not nullify all relevant systemic and structural factors that shape labor and delivery outcomes; provider racial bias and other barriers to care may continue to limit racialized women's access to VBACs. Bearing this in mind, providers should endeavor to apply a person-centered approach, talk with patients about their desire for VBAC, and consider each individual's risks.

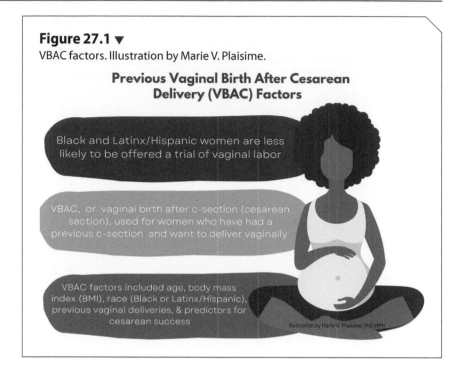

Figure 27.1 ▼
VBAC factors. Illustration by Marie V. Plaisime.

Previous Vaginal Birth After Cesarean Delivery (VBAC) Factors

Black and Latinx/Hispanic women are less likely to be offered a trial of vaginal labor

VBAC, or vaginal birth after c-section (cesarean section), used for women who have had a previous c-section and want to deliver vaginally

VBAC factors included age, body mass index (BMI), race (Black or Latinx/Hispanic), previous vaginal deliveries, & predictors for cesarean success

Illustration by Marie V. Plaisime, PhD MPH

BMI

BMI is a tool used to measure adiposity, or body fat. It considers an individual's height and weight to determine how likely that person is to experience various health outcomes, including heart disease, hypertension, and maternal morbidity and mortality. BMI is calculated by dividing a patient's weight in pounds or kilograms by height in inches or meters squared (CDC, 2022). Current BMI categories for adults age 20 and older include underweight (below 18.5), healthy weight (18.5–24.9), overweight (25.0–29.9), and obesity (30.0 and above). The BMI tool is widely used across many specialties and practices to determine eligibility for certain health services. Because it has no cost, the use of BMI in risk assessment has been implemented across many interventions and medical evaluations—it is intrinsically connected to our understanding of health and well-being. As a result, BMI has implications for the health resources people access.

Although viewed as beneficial, inexpensive, and seemingly neutral, the BMI tool was not originally intended to measure the distribution of body fat, muscle tone, or bone density. In the 19th century, Adolphe Quetelet, a Belgian sociologist, mathematician, and statistician, created a tool to assess ideal human attributes of "the average man." He created "ideal" measurements and deviation measurements relative to average white, male bodies. Metropolitan Life Insurance Company created the BMI cut points to determine who was the least risk to insure. In 1972, Ancel Keys, a researcher whose primary population of focus also was white men, recommended the Quetelet tool as the best way to measure body fatness and obesity, renaming it the body mass index. This brief history demonstrates that the BMI tool is rooted in racist and misogynoir practices.[9] The continued use of BMI must be critically evaluated.

Given the stigmatization of weight, there are implications of being categorized as "obese." People in this category typically are found to have worse health outcomes than people with "average" body weights. Current conventions suggest that obese individuals are at increased risk of worse health outcomes solely related to their weight. But this is not the complete picture, because obesity is a complex disease. When healthcare providers rely solely on the BMI, they may ignore or not provide quality care to individuals they perceive as obese,[10] and people of color who are seen as obese face additional discrimination in clinical settings.[9] As a result of this mistreatment, one poor outcome is that obese people may avoid visiting the doctor or may delay seeking medical attention.[11]

When we consider the relationship between BMI and maternal health, we see that women with higher BMIs are at increased risk of maternal morbidity and mortality.[12] The relationship between BMI and race makes maternal health outcomes more nuanced for racialized communities. Black women and birthing people are more likely to be categorized as overweight and obese.[13] This means that when they become pregnant, in addition to the discrimination they experience because of their race, they also face mistreatment because of their weight, which has implications for their pregnancies and deliveries. While the term *obese* is used by providers to describe patients, it also stigmatizes individual bodies. The term mischaracterizes risk, potentially affecting healthcare and health outcomes.

Although there are ongoing conversations and debates about the use of BMI, there is no consensus about a solution. Some researchers argue for updates to the BMI cut points, while others suggest that providers should instead carefully consider how and when they use BMI to assess a patient's health.[9] There are better data points, such as the social determinants of health, for assessing overall health. Evaluating the structural factors that affect health, such as access to green spaces and healthy food options, provides more relevant data.

The CDC continuously notes that Black, Latinx/Hispanic, and Indigenous communities are more likely to be obese and to suffer from associated risks. Still, we must interrogate these conclusions and recognize the underlying relationships between race, weight, and health. When determining care for a pregnant person, providers should look to lab results and people's lived experiences rather than rely solely on BMI to assess risk for health conditions like hypertension, preeclampsia, and gestational diabetes.

CONCLUSIONS AND CONSIDERATIONS FOR RESEARCHERS

The VBAC algorithm and BMI are just two examples of data tools based on bad data and racist ideas. We have made progress in addressing race-related maternal health disparities, but the gap persists and has grown worse during the COVID-19 pandemic. Some of the work yet to be done includes examining the data and data tools we use to answer research questions, to make health recommendations, to inform policies, and to evaluate interventions. With a growing understanding of the ways race has been incorrectly used to develop data and data tools, maternal healthcare providers, researchers, advocates, and evaluators must be cautious about selecting data—it is imperative that an antiracist and equity lens be applied to this work.

Researchers must critically assess and explore the origins of the data measures they plan to use. In recent decades, for example, individuals often have used race as a proxy for poverty. This flawed inclusion of race as a data point has implications for data collection and conclusions. Structural factors, such as geographic location and the social environment, provide more relevant information for a patient's health.[14] For example, research shows that residential location, age, marital status, and history of incarceration are associated with future risk of preterm births.[15] In her work about maternal health, Dr. Brittney Francis, a social epidemiologist, argued for investigating how social and structural factors, such as the built environment, contribute to maternal health.[16]

Before research begins, investigators should think deeply about which data and measures will produce high-quality results. Here are some questions to guide that process:

1. How do I define race in my research question and project? Why am I including it?
2. What are the origins and histories of the data measures I want to use?
3. If I want to do secondary data analysis, how were the data collected (e.g., through self-report or from an electronic medical record)?
4. If data measures previously have been associated with race, what was the association?
5. How has the race-based association been described? (For example, Black women have higher BMIs than women of other races, but this association is related to their lack of access to healthy food options and healthy public spaces.)
6. Can I include structural measures (racism, as an example) that better assess outcomes?

REFERENCES

1. Jones CP. Levels of racism: a theoretic framework and a gardener's tale. *Am J Public Health*. 2000;90(8):1212–1215. doi:10.2105/ajph.90.8.1212.

2. Vyas DA, Eisenstein LG, Jones DS. Hidden in plain sight—reconsidering the use of race correction in clinical algorithms. *N Engl J Med*. 2020;383(9):874–882. doi:10.1056/NEJMms2004740.

3. Hoyert D. Maternal mortality rates in the United States, 2020. https://dx.doi.org/10.15620/cdc:113967. Published online 2022.

4. Zandvakili F, Rezaie M, Shahoei R, Roshani D. Maternal outcomes associated with caesarean versus vaginal delivery. *J Clin Diagn Res*. 2017;11(7):QC01–QC04. doi:10.7860/JCDR/2017/24891.10239.

5. March of Dimes. March of Dimes peristats: delivery method. https://www.marchofdimes.org/peristats/data?lev=1&obj=1&reg=99&slev=1&stop=355&top=8. Published January 2022. Accessed November 29, 2022.

6. Gilbert SA, Grobman WA, Landon MB, et al. Lifetime cost-effectiveness of trial of labor after cesarean in the United States. *Value Health*. 2013;16(6):953–964. doi:10.1016/j.jval.2013.06.014.

7. Childbirth Connection. What every pregnant woman needs to know about cesarean birth. 2016. https://www.nationalpartnership.org/our-work/resources/health-care/maternity/what-every-pregnant-woman-needs-to-know-about-cesarean-section.pdf.

8. Rubashkin N. Why equitable access to vaginal birth requires abolition of race-based medicine. *AMA J Ethics*. 2022;24(3): E233–E238. doi:10.1001/amajethics.2022.233.

9. Stern C. Why BMI is a flawed health standard, especially for people of color. *Washington Post*. May 5, 2021. https://www.washingtonpost.com/lifestyle/wellness/healthy-bmi-obesity-race-/2021/05/04/655390f0-ad0d-11eb-acd3-24b44a57093a_story.html.

10. Huizinga MM, Cooper LA, Bleich SN, Clark JM, Beach MC. Physician respect for patients with obesity. *J Gen Intern Med*. 2009;24(11):1236–1239. doi:10.1007/s11606-009-1104-8.

11. Alberga AS, Edache IY, Forhan M, Russell-Mayhew S. Weight bias and health care utilization: a scoping review. *Prim Health Care Res Dev*. 2019;20:e116. doi:10.1017/S1463423619000227.

12. Frey HA, Ashmead R, Farmer A, et al. Association of prepregnancy body mass index with risk of severe maternal morbidity and mortality among Medicaid beneficiaries. *JAMA Netw Open*. 2022;5(6):e2218986–e2218986. doi:10.1001/jamanetworkopen.2022.18986.

13. US Department of Health and Human Services Office of Minority Health. Obesity and African Americans. https://minorityhealth.hhs.gov/omh/browse.aspx?lvl=4&lvlid=25. Published 2020. Accessed November 30, 2022.

14. Bailey ZD, Krieger N, Agénor M, Graves J, Linos N, Bassett MT. Structural racism and health inequities in the USA: evidence and interventions. *Lancet*. 2017;389(10077):1453–1463. doi:10.1016/S0140-6736(17)30569-X.

15. Sealy-Jefferson S, Butler B, Price-Spratlen T, Dailey RK, Misra DP. Neighborhood-level mass incarceration and future preterm birth risk among African American women. *J Urban Health*. 2020;97(2):271–278. doi:10.1007/s11524-020-00426-w.

16. Butler B, Gripper A, Linos N. Built and social environments, environmental justice, and maternal pregnancy complications. *Curr Obstet Gynecol Rep*. 2022;11(3):169–179. doi:10.1007/s13669-022-00339-2.

Chapter 28

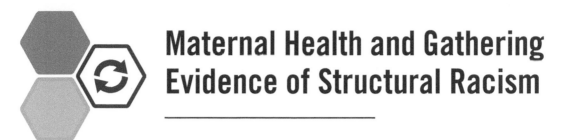

Maternal Health and Gathering Evidence of Structural Racism

LAURI ANDRESS

INTRODUCTION

Persistent disparities in maternal health outcomes are a long-standing public health crisis in the United States.[1] Moreover, decades of evidence documenting US inequities in maternal health outcomes demonstrate that babies born to Black mothers stand a greater chance of dying in the first year of life compared with babies born to white mothers. In fact, Black women are three times more likely to experience pregnancy-related morbidity or mortality compared with white women.[2] What makes this ongoing public health crisis especially hard to unravel is that many of the thought leaders responsible for shaping the marketplace of ideas, including research, public policy, and print and electronic media, remain reluctant to identify structural racism as a significant social factor and root cause that influences poor maternal health outcomes for Black women.[3]

Many of today's public health strategies and medical practices use theories, frameworks, and models, which help shape our understanding of population health outcomes and yet fail to account for contextual, nonmedical factors, such as structural racism. The omission of structural racism is particularly important in the field of maternal health, as Black women's lived experiences of persistent, multigenerational, and daily occurrences of structural racism contribute to maternal outcomes. Acknowledging and understanding structural racism through these experiences could help identify key factors able to influence public health strategies and healthcare practices.[4]

One way to begin to increase the likelihood that structural racism is recognized as a prominent factor influencing disparities is to acknowledge that the topic is not just about science but is also driven by societal values and ideals that structure community narratives, discourse, and standards. Intentional

Lauri Andress, *Maternal Health and Gathering Evidence of Structural Racism* In: *The Practical Playbook III*. Edited by: Dorothy Cilenti, Alisahah Jackson, Natalie D. Hernandez, Lindsey Yates, Sarah Verbiest, J. Lloyd Michener, and Brian C. Castrucci, Oxford University Press. © de Beaumont Foundation 2024. DOI: 10.1093/oso/9780197662984.003.0028

efforts aimed at changing the narratives and discourse surrounding maternal and infant health disparities will help alter public health and medical theories, frameworks, and models so that structural racism becomes a fundamental factor that informs and explains the documented, historically unjust gaps between US-born Black and white mothers.

Another way to influence understanding consistent with narrative and discourse change is to collect qualitative data that measure and capture structural racism and its impact on the lived experiences of US-born Black women and other historically vulnerable groups. This kind of data would offer a feasible, promising approach for advancing current strategies to address the complex range of societal, material, and psychosocial inequities that differentially affect the lived experiences of women based on race and ethnicity.

This chapter has two aims: (1) to highlight mechanisms and theories that ground racism as a social process portrayed by a pathway that starts with an emotional/psychological experience and results in harmful physiological maternal health outcomes[5,6] and (2) to describe data-collection methodologies that allow public health researchers to understand the effect of structural racism in maternal health outcomes. Through broader theories, models, and frameworks, and through collection of other forms of data, public health and clinical interventions, which are often developed based on this knowledge, can better account for structural racism as a driver of inequities.

It is important to note that because most of the epidemiological research cited in this chapter deals with US-born Black women, the chapter initially speaks to experiences of structural racism for this population. Later, through descriptions of causal mechanisms and qualitative methods, the chapter demonstrates not only ways to expand causal explanations for maternal health disparities but also how other socially marginalized populations may be incorporated into work on structural discrimination, stigmatization, racism, and maternal health outcomes.

THEORIES, MODELS, AND EXPLANATIONS OF HOW RACISM SHAPES INEQUITIES IN MATERNAL AND INFANT HEALTH

Studies from many disciplines explore how structural racism undermines the health of Black people.[7,8] In this research, structural racism commonly refers to the totality of ways in which societies foster racial discrimination through mutually reinforcing systems that deny opportunities and resources to Black people and simultaneously benefit white people.[9] Several groundbreaking theories have helped shed light on how factors outside the body—like structural racism—can become part of the biological equation and operate to damage Black peoples' health.

While individual lifestyle decisions shape health, there is currently enough accumulated evidence to demonstrate a relationship between population health and systemic, institutional, social, and structural factors. Understanding the dynamic relationships between population health and these factors is key to finding solutions to health disparities.[10,11] More specifically, it is the concept of *embodiment* that explains how external physical and social worlds are taken in and expressed in human biology.[4,12-18] In this theory, place is not just a dot on a map but also a set of social processes, relationships expressed as systems and institutions that get under the skin to eventually shape population health.[19,20]

These ideas from public health facilitate characterizations of health as a composition of both human biology and social processes. This stands in stark contrast to medicine's privileging of models, theories, and narratives asserting that good and poor health originate from a body unmoored, floating in space with no connection to context, historical trajectories, and social processes, such as structural racism.[18,21]

Additional research has also explored the association between trauma, defined as structural racism experienced by Black women during pregnancy, and subsequent adverse birth outcomes.[22-26] These studies emphasize the relationship between trauma (i.e., structural racism causing maternal psychosocial and sociodemographic stress) and the biological pathways that lead to adverse birth outcomes.[27-30]

Additionally, while structural racism is thought to affect maternal health during pregnancy, it is also recognized as a contributing factor to the health of historically vulnerable people throughout their lives.[8,31] That structural racism operates across a woman's existence is captured in the life-course approach, which theorizes that health is the sum of our experiences from childhood through adulthood. This perspective leverages theories that demonstrate how current health embodies exposures to historical, physical, environmental, and psychosocial factors. These exposures, which occur over a lifetime, not only have an aggregate and direct impact on an individual but can affect future generations who have not had direct contact or personal encounters with the same traumas. Based on this idea, the trauma caused by structural racism experienced across generations (or the life course) of US-born historically vulnerable groups becomes embodied, affecting the maternal health of those generations.[5,32,33]

Two influential ideas—the weathering hypothesis and allostatic load (AL) theory—help explain how structural racism harms both US-born Black women and birthing people who also experience discrimination. The theories open the door to understanding why Black birthing people have worse health outcomes than white birthing people.[16] The weathering hypothesis posits that cumulative and stress-mediated wear and tear at the cellular level speed up biological aging. This contributes to dysregulation or exhaustion of important body systems, the early onset of chronic diseases and health-induced disability, and excess mortality. An existing and ever-growing body of evidence shows that US-born Black people experience higher levels of trauma and anxiety across their lives and from generation to generation because of structural racism. Based on the weathering hypothesis, the trauma caused by structural racism results in Black people's being biologically older than white people of the same chronological age.[6]

AL theory explains the effects of structural racism on Black people and quantifies how human exposure to trauma leads to wear and tear on the body. Allostatic load is defined as the cumulative toll of ongoing stressful events and life conditions on multiple body systems.[5,6]

Taken together, the life-course perspective, weathering hypothesis, and AL theory help us understand how structural racism harms health, starting with marginalized groups that live through experiences of discrimination and stigmatization. Yet these theories and relevant factors have not been incorporated into public health data sets or health research. There are several reasons why. First, there is no standard, universal measure for structural racism.[6,8,26,34,35] Although there have been efforts to quantify structural racism, the most common measures capture one aspect of racism and do not account for the multiple, layered ways that racism affects health. Researchers have noted that the most common measures of structural racism fall into one of the following domains: residential neighborhood/housing, perceived racism in social institutions, immigration and border enforcement, political participation, socioeconomic status, criminal justice, and workplace environment.

Second, healthcare and public health research methods historically are based in disease-specific theories. Such theories may miss or underestimate the total impact of social factors like structural racism. As a result, public health data sets based on these theories will not include more robust measures of racism as a social process and will instead focus on other discrete social determinants of health, such as income, employment status, and education level. Although these measures are related to racism, by themselves they don't fully account for the upstream social processes of structural racism that occur from encounters inflicted over time.

Finally, current policies and practices are primarily focused on investments in healthcare and reducing risky, individual-level behaviors. This may limit the ability of public health organizations to incorporate measures of structural racism in their data sets. Although investments in healthcare are important, investments focused on reducing the social inequities behind health problems can better prevent multiple negative health conditions.

As public health analysts and epidemiologists grapple with these challenges and consider how to better incorporate the life-course perspective, weathering hypothesis, and AL theory into existing theories, they should explore other ways of studying and acquiring knowledge about human behavior, social processes, and interactions between place and health. This opens the door to the use of qualitative methods that demonstrate the embodiment of structural racism as a set of social processes and relationships.

MEASURING STRUCTURAL RACISM USING QUALITATIVE METHODS

The use of qualitative methods presents one of the best options for exploring whether and how structural racism, as a set of social processes and relationships, triggers biological mechanisms that affect the health of Black women and birthing people. More important for public health, qualitative methods can respond to ongoing and yet urgent demands for evidence and immediate strategies that address structural social processes and outcomes based on race, ethnicity, and/or socioeconomic position that manifest as the loss of opportunities and resources through the unjust and unfair application of programs, regulations, and public policies.

Qualitative evidence representing lived experiences reveals unjust occurrences, making it easier to prioritize social justice values and narratives that challenge inequity. The lived experiences speak to, and promote, social justice values by centering them as a driver of public policy able to confront (and possibly overcome) marketplace justice, which typically features limited government protection and individual freedom at the expense of concern for the common good and one's fellow human beings.

Qualitative research can also supply vivid descriptors of lived experiences and rich information that reveals the chronic distress and anxiety from both generational and daily encounters with structural racism, by allowing people closest to the reality to describe how it affects their lives.[36,37]

Additional benefits of qualitative research are its methodological characteristics that amplify the context of lived experiences and the constructs that intersect to represent a phenomenon, rather than relying on the typically predetermined variables researchers assume are impactful.[38] Qualitative methods may provide a more nuanced, in-depth exploration of factors that show up as social processes so that the breadth of the topic takes precedence over health-related requirements to take up disease-focused topics using quantitative methods that must define and validate measurable variables.

Importantly, qualitative research helps to avoid medicalization, which is described as the process and outcome of human problems' entering the jurisdiction of the medical profession, or a process where everyday experiences fall under the influence of medical authority and supervision.[39]

Medicalized discourses and narratives make it harder to view experiences of structural racism as part of the causal equation. In this case, theories, strategies, and analytical frameworks view the poor health outcomes of Black women and birthing people as problems with their bodies, the lack of particular healthcare services, or, if considering adverse experiences, trauma—defined as emotional problems that may be solved through psychotherapy and better coping skills.[39,40] Medicalized discourses and frameworks tend to exclude social and structural causal factors related to inequities in maternal health outcomes between US-born white women and historically vulnerable groups, including US-born Black women and birthing people.

A variety of qualitative methods may be used to better explore structural racism. One method that can help highlight whether, and how, US-born Black women and birthing people experience structural racism is use of ethnographic findings that provide a thick description of daily and multigenerational encounters with racist systems. In addition to recording the fact and appearance of what a person does, thick description is transparent about the researcher's efforts to assist readers by ascribing context, emotion, and the maze of social relationships that join persons to one another.[41] Thick description also invokes emotionality, intentionality, and the sense of feelings a person has centered in, or concerned with, oneself. Inserting history into experience and establishing the significance of an experience, or the sequence of events for the person or persons, as thick description does, makes it easier to sense the voices, feelings, actions, and meanings of interacting individuals.[42] Thick description is meant to allow readers to digest the findings and determine whether they would have come to the same interpretive conclusions as the researcher.[41] Additional examples of novel qualitative research methods used in maternal health can be found in Chapter 29.

One other point relates to this chapter's narrow portrayal of US-born historically vulnerable groups experiencing structural racism: At issue are research theories on the "Hispanic paradox" and "healthy immigrant effect," theories that seem to suggest that non-US-born people of color may not experience structural racism because they have been shown to have better health outcomes.[43,44]

However, there is a way forward to expand the evidence base on groups experiencing structural racism. In prioritizing the social processes of structural racism and pathways that start from emotional/psychological uptake of racist experiences, qualitative methods could be used to capture lived experiences and explore interactions between non-US-born people of color using theories on embodiment, AL, and weathering.

CONCLUSION

Medicine's preservation of models, theories, and narratives that frame health in reference to the body prioritizes the notion that good and poor health originate in the body, with no connection to context, historical trajectories, and social processes. Moreover, medicine's continued triangulation of race, bodies, and culture implicitly cements the widely disproven, unacceptable notion of race as a biological phenomenon and physical appearance and bodies as the sole explanatory variables for culture.

In seeking only quantitative evidence of structural racism, we run the risk of reifying these outdated ideas and missing out on newer explanatory models that account for the embodiment of race and racism as social processes external to the body that shape the health of historically vulnerable groups.

Qualitative methods and resulting data demonstrating lived experiences of historically marginalized groups overcome the limitations we face in developing practices, policies, and studies that measure structural racism. Furthermore, qualitative methods can facilitate the creation of immediate and future strategies that support structural changes and direct public health in any number of ways, including:

- Creation of initiatives that facilitate community organizing, empowerment, and development of a unified narrative leading to social movements where groups employ nonmedical frames that elucidate how social processes, such as historical practices of racism, affect the health of US-born Black women and birthing people.
- Development of vivid, impactful evidence to support immediate changes in structures and public policies that address inequities in maternal health outcomes.
- Generation of directions for future antiracism research that uses biomedical measures and methods of data collection to address maternal health inequities.
- Development of evidence that posits how experiences of structural racism affect other groups beyond US-born historically vulnerable groups.

The world can change according to the way people experience it, see it, and speak about it.[45,46] If we use methods that reveal reality as less of a set of facts and more as an outcome relative to who we are, then we can collect the evidence needed to change the social processes that engender structural racism and poor maternal health outcomes experienced by Black birthing people.[47-49]

REFERENCES

1. Petersen E, Davis N, Goodman D, et al. Racial/ethnic disparities in pregnancy-related deaths—United States, 2007–2016. 2019. http://dx.doi.org/10.15585/mmwr.mm6835a3.

2. Hoyert D. Maternal mortality rates in the United States, 2020. https://dx.doi.org/10.15620/cdc:113967. Published online 2022.

3. Castle B, Wendel M, Kerr J, Brooms D, Rollins A. Public health's approach to systemic racism: a systematic literature review. *J Racial Ethn Health Disparities*. 2019;6(1):27–36. doi:10.1007/s40615-018-0494-x.

4. Bailey ZD, Krieger N, Agénor M, Graves J, Linos N, Bassett MT. Structural racism and health inequities in the USA: evidence and interventions. *Lancet*. 2017;389(10077):1453–1463. doi:10.1016/S0140-6736(17)30569-X.

5. O'Campo P, Schetter CD, Guardino CM, et al. Explaining racial and ethnic inequalities in postpartum allostatic load: results from a multisite study of low to middle income women. *SSM-Popul Health*. 2016;2:850–858.

6. Geronimus AT, Hicken MT, Pearson JA, Seashols SJ, Brown KL, Cruz TD. Do US Black women experience stress-related accelerated biological aging? A novel theory and first population-based test of Black–white differences in telomere length. *Hum Nat*. 2010;21(1):19–38. doi:10.1007/s12110-010-9078-0.

7. Homan PA, Brown TH. Sick And Tired Of Being Excluded: Structural Racism In Disenfranchisement As A Threat To Population Health Equity. *Health Aff*. 2022;41(2):219–227. doi:10.1377/hlthaff.2021.01414.

8. Hardeman RR, Homan PA, Chantarat T, Davis BA, Brown TH. Improving the measurement of structural racism to achieve antiracist health policy. *Health Aff*. 2022;41(2):179–186. doi:10.1377/hlthaff.2021.01489.

9. Adams C, Thomas SP. Alternative prenatal care interventions to alleviate Black–white maternal/infant health disparities. *Sociol Compass*. 2018;12(1):e12549.

10. Hansen H, Braslow J, Rohrbaugh RM. From cultural to structural competency—training psychiatry residents to act on social determinants of health and institutional racism. *JAMA Psychiatry*. 2018;75(2):117–118. doi:10.1001/jamapsychiatry.2017.3894.

11. Hansen H, Metzl J. Structural competency in the U.S. healthcare crisis: putting social and policy interventions into clinical practice. *J Bioeth Inq*. 2016;13(2):179–183. doi:10.1007/s11673-016-9719-z.

12. Krieger N. Proximal, distal, and the politics of causation: what's level got to do with it? *Am J Public Health*. 2008;98(2):221–230. doi:10.2105/AJPH.2007.111278.

13. Krieger N. Public health, embodied history, and social justice: looking forward. *Int J Health Serv*. 2015;45(4):587–600.

14. Krieger N. Theories for social epidemiology in the 21st century: an ecosocial perspective. *Int J Epidemiol*. 2001;30(4):668–677. doi:10.1093/ije/30.4.668.

15. Krieger N. Embodiment: a conceptual glossary for epidemiology. *J Epidemiol Community Health*. 2005;59(5):350–355. doi:10.1136/jech.2004.024562.

16. Krieger N. Epidemiology and the web of causation: has anyone seen the spider? *Soc Sci Med*. 1994;39(7):887–903. doi:10.1016/0277-9536(94)90202-x.

17. Petteway R, Mujahid M, Allen A. Understanding embodiment in place-health research: approaches, limitations, and opportunities. *J Urban Health*. 2019;96(2):289–299. doi:10.1007/s11524-018-00336-y.

18. Andress L, Purtill MP. Shifting the gaze of the physician from the body to the body in a place: a qualitative analysis of a community-based photovoice approach to teaching place-health concepts to medical students. *PLOS One*. 2020;15(2):e0228640. doi:10.1371/journal.pone.0228640.

19. Fullilove MT. *Root Shock: How Tearing up City Neighborhoods Hurts America, and What We Can Do about It*. New York, NY: New Village Press; 2016.

20. Fullilove MT. *Urban Alchemy: Restoring Joy in America's Sorted-out Cities*. New York, NY: NYU Press; 2013.

21. Garner S. *Racisms: An Introduction*. Thousand Oaks: SAGE; 2017.

22. Li Y, Rosemberg M-AS, Seng JS. Allostatic load: a theoretical model for understanding the relationship between maternal posttraumatic stress disorder and adverse birth outcomes. *Midwifery*. 2018;62:205–213. doi:10.1016/j.midw.2018.04.002.

23. Geronimus AT, Pearson JA, Linnenbringer E, et al. Weathering in Detroit: place, race, ethnicity, and poverty as conceptually fluctuating social constructs shaping variation in allostatic load. *Milbank Q*. 2020;98(4):1171–1218. doi:10.1111/1468-0009.12484.

24. Jutte DP, Miller JL, Erickson DJ. Neighborhood adversity, child health, and the role for community development. *Pediatrics*. 2015;135 Suppl 2:S48–S57. doi:10.1542/peds.2014-3549F.

25. Leimert KB, Olson DM. Racial disparities in pregnancy outcomes: genetics, epigenetics, and allostatic load. *Curr Opin Physiol*. 2020;13:155–165.

26. Wallace ME, Harville EW. Allostatic load and birth outcomes among white and Black women in New Orleans. *Matern Child Health J*. 2013;17(6):1025–1029. doi:10.1007/s10995-012-1083-y.

27. Wallace ME, Green C, Richardson L, Theall K, Crear-Perry J. "Look at the whole me": a mixed-methods examination of Black infant mortality in the US through women's lived experiences and community context. *Int J Environ Res Public Health*. 2017;14(7):727. doi:10.3390/ijerph14070727.

28. Wallace M, Crear-Perry J, Richardson L, Tarver M, Theall K. Separate and unequal: structural racism and infant mortality in the US. *Health Place*. 2017;45:140–144. doi:10.1016/j.healthplace.2017.03.012.

29. Nuru-Jeter A, Dominguez TP, Hammond WP, et al. "It's the skin you're in": African-American women talk about their experiences of racism—an exploratory study to develop measures of racism for birth outcome studies. *Matern Child Health J*. 2009;13(1):29–39. doi:10.1007/s10995-008-0357-x.

30. Lu MC, Kotelchuck M, Hogan V, Jones L, Wright K, Halfon N. Closing the Black–white gap in birth outcomes: a life-course approach. *Ethn Dis*. 2010;20(1 suppl 2):S62–S76.

31. Egede LE, Walker RJ. Structural racism, social risk factors, and Covid-19—a dangerous convergence for Black Americans. *N Engl J Med*. 2020;383(12):e77.

32. Jones NL, Gilman SE, Cheng TL, Drury SS, Hill CV, Geronimus AT. Life course approaches to the causes of health disparities. *Am J Public Health*. 2019;109(suppl 1):S48–S55. doi:10.2105/AJPH.2018.304738.

33. Theall KP, Francois S, Bell CN, Anderson A, Chae D, LaVeist TA. Neighborhood police encounters, health, and violence in a Southern city: study examines neighborhood police encounters, health, and violence in New Orleans, Louisiana. *Health Aff*. 2022;41(2):228–236.

34. Groos M, Wallace M, Hardeman R, Theall KP. Measuring inequity: a systematic review of methods used to quantify structural racism. *J Health Dispar Res Pract*. 2018;11(2):13.

35. Adkins-Jackson PB, Chantarat T, Bailey ZD, Ponce NA. Measuring structural racism: a guide for epidemiologists and other health researchers. *Am J Epidemiol*. 2022;191(4):539–547. doi:10.1093/aje/kwab239.

36. McInnes RJ, Chambers JA. Supporting breastfeeding mothers: qualitative synthesis. *J Adv Nurs*. 2008;62(4):407–427. doi:10.1111/j.1365-2648.2008.04618.x.

37. Chambers BD, Arabia SE, Arega HA, et al. Exposures to structural racism and racial discrimination among pregnant and early post-partum Black women living in Oakland, California. *Stress Health*. 2020;36(2):213–219. doi:10.1002/smi.2922.

38. Prosek EA, Gibson DM. Promoting rigorous research by examining lived experiences: a review of four qualitative traditions. *J Couns Dev*. 2021;99(2):167–177.

39. Conrad P. Medicalization and social control. *Annu Rev Sociol*. 1992;209–232.

40. Crawford R. Healthism and the medicalization of everyday life. *Int J Health Serv*. 1980;10(3):365–388.

41. Ponterotto JG. Brief Note on the Origins, Evolution, and Meaning of the Qualitative Research Concept Thick. *TQR*. 2006;11(3):6.

42. Denzin NK. *Interpretive Interactionism*. Vol 16. Thousand Oaks: SAGE; 2001.

43. Teitler JO, Hutto N, Reichman NE. Birthweight of children of immigrants by maternal duration of residence in the United States. *Soc Sci Med*. 2012;75(3):459–468.

44. Markides KS, Rote S. The healthy immigrant effect and aging in the United States and other Western countries. *Gerontologist*. 2019;59(2):205–214.

45. Angouri J. Quantitative, qualitative or both? Combining methods in linguistic research. *Res Methods Linguist*. 2010;1:29–45.

46. Wodak R. Critical linguistics and critical discourse analysis. *Discursive Pragmat*. 2011;8:50–70.

47. Dorfman L. Studying the news on public health: how content analysis supports media advocacy. *Am J Health Behav*. 2003;27(1):S217–S226.

48. Dorfman L, Krasnow ID. Public health and media advocacy. *Annu Rev Public Health*. 2014;35(1):293–306.

49. Lynch J, Gollust SE. Playing fair: fairness beliefs and health policy preferences in the United States. *J Health Polit Policy Law*. 2010;35(6):849–887.

Chapter 29

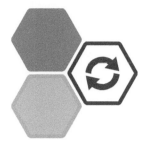

Using Narrative Medicine and Longitudinal Qualitative Research to Examine Maternal Health Outcomes

BURCU BOZKURT

DEFINING NARRATIVE MEDICINE AND LONGITUDINAL QUALITATIVE RESEARCH

Grounded in the social sciences, narrative medicine is a qualitative approach of collecting and disseminating stories from people to enhance our understanding of an illness, condition, or patient experience.[1,2] These narratives primarily center the patient and the patient's experience and context, rather than the physician or other dominant voices in the medical establishment.[3] Narrative medicine is unique in that it has two different applications that can be combined or used separately. Narrative medicine may be used as a qualitative research method to better understand patient experiences in medical practice; it also is commonly used as a model for physician–patient communication, patient advocacy, and medical education.[3,4] For example, hospitals may offer narrative medicine programs to groups of patients to help them claim their illnesses and promote healing, while simultaneously improving healthcare providers' understanding of patients' lived experiences and emotional needs. In addition, narrative writing has become a common offering in medical schools to strengthen the self-awareness and empathetic capacity of trainees.

Longitudinal qualitative research (LQR) uses sequential interviews with participants to investigate time-varying, dynamic processes.[5] The premise of LQR, which may incorporate ethnographic approaches, is to understand how and why a phenomenon or behavior changes across time.[6] This method can strengthen our understanding of transitions or developmental and behavioral changes along the life course.[6]

NARRATIVE MEDICINE AND LQR AS PIVOTAL TOOLS IN MATERNAL HEALTH RESEARCH

While qualitative studies are used for a wide array of research questions and take many forms, narrative medicine and LQR exemplify two distinct approaches to gathering evidence. Narrative medicine often complements the evidence from randomized controlled trials; LQR can provide in-depth insights into contextual aspects of critical transitions or time periods that would be harder to glean from traditional cross-sectional qualitative or quantitative methods. Since there are multiple transitions across the maternal life course, LQR has the potential for broader application in maternal health services research.

Both methods require a fundamental shift in perspective about how evidence is traditionally conceptualized and created. While narrative medicine and LQR are not widely used in maternal health, they are promising ways to advance our understanding of the lived experiences, contexts, and trajectories of women and birthing people and for improving programs, policies, and interventions.

FITTING THE RIGHT RESEARCH QUESTION TO NARRATIVE MEDICINE AND LQR

Both qualitative approaches provide contextually rich and multifaceted insights about people and phenomena of interest and can be used effectively to answer certain research questions. Because narrative medicine is intertwined with everyday medical practice and uses stories as a tool to gather data on a patient's experience of illness, it can be studied as an intervention or used as a research tool. As an intervention, narrative medicine can be combined with evidence-based medicine to increase empathy and strengthen clinical practice by helping physicians better meet patients where they are.[4] Previous research has focused on narrative medicine as the primary intervention to evaluate whether it is useful in promoting positive outcomes in certain groups of patients.[7] An example of a question that could use narrative medicine as an intervention is: Does narrative medicine help decrease the mental health burden of birthing people who have experienced birth trauma?

Narrative medicine may also be a method for collecting data from patients. As an example, one study used narrative medicine as a qualitative method to investigate the experiences of women who became pregnant after a liver transplant.[8] Other researchers used narrative medicine to explore psychological challenges couples face after using assisted reproductive technology to become pregnant.[9] Research questions proposing to use narrative medicine should focus on the voices and language of patients and their engagement with their providers, their test results, and the health and social systems around them.

Researchers proposing to employ LQR should mainly be concerned with the question of time, particularly how a person or phenomenon of interest changes across time. For example, investigators used LQR methods to explore psychosocial factors that may influence breastfeeding discontinuation two weeks postpartum.[10] Another study used an LQR design to examine the challenges that HIV-positive women face at different stages of early infant feeding.[11] Both studies explored behavior across time, particularly in the early postpartum period, a critical transition point. Investigators thus have two main considerations in posing a question with the application of LQR: how to define time (days, weeks, months), and how to define change. How often a researcher collects data and the questions used to ascertain change (or lack of change) will depend on the focus of the study.

ETHICAL CONSIDERATIONS IN THE APPLICATION OF NOVEL QUALITATIVE METHODS

Robust adherence to ethical best practices in research is vital in planning studies involving narrative medicine and LQR, especially because these approaches are well suited to investigating phenomena in underserved populations (such as birthing people and minoritized populations) who may need special protections.

Particularly in narrative medicine, a primary ethical consideration is the use of data with intention other than treatment, which may lead to harm.[1] Because narrative medicine may be used as an intervention, a research tool, or in a combined manner, researchers must explain to all stakeholders how they will use the technique and how that may affect the way the narratives are used and disseminated.

For studies using an LQR approach, informed consent is profoundly important. Because of the longevity of LQR studies, informed consent is not a one-time procedure but rather an ongoing process.[5] In our LQR postpartum study at the University of North Carolina at Chapel Hill, we found that, over time, participants would sometimes forget the objective of the study. A dedicated consent conversation prior to each interview, as well as staying in touch between interviews, was important for ensuring that participants could appropriately provide consent.

Both narrative medicine and LQR may generally involve a smaller number of participants than more common qualitative approaches. With both methodologies, efforts must be made to maintain confidentiality, especially in an era when technological data collection is common. Because both approaches require someone capturing, analyzing, and disseminating data, researchers should examine their own biases and experiences and make sustained commitments to participants about the intended use of their data. Explicitly acknowledging reflexivity and power in qualitative research is becoming an important part of presenting research methodologies, and such reflexivity plays a particularly important role in implementing both narrative medicine and LQR. For example, in our study with Black women, it was important to acknowledge that the research was being led and conducted by a scholar with white-skin privilege. Putting that acknowledgment front and center, along with a commitment to respect participants' judgment in discussing as little or as much as they choose to disclose, was important in establishing social accountability and rapport with them.

At the heart of these methods is their reliance on trusting relationships to capture an honest and comprehensive understanding of patients and their experiences. This is particularly important when conducting LQR, as it requires long-term engagement. As a result, both approaches present researchers with a critical opportunity to build and sustain long-term community relationships and coalitions that set the foundation for equitable relationships between investigators and the communities at the center of the inquiry.

RESEARCH DESIGN IN NARRATIVE MEDICINE AND LQR

Research participants in narrative medicine and LQR are selected based on their shared experience of the phenomenon of interest.[6] There are several components of research design for investigators to consider, including:

- Purposive sampling
- Key research design decisions (including the type of clinical setting in which to conduct the study)
- How to recruit participants
- How, and in which format, to gather data (interviews or written prose, for example)
- Whether to involve participants in developing the research design and tools

In narrative medicine, selection of the type of data to be gathered (observation, written prose, interviews with individuals and/or group sessions) may influence both who is recruited to participate in the study and the research setting. Investigators may choose to recruit participants with a shared illness across sociodemographic domains to better diversify the study sample. Individuals like close family, friends, and other caregivers may also be recruited for their valuable insight into the lived experience and context of an illness. While data saturation is harder to discern in narrative medicine, researchers should aim for getting as comprehensive a picture as possible from study participants. Furthermore, narrative medicine ultimately focuses on the interaction between a healthcare professional and a patient via the patient's story. Given this focus, it is important to carefully listen to the realities and perceptions of study participants. Important questions of power—who has control over the narrative, for example, or how researchers are positioned relationally to study participants throughout data collection—must be answered before and throughout data collection and analysis.

Designing LQR research necessitates specifying how frequently data should be collected from the same participants. This method does not limit the unit of analysis to single individuals and may include focus groups, field notes, and other data sources.[6] Researchers should thoughtfully select the duration between interview periods, which should be clinically significant as well as implementable. Determining the right number of participants to recruit for LQR studies includes accounting for potential data saturation and potential attrition of participants.[5] LQR research design relies on the ongoing engagement and willingness of participants across time, which can be facilitated through partnerships and meaningful engagement with the participants' community.[6] Box 29.1 summarizes the deliberate approach to recruitment and sampling

Box 29.1 | An Example of LQR Research Design Used to Examine How the Postpartum Experiences of Black Women in North Carolina Change Over Time

We chose to interview both Black postpartum women and birth workers, individually. We made this decision because we believed individuals might be inclined to offer more insights around their postpartum transition and care in a nongroup, confidential setting. We chose to conduct three sequential interviews, four to six weeks apart, with Black women during their postpartum year. This allowed us to capture changes in individual trajectories and to gain insight into longitudinal healthcare processes. While the study captured at most three to four months of participants' postpartum year, we purposefully chose shorter data-collection intervals to limit recall bias and to prioritize participant retention, and because this design aligned with the exploratory nature and small scope of our study. We supplemented the data from the postpartum women with an additional ten interviews with obstetricians/gynecologists and other birth workers.

To address attrition concerns, we provided tiered financial incentives, with increasing amounts for each subsequent interview. This strategy, combined with building rapport during interviews and checking in between interviews, was successful in retaining participation.

We leveraged informal partnerships with doula networks to recruit interested mothers and found that potential participants referred by partner doulas were more likely to be interested in participating for the duration of the study than mothers contacted using other recruitment techniques. Throughout the study, we compared thematic insights from individual postpartum trajectories to thematic domains gleaned from interviews with birth workers.

Our interview guides incorporated both discrete and recurring questions across time. Recurring questions across the three interviews focused on ascertaining change in postpartum participants' perceived social support, as well as in their physical health, psychosocial needs, and their experiences navigating the healthcare system. Discrete questions included specific follow-up items for prior interviews to gain greater insight into participants' unique contexts and social environments.

in our longitudinal qualitative study of Black postpartum women in North Carolina. LQR research design should also incorporate ways to triangulate and validate data across time as data are collected. This could include comparing findings from one set of interviews to another, midstream audits, or validity checks to ensure that investigators are on the right track. Conducting an exit interview with each participant will also help ensure validity.[5]

ANALYSIS IN NARRATIVE MEDICINE AND LQR

As with any qualitative methodology, an analytic approach should be devised and modified for specific research questions using narrative medicine or LQR. Applying a theoretical framework or a list of analytic objectives may assist in organizing the data in the study's early stages.

Analysis for studies that utilize narrative medicine is similar to analysis for traditional qualitative studies with one-off interviews and consists of transcription, thematic analysis via coding, and triangulation or validation checks. Narratives may be complemented with clinical records, participant surveys, and data from others in participants' care environment. Prior research leveraging narrative medicine as a methodological approach has used "illness plots" to guide narratives chronologically and to identify change over time.[12] The illness plots are characterized by evocative and open words that facilitate more individual expression.[12,13] Throughout analysis and data interpretation, it is paramount that researchers place an emphasis on centering the lived experiences of participants as legitimate evidence.

Due to the layered and time-variant nature of longitudinal data, analyses for LQR studies also are layered and complex. Recurrent cross-section and trajectory analyses are the two tools primarily used to evaluate the data. Recurrent cross-sectional analysis investigates themes and changes across time at the level of the entire study sample. This type of analysis is more useful for studies looking at before/after questions, or how group-level beliefs change over time.[14] Trajectory analysis focuses on changes over time for an individual or small groups of individuals. For example, in our postpartum LQR study, by following the trajectories of the same cohort of postpartum women and birthing people across time, we found that the factors influencing their perceived social support varied across time. These insights would not have surfaced if the study had used cross-sectional analysis. Based on the research question, investigators may choose to review and analyze data from prior interviews before conducting subsequent ones. In these cases, analysis of future data should be informed by previous data to tie in relevant themes and insights from one interview to the next. Prior to coding interviews, indexing the text to allow for chronological organization is pivotal.[5] Coding and thematic analysis in LQR likely will be complemented by other analytic tools, such as change memos, framework analyses that summarize themes within and across participants at

Figure 29.1 ▼
Key considerations for narrative medicine and LQR.

1. **Leverage community partnerships and social networks to recruit participants.** Narrative medicine and LQR can be further enriched by the voices of community members informing research projects. Aside from using community partnerships and social networks for recruitment, researchers should find ways to engage participants and communities throughout the process to triangulate and validate data instruments, findings, and interpretations.

2. **Plan ahead.** Aspects of narrative medicine and LQR can be labor-intensive and complex. Researchers should incorporate more time than for traditional qualitative data collection to recruit participants, collect data, and iterate research instruments and to allow for data analysis between data collection waves.

3. **Be thoughtful stewards of the data.** Both narrative medicine and LQR present unique data analysis and interpretation challenges. However, these should be seen as potential opportunities for investigators to be transparent in their reflexivity and thoughtful about who ultimately holds the power and the control over collected narratives in the research relationship.

4. **Ensure consistency in analytic approaches with these methods.** While there is certainly room in both methods for standard qualitative thematic analysis, there is additional need for proactive adoption of data management and analytic tools, particularly in LQR, to facilitate ongoing analysis throughout data collection.[1] Consistency from the beginning will ensure a robust approach.

different points in time, cross-sectional profiling, and case histories, among others.[5,6,15-17]

RECOMMENDATIONS FOR FUTURE ACTION

Narrative medicine and LQR are promising methods that stakeholders invested in maternal health can adopt to gain context about the lived experiences of birthing people. These approaches are especially useful in providing more nuanced context and social understandings of underserved or minoritized populations affected by health inequities. Figure 29.1 summarizes four key considerations for those interested in implementing these methodologies.

There is immense potential in growing and improving use of qualitative approaches in maternal health scholarship to improve policies, programs, and interventions that aim to better serve women, children, and families.

REFERENCES

1. Charon R. *Narrative Medicine: Honoring the Stories of Illness*. Oxford, England: Oxford University Press; 2006.

2. Marini MG. *Narrative Medicine: Bridging the Gap between Evidence-Based Care and Medical Humanities*. London, England: Springer International Publishing; 2016.

3. Kalitzkus V, Matthiessen PF. Narrative-based medicine: potential, pitfalls, and practice. *Perm J.* 2009;13(1):80–86. doi:10.7812/TPP/09.996.

4. Charon R. The patient–physician relationship. Narrative medicine: a model for empathy, reflection, profession, and trust. *JAMA.* 2001;286(15):1897–902. doi:10.1001/jama.286.15.1897.

5. Saldaña J. *Longitudinal Qualitative Research: Analysing Change Through Time.* Lanham, Maryland: Rowman & Littlefield; 2003.

6. Tuthill EL, Maltby AE, DiClemente K, Pellowski JA. Longitudinal qualitative methods in health behavior and nursing research: assumptions, design, analysis and lessons learned. *Int J Qual Methods.* 2020;19:10.1177. doi:10.1177/1609406920965799.

7. Fioretti C, Mazzocco K, Riva S, Oliveri S, Masiero M, Pravettoni G. Research studies on patients' illness experience using the narrative medicine approach: a systematic review. *BMJ Open.* 2016;6(7):e011220. doi:10.1136/bmjopen-2016-011220.

8. Donzelli G, Paddeu EM, D'Alessandro F, Nanni Costa A. The role of narrative medicine in pregnancy after liver transplantation. *J Matern Fetal Neonatal Med.* 2015;28(2):158–161. doi:10.3109/14767058.2014.906578.

9. Smorti M, Smorti A. Medical successes and couples' psychological problems in assisted reproduction treatment: a narrative based medicine approach. *J Matern Fetal Neonatal Med.* 2013;26(2):169–172. doi:10.3109/14767058.2012.722728.

10. Jardine EE, McLellan J, Dombrowski SU. Is being resolute better than being pragmatic when it comes to breastfeeding? Longitudinal qualitative study investigating experiences of women intending to breastfeed using the Theoretical Domains Framework. *J Public Health.* 2017;39(3):e88–e94. doi:10.1093/pubmed/fdw073.

11. Doherty T, Chopra M, Nkonki L, Jackson D, Persson LA. A longitudinal qualitative study of infant-feeding decision making and practices among HIV-positive women in South Africa. *J Nutr.* 2006;136(9):2421–246. doi:10.1093/jn/136.9.2421.

12. Reid K, Soundy A. A qualitative study examining the illness narrative master plots of people with head and neck cancer. *Behav Sci.* 2019;9(10):110. doi:10.3390/bs9100110.

13. Ragusa L, Crino A, Grugni G, et al. Caring and living with Prader-Willi syndrome in Italy: integrating children, adults and parents' experiences through a multicentre narrative medicine research. *BMJ Open.* 2020;10(8):e036502. doi:10.1136/bmjopen-2019-036502.

14. Grossoehme D, Lipstein E. Analyzing longitudinal qualitative data: the application of trajectory and recurrent cross-sectional approaches. *BMC Res Notes.* 2016;9:136. doi:10.1186/s13104-016-1954-1.

15. Barrington C, Rosenberg A, Kerrigan D, Blankenship KM. Probing the processes: longitudinal qualitative research on social determinants of HIV. *AIDS Behav.* 2021;25(suppl 2):203–213. doi:10.1007/s10461-021-03240-w.

16. Thomson R. The qualitative longitudinal case history: practical, methodological and ethical reflections. *Soc Policy Soc.* 2007;6(4):571–582. doi:10.1017/s1474746407003909.

17. Lewis J. Analysing qualitative longitudinal research in evaluations. *Soc Policy Soc.* 2007;6(4):545–556. doi:10.1017/S1474746407003880.

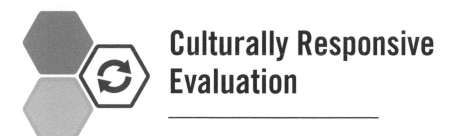

Chapter 30

Culturally Responsive Evaluation

KIMBERLEY BROOMFIELD-MASSEY, RAKIAH ANDERSON,
CALONDRA TIBBS, AND CHRISTINE TUCKER

INTRODUCTION: CENTERING EQUITY IN MATERNAL HEALTH

As maternal health professionals, we know that maternal morbidity and mortality are serious public health issues. This is especially true for Black women, who are two to three times more likely to die of pregnancy-related causes than white women.[1] We also know that what works for Black women in rural Alabama, for example, may not be suitable for Indigenous women in the Lumbee region of North Carolina. Practitioners must apply "the right program or service, at the right time, for the right people, under the right set of conditions,"[2] which means what the field is starting to understand as equitable approaches in maternal health. The more we understand the unique attributes of a community—its strengths, challenges, history, culture, access to resources, and broader social determinants of health that influence differences in maternal outcomes—the more we can strategically implement and evaluate programs, policies, and other efforts aimed at responding to, preventing, and reducing poor maternal health outcomes.

Program evaluation is the systematic "collection of information about the activities, characteristics, and outcomes of programs for use by specific people to reduce uncertainties, improve effectiveness, and make decisions with regard to what those programs are doing and affecting."[3] For example, an evaluation of a program to promote breastfeeding in the African American community may collect demographic data on program participants to understand whether the program is reaching the intended target population and may ask program participants about their experience with the program to ensure that the program being delivered is high quality and that its intended benefits are being

Kimberley Broomfield-Massey, Rakiah Anderson, Calondra Tibbs, and Christine Tucker, *Culturally Responsive Evaluation*
In: *The Practical Playbook III*. Edited by: Dorothy Cilenti, Alisahah Jackson, Natalie D. Hernandez, Lindsey Yates, Sarah Verbiest, J. Lloyd Michener, and Brian C. Castrucci, Oxford University Press. © de Beaumont Foundation 2024.
DOI: 10.1093/oso/9780197662984.003.0030

realized. Evaluation is more than a tool to help program managers strengthen the quality of their programs; it can also help communities determine whether a program is the right fit for them or if it has had the desired effects. Engaging communities in evaluation and the decision-making process of public health interventions ensures that programs are implemented based on the needs and desired outcomes of the community. Community engagement in evaluation also provides context to the cultural and health-equity-related nuances that can affect successful implementation of programs to improve maternal health outcomes.

This chapter focuses on culturally responsive evaluation (CRE), one of many evaluation frameworks, and provides examples of how to use the CRE approach to ensure that communities are at the center of evaluation. The chapter describes why local data are an important part of program evaluation, explains how CRE can be leveraged to center the community in the evaluation of maternal health efforts, and provides an overview of the CRE process. For each evaluation step, the chapter includes evaluators' reflections about real-world application of CRE strategies to the maternal health field. Finally, the chapter provides a link to an assessment tool to help researchers get started using CRE in their own evaluations.

PROBLEM: ACCESS TO RELEVANT MATERNAL HEALTH DATA AT THE COMMUNITY LEVEL

To effectively evaluate a program or service, it is essential that relevant data and information are made available about program implementation, services provided, and outcomes for program participants. Examples of data include demographic information about participants, processes used to recruit and retain participants, and measures and indicators collected about the health status or outcomes of participants. The data are used to inform whether a program was implemented as intended and to assess the outcomes of the program. Although data and information are critical to understanding the effectiveness of programs, there are several challenges to ensuring that data are available at the community level for use in program evaluation. Some of the challenges include:

- *Negative perceptions of research and evaluation.* Some communities may not participate in research or program evaluation efforts because historically they have not had data returned to the community or were left out of decision-making activities related to the data. Another significant contributor to low community participation in research and evaluation or sharing of data is the historical dismantling of trust between communities and researchers rooted in racist or discriminatory beliefs and practices. Examples include unethical experimentation and research on Black, Indigenous, and Hispanic/Latinx communities, systematic classification of some people as inferior, and discriminatory care and treatment practices based on poor research practices.[4]

- *Limited availability of local data.* Most data on maternal health, such as vital statistics from the Centers for Disease Control and Prevention (CDC) and PRAMS (Pregnancy Risk Assessment Monitoring System) data, are not publicly or readily available at the county, city, or ZIP Code levels and may have a two-year lag from time of collection to public accessibility. (For more information about state and federal maternal health data, see Chapter 25.) This limits the ability of maternal health programs to adjust services based on health outcomes. Accessing medical records data from a health system is difficult because of HIPAA (Health Insurance Portability and Accountability Act), which protects sensitive patient data and data use agreements. This creates a challenge to understanding the circumstances for maternal health outcomes and how to make program or community-level changes to address these issues directly. Without easily accessible secondary data, or data that have been previously gathered that can be accessed by researchers and evaluators, program evaluators are left to collect their own local data.
- *Small numbers.* When local data are available, unless they are collected in larger or urban metropolitan areas, the numbers are usually small, making it hard to see trends over time. To protect privacy, data may be prohibited from being displayed. Strategies to address small numbers, such as grouping together several years of data to stabilize rates or grouping together smaller demographic samples, make it difficult to understand how trends are changing over time or how a certain group is faring after an intervention.
- *Lack of standard, shared measurement across organizations.* Creating a shared measurement system across local organizations can be challenging, and comparing maternal health outcomes across communities and programs may not effectively reflect where interventions are needed. Lack of investment in public health has left many areas without a strong infrastructure for quickly collecting and using data to inform decision-making, enhance care delivery, and reduce maternal health disparities.

To ensure that efforts to reduce disparities in maternal outcomes or to improve overall maternal health are successful, there is a need for communities to have access to data, to contribute to local data collection, and to be included in decision-making. Although communities may not be familiar with jargon related to measurement and collection of data, community-based organizations and people with lived experiences know best how to meet their community's needs. Equipping communities with relevant data can help them to prioritize their needs, to understand where services are most essential, to apply for grant funding, and to measure the impact that programs and services have on maternal health outcomes. Ensuring that communities have access to data can foster community trust with researchers and evaluators (who may not be members of the community) and can help the community to own solutions for addressing issues important to them, including racial disparities in maternal mortality. Thus, a shift in power from those who traditionally have access to data and decision-making (researchers, governmental organizations, and funders) to those in the community (community members and community-based organizations) will advance maternal health efforts at the community level. This opens possibilities for communities to be fully engaged in evaluation and to be more willing to share data and information that can potentially help improve health outcomes for all.

Using a CRE approach is one way to support evaluation that leverages community and program assets (data) and to influence efforts to improve maternal health outcomes and reduce disparities. Grounding program evaluation in a culturally responsive framework can improve the validity of data, help determine which programs are benefiting the community, and lead to real change in local maternal health efforts.

SOLUTION: AN EVALUATION APPROACH THAT CENTERS CULTURE AND COMMUNITY

CRE calls explicit attention to culture and cultural context as integral to producing quality, useful, credible, and valid information to effectively advance the goals of a community, to serve the needs of its people, and to inform decision-making that improves outcomes. With better decision-making that serves the needs of people, CRE fosters a climate for social justice and systemic change.

In CRE, the terms *culture* and *cultural context* refer both to the evaluator(s) and the person(s)/program/policy being evaluated. Before engaging in an evaluation, a culturally responsive approach calls for dedicated time to reflect on the culture, cultural competence, and cultural context of the evaluator(s) and the person(s)/program/policy being evaluated.

Definitions: Important Concepts in CRE

The term *culture* refers to norms, traditions, histories, shared behavior, values, ways of knowing, and customs common to a particular group or society.[5]

It is essential that evaluators reflect on their cultural experiences and their respect, understanding, and connection to the cultural experiences of individuals affected by the program, policy, or other focus of the evaluation. This reflection is rooted in *cultural competence*, "a set of skills, both academic and interpersonal, that recognizes the importance of cultural differences and similarities within, among, and between groups."[6] Cultural competence is an ongoing and continuous learning process, and cultural competence in one community or population does not mean competence in another.

The term *cultural context* describes the circumstances that situate the evaluation and the program or policy being evaluated, such as the history of the community, policy, power dynamics, resources, perceptions, or any set of factors and how they affect the evaluation.[6]

In their work on CRE, Kirkhart and Hopson highlighted intersectionality in the discussion of culture, cultural competence, and cultural context. The term *intersectionality* was coined by Kimberlé Crenshaw, but the concept originated with feminist scholars of color, such as Sojourner Truth. Intersectionality is the idea that various aspects of our identity—race, ethnicity, language, gender, age, religion, sexual orientation, disability, social class, geographic location—overlap and influence our experience of oppression or privilege in different societal systems.[7] Applying an intersectional lens to program evaluation emphasizes the dynamic and interdependent nature of identities and emphasizes the importance of power relations based on those identities.[8,9]

HOW DO I USE CRE?

CRE is akin to other evaluation frameworks, such as the CDC's Framework for Program Evaluation in Public Health.[10] What distinguishes CRE is how evaluators engage in, and carry out, the evaluation steps that promote critical reflection and the intentional focus of centering culture in all phases of an evaluation. Figure 30.1 depicts the nine steps in the CRE framework.

Implementing the tenets of CRE is rewarding; however, it may force academics outside of their comfort zone. It requires the evaluator (or evaluation team) to enter a space with humility and a willingness not only to share control of the evaluation but also, in many ways, to relinquish power. It requires the evaluation team to recognize all stakeholders as experts and to engage in collaborative discourse. In many cases, implementing the CRE framework will be easier for program staff than for "academically trained professionals."

To support inclusion of CRE in program and policy evaluation, each of the nine steps is discussed below, along with key points taken from the work of Hood et al[11] and a list of references for more in-depth information and scholarship on CRE.[11] Each description also includes an evaluator's reflection on real-world application of CRE strategies to the field of maternal health. Although the components of CRE do not happen linearly, these reflections provide context for evaluating programs focused on eliminating maternal health disparities.

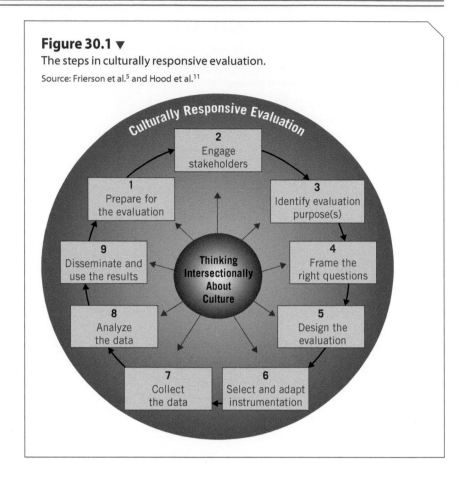

Figure 30.1 ▼

The steps in culturally responsive evaluation.

Source: Frierson et al.[5] and Hood et al.[11]

Step 1. Prepare for the Evaluation

- Evaluators have a responsibility to educate themselves on the context.
- Evaluators must reflect on and name their own assumptions, experiences, and biases related to the evaluation contexts and cultures.
- The evaluation team should have a connection to the lived experience of the community and contexts.

Reflection from the Field

As an evaluator, it is always important to reflect and check all assumptions at the door. Uninformed evaluators and teams may take phenotypic similarities for granted. For instance, each evaluator must acknowledge the socioeconomic, demographic, and regional differences of the communities they work in. This means learning the culture and demographics of both the organization and the community; being clear about your own assumptions and biases; watching and listening to learn, understand, and appreciate the expertise of the organizational staff; and understanding staff roles in the organization and the community at large. This is necessary for the leader of the evaluation team as well as for each team member.

Box 30.1 | Example of Preparing for the Evaluation

I had to learn that "All skin folk ain't kinfolk," which simply means that although one can share the same race, skin color, or even the community of those with whom one works, there may be distinct differences in culture and values. — Chapter coauthor Kimberley Broomfield-Massey

Step 2. Engage Stakeholders

- Respectfully enter the community.
- Make agreements around trust and respect for the process.
- Listen to stakeholders' concerns and involve them in the process.
- Spend ample time building relationships through continuous and ongoing engagement at a level that is meaningful and appropriate to stakeholders.

Reflection from the Field

While paying attention to your own attitudes and biases, and those of your team, it is also important to approach the space with authenticity, to show respect, and to grow trust in the communities and organizations you work with. As relationships and trust grow, so does interest in the importance of evaluation and the evaluation team's role in the organization. Engagement means that all stakeholders are a part of the evaluation team and all members have a voice in the evaluation. Learn from one another to avoid mistakes or mishaps, develop mutual respect for each member's contributions, and have a shared understanding of how you will work collaboratively to move the work forward.

Collaborating with all stakeholders on a logic model is one way to help create consensus among program administrators, program staff, and program participants about the theory of the change that this program will induce among participants. It also allows the group to center equity, community needs, and funder requirements in the overall program evaluation. At the end of the process, the team and organization walk away with a logic model, which gives one big picture, gets everyone on the same page, helps to establish buy-in, and ensures stakeholder engagement throughout the next steps.

Step 3. Identify Evaluation Purpose(s)

- The purpose of the evaluation should be rooted in social justice and ultimately benefit the community.
- The purpose of the evaluation should be clearly laid out for the mutual understanding of all stakeholders.
- Provide opportunities for ongoing feedback and information-sharing about the purpose with stakeholders.

> ### Box 30.2 | Example of Engaging Stakeholders
>
> When I have engaged colleagues working with stakeholders, I have had to have difficult conversations with white or other team members about understanding and respecting the culture and other social norms of the communities we serve. For example, I have shared that a "check-in," some way of connecting to one another personally before starting with the formal agenda, was a part of every meeting and that diving straight into the agenda was considered rude and off-putting for some communities. — Chapter coauthor Kimberley Broomfield-Massey

Reflection from the Field

It is important to create consensus about the purpose of the evaluation from all perspectives, including funders, staff, and participants. This means translating evaluation concepts and processes into clear, simple language that is not intimidating, yet not so simplistic that people are insulted. Developing the evaluation purpose is meant to be collaborative; each stakeholder should contribute to the process to ensure that outcomes are used in decision-making that benefits the organization and the community served by the program or policy.

Step 4. Frame the Right Questions

- Create dialogue with, and among, stakeholders to craft the right questions.
- Be explicit about whose interests and values are represented in the questions.
- Consider what evidence will be accepted as credible.
- Ensure that questions address issues of social justice, equity, and opportunity.

Reflection from the Field

Once the purpose of the evaluation is established, creating the right evaluation questions can be an interesting, collaborative, and fun process. As a general guideline, evaluations should have at least two or three key questions, but no more than ten, so that the evaluation can focus on the questions that meet the overall purpose. While the funder may require certain evaluation questions, it is important to identify questions that align with the questions that community members are intent on learning about or questions program staff need information on to make programming decisions. Asking who the evaluation will serve is an important step and an often-overlooked opportunity.

Step 5. Design the Evaluation

- Determine which data will answer which questions.
- Stay attentive to the cultural congruence of data-collection procedures.

- Be transparent about what data are being collected.
- Develop agreements with stakeholders on data ownership.

Reflection from the Field

After evaluation questions are framed, map out the best data to answer the questions. Often, it can be more affordable to use secondary data or data that are already available and not necessarily collected directly from program participants. Such data can provide important context to what else may be going on in a community, in addition to the program that you are evaluating. Employing secondary data might include using US Census data to obtain demographic information about the community served or using the CDC's vital statistics birth data to understand maternal health issues for the community. For communities seeking to provide context for program implementation, it may be important to have a better understanding of what other maternal, social, and mental health programs are available for women during the perinatal period, as an indicator of opportunities to prevent maternal death. This will provide richer context for the diversity of a community, availability of services in a community, and clearer understanding of how these factors influenced efforts to affect maternal health outcomes.

Arrangements should be made to ensure that data are collected and used in a manner that is culturally appropriate and reflects the purpose of the evaluation. A culturally responsive approach means hearing from participants of a program about their experience and satisfaction with the program. This may require having interpretation or translation services in multiple languages to ensure that all constituents of a program are heard.

When collecting data from the community, it is crucial that agreement be established up front on what data will be collected and on how the data are collected, used, and owned to make sure the process remains in step with the needs of the organization and community. Keeping in mind that evaluation is a process done with an organization or community, the data should be solely or jointly owned by the organization or community.

Step 6. Select and Adapt Instrumentation

- Ensure that data collection instruments are culturally appropriate.
- Be attentive to language and nonverbal communication.
- Align instruments with stakeholder agreements.

Reflection from the Field

This is where the "experts" must take a back seat. Evaluators should choose a few tools they think are appropriate and then discuss with frontline staff whether the instruments are appropriate based on stakeholder literacy and the context in which the instrument will be administered. Modification of surveys and tools creates a win–win situation for the evaluator and program, resulting in more valid data. When using new or modified tools, it is also important to pilot instruments to ensure that they capture what you intend to measure.

Step 7. Collect the Data
- Prioritize respect.
- Ensure that the pace of data collection is appropriate, flexible, and adaptive to respondents' needs.
- Help data collectors to see themselves as an instrument—acknowledging how biases, assumptions, and subjectivities can shape data collection.

Reflection from the Field

Building strong relationships in the design of an evaluation, through a collaborative and transparent process, will help data collection go more smoothly. Frontline staff typically are responsible for data collection. These staff members may be apprehensive at the start of the process, and taking time to consider their constraints and knowledge can help gain their support. Creating buy-in builds interest in the findings among frontline staff and encourages them to dedicate time for posttest data collection and focus groups as part of program implementation. Garnering buy-in also leads to evaluation of pretest and posttest instruments, follow-up and satisfaction survey collection, and participant story collection being built into day-to-day program structure. When stakeholders are involved all along the way, it creates a sense of curiosity so that data collection becomes easier and more useful in decision-making. Pushing people too hard to collect a large amount of data that they may not agree are relevant can create inaccurate or questionable data.

Step 8. Analyze the Data

- "Data do not speak for themselves; they are given voice by those who interpret them."[11]
- Involve stakeholders in data-interpretation "member checks,"[12] a common practice in qualitative research where you share findings with participants and obtain their feedback on interpretation of findings to improve the credibility and accuracy.
- Disaggregate data to explore how the program affects each stakeholder differently.
- Notice which pieces of data are given more weight, and why.

Reflection from the Field

While the evaluation team might conduct the pretest and posttest analyses and/or analyze focus group data, interpretation of the data can happen collectively through a facilitated process. Holding "meaning-making" sessions, a facilitated process to share preliminary findings with stakeholders, can help the evaluator and community understand and interpret the findings and generate action steps or recommendations from the data. It can also highlight what outcomes are important to program participants, which may be very different from outcomes that are important to the funder or the organization. Evaluators should keep in mind how data will be interpreted by the various groups of stakeholders. Outlining clear statements about the results of, limitations of, and even challenges in the data-collection process also helps to frame expectations of the data and how they can be used to shape the program.

Step 9. Disseminate and Use the Results

- Use results to promote equity.
- Determine what information will be shared or safeguarded.
- Involve stakeholders in findings review and the dissemination plan.

Reflection from the Field

Most important in any community-driven evaluation process is the dissemination and use of findings from the program evaluation. As discussed previously, program evaluation succeeds when it is built on a trusting, inclusive, and transparent foundation. While sharing results, any changes or enhancements to the program that are made based on the results should be clearly communicated to all stakeholders. Bear in mind that each stakeholder group may need a different presentation of the evaluation findings and recommendations, depending on the audience (funders or administrators, for example) and use (decision-making or sharing program success, for example). This shows the value of

Box 30.5 | Example of Analyzing and Interpreting Data

There are many group learning activities that an evaluator can use to help guide stakeholders through reflection and dialogue as they review findings. One of our favorite ways to present data and foster dialogue among small groups of diverse stakeholders is using data placemats.[i,ii] Data placemats—large sheets of paper that display evaluation findings—are set at a table like placemats for a meal. After stakeholders review the data on their placemat, they share with the group what they noticed on their sheet, any surprises in the data, factors that may explain the trends, and implications or insights from the findings. Other data analysis and interpretation activities are presented in detail in the guide *Facilitating Intentional Group Learning*. These activities can help the evaluators see which findings are most important to stakeholders, catch mistakes before disseminating the results further, and improve the credibility of the findings. —Chapter coauthor Christine Tucker

REFERENCES

i. Gutierrez E, Preskill H, Mack K. Facilitating Intentional Group Learning: A Practical Guide to 21 Learning Activities. 2017. https://collectiveimpactfo rum.org/wp-content/uploads/2021/12/Facilitating-Intentional-Group-Learn ing.pdf

ii. Pankaj V, Emery AK. Data placemats: a facilitative technique designed to enhance stakeholder understanding of data. In: *New Directions for Evaluation*. Wiley Online Library; 2016:81–93.

the contributions of each of the evaluation participants and creates stronger relationships among the funder, organization, and program participants. Determining how to disseminate and use evaluation results should not wait until the end of the evaluation process. Collaborate with all stakeholders in order to shape the dissemination plan and determine what information will be shared internally or externally about a program's activities.

Most importantly, involve stakeholders to determine how program evaluation results can be used to address maternal health inequities. If the evaluation results are not used in service of equity, trust may be broken, and stakeholders may lose faith in the evaluation team and in future evaluation efforts.

WHERE TO BEGIN: IS MY EVALUATION CULTURALLY RESPONSIVE?

A good starting point for developing culturally responsive evaluations is to identify whether the evaluation team uses principles of cultural competence and equity in its practices. The checklist tool *Is My Evaluation Practice Culturally Responsive?* serves as a point-in-time assessment for evaluators to

Table 30.1	Selected Assessment Items from Is My Evaluation Practice Culturally Responsive?
Cultural Competence of the Evaluator	
At all stages of an evaluation, I examine the potential impact of cultural stereotypes and my own personal biases around race, ethnicity, gender, socioeconomic status, and other individual differences.	
I pay attention to the similarities and differences of life experiences between the evaluation team and members of the target population, and consider how those dynamics might impact the evaluation.	
Cultural Competence of the Evaluation Practices	
Data-collection instruments (i.e., surveys, interview protocols) are selected and adapted to ensure appropriateness for the culture(s) of the people of whom the questions are being asked.	
Data-collection activities that require interaction with community members, consumers, and stakeholders are led by the team members who are best suited to understand the specific cultural context, based on factors such as shared experiences with the target population, knowledge of the target population, and awareness of biases.	
Applying the Lens to Process Evaluation	
I assess the extent to which community stakeholders were actively involved in the planning and implementation of program activities.	
I collect input from program stakeholders about the extent to which the organization is perceived as a credible proponent of diversity, inclusion, and equity.	
Applying the Outcomes to Process Evaluation	
In analyzing and interpreting outcome data, I disaggregate data along demographic lines to identify and assess the extent of differential impacts of the program.	
In assessing program outcomes, I look for any unintended consequences of program activities due to cultural or racial/ethnic issues/context.	

Source: Elam P, Walker W.15

determine "the degree to which their [evaluation] practices incorporate the principles and methods for conducting evaluation through a cultural competence and racial equity lens."[15] The assessment uses a list of 38 questions, across four areas, that allow evaluators to reflect on how often they included culturally competent and racial equity principles in their evaluation activities over the last year. Table 30.1 lists a selection of assessment statements from the tool.

Is My Evaluation Practice Culturally Responsive? supports evaluators who are exploring cultural competency; their own culture, including assumptions, biases, and understanding of different cultures; and how culture is positioned in evaluation activities to produce data that are responsive to community stakeholders.

CONCLUSION

In CRE, it is important for evaluators to think ahead about the ways that communities are affected by programs and how the evaluation will shape decision-making processes. Evaluation should influence decision-making at all levels of a program; thus, the data and information gathered should be from the community affected and not solely "about" the community where a maternal health program is implemented. Accounting for the culture and context of communities in program evaluation means including a diverse range of factors and voices to make decisions about the programs and services that will best support improvements in maternal health and eliminate disparities.

REFERENCES

1. Hoyert DL. Maternal mortality rates in the United States, 2021. NCHS Health E-Stats. 2023. https://dx.doi.org/10.15620/cdc:124678.

2. Agency for Healthcare Research and Quality. Care coordination. https://www.ahrq.gov/ncepcr/care/coordination.html. Published 2018. Accessed December 8, 2022.

3. Patton MQ. *Utilization-Focused Evaluation*. Thousand Oaks, CA: SAGE; 2008.

4. Armstrong K, Ravenell KL, McMurphy S, Putt M. Racial/ethnic differences in physician distrust in the United States. *Am J Public Health*. 2007;97(7):1283–1289.

5. Frierson H, Hood S, Hughes G. A guide to conducting culturally responsive evaluation. In: *The 2002 User-Friendly Handbook for Project Evaluation*. Alexandria, VA: National Science Foundation; 2002:63–73.

6. Kirkhart K, Hopson R. Strengthening evaluation through cultural relevance and cultural competence. Slides and handout from AEA/CDC Summer Evaluation Institute, June 13–16, 2010. https://higherlogicdownload.s3-external-1.amazonaws.com/EVAL/Case Scenario Dialogue for Diversity and Social Change.pdf?AWSAccessKeyId=AKIAVRDO7IEREB57R7MT&Expires=1670520028&Signature=mV%2BBCmbXlkjNHOYgr1I5edqjANU%3D.

7. Crenshaw K. Demarginalizing the intersection of race and sex: a Black feminist critique of antidiscrimination doctrine, feminist theory, and antiracist politics. *Chicago Unbound1989*;1(8). https://chicagounbound.uchicago.edu/uclf/vol1989/iss1/8.

8. Cho S, Crenshaw KW, McCall L. Toward a field of intersectionality studies: Theory, applications, and praxis. *Signs*. 2013;38(4):785–810.

9. McKinzie AE, Richards PL. An argument for context-driven intersectionality. *Sociol Compass*. 2019;13(4):e12671.

10. Centers for Disease Control and Prevention Program Performance and Evaluation Office. Framework for program evaluation. https://www.cdc.gov/evaluation/framework/index.htm. Published 2017. Accessed December 8, 2022.

11. Hood S, Hopson RK, Kirkhart KE. Culturally responsive evaluation. In: Katherine E. Newcomer, Harry P. Hatrey, and Joseph S. Wholey, eds. *Handbook of Practical Program Evaluation*. Hoboken, NJ: Josses-Bass; 2015:281–317. doi:https://doi.org/10.1002/9781119171386.ch12.

12. Birt L, Scott S, Cavers D, Campbell C, Walter F. Member checking: a tool to enhance trustworthiness or merely a nod to validation? *Qual Health Res*. 2016;26(13):1802–1811. doi:10.1177/1049732316654870.

13. Gutierrez E, Preskill H, Mack K. *Facilitating Intentional Group Learning: A Practical Guide to 21 Learning Activites*. Brussels: European Foundation Centre; 2017.

14. Pankaj V, Emery AK. Data placemats: a facilitative technique designed to enhance stakeholder understanding of data. In: *New Directions for Evaluation*. Wiley Online Library; 2016:81–93.

15. Elam P, Walker W. Is my evaluation practice culturally responsive? https://vepimg. b8cdn.com/uploads/vjfnew/4338/content/docs/1619888875is-my-evaluation-pract ice-culturally-responsive-pdf1619888875.pdf. Published online 2021.

Innovations

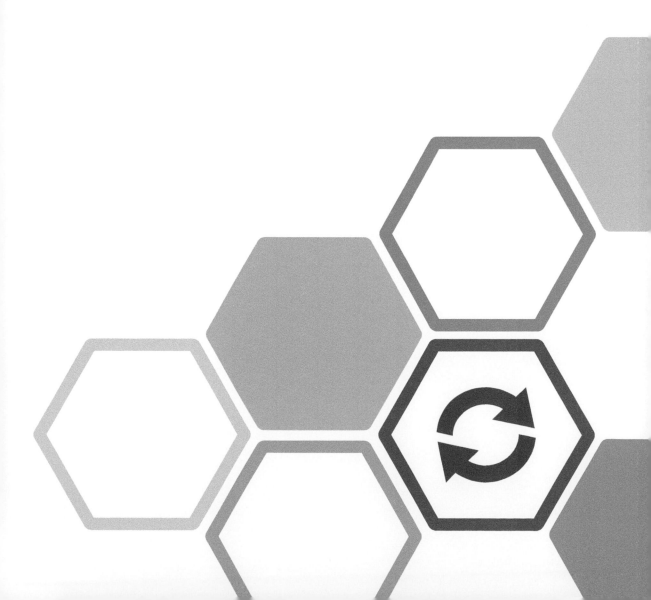

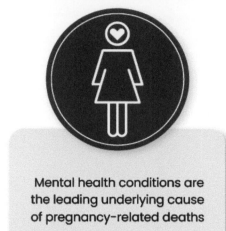

Mental health conditions are the leading underlying cause of pregnancy-related deaths

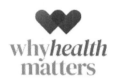

Source: Why Health Matters and Imaginari

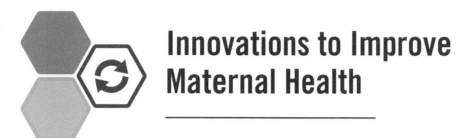

Chapter 31

Innovations to Improve Maternal Health

SARAH VERBIEST AND MONICA BELTRAN

Providing equitable, culturally appropriate, coordinated care across the life course, wherein people are treated with respect and receive quality, evidence-based treatment, is not an innovative concept—it is the way the healthcare system should function. Unfortunately, in the United States, the system was not designed to care for everyone well and is a hodgepodge of state-specific, Westernized, white-dominated, and financially driven approaches to the provision of healthcare services. Furthermore, attention to the needs of women and birthing people is steeped in an American culture of individualism and independence that has led many new parents to navigate this sensitive period in the life of their family with limited resources and supports. We must do better.

The concept of innovation has been popular in thinking about how to approach improving maternal health. In part, its popularity may be driven by the federal Maternal and Child Health Bureau of the Health Resources and Services Administration, which has been releasing calls for proposals for innovative work across their portfolio for several years, including home visiting, serving children with special healthcare needs, the Alliance for Innovation in Maternal Health, the Maternal Health Innovations state grants, and the national Maternal Health Learning and Innovation Center, among many others. Resources to support new ideas and approaches are critically important to the work.

The idea of innovation has broad application. At its most common interpretation, innovation is about something new. One definition is that innovation in maternal health includes developing a new process, policy, product, or program to improve outcomes—changing how something is done to increase quality, efficiency, or effectiveness. This definition leaves room for broad interpretation

Sarah Verbiest and Monica Beltran, *Innovations to Improve Maternal Health* In: *The Practical Playbook III*. Edited by: Dorothy Cilenti, Alisahah Jackson, Natalie D. Hernandez, Lindsey Yates, Sarah Verbiest, J. Lloyd Michener, and Brian C. Castrucci, Oxford University Press. © de Beaumont Foundation 2024. DOI: 10.1093/oso/9780197662984.003.0031

and understanding. For example, something that may be common practice in an urban area may be innovative in a rural area.

As we tackle complex, systemic, interconnected problems that are resulting in deepening and disparate health outcomes, there is an urgent need for new mindsets, approaches, and voices to move the field toward change. This is reflected in the work of Clark et al in their chapter, "Respectful Care and Reproductive Justice as Foundations for Maternal Health Innovation." In the *Practical Playbook II, Building Multisectoral Partnerships That Work*, in their chapter on innovation, Michener and Hunter underscored this point when they wrote about the role communities have in innovation: "Communities are disrupting both as they assert their fundamental ability to set priorities and processes for engagement. In many cases becoming the leaders of change."[1]

Furthermore, innovation can mean a renaissance of practices that have been overlooked or even intentionally shut down—often due to structural racism—and an expansion of our understanding of healthcare teams and community connection. Dillion and Sulaiman spotlight the re-emergence of doulas in their chapter, "The Integral Role of Community-Based Doulas in Supporting Birth Equity," as a key strategy where communities, particularly communities of color, are not supporting/saving birthing people but and have the potential to reshape OB/GYN care. As evidenced here, innovation can be a rediscovery and return to what is vital. Finding the way back to these practices requires innovation, courage, and determination.

The chapter by Harper Tully et al on postpartum care aligns with several of the approaches to innovation as the authors offer models of changes to the way care is delivered, aligning with the chapter by Clark et al, as well as what care is offered, centering the voice of people with lived experience across all processes. Harper Tully et al offer information about new tools, Web sites, and strategies for change.

Innovation can mean using new technology as well as using existing technology in new ways. The COVID-19 pandemic upended the way we work, meet, do research, and provide support, healthcare, and behavioral health services to pregnant and birthing people. The transition to telehealth also opened the doors for access to culturally congruent maternal mental health services for communities who did not have access to it before. The pandemic forced quick change and demonstrated that some of the barriers that hold us back from doing new things (e.g., reimbursement and policy structures) can be broken down quickly. And new technology likewise continues to review structural fault lines around access to resources that can exacerbate disparities unless addressed explicitly and well. In the chapter "Innovations in Virtual Care," deRosset, Neeley, and Palmquist provide an excellent overview of changes, challenges, and transformations in telemedicine and telehealth.

Innovation also means applying a new perspective or lens in looking at, and solving, existing problems. Mental health and substance use disorders are two significant contributors to maternal mortality and morbidity. Neither is a new problem, and both have been exacerbated by the COVID-19 pandemic, economic challenges, concerns about climate change, civil tensions over justice and equity issues, and more. Women are dying—outside of the clinic and hospital setting—due to a lack of screening and support, a shortage of treatment resources, inadequate financial resources, and stigma. While this is a problem for many birthing people, Black and American Indian/Native American women continue to die at rates three to four times higher than those of white women. In Chapter 37, Akbarali et al share strategies from their innovative learning community model to address substance misuse and co-occurring mental health challenges. In Chapter 36, Raines and Davis spotlight new approaches to bridging the gap in perinatal mental health that run from grassroots to telecommunication.

Over time, one can also follow the way that funding tends to focus in "hot topic" areas. While this can be an important catalyst for change, this narrow approach can sometimes be overly restrictive and miss the chance to invest in efforts that take novel, upstream approaches to the work. In the chapter "Women's Health Before, Between, Beyond, and Regardless of Pregnancy," Verbiest, Woodward, and Yates underscore the necessity of investing in new approaches to women's health, including the health of women outside the context of pregnancy. This investment is key because innovation also calls us to look forward to emerging challenges. According to Birth by the Numbers, the death rates for women ages 25 to 34 are increasing exponentially in the United States, with American Indian/Alaska Native women experiencing a 50% increase between 2010 and 2019.[2] Furthermore, changes in access to the full reproductive suite of services, including abortion care, are likely to continue to challenge current strategies for improving women's and birthing people's health and well-being.[1]

As Mitchener and Hunter emphasized, "Not all innovation is effective—it must be married to the need it addresses, be evaluated and be connected to the community." This is especially important, because the "shiny new thing" has the potential to take us off course from addressing equity, away from community, and off focus from the necessary work at hand. As we've seen in history, there have been "innovations" in OB-GYN care that have caused harm and new "community" initiatives that have driven deep wedges between healthcare and community because they were not grounded in equity.

Innovation requires new perspectives and creative approaches, which are more likely to come from teams that have diverse perspectives, experiences, and identities. Teams and organizations also need to be open to collaborating on solutions with the communities they serve. We believe that increased representation of people of color in leadership roles and engagement of community partners at all levels will spark a new wave of innovation. Imagine the possibilities they bring to this work! New ways of working need to include intentional design and support systems to make way for these voices and ideas.

We believe that innovation and change in maternal health needs reproductive justice organizations, maternal and child health organizations, and programs that address social determinants of health to find common ground and to align interests toward collective impact. Innovation extends to whom we bring together and how. The pandemic, new civil rights movement, major policy changes, climate change, and the economy signal that there will not be a "return to normal" as people may have hoped in 2020. There is even a growing understanding that the "normal" of the past was in fact not healthy or right for many people. Leaders, public practitioners, healthcare providers, community leaders, and all of us are living in transformational times. Let us work together to innovate for change!

REFERENCES

1. Michener JL, Hunter EL. Overview—innovation: enhancing coordinated impact through new roles and tools. In: Michener JL, Castrucci B, Bradley DW, et al, eds. *The Practical Playbook II: Building Multisector Partnerships That Work*. New York, NY: Oxford University Press; 2019:231–234.

2. DeClercq G. The contemporary challenge of maternal mortality in the US. Birth by the Numbers. https://www.birthbythenumbers.org. Accessed June 16, 2022.

Chapter 32

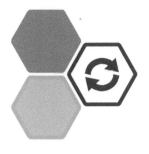

Respectful Care and Reproductive Justice as Foundations for Maternal Health Innovation

AJA CLARK, PHOEBE WESCOTT, AMY USHRY, KIARA CRUZ, CHRISTIE ALLEN, AND INAS-KHALIDAH MAHDI

INTRODUCTION

This chapter discusses opportunities for improved care for communities that have sustained historical and ongoing harm by the medical establishment. The chapter presents a brief rationale for innovation in maternal healthcare delivery, particularly the need for dignity, respect, and acknowledgment of the historical and ongoing medical mistreatment, disrespect, abuse, and reproductive oppression burdening Black birthing people. The chapter revisits reproductive justice as a broad framework and respectful care as a practical strategy to shift the culture of maternal healthcare systems toward improving quality of care and reducing bias and inequities among Black birthing people. Examples of successful community–clinical partnerships and other innovative programs are highlighted, including tools to pursue structural shifts toward optimizing maternal health in communities.

THE LEGACY AND IMPACT OF RACISM IN MATERNAL HEALTH

Practical conversations about the current state of maternal health in the United States require acknowledgment of the historical and contemporary presence of racism and the role of power in modern obstetrics and gynecology. The maternal health system in the United States was constructed at a time when it was

Aja Clark, Phoebe Wescott, Amy Ushry, Kiara Cruz, Christie Allen, and Inas-Khalidah Mahdi, *Respectful Care and Reproductive Justice as Foundations for Maternal Health Innovation* In: *The Practical Playbook III*. Edited by: Dorothy Cilenti, Alisahah Jackson, Natalie D. Hernandez, Lindsey Yates, Sarah Verbiest, J. Lloyd Michener, and Brian C. Castrucci, Oxford University Press. © de Beaumont Foundation 2024. DOI: 10.1093/oso/9780197662984.003.0032

acceptable to disregard the lives of Black women and birthing people. This lack of regard for Black life unfortunately persists today and is evident in the racial health disparities related to birthing outcomes in the United States. For more information about the history of race and obstetrics, see the report, "Reversing the U.S. Maternal Mortality Crisis," released by the Aspen Health Strategy Group in 2021.[1]

A violent link exists between Black birthing people, the plantation economy, and the nation's current maternal healthcare system. In 2017, Dr. Deirdre Cooper Owens illuminated the complex relationship that emerged between the burgeoning field of gynecology, Black birthing people, and slaveholders in the 1800s.[2] Following the decision by Congress in 1808 to ban trafficking of African people into the United States, slaveholders endeavored to maintain the reproductive capacity of enslaved Black birthing bodies. Concurrently, the white male-dominated field of obstetrics and gynecology was forming, seeking a surplus of bodies from which to gain experience, to design new procedures, and to learn how to correct gynecological disorders common at the time. Prior to the emergence of what would become the field of obstetrics and gynecology, Black midwives were the primary caregivers for enslaved birthing people, and midwives drew on generational knowledge and traditions of care rooted in their places and communities of origin. It is ironic that many of the maternal health interventions being proposed today are adjacent to the holistic care that the Black midwives provided to their communities, although recognition of the resemblance is often missing.

In the early phases of the field of obstetrics and gynecology, physicians and slaveholders often collaborated on the medical treatment provided to Black birthing people. As one can imagine, this triad rendered enslaved Black birthing people silent and subject to experimentation at the hands of practitioners who sought scientific legitimacy and support from the dominant social group.[2]

Why is the history of a field that began in the 1800s relevant today? The legacy of early practices of devaluation, dehumanization, and abuse continues as Black women are routinely silenced, neglected, abused, and harmed in their interactions with the maternal healthcare system. Transforming medical and public health institutions requires innovation to disrupt tacit support for this mistreatment and abuse. There can be no contemporary innovation without the inclusion of the historical record.

According to the Centers for Disease Control and Prevention, in the United States, Black women are three times more likely than white women to experience pregnancy-related death.[3] In addition to the differential power dynamics embedded in obstetrics and gynecology, structural racism has also been identified as a fundamental contributor to health disparities. Structural racism includes the racial biases inside institutional and governmental policies, laws, and norms that systematically affect the lives of Black people and other people of color. Decades of narratives sought to blame Black communities[4]—namely,

Black mothers—for poor Black maternal and infant health outcomes. The maternal health community now seeks to confront, and in some places correct, how the social determinants of health, such as housing, transportation, wages, access to healthcare, and more, come together in a matrix that can either severely limit or pose no resistance to someone's ability to reach their highest potential of health.

Beyond structural racism, personal and individual manifestations of racism, such as microaggressions and bias, fuel disrespect in labor and delivery care in the United States.[5] Despite evidence of such mistreatment and bias, providers and health-system leaders have limited holistic frameworks and practical tools for examining patients' experiences through the lens of historical reproductive oppression and racism.

REPRODUCTIVE JUSTICE: A FRAMEWORK FOR WELL-BEING AND HEALTH

SisterSong, a national organization focused on reproductive justice, defines reproductive justice as "the human right to maintain personal bodily autonomy, [to] have children, not [to] have children, and [to] parent the children we have in safe and sustainable communities."[6] Reproductive justice pointedly centers and is led by those who are experiencing a disproportionate amount of harm from systemic forces.[7] Reproductive justice is innovation! It brilliantly asserts that those who are experiencing vulnerability based on race, class, sex, gender, sexuality, or ability are the most equipped to address their circumstances. This means that in seeking to implement innovative methods to address inequities in the US maternal health system—and consequently abroad—communities experiencing the most harm should be centered, resourced, and leading the efforts toward innovation and culture shifts. Communities must be responsibly and ethically integrated into the care that they receive. To do this, those currently possessing disproportionate amounts of systemic and interpersonal power, namely medical providers and systems, must be willing to participate in an appropriate redistribution of power. It is time for actors in the maternal healthcare system to center the needs, autonomy, and desires of the communities it has harmed in order to realize a future where every Black mama and birthing person, their babies, and their villages thrive.

Strategies to Operationalize Reproductive Justice

Understanding the historical shifts from predominantly midwife-attended birth to predominantly physician-attended birth in this country is fundamental for analyzing the various reforms in maternity care models and their impact on maternal and infant health.[4] Historically and cross-culturally, women have been attended to, and supported by, other women during labor and birth. However, in hospitals worldwide, continuous support during labor has become the exception rather than the routine, with physician-provided care as the most common maternity care model in the United States.[6] Because obstetric care focuses on preventing, diagnosing, and treating pregnancy and birth complications, training in this model does not typically focus on skills to support the natural progression of an uncomplicated birth. The traditional fee-for-service model incentivizes providers to increase the volume of services without addressing quality and outcomes.[7]

Core Principles of the Reproductive and Sexual Health Equity Framework

Created by a group of reproductive justice leaders, maternal and child health experts, and reproductive health researchers and practitioners, the Reproductive and Sexual Health Equity Framework is an approach to achieving the highest level of health for all people and addressing inequities in health outcomes by centering people's reproductive and sexual health needs.[8] Principles of the framework include centering the needs of, and redistributing power to, communities; having clinical and public health systems acknowledge historical and ongoing harms related to reproductive and sexual health; and addressing root causes of inequities.[8]

The Cycle to Respectful Care framework is an example of how organizations can operationalize the core principles of the Reproductive and Sexual Health Equity Framework. Elevating Black birthing people's experiences and their interpersonal interactions, as well as understanding the social and structural context, are critical to the development of programs and policies to prevent and eliminate maternal outcome disparities.

Cycle to Respectful Care Framework

Disrupting America's maternal health crisis begins with acknowledging that structural racism affects Black birthing people and proposing a new standard of care that honors trust, autonomy, Blackness, equity, and responsiveness. In partnership with community-based organizations (CBOs), focus groups were held by the National Birth Equity Collaborative to illuminate the hospital birthing experiences of Black birthing people across the United States.[9] CBO leaders helped recruit, co-facilitate, analyze the data, and develop the framework. CBO leaders also determined that the key elements of a respectful care framework must address racism, promote the ongoing growth and development of healthcare workers, and center the experiences of Black birthing people. The Cycle to Respectful Care acknowledges the development and perpetuation of biased healthcare delivery while providing a solution for dismantling the providers' socialization that results in biased and discriminatory care. The Cycle to Respectful Care is an actionable tool for freeing patients, by way of their healthcare providers, from biased practices and beliefs, structural and institutional racism, and policies that perpetuate racism.

Accordingly, the Cycle to Respectful Care framework combines theory, analysis, and experiences of Black mothers across the United States (see Figure 32.1). The primary audience for the framework is physicians, nurse midwives, and nurses, because birthing people's care experiences are highly influenced by these individuals. Although this framework was written for the direct use of traditionally/academically trained medical professionals, it can be used by any healthcare professional who serves Black birthing people in their reproductive life course and who has a vested interest in improving maternal health experiences and outcomes.

Figure 32.1 ▼

National Birth Equity Collaborative Cycle to Respectful Care.

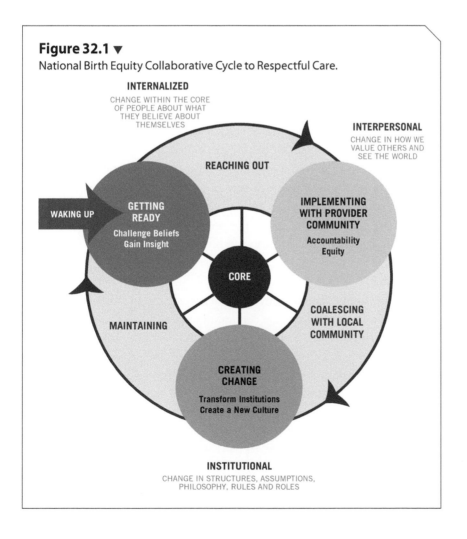

Integrative Models for Maternity Care Delivery

As new approaches are explored for addressing long-standing inequitable maternity outcomes in the US healthcare system, we must examine root causes—racism, unfair structural distribution of power, and neglect of women's lived experiences.[10] To overcome these inequities, the focus has shifted to holistic models of care using a reproductive justice framework to create clinical–community linkages. According to the Black Mamas Matter Alliance, holistic maternity care addresses gaps and provides care that is accessible, affordable, confidential, safe, and trauma-informed; centers Black women and families; and is patient-centered and patient-led.[11] Using these models in maternity care is critical for developing sustainable and scalable paths from the clinical environment to community-based resources and services.[13,14] Moving forward, the field must shift to incorporating reproductive justice frameworks like those mentioned above that center on community-led approaches to improve maternal health outcomes.

An important first step in incorporating innovative models for maternal care delivery is an organizational birth-equity assessment. Equity assessments provide baseline knowledge for organizations' capacity to achieve birth equity, no matter where they begin the journey. *Birth equity*, a term coined by Dr. Joia Crear-Perry, founder and president of the National Birth Equity Collaborative, is the assurance of the condition of optimal birth for all people, with a willingness to address racial and social inequities in a sustained effort.[15] Results from a birth-equity assessment help identify the capacity for equity, priority action areas, organizational policies and practices, and localized structural determinants of health, while also centering the voices of those who are most marginalized. By committing to a thorough review and reflection of harmful practices, an organization is better positioned to direct resources, to modify practices and policies, and to allocate funding to drive action for birth equity.

Holistic Care Models

Holistic care models for maternity care can provide a guide for healthcare systems that seek to incorporate the community voice into their practice. The JJ Way® is a patient-centered model for care to reduce adverse maternal and newborn health outcomes. Created by Jennie Joseph, British-trained midwife, and founder and director of the Commonsense Childbirth Easy Access Clinic in Orlando, Florida, the model not only uplifts the patient's voice but also supports the inclusion of the patient's family/support group as a critical part of prenatal visits. The clinics do not turn away patients if they have no insurance coverage or cannot pay.[16] The JJ Way® provides patients with navigators to guide patients through the healthcare system and provides personalized care plans based on an individual's needs. An evaluation of the program in 2017 showed that those who received maternity care using the JJ Way® had better birth outcomes and lower preterm birth rates than women in the county and the state of Florida. Ultimately, the JJ Way® completely removed preterm birth disparities and reduced low-birth-weight outcomes for marginalized populations.[16]

With the goal of improving maternal health outcomes in the United States, the Alliance for Innovation on Maternal Health Community Care Initiative (AIM CCI) seeks to expose and address racial inequities and to create a more standardized approach to incorporating equitable frameworks in communities and health systems. Under the leadership of the National Healthy Start Association and funded by the Health Resources and Services Administration, AIM CCI partners with community-based organizations to create coordinated quality-improvement initiatives to build linkages between communities and healthcare systems' implementation of non-hospital-focused bundles in selected pilot sites. The bundles are a set of evidence-based practices that, when implemented consistently, can improve maternal health outcomes. They aim to address needs and priorities in community and outpatient settings by identifying birthing people's pregnancy and postpartum experiences and community perspectives on how to attain equity.[18] Findings from the project will inform recommendations to strengthen clinical–community linkages in local programming.

While no one innovative clinical–community intervention will eliminate all health inequities, the opportunities just described can help in dismantling long-standing inequitable outcomes, resetting imbalances in power, and designing a holistic maternal health system. Maternal health outcomes can be improved when health systems and communities have aligned action steps toward equity.[11]

MODELS FOR INNOVATION

Clinical and Community Care

Models of clinical medical care and community care delivery (see Figure 32.2) require integration and infusion with the core concepts of reproductive justice to achieve sustainability and to address the disparities noted above. A model of care delivery that educates and trains people strongly influences approaches to care and everyone's understanding of the boundary, scope, and role of who is providing care.[17] When considering the need for integration of care models in innovation, it is important to understand the models that people use and their potential impacts.

Medical care is disease-focused, and the medical care provider primarily responds to symptoms, conditions, and health deficits. Little room is left in the medical model to consider social, psychological, or behavioral elements that drive health. Community care models focus on health promotion and beliefs of populations, including integration of needs, holistic approaches to the assessment of health-affecting behaviors, and strengths-based interventions.[18] While community care uses person-centered approaches, it does not have access

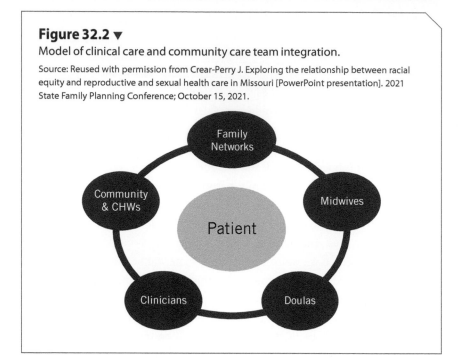

Figure 32.2 ▼
Model of clinical care and community care team integration.

Source: Reused with permission from Crear-Perry J. Exploring the relationship between racial equity and reproductive and sexual health care in Missouri [PowerPoint presentation]. 2021 State Family Planning Conference; October 15, 2021.

to the materials, skills, and operational processes to address acute health crisis conditions that affect morbidity and mortality.

The nature of these models and their influence on how maternal care is delivered create barriers to innovation. A rejection of the medical model by communities who have been marginalized or harmed by this type of model and resulting care is understandable. Complete rejection of the model, however, creates serious risk of harm and lack of safety for the people who need that care. Exclusion of community care approaches, on the other hand, results in medical care that fails to account for personal autonomy and strategies that would be most meaningful for those seeking care and for their health outcomes.

Integration is possible and can be fostered by reproductive justice. One example of reproductive justice used in a medical model is the patient-centered contraceptive counseling guidance from the American College of Obstetricians and Gynecologists (ACOG). This guidance states that because contraception can be fundamental to an individual's health and wellness, counseling to support decision-making must be offered with an intentional application of a patient-centered reproductive justice framework. Specifically, this should acknowledge historical and current-day reproductive maltreatment of people of color and other marginalized individuals, recognize counselor bias, and prioritize a patient's values and lived experiences.[19]

Because of the harm created by the lack of integration of these models, it is critical that best practices in integration are honored through the lens of reproductive justice in maternal care. Here, best practices include shared decision-making and informed consent, reshaping of the traditional care team model, risk assessment for the appropriate level and placement of care, and development of tools and resources to support the work.

Shared Decision-Making and Informed Consent

To foster care environments in which clinical medicine and communities are integrated, an underlying foundation of trust and respect must be established. Building informed consent and shared decision-making into medical culture helps lay that foundation. According to ACOG's Committee Opinion on Informed Consent and Shared Decision-Making in Obstetrics and Gynecology,

> Informed consent is a practical application of the bioethics principle of respect for patient autonomy and self-determination as well as the legal right of a patient to bodily integrity. The goal of the informed consent process is to provide patients with information that is necessary and relevant to their decision-making (including the risks and benefits of accepting or declining recommended treatment) and to assist patients in identifying the best course of action for their medical care.[20]

Shared decision-making provides a patient-centered approach to the informed consent process. With this approach, clinicians share and discuss the potential risks and benefits of treatment options with individuals seeking care. In turn, the individuals are encouraged to express the values and priorities that influence their medical decision-making and inform the treatment plan. This allows individuals to receive personalized information about treatment options, thus supporting their ability to make autonomous decisions.[21]

In fast-paced clinical environments, providers may find it challenging to balance the shared decision-making process with the need for decisive action in certain scenarios. The skills needed to provide comprehensive, compassionate counseling on medical decision-making are not often taught. Additionally, the power dynamic in modern-day clinical encounters favors the provider as the source of knowledge and expertise. Patients' expertise and knowledge of their bodies are not always respected or valued. Acknowledging these factors creates space for both clinicians and community members to recognize the real-life barriers that inhibit consistent and optimal use of these best practices. In spite of these barriers, informed consent and shared decision-making are not optional when seeking to foster care environments built on mutual trust and respect. Integrating clinical medicine and communities may provide an innovative approach to building these skills. Often, stakeholders across disciplines and within communities have expertise in how to provide counseling, facilitate meaningful conversations among community members, and link individuals to local resources. Leveraging these and other community strengths can be valuable in helping shift the culture of medicine to one that entrenches shared decision-making.

Models of care must include shared decision-making and open, transparent conversations about risk between medical and community-based care systems while avoiding fear tactics to drive choices. In an environment where models of care are fully integrated for the benefit of those they serve, the assessment of risk is standard and clear. Where care should, and can, be optimally provided is a primary aspect of equitable and respectful care and is key throughout the lifespan continuum of maternal and child healthcare. This need was discussed in a report by the National Academies of Sciences, Engineering, and Medicine: "Studies suggest that home and birth center births may be as safe as hospital births for low-risk women and infants when they are part of an integrated and regulated system." The report highlighted the lack of true integration in the majority of current regional and national structures.[22] At times, providing equitable and respectful care may involve the recognition that a provider or setting is not optimal for meeting a person's health and wellness needs.

Reshaping the Care Team

The composition of the clinical care team varies across medical settings depending on staffing resources and organizational norms. At a minimum, the care team in the setting of maternal health traditionally includes the medical professionals involved in providing treatment over the course of an individual's prenatal, birth, and postpartum experiences. Reshaping perspectives on the composition of care teams allows for communities and clinical medicine to become more fully integrated. This may start with considering a broader range of multidisciplinary professionals who enhance and optimize obstetric care. For example, midwives provide prenatal, birth, and postpartum care in multiple settings, including at home, in a birth center, and in hospitals.[21] While studies show that integration of midwifery care results in positive outcomes, such as lower rates of cesarean deliveries, preterm births, and low-birth-weight infants,[21,23] only fewer than 10% of births in the United States are delivered by certified nurse midwives.[21,24] This imbalance is the result of a historical shift toward a primarily biomedical birth model. Prior to the rise of physician-attended births in the late 1800s through early 1900s, most births in the United States were attended by midwives. As the field of obstetrics and gynecology moved toward the biomedical model, medical professionals erroneously argued that midwives, particularly Black midwives serving rural communities, were primarily responsible for high infant and maternal mortality. This push to delegitimize midwifery care resulted in a power shift toward primarily physician-attended birth.[25] By seeking ways to expand the integration of midwives and other multidisciplinary professionals often excluded in care teams, health systems can advance innovation and create a power shift that allows patients to benefit from holistic care models.[26]

Including individuals who are seeking care as respected members of their own care team is also critical for improving patient safety and for upholding a culture that promotes shared decision-making. Full inclusion means that an individual's concerns, goals, priorities, and input are listened to and valued by all team members. In addition, all treatment options and medical procedures are explained to the individual using a comprehensive, culturally appropriate approach. Discussions should include the individual's self-identified support network and community to the extent the individual prefers. This may include, but is not limited to, partners, family, friends, spiritual support persons, doulas, patient navigators, or other community health workers.

Doulas and other community health workers are trained to provide emotional, psychosocial, and educational support to individuals during the prenatal, birth, and postpartum time frames.[20,25] Studies show that including doulas as respected members of the care team may improve health outcomes, including decreasing the likelihood of birth complications and increasing the likelihood of breastfeeding.[21,27] Although studies support the efficacy of doula services, especially for those in historically marginalized communities, low reimbursement rates for doula services remain a barrier to doulas' becoming more fully included in care teams.[21,28,29] Innovative models for reimbursing doulas and community health workers are a critical need in order to reshape and enhance care teams.

Recommendations for Maternal Health Practitioners and Healthcare Systems

Selecting Quality Improvement Frameworks

- Acknowledge long-standing inequitable outcomes in the US healthcare system due to racism, unfair structural distribution of power, and neglect of women's lived experiences.
- Apply relevant frameworks for quality improvement that incorporate a community's lived experiences and historical treatment in care systems. Utilize frameworks developed by Black women, birthing people, and the affected communities.
- Examine an organization's power structure and consider methods to shift the power balance to birthing communities. Center patients in a manner that prioritizes their perspectives and acknowledges the appropriate risk.
- Expand opportunities to explore integrative care models. Expand models of equity to encompass those that center on birthing populations with the poorest outcomes.

Practical Tools

- Conduct objective, rigorous assessment to collect and analyze population perspectives, organizational climate for equity, and practices and policies that hinder birth equity.

- Identify and prioritize collaboration with local community advisory boards that uplift patient experiences in a healthcare system.
- Include all levels of staff on the health system's quality improvement committee to include all touchpoints for birthing people, including but not limited to, hospital and health system administrators, physicians, obstetric nurses, midwives, and front desk staff.
- Align short- and long-term health-system goals for maternal health outcomes with respectful care and reproductive justice frameworks that require commitment, integrity, and community accountability.
- Train staff on shared decision-making practices and ensure that support efforts include ongoing checks for power imbalances in the patient's care interactions.

Fostering Integration

To foster best practices in integration, materials and resources should be developed to dismantle existing processes that have negative impacts, to augment existing strengths, and to foster innovation in care. Examples of resources include:

- Creation of a guide for providers and practitioners on the concepts of reproductive justice, respectful maternity care, and other types of patient-centered care provision.
- Creation of care spaces that welcome and integrate community members into clinical shared decision-making.
- Reshaping of care teams to incorporate a broader array of patient supports that represent a holistic approach to care, including the patient, family members, doulas, midwives, spiritual supports, and community-based health workers.
- Facilitation of provider training and development of corresponding materials to improve overall patient–provider communication.

CONCLUSION

Innovation in maternal healthcare necessitates a shift in the dominant culture of healthcare practice and provision. While innovation has typically represented new, cutting-edge practices, the historical carryovers in the US healthcare system require a return to simpler, patient-centered, integrated strategies that allow a better response to the long-standing and ongoing impacts of structural racism. Maternal healthcare has been emphasizing distinct values that unfortunately center the healthcare system over community and clinicians over patients. Therefore, retrofitting values in the health system will require a concerted effort toward more just, respectful, and innovative approaches to care. The innovations and integrations suggested here will help move the field toward dignified and respectful improvement in care and well-being for those most affected by poor maternal health outcomes.

REFERENCES

1. Aspen Health Strategy Group. Reversing the U.S. Maternal Mortality Crisis. The Aspen Institute. Published April 22, 2021. https://www.aspeninstitute.org/wp-cont ent/uploads/2021/04/Maternal-Morality-Report.pdf

2. Cooper Owens D. *Medical Bondage: Race, Gender, and the Origins of American Gynecology*. Athens, GA: University of Georgia Press; 2017.

3. Centers for Disease Control and Prevention. Working together to reduce Black maternal mortality. https://www.cdc.gov/healthequity/features/maternal-mortality/ index.html. Published 2021. Accessed January 31, 2022.

4. Scott KA, Britton L, McLemore MR. The ethics of perinatal care for Black women: dismantling the structural racism in "mother blame" narratives. *J Perinat Neonatal Nurs*. 2019;33(2):108–115. doi:10.1097/JPN.0000000000000394.

5. Goode KL. *Birthing, Blackness, and the Body: Black Midwives and Experiential Continuities of Institutional Racism* [master's thesis]. New York: City University of New York; 2014.

6. SisterSong. Reproductive justice. https://www.sistersong.net/reproductive-justice. Accessed January 31, 2022.

7. Ross L, Solinger R. *Reproductive Justice: An Introduction*. Oakland: University of California Press; 2017.

8. Hodnett ED, Gates S, Hofmeyr GJ, Sakala C. Continuous support for women during childbirth. *Birth*. 2003;32(1):72–72. doi:10.1111/j.0730-7659.2005.00336.x.

9. Crockett A, Heberlein EC, Glasscock L, Covington-Kolb S, Shea K, Khan IA. Investing in CenteringPregnancy™ group prenatal care reduces newborn hospitalization costs. *Womens Health Issues*. 2017;27(1):60–66.

10. Dehlendorf C, Akers A, Borrero S, et al. Evolving the preconception health framework. *Obstet Gynecol*. 2021;137(2):234–239. doi:10.1097/ aog.0000000000004255.

11. Bey A, Brill A, Porchia-Albert C, Gradilla M, Strauss N. Advancing birth justice: community-based doula models as a standard of care for ending racial disparities. Ancient Song Doula Services, Village Birth International, Every Mother Counts; 2019. https://everymothercounts.org/wp-content/uploads/2019/03/Advancing-Birth-Justice-CBD-Models-as-Std-of-Care-3-25-19.pdf.

12. Muse S, Dawes Gay E, Doyinsola Aina, A, et al. Setting the standard for holistic care of and for Black women [Black paper]. Black Mamas Matter Alliance; 2018. https://black mamasmatter.org/wp-content/uploads/2018/04/BMMA_BlackPaper_April-2018.pdf.

13. Centers for Disease Control and Prevention. Community–clinical linkages for the prevention and control of chronic diseases: a practitioner's guide. 2016. https://www. cdc.gov/dhdsp/pubs/docs/ccl-practitioners-guide.pdf.

14. Agency for Health Care Research and Quality. Clinical–community linkages. https://www.ahrq.gov/ncepcr/tools/community/index.html. Published 2011.

15. National Birth Equity Collaborative. Solutions. http://birthequity.org/about/birth-equity-solutions/. Published 2018.

16. Center for American Progress. Eliminating racial disparities in maternal and infant mortality. 2019.https://www.americanprogress.org/article/eliminating-racial-disp arities-maternal-infant-mortality/.

17. Farre A, Rapley T. The new old (and old new) medical model: four decades navigating the biomedical and psychosocial understandings of health and illness. *Healthcare (Basel).* 2017;5(4):88. doi:10.3390/healthcare5040088.

18. Alliance for Innovation on Maternal Health Community Care Initiative. https://www.aimcci.org. Accessed January 28, 2022.

19. Linkpas.com. Nursing model vs. medical model (similarities & differences). https://linkpas.com/nursing-vs-medical-model. Published 2020. Accessed January 22, 2022.

20. Ruralhealthinfo.org. The Health Belief Model—Rural Health Promotion and Disease Prevention Toolkit. https://www.ruralhealthinfo.org/toolkits/health-promotion. Accessed January 22 2022.

21. American College of Obstetricians and Gynecologists. Patient-Centered Contraceptive Counseling Committee Statement. https://www.acog.org/clinical/clinical-guidance/committee-statement/articles/2022/02/patient-centered-contraceptive-counseling. Published 2022. Accessed January 28, 2022.

22. Informed consent and shared decision-making in obstetrics and gynecology: ACOG Committee Opinion, Number 819. *Obstet Gynecol.* 2021;137(2):e34–e41. doi:10.1097/aog.0000000000004247.

23. Zephyrin L, Seervai S, Lewis C, Katon J. Community-based models to improve maternal health outcomes and promote health equity. Commonwealth Fund. https://www.commonwealthfund.org/publications/issue-briefs/2021/mar/community-models-improve-maternal-outcomes-equity. Published 2021. Accessed January 24, 2022.

24. National Academies of Science, Engineering, and Medicine. No hospital, birth center, or home birth is risk-free — but better access to care, quality of care, and care system integration can improve safety for women and infants during birth, says report. https://www.nationalacademies.org/news/2020/02/no-hospital-birth-center-or-home-birth-is-risk-free-but-better-access-to-care-quality-of-care-and-care-system-integration-can-improve-safety-for-women-and-infants-during-birth-says-report. Published 2020. Accessed January 22, 2022.

25. Sandall J, Soltani H, Gates S, Shennan A, Devane D. Midwife-led continuity models versus other models of care for childbearing women. *Cochrane Database Syst Rev.* 2016;(4):CD004667. https://pubmed.ncbi.nlm.nih.gov/27121907/.

26. Vedam S, Stoll K, MacDorman M, et al. Mapping integration of midwives across the United States: impact on access, equity, and outcomes. *PLOS One.* 2018;13(2):e0192523. doi:10.1371/journal.pone.0192523.

27. Morrison SM, Fee E. Nothing to work with but cleanliness: the training of African American traditional midwives in the South. *Am J Public Health.* 2010;100(2):238–239. doi:10.2105/AJPH.2009.182873.

28. Ellmann N. Community-based doulas and midwives: key to addressing the U.S. maternal health crisis. https://www.americanprogress.org/article/community-based-doulas-midwives/. Published 2020. Accessed January 24, 2022.

29. Gruber KJ, Cupito SH, Dobson CF. Impact of doulas on healthy birth outcomes. *J Perinat Educ.* 2013;22(1):49–58. doi:10.1891/1058-1243.22.1.49.

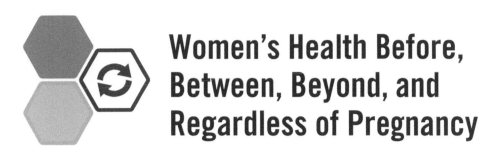

Women's Health Before, Between, Beyond, and Regardless of Pregnancy

SARAH VERBIEST, SUZANNE WOODWARD, AND LINDSEY YATES

INTRODUCTION

A woman's health and well-being are the foundations of maternal health. From a life course perspective, a person's health from adolescence through adulthood sets the stage for health during pregnancy, childbirth, and postpartum, in addition to aging well over time. Providing quality healthcare to women means providing care to a large and diverse group over several decades of their lives. To achieve this goal, innovation in public health and clinical care is essential. This chapter highlights a range of digital and social innovations that have helped to fill important gaps in women's health while also addressing some racial inequities in care. The chapter addresses some new technologies and changes to language that can better support women's well-being. It also offers some strategies for improving primary care for women and concludes with recommendations to the field.

First, though, the limitation of the term *women's health* must be acknowledged. The health status and needs of other individuals with a uterus must also be prioritized because of their unique requirements. This is particularly true for nonbinary people and transgender men, who are positioned at the intersection of other historically marginalized identities. The use of the word *woman* in this chapter seeks to include these people, although the term is limited.

BACKGROUND

Women's health in the United States has traditionally been conceptualized in relation to an individual's status as a potential or current mother, or as a pregnant

Sarah Verbiest, Suzanne Woodward, and Lindsey Yates, *Women's Health Before, Between, Beyond, and Regardless of Pregnancy* In: *The Practical Playbook III*. Edited by: Dorothy Cilenti, Alisahah Jackson, Natalie D. Hernandez, Lindsey Yates, Sarah Verbiest, J. Lloyd Michener, and Brian C. Castrucci, Oxford University Press. © de Beaumont Foundation 2024. DOI: 10.1093/oso/9780197662984.003.0033

person. However, women's health should be prioritized not only because it is associated with better maternal health outcomes but also because it is essential to women first and foremost as individuals. Many biopsychosocial conditions that influence health also affect a person's ability to conceive and have good birth outcomes. For example, fairly common conditions like uterine fibroids, endometriosis, and polycystic ovarian syndrome are strongly associated with infertility, subfertility, and poor maternal health outcomes, such as gestational diabetes and pregnancy hypertensive disorders.[1-3] Chronic health conditions, such as hypertension, diabetes, and heart disease, affect a woman's quality of life across her life span and also contribute to a higher risk of maternal mortality and morbidity if she decides to bear children.[4]

Although women's access to preventive healthcare improved under the Affordable Care Act, not all states have expanded Medicaid, and access to other essential healthcare services, like abortion care, continues to be limited in various states since the overturn of *Roe v Wade*.[5] The health conditions and issues around access to care disproportionately affect women of color because of the dual impacts of systemic racism and sexism that limit access to health-promoting resources—such as quality preventive healthcare and chronic condition management—and increase stress. Women who receive quality care and support when they are not pregnant can reduce risks to their lifelong health and improve their chances of reaching their personal reproductive goals.

In addition to physical health, mental health is essential to overall well-being. An increasing number of women report mental health concerns. These problems have been exacerbated during the COVID-19 pandemic, with more women reporting poor mental health status compared to men.[6] Further, recent data show that while almost one-fifth of young adults age 18 to 25 had a mental illness in the past year, two-thirds of this group and almost half of all people with a serious mental illness did not receive treatment.[7] Increasing access to mental and behavioral healthcare, particularly for those in rural areas and for those who are underinsured or have no insurance, is essential for women to reach and maintain optimal quality of life.

For women desiring to become pregnant, preconception care is still the exception and not part of routine primary care. Using 2009 PRAMS data from the Centers for Disease Control and Prevention (CDC), Robbins et al[8] reported that only one in five women reported preconception counseling before her last pregnancy. This is likely due to patient-level barriers (e.g., not knowing about, or not choosing to seek, care prior to pregnancy) and provider-level barriers (e.g., not knowing about, or not choosing to provide, preconception care).[8] In a study of over 25,000 ambulatory healthcare visits of reproductive-age women across the United States, Bello et al found that, despite CDC recommendations, less than 15% of the visits included preconception or contraceptive services, regardless of medical comorbidities and physician specialty.[9]

DIGITAL INNOVATION

Digital technology and social media can help address health inequities by eliminating some health information barriers. Online platforms and tools have streamlined and advanced the way people are able to think about and manage their health. From using social media to engage with others about specific health topics, to tracking all aspects of health from a smartphone, and using telehealth, healthcare is now available in the palm of the hand.

Social Media and Content Creation

People who are white, Black, and Hispanic have similar rates of smartphone ownership, with people in minority groups more likely than white people to use their phones to look up information about health conditions and educational content.[10] Furthermore, over 88% of young adults are engaging with at least one social media site (e.g., Facebook, Instagram, Twitter, TikTok).[11] Pew Research analyzes and reports annual social media consumption in the United States and has found that different age groups and communities use various social media channels in different ways and for different purposes. For example, people age 30+ are more likely to use Facebook, while people < 30 years old use platforms like Snapchat or Instagram every day.[12] Thus, the strategies used to reach different populations need to be data-driven and tailored to the way people want to receive health messages on their social media platforms. Organizations need to listen to, to understand, and to collaborate with the women they want to serve so that the language, imagery, tone, and delivery format used resonate with that group.

While public health professionals are making efforts to share health messages online, reaching target audiences takes investment in social listening and understanding, content creation, and promotion. For example, updates to social media algorithms and emphasis on user-generated content, such as TikTok and Instagram Reels, mean that more efforts are needed to reach young adults. Regularly posting messages is not enough; taking the time to interact with followers is essential. Facebook, Instagram, and Twitter have made it easier for organizations to interact using livestreaming and 24-hour Instagram stories. Accounts can now interact in real time using different techniques, such as asking poll or quiz questions, joining conversations using stickers, GIFs, or hashtags, and sharing clickable links. There are free applications to create graphics and videos.

Social media platforms also are rapidly moving toward captioned video clips and relying on the "explore" pages to help audiences better identify and engage with meaningful content. Across social media channels, each platform analyzes the type of accounts and posts the user engages with on the channel and has an algorithm that optimizes the type of content the user might like to see.[13] The algorithm shows more, or less, of a specific type of content based on how much the user interacts with that content type. The explore page is a roundup of stories, videos, posts, and products that a social media site believes a user might like to view. For example, if a user frequently engages with accounts or posts focused on yoga, the user's explore page will include more yoga-focused content. Users are also able to curate their explore pages based on their preferences. The good news: You no longer need millions of followers to show up on someone's explore page. It is very important, however, to share the right type of content at the right time, with the focus audience in mind. Hashtags are another way to see what people are saying about specific topics, linking micro-communities of people. Using specific hashtags allows accounts to listen to, and engage with, their target audiences on a particular topic (e.g., #InvisibleIllness).

Emphasis on user-generated content, specifically graphics and video, makes authentic community collaboration more vital than ever, and engaging people who reflect the target audience in developing content is a must.[14] People want to see real faces, real bodies, and realistic messages from people who reflect the community they trust. Representation and equity also are important when it comes to sharing content that is relatable and busts myths and stereotypes. It is vital that organizations attribute social media posts to the original content creators. Specifically, white-led organizations often appropriate content from people of color without permission or without giving appropriate credit. As one way to address this issue, Instagram has created tags to give Black content creators recognition.[15] A best practice is to directly ask creators for permission to repost their multimedia/message. Social media channels have created ways for groups to better cite their user-generated content, such as directly sharing a clickable post or combining account names for co-created content. Content curators work hard on their content and to build their following, so it is always best to directly engage with them about your ideas for sharing their work.

The Show Your Love wellness campaign is an example of an initiative that seeks to advance the health of women of reproductive age through dissemination of expert-written online resources on social media.[16] The Show Your Love community was built by young adults who wanted to share their health stories and encourage others to join them on a wellness and learning journey. The Show Your Love team collaborated with health ambassadors across the United States, including preconception peer educators, to showcase their experiences and stories on various health topics and to build a community of people working to change the narrative on self-care and healthy bodies. The strategy was to collaborate with content creators who reflected the campaign's target audiences and to support their health messaging for others to engage and learn with.

The Show Your Love team also partnered with health providers to share facts about health topics online. For example, Dr. Charis Chambers, also known as @ThePeriodDoctor, has many popular videos that model for people with a uterus how to talk with providers about managing health and common concerns. Dr. Chambers provides key information about anatomy, periods, and gynecological health, and she often role-plays the patient in the videos to demonstrate how patients might advocate for themselves in various health-care settings.[17] There are many health professionals and providers willing to collaborate with organizations, and many of them already use social media to combat misinformation and to share health information. Sharing of online health information has made space for diverse voices and expanded accessibility through video captions, autotranslation of captions, flagging of content that may include incorrect facts, requiring certain accounts/facts to be verified, and more.

Thankfully, social media channels are creating new ways for organizations to engage with their focus audience. There are several tools to assist with creating engaging content, including free support tools, easy-to-use video and audio recorders, and sites that help queue up messages and manage data analysis. With Internet access, anyone can now be a content creator. Figure 33.1 elevates several key points from a conversation with Dr. Chambers during the Future Forward National Convening of Equity-Centered Women's Wellness in September 2021. The fifth national gathering on preconception health, held virtually, used graphic facilitation, panels, Jamboard, and active social media engagement to elevate conversations on the future of preconception and women's wellness, to challenge the language that is used, and to highlight the potential of national programs like Title V.

The Power of the Smartphone

In the United States, 85% of people own a smartphone, and there now are activity trackers accessible through Apple or Android platforms, meaning that people can collect their health data each day using their phone, without needing a separate device or app.[18] In addition, there are thousands of digital apps that support health knowledge and management. Examples include menstrual cycle or fertility trackers, such as Fertility Frame and Cycle; food preparation and counting tools, such as MyFitnessPal; anxiety and sleep trackers, such as the ReachOut Breathe app and the Calm app, respectively; and meditation and motivation apps like Shine and Insight Timer. The available apps even include tracking tools for specific health conditions. Some digital apps can link to a smartphone dashboard or share information with a health provider. Others are designed by people of color for people of color, among them Health in Her Hue, the Black Women's Health Imperative, SheMatters, Meet Mae, OurCultureCare, Shine, Ayana, and the Safe Place. While more evidence is needed about the efficacy of mobile health apps, apps for certain topics have been shown to be beneficial, including those for medicine adherence, mental health, and nutrition/fitness tracking.[11,19] Many of these apps are free or have limited fees. Providers should talk with their patients about which apps they use and steer them toward apps and programs that fit their care plan or help to answer relevant health questions.

Beyond mobile health applications, online resource hubs with mobile-friendly design are crucial for building engagement and awareness of topics and resources. Approximately 61% of people view Web sites from a mobile phone or tablet rather than a desktop,[18] so it is important to build mobile-responsive Web sites and e-newsletters that are accessible and easier to find when searching on Google and other search engines. Rather than asking a user to download an app, organizations can create mobile-friendly online resource centers that smartphone users can bookmark and refer to. Providers often hand patients a printout to read about their health, but many prefer to refer patients to Web sites to learn more. This can include the use of QR codes that patients scan during their office visit.

Telehealth and Getting Local

COVID-19 pushed telehealth to the forefront of healthcare.[20] In fact, in a recent survey, 80% of respondents reported that they prefer to use digital communications, such as online messaging and virtual appointments, with their healthcare providers.[21] Telehealth has opened doors to reach many different people using different venues. Companies and policies are moving to address broadband and connection issues for people unable to access stable Internet, such as homeless and rural populations. Digital platforms, such as Google and social media, allow organizations to reach people through geographic mapping to share health messages and to encourage engagement with their health sites. The outreach can be done using state, county, or ZIP Code—even right down to storefront location. Many sites, such as https://findahealthcenter.hrsa.gov/ and https://www.bedsider.org/find-health-care/clinics, allow people to find care nearby. By inserting their ZIP Code, users can find clinic resources, such as federally qualified health centers and Title X clinics, to access care, regardless of insurance status.

SOCIAL INNOVATIONS

In addition to digital innovations, social innovations in women's health have also blossomed over the past decade. In this chapter, the term *social innovations* means innovations that focus on direct communication and care for women and birthing people regarding their health. These innovations are transforming how we interact with people about their reproductive health across their life span, whether they choose to become parents or not. This section focuses on language and primary care as two types of social innovations.

Messaging and Language

While there are more innovative ways to share health information, we are in the early stages of changing the language to make health information more accessible to more people. The improvements in the narrative are just as important as improvements in technology. There has been an increased call to use messaging and language that centers reproductive justice. Coined in 1994 by a collective of Black women, the term *reproductive justice* combines ideals from the reproductive rights and social justice movements.[22] The key principles of reproductive justice are: (1) the right to bodily autonomy, (2) the right to decide when to have and not to have children, (3) the right to parent children how you desire, and (4) the right to raise children in safe and sustainable communities.[23] The reproductive justice framework uses language that values each person's unique reproductive goals and highlights how various systems of oppression can influence an individual's reproductive health. In using such language, providers, policy makers, and influencers can better prioritize individuals' well-being and acknowledge the systemic factors that influence individuals' health decision-making.

One field in which language continues to evolve is preconception healthcare. Preconception health is the physical, emotional, and social health of people during their reproductive years and includes interventions that can help identify and modify challenges to a person's well-being and future pregnancy (if desired).[24] Historically, messaging around preconception health has been limited to helping people understand how their health and healthcare decisions affect a future pregnancy, and it has been most appropriate for people who are seeking to become pregnant in the near future. Those not currently interested in becoming pregnant were often left out or not well served by this messaging. This change represents an important shift in the language and messaging used in the preconception health field. Figure 33.2 depicts a reflective dialogue on the topic of messaging around health, wellness, and care. This graphic is another image that emerged from the Future Forward 2021 National Convening of Equity-Centered Women's Wellness.

Wellness programs have capitalized on these shifts in language and adopted them in their quest to create community and focus on women's health. One example is GirlTrek, the largest public health nonprofit organization centering the health and well-being of Black women and girls. Founded by Black women,

Figure 33.2 ▼

Vision forward, new ideas for advancing an equity-aligned approach to wellness and well-being.

Source: Future Forward National Convening on Equity-Centered Wellness, 2021. https://befo reandbeyond.org/wp-content/uploads/2021/09/9_Vision-Forward.png. Licensed under CC-BY-ND. Accessed December 6, 2022.

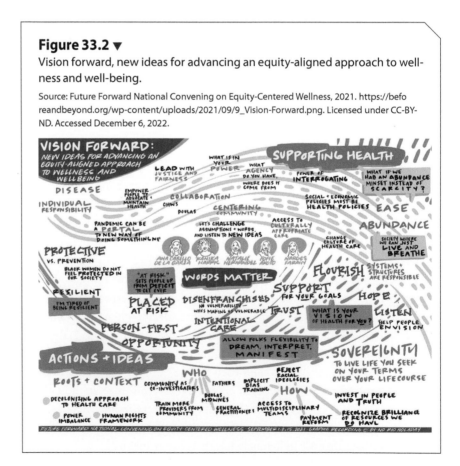

GirlTrek uses walking as one tool to enhance the health of communities. Some of the language used by GirlTrek organizers includes a focus on "healing," "transformation," and "self-care," encouraging women to prioritize their health to reach their most fulfilled lives. In part because of the purposeful use of language, GirlTrek has more than one million women committed to walking and improving their own health.[25]

Improving the Well Woman Primary Care Visit

Primary care is not necessarily an "innovation," but the evolution in thinking about this care as a key component of women's health is innovative. Primary care is essential in making sure people have the information and support they need to achieve their reproductive goals. A study examining clinical practice in the state of Delaware, for example, found that, despite their beliefs about the importance of offering preconception care, many primary care providers were not consistently offering it.[26] Another study found that, overall, only 55% of providers reported "frequently providing preconception care."[27] The reasons for this gap are multifaceted, but there are emerging innovations that provide new guidance about the contents of preconception care and quality indicators.

On March 1, 2016, the American College of Obstetricians and Gynecologists (ACOG) launched the Women's Preventive Services Initiative. In collaboration with the US Department of Health and Human Services, Health Resources and Services Administration (HRSA), ACOG is engaging a coalition of national health professional organizations and consumer and patient advocates with expertise in women's health across the life span to develop, review, and update recommendations for women's preventive healthcare services. This includes the HRSA-sponsored "Women's Preventive Services Guidelines." The recommendations are helping ensure that women receive a comprehensive set of preventive services free of copayment, coinsurance, or deductible.[28]

In January 2022, the National Preconception Health and Health Care Initiative, currently supported by the schools of social work and medicine at the University of North Carolina at Chapel Hill, launched a series of training modules for healthcare workers to guide clinicians in providing respectful, quality preconception and interconception care for women. The redesigned modules are centered on advancing equity and reproductive justice. The Before and Beyond Web site houses many resources, such as a women's health practice bulletin and sample screening tools, for clinicians and public health professionals working to improve preconception and preventive care. People can access key publications, sign up for biweekly email updates, and more.[29] The initiative also relaunched the wellness section of the Show Your Love Today Web site. Among other things, it enumerates the social determinants of health that make accessing health-promoting resources more difficult for people who are financially challenged and people with minoritized identities. Box 33.1 describes

Box 33.1 | The Preconception Collaborative Improvement and Innovation Network (CoIIN)

Recognizing the importance of preventive care visits and preconception health, the US Department of Health and Human Services, Health Resources and Services Administration (HRSA), Maternal and Child Health Bureau (MCHB) funded a project to develop, implement, and disseminate a woman-centered, clinician-engaged, community-involved approach to the well-woman visit. The goal was to improve the preconception health status of women of reproductive age, particularly low-income women and women of color. The Collaborative for Maternal and Infant Health at the University of North Carolina at Chapel Hill partnered with Title V leaders in California, Delaware, Oklahoma, and North Carolina. Each state team engaged multiple clinic and site partners to assist in the development and implementation of their project. Many sites provide services to low-income women and minority women served by community-based groups (e.g., Healthy Start).

There are many areas of improvement for preventive care—from basic access to the visit to appropriate referral for needed follow-up services and everything in between. The ability to follow through on provider recommendations is connected to the social determinants of health and equity, including access to safe places to exercise, affordable food, and a work schedule that supports adequate rest. Structural and historic racism not only hinder access to needed resources but layer stress and anxiety on individuals of color who must deal with the impact on a daily basis. This project could not cover all areas and focused on one, actionable piece of the mosaic - maximizing the clinical encounter by developing patient-centered screening tools and educational materials. The project also provided training to sites on respectful, quality care and the context of women's lives.

Partners utilized Human-Centered Design (HCD) informed approaches and quality improvement methodology to develop patient-centered visit screening tools. The HCD-informed approach initiated the development of the screening tool with the end-users (patients and providers). State teams and their site/clinic partners worked together over a three-year timeframe to create and implement preventive screening tools, testing and refining the tool and screening process and engaging the perspectives of the population being served and members of their teams. State team members expressed a strong commitment to this work, "It's been a passion of my work," "this is where my heart is," and, "[this] goes back to my roots."

One team member said, "This was an opportunity to leverage the experience of creating a well-woman tool, share it, learn from it, and leverage it with many other partners across the country." Team members spoke of the ways the project brought together many partners (medical providers, care coordinators, peer educators, community-based organizations, and patients) to propel the work forward. The perspectives of patients are foundational. One team member said, "[The key partners] have helped us engage women . . . they have helped us stop and pause, make us aware of what is going on, and help us to do better." Another added, "[Patients] gave us a lot of feedback . . . they are a part of this collaboration and partnership. They helped us make changes that made things much more user friendly." Another team member added,

> **Box 33.1 | Continued**
>
> This was not a top-down approach, this was done by the community, this was done with clinical support staff, and everybody was involved in the design of this...this also allowed us to realize that what we brought to the table is not actually what the client wanted, even if we thought it was great. What we completed is not what we envisioned . . . but in the end we have what the client wanted.
>
> Another team member spoke to the success of standardizing the discussion of pregnancy intention across sites: "It is now a standard that every clinician and every resident incorporates into their visit . . . before it was something that was done ad hoc or by a passionate clinician, but now it is happening routinely in how we care for women." Someone else added: "[we have found] women feel they are getting more from their visits than they were before . . . they are going out with more information even though they might not have come in to talk about family planning." All state teams highlighted two similar successes; first, the focus of preconception healthcare has shifted from an OBGYN issue to a primary care issue. One team member explained: "There's been a [movement] from being 'aware' to being 'committed' . . . there's an overall commitment to women's health. Women are more than just their breasts or uterus . . . we're looking overall at women's health, not just their contraception or if they are choosing to become a mother." Second, that the process of listening to women and co-designing preventive visit screening tools was innovative and essential. One team member stated, "This journey has helped us empower women in [our state] in their personal health and we're really working together with [patients] to do that."

a four-state project that focused specifically on developing screening tools to support a person-centered wellness visit.

CONCLUSION AND CALL TO ACTION

The strategies outlined in this chapter provide some examples of ways to improve women's health and address racial inequities in care. Digital innovations have revolutionized how we access health information and support women, particularly women of color, to focus on health issues relevant to them. Thoughtful messaging and the use of positive language help create community and prioritize women's well-being. There also is an opportunity to improve women's health through primary healthcare and preconception health tools. Achieving equitable health outcomes requires a focus on women's equitable healthcare and outcomes. Since 2005, ACOG, CDC, the American Academy of Family Physicians, and other national professional organizations have recommended

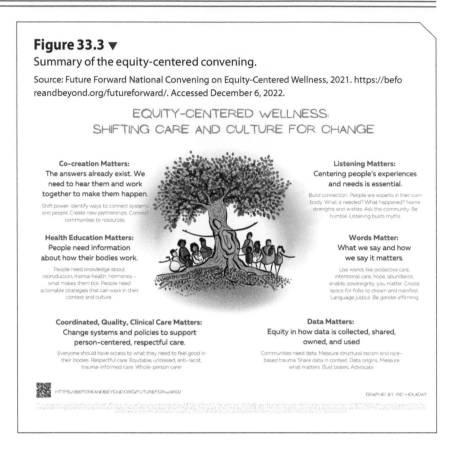

Figure 33.3 ▼
Summary of the equity-centered convening.
Source: Future Forward National Convening on Equity-Centered Wellness, 2021. https://befo reandbeyond.org/futureforward/. Accessed December 6, 2022.

that strategies to improve maternal health focus upstream on women's pre-pregnancy health.[24,30] The time has come for a focus on women's health as the foundation of maternal health. There are broadening approaches to women's health, and there is more space for innovation, strategy, and creativity to address it. Figure 33.3 shows strategies for shifting care and creating a culture for change in advancing equity-centered wellness. This work reflects the perspectives of a very diverse group of people who presented and shared during the 2021 Future Forward National Convening of Equity-Centered Women's Wellness. An ar-chive of the informative recorded conversations from those sessions can be found at https://beforeandbeyond.org/futureforward/.

Everyone can be part of supporting change and innovation in improving women's health and well-being. The dividends are priceless. To better achieve these goals, listed here are specific activities that can be undertaken by organiza-tions and funders/venture capitalists (VCs) invested in women's health.

Women's Healthcare Organizations
- Make an effort and invest in personnel who can help craft and share digital content. Including this focus as a standard line item in budgets

and implementation plans will be key for organizations that are focused on reaching more clients and strengthening their infrastructure.

- Work with focus audiences to incorporate language that is authentic to their needs and experiences and that is grounded in reproductive justice.
- Encourage, train, and support providers in speaking with patients about chronic health conditions. The use of preventive health screening tools and other resources helps systematize shared decision-making and focuses on women's health beyond pregnancy.

Funders/VCs

- Invest in both content creators and entrepreneurs focused on developing innovative resources for women. The women's health sector is growing and is expected to be worth more than $58.24 billion by 2030,[31] but investment in this area lags investment in other digital health resources, making up less than 5% of investment in this space.[32]
- Support a diversity of resources that recognize the diversity of the market to be served. Women are not a monolith, and their healthcare needs are not singular. Although much investment has focused on women's menstruation and fertility, they comprise only a small portion of women's health. Resources focused on helping women address other health concerns are needed.
- Fund content spearheaded by and featuring Black, Indigenous, Asian, Latina, and other women of color. Because of inequities and disparities in healthcare rooted in systemic racism and other forms of oppression, women of color may benefit most from these innovations and should help lead their development.
- Invest in, and support the use of, preventive tools and resources that providers can use as part of their care for women.

ACKNOWLEDGMENT

We would like to thank Erin McClain, MA, MPH, for reviewing an early draft of this chapter and providing feedback.

REFERENCES

1. Chen Y, Lin M, Guo P, et al. Uterine fibroids increase the risk of hypertensive disorders of pregnancy: a prospective cohort study. *J Hypertens*. 2021;39(5):1002–1008. doi:10.1097/HJH.0000000000002729.

2. Yu H-F, Chen H-S, Rao D-P, Gong J. Association between polycystic ovary syndrome and the risk of pregnancy complications: a PRISMA-compliant systematic review and meta-analysis. *Medicine (Baltimore)*. 2016;95(51):e4863–e4863. doi:10.1097/MD.0000000000004863.

3. Breintoft K, Pinnerup R, Henriksen TB, et al. Endometriosis and risk of adverse pregnancy outcome: a systematic review and meta-analysis. *J Clin Med*. 2021;10(4):667. doi:10.3390/jcm10040667.

4. Nelson DB, Moniz MH, Davis MM. Population-level factors associated with maternal mortality in the United States, 1997–2012. *BMC Public Health*. 2018;18(1):1007. doi:10.1186/s12889-018-5935-2.

5. KFF. Abortion in the United States dashboard. KFF Web site. https://www.kff.org/womens-health-policy/dashboard/abortion-in-the-u-s-dashboard/#state. Accessed July 29, 2022.

6. Panchal N, Kamal R, Cox C, Garfield R. The implications of COVID-19 for mental health and substance use. https://www.kff.org/coronavirus-covid-19/issue-brief/the-implications-of-covid-19-for-mental-health-and-substance-use/. Published February 10, 2021.

7. Bonnie RJ, Stroud C, Breiner H, eds. *Investing in the Health and Well-Being of Young Adults*.Washington, DC: National Academies Press; 2015. doi:10.17226/18869.

8. Robbins CL, Zapata LB, Farr SL, et al. Core state preconception health indicators—Pregnancy Risk Assessment Monitoring System and Behavioral Risk Factor Surveillance System, 2009. *MMWR Surveill Summ*. 2014;63(3):1–62.

9. Bello JK, Rao G, Stulberg DB. Trends in contraceptive and preconception care in United States ambulatory practices. *Fam Med*. 2015;47(4):264–271.

10. Anderson M. Racial and ethnic differences in how people use mobile technology. https://www.pewresearch.org/fact-tank/2015/04/30/racial-and-ethnic-differences-in-how-people-use-mobile-technology/. Published April 15, 2015.

11. Huo J, Desai R, Hong Y-R, Turner K, Mainous AG III, Bian J. Use of social media in health communication: findings from the Health Information National Trends Survey 2013, 2014, and 2017. *Cancer Control*. 2019;26(1):1073274819841442. doi:10.1177/1073274819841442.

12. Auxier B, Anderson M. Social media use in 2021. https://www.pewresearch.org/internet/2021/04/07/social-media-use-in-2021/. Published April 7, 2021. Accessed May 17, 2022.

13. O'Brien C. How do social media algorithms work? https://digitalmarketinginstitute.com/blog/how-do-social-media-algorithms-work. Published January 19, 2022. Accessed May 17, 2022.

14. Nosto. Bridging the gap: consumer & marketing perspectives on content in the digital age. Nosto Web site. 2019. https://www.nosto.com/wp-content/uploads/2019/02/Data-Report-2019-FINAL-FINAL.pdf.

15. TheGrio Staff. Instagram introducing tags that give Black content creators recognition. TheGrio Web site. 2022. https://thegrio.com/2022/03/08/new-instagram-tag-black-content-creators-recognition/. Published March. Accessed May 17, 2022.

16. Show Your Love Today. https://showyourlovetoday.com/. Published 2022. Accessed May 17, 2022.

17. Chambers C. @theperioddoctor. https://www.instagram.com/theperioddoctor/. Accessed May 17, 2022.

18. Pew Research Center. Mobile fact sheet. Pew Research Center Web site. https://www.pewresearch.org/internet/fact-sheet/mobile/. Published April 7, 2021. Accessed May 17, 2022.

19. Gardiner A. Health apps are popular, but do they really improve our health? MDLinx website. https://www.mdlinx.com/article/health-apps-are-popular-but-do-they-really-improve-our-health/5an1dtuXNobd3cnMFxkbuB. Published May 20, 2021. Accessed May 17, 2022.

20. Bestsennyy O, Gilbert G, Harris A, Rost J. Telehealth: a quarter-trillion-dollar post-COVID-19 reality? McKinsey & Company website. https://www.mckinsey.com/industries/healthcare-systems-and-services/our-insights/telehealth-a-quarter-trillion-dollar-post-covid-19-reality. Published July 9, 2021. Accessed May 17, 2022.

21. Gordon D. New survey shows consumers expect better healthcare experiences—but are often disappointed. Forbes website. https://www.forbes.com/sites/debgordon/2021/12/07/new-survey-shows-consumers-expect--better-healthcare-experiences-but-are-often-disappointed/?sh=46f169e473f6. Published December 7, 2021. Accessed May 17, 2022.

22. Ross L, Solinger R. *Reproductive Justice: An Introduction*. Oakland: University of California Press; 2017.

23. SisterSong Women of Color Reproductive Justice Collective. Reproductive justice. SisterSong Web site. https://www.sistersong.net/reproductive-justice. Accessed October 8, 2020.

24. Johnson K, Posner SF, Biermann J, et al. Recommendations to improve preconception health and health care—United States. A report of the CDC/ATSDR Preconception Care Work Group and the Select Panel on Preconception Care. *MMWR Recomm Rep*. 2006;55(RR-6):1–23.

25. GirlTrek. https://www.girltrek.org/. Published 2022. Accessed May 17, 2022.

26. Kukreja R, Locke RG, Hack D, Paul DA. Knowledge of preconception health care among primary care physicians in Delaware. *Del Med J*. 2012;84(11):349–352.

27. Robbins CL, Gavin L, Carter MW, Moskosky SB. The link between reproductive life plan assessment and provision of preconception care at publicly funded health centers. *Perspect Sex Reprod Health*. 2017;49(3):167–172. doi:10.1363/psrh.12030.

28. Women's Preventive Services Initiative (WPSI). About WPSI. WPSI website. https://www.womenspreventivehealth.org/about/. Published 2018. Accessed May 17, 2022.

29. National Preconception Health and Health Care (PCHHC). Before, Between & Beyond Pregnancy. www.beforeandbeyond.org. Published 2022. Accessed March 17, 2022.

30. Frayne DJ. Preconception care is primary care: a call to action. *Am Fam Physician*. 2017;96(8):492–494.

31. Women's health market size worth $58.24 billion by 2030. Grand View Research website. https://www.grandviewresearch.com/press-release/global-womens-health-market. Published April 2022. Accessed May 17, 2022.

32. DeSilva A, Krasniansky A. Building comprehensive women+ digital health: eight sectors serving women+ needs. Rock Health website. https://rockhealth.com/insights/building-comprehensive-women-digital-health-eight-sectors-serving-women-needs/. Published September 27, 2021.

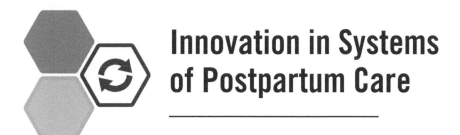

Chapter 34

Innovation in Systems of Postpartum Care

KIMBERLY D. HARPER, NKECHI U. CHARLES, AMELIA N. GIBSON, AND KRISTIN P. TULLY

INTRODUCTION

The postpartum period is a critical part of the life course for mothers and birthing people. The care they receive can affect their health trajectories for the remainder of their lives. In the United States, postpartum maternal deaths account for more than half (52%) of pregnancy-related deaths. Among these deaths, infection is the leading cause within 42 days postpartum, followed by cardiovascular problems. Mental health conditions are the leading cause of maternal mortality between 43 days and one year postpartum.[1] Critically, many maternal deaths are preventable. This calls attention to the urgent need to improve systems of postpartum care to prevent mortality, to reduce complications, and to improve conditions for birthing parents' health and wellness.

The fragmented nature of US healthcare translates into postpartum services that are largely inaccessible and ineffective. "Soon after delivery," Cohen and Daw (2021) wrote, "patients face a multidimensional postpartum 'cliff,' including insurance interruptions, incomplete handoffs between obstetrician-gynecologists and other healthcare providers, and limited monitoring and accountability for the quality of healthcare services."[2] Uncoordinated postpartum care and exclusion of community organizations from the system of care, they explained, forces birthing people to navigate postpartum transitions without support. At the national level, this lack of patient-centered postpartum support exacerbates many of the problems and inequities in healthcare practices during pregnancy.[2]

Intentionally restructuring and expanding systems of postpartum care are imperative for better meeting patient needs and thereby improving their postpartum outcomes. The structure and quality of care drive health outcomes

Kimberly D. Harper, Nkechi U. Charles, Amelia N. Gibson, and Kristin P. Tully, *Innovation in Systems of Postpartum Care*
In: *The Practical Playbook III*. Edited by: Dorothy Cilenti, Alisahah Jackson, Natalie D. Hernandez, Lindsey Yates, Sarah Verbiest, J. Lloyd Michener, and Brian C. Castrucci, Oxford University Press. © de Beaumont Foundation 2024.
DOI: 10.1093/oso/9780197662984.003.0034

through pregnancy, childbirth, postpartum, and beyond. Innovators in the postpartum space at local, state, and national levels have been implementing initiatives to "renovate" the postpartum period. This chapter highlights strategies and interventions that are reclaiming and reshaping postpartum care in the United States. Selected strategies include integration of multidisciplinary teams into the perinatal care continuum, standardization of clinical processes, improvement of patient–healthcare team communication, and recognition and uplift of community leadership.

"RENOVATING" POSTPARTUM CARE

Postpartum health outcomes reflect access to, and acceptability of, healthcare services, and the quality of those services varies across US institutions.[3] The process is working for some—those with privilege to navigate and advocate for themselves—but other people are being harmed or underserved. The postpartum care system and services are structured around medical specialists and addressing specific health topics, rather than person-centered care or a focus on the parent–infant dyad. This approach can, and should, be modified.

To achieve more consistent, equitable, and supportive care, quality improvement efforts should center those who are served, identify a patient's intersecting needs, and explicitly strive to enact holistic care. This type of meaningful engagement for health equity requires that all stakeholders be involved in the development and implementation process. The inequitable and unjust outcomes that flow from US healthcare institutions indicate that care practices and, perhaps, the rules of collaboration do not work the same way for everyone. Being open and honest in how we work together is important to authentically connect and commit to partnership in ways that facilitate honest evaluation of opportunities. In this way, we can determine the components of systems that are working—and for whom. This clarity is needed to improve quality and justice in healthcare.

Critically assessing current frameworks and values in postpartum care is foundational for innovation. There is an opportunity to move from individual-driven problem identification and physician-centered care models to community-informed perinatal and reproductive healthcare (PRH) models.[4] Community-informed PRH models, rooted in the reproductive justice framework, aim to meet the individual and community-identified needs of Black birthing people in a collaborative, transparent, and reciprocal manner.[4] The Cycle to Respectful Care is a framework that focuses on continually strengthening systems by centering individual needs and eliminating structural and interpersonal contributors to healthcare disparities.[5] The model outlines community-centered considerations for continually moving through seven steps toward respectful care: waking up (data collection and analysis), getting ready (examination of personal beliefs and worldviews), reaching out to stakeholders, implementing with the provider community, coalescing with the local community, creating change, and maintaining. Stakeholder partnership occurs throughout to center community needs and to ensure fidelity to centering the experiences of Black birthing people.[5]

The Cycle to Respectful Care can be used as a guide to assess quality healthcare metrics, such as postpartum visit attendance. In this type of collaborative approach, stakeholders lead in both the "problem space" and the "solution space."

Collaborative definition of postpartum care priorities can be achieved by listening to what is most important to mothers and birthing people, their companions, and their healthcare team members at the patient's various healthcare touchpoints. In this example, doing so might lead to a postpartum measure of success more meaningful than postpartum visit attendance, because access to care is shaped by expectations, experiences, and consideration of trade-offs.[15] Low rates of visit attendance might be a symptom of a problem, not the primary issue. Being open to identifying the root causes of inequities in healthcare is key to uplifting the facilitators of positive health outcomes—such as engagement with recommended healthcare visits—and addressing the real barriers—such as the healthcare system as a place of last resort rather than a source of ongoing support.

INNOVATION THROUGH MULTIDISCIPLINARY TEAMS

The present standard of US maternity care positions the comprehensive postpartum follow-up appointment as the endpoint of obstetric services, with transition to primary care. ACOG Committee Opinion No. 736 described innovations to postpartum practice that provide ongoing support around the postpartum visit with other coordinated, routine services that engage with mothers and all birthing people, families, and communities. The ACOG document included additional mechanisms for assessing women's health needs after birth, such as home visits, phone support, text messages, remote blood pressure monitoring, and app-based support. Team-based wraparound services can offer more individualized and accessible support to meet needs.[6] As part of more connected and person-focused postpartum services, effective coordination of care (sometimes referred to as "transitions of care") is critical. Innovation in this space includes integration of community health workers, patient navigators, postpartum doulas, and other such professionals. These caregivers can offer multidisciplinary coordination for patient care and build technical and interpersonal pathways for smoother care transitions across the maternity care timeline and interconception care.

The postpartum discharge transition bundle from the Alliance for Innovation on Maternal Health provides recommendations to support the transition from inpatient care to postpartum discharge and follow-up.[7] This open-access ACOG guidance outlines five interrelated components of quality care: readiness, recognition and prevention, response, reporting/systems learning, and respectful, equitable, and supportive care. The patient safety bundle focuses on preparation of every unit, every provider, and every healthcare team member to offer the best care for every patient and encounter. That means the benchmark for quality care is 100%. One of the bundle components highlights multidisciplinary, coordinated teams. Members include postpartum persons, their identified personal support network, and healthcare teams. These teams may also include community-based, state, or public health agencies. These integrated teams are positioned as the most appropriate for developing and implementing postpartum screenings, determining trauma-informed protocols, and maintaining referral resources. They are intended to facilitate timely, equitable postdischarge care and identification of resources.

An example of multidisciplinary teamwork for improved recognition and response to postpartum health needs is the I Gave Birth project. This work was funded by the Enhancing Reviews and Surveillance to Eliminate Maternal Mortality grant from the Centers for Disease Control and Prevention (CDC). The project is an example of a multidisciplinary initiative focusing on increasing awareness of complications and risk factors associated with the postpartum period and taking prompt action to address them. Vidant Medical Center (a Level IV birthing facility in eastern North Carolina that averages about 4,000 deliveries annually), in partnership with the UNC Collaborative for Maternal and Infant Health, conducted a pilot initiative to educate healthcare team members, patients, and families on maternal health warning signs.

The collaborators intentionally connected with community partners and professionals working in a variety of settings, including emergency departments, neonatal intensive care units, outpatient doctors' offices, health departments, urgent care centers, pediatric offices, and home visiting programs. For the duration of the project, all individuals in the area who delivered at or after 20 weeks' gestation received postnatal maternal warning signs training and an "I gave birth" wristband. They were invited to wear the band for at least six weeks postpartum, with special considerations and processes developed for people with perinatal loss or adoption. Additionally, family members, support people, and other people from local communities were given training and information on the purpose of the wristband and how to support the wearer in the event of an emergency. Once the initiative was successfully integrated into the standard workflow at Vidant Medical Center, it was rolled out to birthing facilities in the Vidant Health System and to surrounding facilities in a 21-county radius. This type of work to strengthen community awareness of postpartum maternal health warning signs helps fortify the "village watch" by (1) equipping communities to recognize the need for timely postpartum treatment or care and

(2) disseminating the knowledge needed to support new mothers and birthing people when they experience postpartum complications.

Another initiative that raises awareness of urgent maternal health warning signs is the CDC Hear Her campaign (cdc.gov/hearher/). The CDC materials highlight concerning health symptoms during and after pregnancy and offer tools for improved communication between patients and their healthcare providers.[8] The primary objectives of the campaign include increasing awareness of serious pregnancy-related complication and warning signs, preparing birthing people and their supports to raise concerns, encouraging important health communication, and providing tools for potentially lifesaving conversations.

Pairing an initiative like the I Gave Birth bracelet project and the CDC's Hear Her Campaign is an example of building pathways with supportive wraparound systems to facilitate better maternal perinatal healthcare and outcomes.

STANDARDIZATION OF CLINICAL PRACTICES AS AN INNOVATION

Preventive healthcare practices, such as screening for postpartum risk factors, proactive scheduling for postpartum visits and/or specialty care, and linking to community services/resources, can be integrated as standards of care. The standardization of processes like discharge planning, postpartum visit templates, and workflows can help to ensure care quality and equity.

The Maternal and Infant Assessment and Follow-up Plan is an example of standardization as an innovation.[9] This nurse-initiated assessment is documented in a patient's electronic health record and includes vital sign trends, behavioral observations, postpartum assessments, and normal newborn assessments. The assessments integrate care plans and educational content for infant and postpartum care into postpartum visits based upon individual needs. A follow-up plan is created at the completion of each assessment. Follow-up recommendations and referrals are entered to support a smooth transition of care. For instance, nurse home visitors might identify a need for appointments with a mental health practitioner. The plan will notify mental health providers within the community to complete follow-up assessments. Some communities have integrated access to community health workers and doulas to provide additional follow-up as needed. The model is best implemented when integrated into systems that are multidisciplinary and have strong connections and collaborations with community-based, state, and public health agencies that support mothers and birthing parents. Such a system, with standardized processes to ensure connection to resources and support while navigating the postpartum transition, can have a major impact.

The postpartum appointment handout is an innovative tool for supporting transitions of care.[9] The handout document is completed prior to the postpartum appointment by the healthcare team and the patient. After discussing patient needs, the healthcare team arranges for follow-up appointments and provides the information at discharge. The handout helps streamline scheduling for both postpartum and newborn appointments and can be placed on the home refrigerator as a reminder. Expanding scheduling options to be inclusive of both in-person and telemedicine visits is one method of developing individualized care. Integrating systems that can produce equitable, tailored care should be a priority.

The Ready, Set, Baby curriculum developed by the Carolina Global Breastfeeding Institute, in the Gillings School of Global Public Health at UNC Chapel Hill, is an innovation that can support standardized clinical practice for breastfeeding education. The information is aimed at the patient and family and the curriculum provides tools for healthcare professionals to use in addressing topics with pregnant people. Content addresses breastfeeding "basics," components of healthy pregnancies, early postpartum experiences consistent with Baby Friendly Hospital Initiative practices, the postpartum transition from inpatient to home, and aspects of return to work or school. There also is a section for partners. The open-access Web site is readysetbabyonline.com, and there are flip-chart materials for individual or group counseling (sph.unc.edu/cgbi/ready-set-baby/, with content in multiple languages). Ready, Set, Baby has shown that conversation-based education is effective,[10-12] and a systematic review[13] of prenatal breastfeeding education identified the importance of combining education with interpersonal support and involvement of the birthing parent's companions or family.

Another patient-centered model of care that promotes preventive healthcare practices is the JJ Way®. According to Commonsense Childbirth, creator of the JJ Way®, every parent who chooses to give birth wants a healthy baby and every parent deserves one.[14] The model has proven effective in reducing disparities and improving outcomes. Parents and family supporters are invited to participate in each prenatal and postpartum visit. Using a team approach, each staff member is integral to the care provided to families. Key components of this delivery model include prenatal bonding through respect, support, education, encouragement, and empowerment. This cost-effective model can be replicated and adapted to fit any practice; additional information is at commensensechildbirth.org.

INNOVATION THROUGH MEANINGFUL COMMUNICATION

Effectively communicating about the postpartum period is critical. In particular, quality patient–provider communication can establish rapport and security for mothers and birthing parents in the clinical relationship.[15-17] However, reports of maternity care experiences suggest that patient–provider communication is falling short,[17-19] especially as mothers and birthing parents enter the postpartum period.[20] A community-based participatory study on Black maternal health identified mother–provider communication as "an important aspect that affected their experiences and led to both positive interaction and outcomes, or created a negative experience that affected them emotionally and physically."[21] Strengthening communication has the potential to improve postpartum health and wellness.

Postpartum communication tools should be patient-centered in content and use. This can be achieved by engaging with new parents to identify their postpartum health information needs and their preferred way to receive the information (e.g., format, timing). The 4th Trimester Project at UNC Chapel Hill implemented this strategy through its collaboration with postpartum parents to develop open-access Web sites and to codesign postpartum tools in English and Spanish. The project was funded by the Patient-Centered Outcomes Research Institute to determine priority postpartum health topics from maternal perspectives and to identify how those needs could be met through coordination and strengthening of systems of healthcare and societal support.

Researchers from UNC Chapel Hill partnered in the project with Family Connects, a nurse home-visiting program at Duke University, and SisterSong Women of Color Reproductive Justice Collective to engage postpartum parents and clinicians from the Triangle region of North Carolina.[22,23] Many participants reported that the comparative lack of information and communication about postpartum topics compared to pregnancy- and birth-related details left birthing parents unaware and unprepared for common postpartum challenges (e.g., pelvic floor recovery).[22,23] The 4th Trimester Project leveraged complementary expertise from nursing, information science, midwifery, and communications with support from the Global Health Foundation to codesign the open-access Websites NewMomHealth.com (in English)[24] and SaludMadre.com (in Spanish).[25] The sites provide low-literacy, positive, and clear information for expecting and postpartum families. There also is a dedicated section for healthcare team members that aims to improve patient–provider communication and education about the postpartum period. The section provides guidance to healthcare providers about how to integrate postpartum tools into clinical care for patient education, for care planning, and for promoting more patient-centered postpartum visits.

The Postpartum Visit Checklist, for example, is a two-page document that is patient-centered in content and design.[26] Patients are given blank space to write down questions and can indicate their postpartum concerns from a list of postpartum topics and whether they have a specific question or concern or would like more information or a referral. Topics include physical recovery, self-care, infant feeding and care, family planning, and staying well.

The team also developed the 4th Trimester Project Postpartum Toolkit,[27] a compilation of one-page information sheets for healthcare providers about how to use postpartum care materials designed to prepare their patients for the postpartum period and facilitate quality postpartum care. The Postpartum Visit Checklist one-pager gives healthcare providers the why, when, and how for introducing the tool to patients and their family members. This instructional design is consistent across all the one-page information sheets. The Birthing Parent Health and New Baby Health one-pagers are highlight tools designed to enhance prenatal preparation for the postpartum period, prioritizing content that is most important for patients and their families (e.g., postpartum warning signs, newborn care).

RECOGNIZING AND UPLIFTING COMMUNITY LEADERSHIP

Community-based organizations and community-led interventions play vital roles in building systemic capacity to improve postpartum care at the local, state, and national levels. Nonprofit organizations like Atlanta-based Reaching Our Sisters Everywhere (ROSE)[28] work to reduce breastfeeding disparities among African American women throughout the country. ROSE's mission is to enhance, encourage, support, promote, and protect breastfeeding. The organization combines evidence-based and community-engaged participatory research to inform policy, to educate community members about breastfeeding, to build interdisciplinary public learning spaces, and to expand access to lactation support. Through outreach, education, and technical assistance to prenatal care providers and delivery centers, ROSE promotes practices and policies that support equity, diversity, and community engagement. ROSE's Breastfeeding Summits facilitate meaningful conversation among national funding agencies, academic researchers, local communities, nonprofit organizations, and businesses that serve postpartum people.

Communicating and connecting with communities are ever-evolving. Finding the pathways to connect authentically and with intention can be difficult without trusted platforms. Dr. Shalon's Maternal Action Project (MAP)[29] is dedicated to increasing awareness of the Black maternal health crisis and promoting evidence-based strategies that improve health outcomes. Utilizing the four pillars of storytelling, empowerment, community-building, and education, the MAP team seeks to build strategic partnerships and to move the needle to improve outcomes. The team uses Believe Her, an anonymous peer-support app dedicated to providing education and connection, to provide a pathway to connect Black mothers, birthing people, and families. This platform lets members share stories, receive support, and identify educational resources.

The Irth app[30] ("Birth, but we dropped the B for bias") helps Black and Brown women and birthing people have a more safe and empowered pregnancy. The platform uses qualitative experiences from Black and Brown consumers and translates it into quantitative data to identify patterns and behaviors in hospital settings. The data are leveraged to push for social change.

Mahmee[31] is a platform that empowers health systems, providers, and allied health professions with the elements essential for care and collaboration that support access to care. Healthcare team members can provide scheduled and on-demand virtual appointments; care plans and sensitive information can be shared and are available to support cross-practice collaboration. Mahmee links in-network physicians and out-of-network ancillary care providers for maternity and pediatric programs.

MEASURING QUALITY FOR ACCOUNTABILITY

Accountability in postpartum care means consistently and reliably tracking measures for timely review and action. In practice, these measures might be patient outcomes from the electronic health record (e.g., health outcomes, postpartum visit attendance, acute-care utilization), patient-reported experiences from surveys or other forms of direct feedback (e.g., satisfaction, comprehension, autonomy in decision-making, institutional trust), clinical safety reports about adverse events or near misses, and process measures of how care was delivered (e.g., wait times, language-concordant care, missed meals during the inpatient stay). Dr. Elizabeth Howell and colleagues at the University of Pennsylvania Health System, for example, recommended creating a dashboard for process measures, including language concordance and cultural sensitivity, to narrow the maternal health disparity gap.[17] Collaborating with mothers and birthing people, families, and communities to identify quality measures helps to effectively improve outcomes.

Cradle Cincinnati was founded in 2012 as a collaborative effort among parents, caregivers, healthcare professionals, and community members with a commitment to reduce infant mortality.[32] This network works across sectors to measurably improve preconception, pregnancy, and infant health. Increasing local data integrity and capacity by standardizing systems of information that allow continuous evaluation of interventions is a primary focus for the organization. More about Cradle Cincinnati is at cradlecincinnati. org/families.

IMPLEMENTING INNOVATIONS

Implementation science offers an effective structure for postpartum innovation. Using a stage-based, structured approach offers the opportunity to determine if an innovation will be sustainable. Focusing on the implementation process will help identify strategies that support successful uptake of an intervention.

An example of clinical innovation guided by implementation science is the Immediate Postpartum Long-Acting Reversible Contraceptive project undertaken in North Carolina Perinatal Region IV.[33] This hospital-based model was developed with the use of implementation science best practices and emphasizes multidisciplinary team-building, identification of champions, use of implementation science at every stage of the process to develop a systematic and replicable strategy, and application of a reproductive justice framework across the project.[33] The innovation, which can be replicated across hospitals, resulted in a systematic, multidisciplinary, and culturally appropriate model for providing immediate postpartum long-acting reversible contraceptives. Leveraging stakeholder partnership is a critical approach for increasing equity and reducing positionality.

CONCLUSION

Innovation in postpartum care is about taking action to change the inequitable processes, systems, policies, and values that lead to poor and disparate outcomes. We might ask ourselves what data or metric indicates effectiveness, and for whom. With any topic or approach in maternal healthcare space, we will be best equipped for success by coming to it with an antiracist lens and to continually strive to determine what matters most, to identify what support looks like, and to evaluate whether goals are achieved. The Cycle to Respectful Care can be used to identify community-driven health processes that can affect maternal mortality and postpartum outcomes. Strategies and interventions that reshape care across the postpartum continuum require effective utilization of multidisciplinary teams, standardized processes, improvements in communication between patients and healthcare teams, and uplift of community leadership.

While these innovations can make a difference in postpartum well-being, some changes that can have major impact are not innovations. For example, access to paid family leave, paid comprehensive medical care, diaper banks, income supports, and food banks have been shown to improve outcomes during the postpartum period. Focusing on integrating and improving access to these services can help mothers and birthing people, their families, and the community to thrive.

REFERENCES
1. Declercq E, Zephyrin L. Maternal mortality in the United States: a primer. Commonwealth Fund; 2020. doi:10.26099/ta1q-mw24.

2. Cohen JL, Daw JR. Postpartum cliffs—missed opportunities to promote maternal health in the United States. *JAMA Health Forum*. 2021;2(12):e214164. doi:10.1001/jamahealthforum.2021.4164.

3. Howell EA, Egorova N, Balbierz A, Zeitlin J, Hebert PL. Black–white differences in severe maternal morbidity and site of care. *Am J Obstet Gynecol*. 2016;214(1):122. e1–e7. doi:10.1016/j.ajog.2015.08.019.

4. Julian Z, Robles D, Whetstone S, et al. Community-informed models of perinatal and reproductive health services provision: a justice-centered paradigm toward equity among Black birthing communities. *Semin Perinatol*. 2020;44(5):151267. doi:10.1016/j.semperi.2020.151267.

5. Green CL, Perez SL, Walker A, et al. The Cycle to Respectful Care: a qualitative approach to the creation of an actionable framework to address maternal outcome disparities. *Int J Environ Res Public Health*. 2021;18(9):4933. doi:10.3390/ijerph18094933.

6. American College of Obstetricians and Gynecologists. ACOG Committee Opinion No. 736: optimizing postpartum care. *Obstet Gynecol*. 2018;131(5):11.

7. American College of Obstetricians and Gynecologists Postpartum Discharge Transition. Alliance for Innovation on Maternal Health. https://saferbirth.org. Published 2021. Accessed May 5, 2022.

8. Centers for Disease Control and Prevention. Hear Her Campaign. https://www.cdc.gov/hearher/index.html. Published February 16, 2022. Accessed May 5, 2022.

9. Havey L. Transitions of care & ACOG AIM postpartum discharge bundle. Paper presented at: NC Maternal Health Innovation Community of Practice; January 27, 2022. https://www.youtube.com/watch?v=gZUmo0xfof8. Accessed May 23, 2022.

10. Palmquist AEL, Parry KC, Wouk K, et al. *Ready, Set, BABY Live* virtual prenatal breastfeeding education for COVID-19. *J Hum Lact*. 2020;36(4):614–618. doi:10.1177/0890334420959292.

11. Parry KC, Tully KP, Hopper LN, Schildkamp PE, Labbok MH. Evaluation of Ready, Set, BABY: a prenatal breastfeeding education and counseling approach. *Birth Berkeley Calif*. 2019;46(1):113–120. doi:10.1111/birt.12393.

12. Parry KC, Tully KP, Moss SL, Sullivan CS. Innovative prenatal breastfeeding education curriculum: Ready, Set, BABY. *J Nutr Educ Behav*. 2017;49(7 suppl 2):S214–S216. doi:10.1016/j.jneb.2017.05.348.

13. Wouk K, Tully KP, Labbok MH. Systematic review of evidence for Baby-Friendly Hospital Initiative Step 3. *J Hum Lact*. 2017;33(1):50–82. doi:10.1177/0890334416679618.

14. The JJ Way®. Commonsense Childbirth Inc. https://commonsensechildbirth.org/the-jj-way/. Accessed June 1, 2022.

15. Thom DH, Campbell B. Patient–physician trust: an exploratory study. *J Fam Pract*. 1997;44(2):169–176.

16. Sheppard VB, Zambrana RE, O'Malley AS. Providing health care to low-income women: a matter of trust. *Fam Pract*. 2004;21(5):484–491. doi:10.1093/fampra/cmh503.

17. Howell EA, Ahmed ZN. Eight steps for narrowing the maternal health disparity gap. *Contemp Obgyn*. 2019;64(1):30–36.

18. Baranowska B, Pawlicka P, Kiersnowska I, et al. Woman's needs and satisfaction regarding the communication with doctors and midwives during labour, delivery and early postpartum. *Healthcare*. 2021;9(4):382. doi:10.3390/healthcare9040382.

19. Attanasio L, Kozhimannil KB. Patient-reported communication quality and perceived discrimination in maternity care. *Med Care*. 2015;53(10):863–871. doi:10.1097/MLR.0000000000000411.

20. Cheng CY, Fowles ER, Walker LO. Continuing education module: postpartum maternal health care in the United States; a critical review. *J Perinat Educ*. 2006;15(3):34–42. doi:10.1624/105812406X119002.

21. Alio AP, Dillion T, Hartman S, et al. A community collaborative for the exploration of local factors affecting Black mothers' experiences with perinatal care. *Matern Child Health J*. 2022;26(4):751–760. doi:10.1007/s10995-022-03422-5.

22. Tully KP, Stuebe AM, Verbiest SB. The fourth trimester: a critical transition period with unmet maternal health needs. *Am J Obstet Gynecol*. 2017;217(1):37–41. doi:10.1016/j.ajog.2017.03.032.

23. Verbiest S, Tully K, Simpson M, Stuebe A. Elevating mothers' voices: recommendations for improved patient-centered postpartum. *J Behav Med*. 2018;41(5):577–590. doi:10.1007/s10865-018-9961-4.

24. 4th Trimester Project. https://newmomhealth.com. Accessed June 1, 2022.

25. Proyecto 4to Trimestre. https://www.saludmadre.com. Accessed June 1, 2022.

26. 4th Trimester Project. Postpartum visit checklist. NewMomHealth.com. https://newmomhealth.com/postpartum-tools/postpartum-visit-checklist. Accessed June 1, 2022.

27. 4th Trimester Project. Postpartum Toolkit. https://newmomhealth.com/postpartum-toolkit. Accessed June 1, 2022.

28. Reaching Our Sisters Everywhere (ROSE). About us. https://breastfeedingrose.org/about/. Published May 7, 2021. Accessed May 5, 2022.

29. Dr Shalon's Maternal Action Project. https://www.drshalonsmap.org. Accessed June 1, 2022.

30. Narrative Nation. IRTH. https://irthapp.com/. Accessed June 1, 2022.

31. Mahmee. https://www.mahmee.com/about. Accessed June 1, 2022.

32. Cradle Cincinnati. Staff & subcommittees. https://www.cradlecincinnati.org/subcommittees/. Published 2021. Accessed June 1, 2022.

33. Harper KD, Loper AC, Louison LM, Morse JE. Stage-based implementation of immediate postpartum long-acting reversible contraception using a reproductive justice framework. *Am J Obstet Gynecol*. 2020;222(4S):S893–S905. doi:10.1016/j.ajog.2019.11.1273.

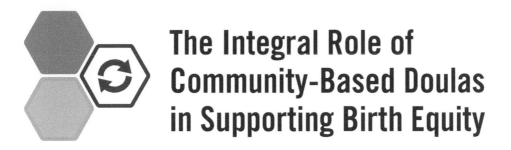

Chapter 35

The Integral Role of Community-Based Doulas in Supporting Birth Equity

TWYLLA DILLION AND ZAINAB SULAIMAN

INTRODUCTION

A disproportionate number of birthing people of color, especially women, suffer poor maternal health outcomes, are at increased risk of experiencing traumatic birth experiences, frequently undergo medical interventions during childbirth, and suffer from high maternal mortality rates.[1] In the United States, research suggests that birthing people of color increasingly report negative interactions with maternity care providers because of their race, ethnicity, or language.[2] Such negative interactions, coupled with an increasing maternal mortality rate among Black birthing people, are a direct result of structural racism and a history of racism in the healthcare system.

Doulas, named using the ancient Greek word meaning "someone who serves," are trained companions who support birthing people and their families. Doulas provide continuous, one-on-one care and evidence-based information, physical support, and emotional support to birthing persons and their partners prenatally, at birth, and postpartum. Academic research has repeatedly shown what doulas and those they serve already know: birthing people matched with formal doula support were less likely to have a low-birth-weight baby, were less likely to have birth complications, and were more likely to initiate breastfeeding than people without this support.[3]

Traditionally, doulas provide support before, during, and shortly after childbirth and are typically independent business practitioners who directly bill families for their services. The support provided by doulas has existed throughout

Twylla Dillion and Zainab Sulaiman, *The Integral Role of Community-Based Doulas in Supporting Birth Equity* In: *The Practical Playbook III*. Edited by: Dorothy Cilenti, Alisahah Jackson, Natalie D. Hernandez, Lindsey Yates, Sarah Verbiest, J. Lloyd Michener, and Brian C. Castrucci, Oxford University Press. © de Beaumont Foundation 2024. DOI: 10.1093/oso/9780197662984.003.0035

Box 35.1 | Key Differences between Community-Based Doulas and Traditional, Non-Community-Based Doulas

Community-Based Doulas	Traditional, Non-Community-Based Doulas
Community-based doula programs add multiple prenatal and postpartum home visits, referrals to comprehensive support, and additional resources to the services typically provided by a traditional doula.	Standard or traditional doula training typically prepares doulas to work as independent doulas immediately after their training.
Community-based doulas are prepared to provide, and skilled at providing, culturally competent, trauma-informed, social, emotional, and informational support to their clients.	Traditional doulas often do not receive ongoing supervision or mentorship, as is common in community-based programs.
Collaboration with other healthcare and social service providers is undertaken when necessary, including transportation; housing; alcohol, tobacco, and other drug (ATOD) cessation; WIC; SNAP; and intimate partner violence resources.	Traditional doula training often lacks historical, educational, and cultural context on how race, institutional and interpersonal bias, and other social determinants play an integral role in birth disparities affecting communities of color.
Referrals and assistance are provided for obtaining appropriate social support services and follow-up (including WIC, housing, case management) and community-based healthcare systems that promote the advancement of the pregnant person and community.	Doulas are trained in an entrepreneurial private practice framework that differs in purpose and mission from community-based doula work.
Assistance is provided in preparing for, and carrying out, a pregnant person's plans for their childbirth that affirms their identities.	
Community-based doula programs also provide peer-to-peer mentorship, support, professional development, and continuing education opportunities for doulas.	

Source: Bey A, Brill A, Porchia-Albert C, Gradilla M, Strauss N. Advancing birth justice: community-based doula models as a standard of care for ending racial disparities. Ancient Song Doula Services, Village Birth International, Every Mother Counts. https://everymotherrcounts.org/wp-content/uploads/2019/03/Advancing-Birth-Justice-CBD-Models-as-Std-of-Care-3-25-19.pdf. Published March 25, 2019.

history in informal ways, including familial and village support throughout the world. Therefore, doulas are not an "innovation," but the recognition of their value and importance is a renaissance of sorts. In many cases, informal support has not received the recognition it deserved because of racism, classism, and the medicalization of birth, which excludes community-based support. Researchers have found that interactions and outcomes improve when doctors and patients share a similar race or ethnicity and the physician's implicit biases are reduced. While doulas are nonclinical providers, evidence from clinical care also applies to the importance of shared cultural and lived experiences in the doula–client relationship.

Years of historic disinvestment in Black, Brown, and Indigenous communities has resulted in the need to use a community-based approach to reduce adverse maternal and child health outcomes. These communities confront many structural issues due to social exclusion, including lack of community safety, financial instability, limited free time, social disconnectedness, lack of culturally reflective support, and much else. The community-based doula model addresses disinvestment in these communities by improving the health of birthing families of color and low-income families through support situated in the community. Community-based doulas are a lifeline for Black, Brown, and Indigenous birthing families, offering culturally reflective support during the birthing process for underresourced and marginalized communities where systemic, structural inequities fuel health disparities.

Community-based doulas often are members of the community they serve and utilize an expanded model of traditional doula care. The expanded model of care includes providing a wider array of services through a holistic and multifaceted approach, building ongoing relationships with community members, and sharing lived experience, culture, and language with the communities they serve.[4] Leveraging natural support systems in communities and focusing on wellness and healing are crucial for community-based doula care.[5] Community-based doula models use community strength as scaffolding for program delivery, and this approach rejects the prevailing deficit-based approach used in most clinical settings when supporting underresourced communities. Community-based doulas come from the communities they serve and are aware of community assets; they are individuals who can draw upon their strengths naturally and through their training. Practitioners often have completed multiple doula training models and continuing education. Extensive and ongoing education ensures that these professionals can provide high-touch support for birthing families, including childbirth education, prenatal visits, childbirth and immediate postpartum support, and postpartum visits. This chapter lays out the history and origins of the community-based doula model, the potential for integration into hospital systems, the discourse around government funding to sustain the profession, and a look at future innovation.

CASE STUDY: THE ORIGINS OF THE HEALTHCONNECT ONE MODEL

HealthConnect One (HC One), formerly the Chicago Health Connection, began as a volunteer initiative in 1986 to promote breastfeeding in low-income communities of color. For over three decades, HC One has focused on the importance of peer-to-peer support, respecting race, ethnicity, and the value of every interaction. Operating with the awareness that birth equity is fundamental to racial equity, HC One has established itself as a leading national organization that provides customized coaching, training, technical assistance, and program development for perinatal support workers, including community-based doulas and breastfeeding peer counselors. HC One offers services to maternal and child health partners in underresourced communities across the nation.

In 1995, HC One partnered with the Ounce of Prevention Fund (now Start Early) to develop the Chicago Doula Project, which aimed to integrate intensive prenatal, intrapartum, and postpartum support into existing teen parent services through training and employing community women as doulas. The community-based doula model that evolved from this partnership grew from HC One's foundation of work based on Paulo Freire's Empowerment Education approach. The model ensures that doulas are carefully selected community members whose racial, ethnic, and socioeconomic backgrounds reflect the population they serve. Practitioners are chosen for their capacity to serve as nurturers, role models, and teachers.

The goals of HC One's community-based doula program are:

- To increase the rates of extended and exclusive breastfeeding in communities with low breastfeeding rates.
- To reduce the rates of low birth weight and prematurity, particularly in Black/African American communities.
- To reduce the use of cesarean deliveries among Black/African American and Hispanic individuals unless they are medically necessary.
- To reduce the use of epidurals in favor of alternative pain management techniques.
- To further develop the corps of community health workers in maternal and child health and early learning.

HC One's training approach emphasizes active learning through role-play, bidirectional learning, discussion, and supervised experience in labor and delivery, as well as didactic sessions on pregnancy, childbirth, adolescence, and breastfeeding.

The community-based doula model at HC One is an innovative replication of the train-the-trainer model, where community-based trainers are prepared to train community members as doulas with the HC One curriculum.

This replication model is building and mentoring a large, new national cohort of community-based doulas. The model has five essential components:

1. Employ women who are trusted members of the community of focus.
2. Extend and intensify the role of a doula with families from early pregnancy through the first months postpartum.
3. Collaborate with community stakeholders/institutions and use a diverse team approach.
4. Facilitate experiential learning using popular education techniques and the HC One training curriculum.
5. Value the doula's work with salary, supervision, and support.

As HC One initiates partnerships with community doula organizations, the five essential components are required to ensure that community support is optimized and that the doulas are valued and respected in their learning and work. Program data from the past four years have shown astounding results for Black mothers and babies covered by Medicaid and supported by HC One programs (see Figures 35.1 and 35.2). Between 2017 and 2021, such partnerships

Figure 35.1 ▼

HealthConnect One (HC One) community-based doula national results, 2017–2021. Top: Results for healthy birth weight versus low birth weight among Black non-Hispanic mothers covered by Medicaid. Bottom: Results for preterm.

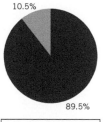

10.5%

89.5%

■ Healthy Birth Weight
■ Low Birth Weight

Low birth weight is two times more likely among non-Hispanic Black mothers than among non-Hispanic white mothers.

Among the sample non-Hispanic Black mothers covered by Medicaid and supported by HC One from 2017 to 2021, the rate of low birth weight was 10.5%, compared to the national rate of 13.9%.

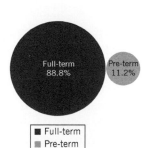

Full-term 88.8% Pre-term 11.2%

■ Full-term
■ Pre-term

Preterm births are 1.5 times more likely among Black non-Hispanic mothers than among white non-Hispanic mothers. Among the sample non-Hispanic Black mothers covered by Medicaid and supported by HC One from 2017 to 2021, the preterm birth rate was 11.2%, compared to the 13.9% rate identified nationally.

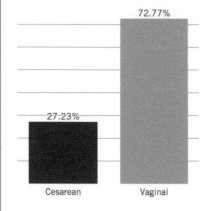

Figure 35.2 ▼

HealthConnect One (HC One) community-based doula national results, 2017–2021, for cesarean versus vaginal deliveries.

Source: National Center for Health Statistics, final natality data. www.marchofdimes.org/peristats. Retrieved May 28, 2021.

72.77%

27.23%

Cesarean   Vaginal

The percentage of cesarean deliveries is **highest among Black women in the United States, at 35.5%.**

Among the sample non-Hispanic Black mothers covered by Medicaid and supported by HC One from 2017 to 2021, 27.2% of births were cesarean deliveries.

had 24.5% fewer babies born with low weight and 19.4% fewer babies born preterm among Black mothers on Medicaid compared with the national average. HC One programming also resulted in 23.4% fewer babies born by cesarean delivery.

Today, HC One focuses on training, integrating, and advocating for breastfeeding peer counselors, community-based doulas, and other community health workers, as well as valuing their work with fair pay. The organization has codesigned programs with over 50 community organizations and nonprofits across 20 states. Since its founder, Rachel Abramson, retired in 2018, the organization has grown and evolved to become a Black-led organization with a primarily Black and Latinx team dispersed across the United States but still based in Chicago. Several examples of HC One's community-based programs are described below.

Open Arms Perinatal Services

Since 1997, Open Arms Perinatal Services in Seattle has provided childbirth support for over 3,900 families. Trained and accredited as an HC One community-based doula site, Open Arms is not hospital-directed or hospital-based. Open Arms utilizes a trusted, community-centered approach that prioritizes each client's unique cultural, linguistic, and emotional needs, and its care is free of charge. The community-based doula approach helps connect families with resources to meet the growing demand for mental health support, housing, transportation, domestic violence services, and legal aid. COVID-19 posed significant challenges in connecting with families, yet Open Arms provided 200 individual lactation support virtual visits. As of 2021, 95% of families served by Open Arms gave birth at full term and healthy birth weight, while 96.3% were breast/chestfeeding at birth and 82% were still breast/chestfeeding at six months.

BirthMatters

With the mission to reduce teen pregnancy through reproductive health education and to empower birthing people (age 24 and under) to raise healthy families, BirthMatters utilizes the community health worker model to provide young birthing families with doulas. The only community-based doula program in South Carolina, the organization offers support in Spartanburg and outlying rural communities. BirthMatters was set in motion in 2007, when it received its first planning grant and began conducting focus groups and visiting existing doula programs. By 2010, its team had supported over 30 mothers and families with birth doula services. That same year, BirthMatters partnered with HC One and replicated the Chicago group's community-based doula program. Since its inception, BirthMatters has completed six community-based doula trainings using the HC One model, and in 2020, the organization successfully underwent a rigorous review with HC One's accreditation team. The BirthMatters team attends 50 births per year, with three community-based doulas on staff, and about 65 families (at time of publication) are enrolled every year. Ninety-two percent of participants served by the organization are Black and all participants are on, or eligible for, Medicaid.

Black Mothers Breastfeeding Association

Detroit has multiple issues with social determinants of health that create a challenging landscape for birthing people, families, and children and stem from a poverty rate of 30.6%. (Detroit is the second-most impoverished city in the country.) The Black Mothers Breastfeeding Association (BMBFA) addresses the sociohistorical context for why breastfeeding has not been a cultural norm in Detroit's African American community. Understanding the effects of slavery, racism, discrimination, biased treatment, and active marketing of formula in disinvested neighborhoods is key to BMBFA's work with community members and professionals. Creating a culture of prenatal care, breastfeeding, and postpartum care to grow healthier babies, mothers, families, and communities, the organization provides families with breastfeeding peer counselors and community-based doulas. Initially trained by HC One utilizing its breastfeeding peer counselors curriculum, BMBFA has been a long-time partner and has augmented its training to include national accreditation through HC One's Community-Based Doula Accreditation Program. The organization's existence in Detroit for over a decade has increased diversity in the peer-to-peer lactation support and community-based doula field by creating a pathway for women and people from the community to better serve the population they mirror.

DOULAS AND HOSPITAL SYSTEMS

In Black, Brown, and Indigenous communities, a doula's shared lived experience and authenticity are crucial. As we work toward increasing the availability of doulas, we need to be mindful not to eliminate the elements of the work that have made community-based doulas effective. Mistakenly, the formalization of doula care often whitewashes the practice, leaning into the medical model that the dominant group developed. Relatability, formation of authentic relationships, and responsiveness to birthing people's needs are key elements of the community-based doula approach that support highly effective care. It is possible for community-based doulas to be included in community clinical care teams and to be reimbursed by Medicaid and private insurance without losing essential elements. The development of community clinical care teams requires a commitment to diversity, equity, inclusion, and the emphasis that birthing people and communities know what they need for better birth outcomes. Clinical-level rigidity in providing doula support is not an ideal approach, as doula support is not clinical care. Instead, healthcare systems and payers must partner with, and learn from, community-based doulas/organizations to understand how the model works and how clinical care and community support can complement each other.

Clinical providers, health systems, and payers must acknowledge that birthing people's decision to have doula support is their right. Doula-supported advocacy in the delivery room mitigates the harm of implicit bias and racism during birth; HC One continues to elevate the need for this advocacy, especially during the global shift of COVID-19 from pandemic to endemic. HC One's national community-based birth worker advocacy and projects centered on systemic change are vital to this work. Community-based doulas serving in hospitals have shared their challenges with acceptance and respect when working in a healthcare team. For doulas to be most effective at providing care and support to birthing families, they must be well valued and able to work collaboratively with physicians, nurses, and other hospital staff. The inclusion of doulas in the healthcare system must also strike a balance between collaboration and autonomy, while promoting patient-centered care.[5]

HC One's ongoing collaboration in Rochester, New York, is an example of how community-based doulas and hospital systems can work together to provide culturally reflective community-based support that involves a community–clinic team. HC One is collaborating with three community-based organizations in this work: Healthy Baby Network, Finger Lakes Community Health, and Finger Lakes Performing Provider System (FLPPS), a not-for-profit organization established in 2014 to improve the healthcare delivery system for the Medicaid population. FLPPS has worked intensively with Rochester-area hospital systems to develop programs focused on improving the quality of care for Medicaid recipients and has as one of its goals improved health and well-being of birthing people and infants. The program will identify and train trusted community members to provide doula services and to help improve prenatal care, to raise breastfeeding rates, to decrease unnecessary medical interventions, to increase positive birth experiences, and to improve parenting skills. To ensure community–clinical collaboration, the project will involve meetings among FLPPS, the lead community-based organizations, and maternal and child health and diversity, equity, and inclusion leadership at both Rochester hospital systems.

ENSURING SUSTAINABILITY—NATIONAL AND STATE-LED EFFORTS ON REIMBURSEMENT

Many community-based doulas have experience working with Black, Brown, and Indigenous communities. These inadequately served communities often have needs and risks that the traditional medical system cannot meet. Doulas build a bridge between birthing families and healthcare systems and support clients in accessing resources. Their unique training and expertise in underserved communities fills a significant gap in care, and these professionals should be appropriately compensated for their expertise. Advocacy around sustainable billing practices that align with the work community-based doulas provide has been ongoing for nearly a decade.

Most traditional doulas make a living by serving clients who can pay out of pocket. While community-based doulas often charge very little (or nothing), they often serve people who are low-income Medicaid beneficiaries who would benefit significantly from free access to doula services. Despite their dedication to serving their communities, community-rooted doulas cannot continue to work for free.

Government funding is essential to sustain community-based organizations that provide peer-to-peer pregnancy, labor, and postpartum support within communities. Community-based doulas should be prioritized and centered in reimbursement structures, as a pathway to reducing inequities and creating a way for all doulas—traditional, community-based, or private—to be covered for the support they offer birthing people. The community-based organizations, which report evidence of improved outcomes, are embedded in their communities and employ doulas who understand the unique needs of their respective populations. Yet Congress has in general been slow to act on maternal health issues, including legislation to expand the doula workforce and to provide sustainable federal funding for this work. Medicaid covers approximately 40% of births nationwide, particularly in communities of color, offering a vital source of coverage for pregnant people and women. State governments have demonstrated leadership by leveraging Medicaid to address poor maternal and child health outcomes.

Several states have proposed legislation, pilot programs, and initiatives to expand doula support and to explore Medicaid coverage of this work.[6] Diversifying doula care to embody the community-based model will ensure that the doula workforce can provide culturally congruent care to Black, Brown, and Indigenous families. It also requires a sustainability pathway that includes training, fee waivers, other incentives to help recruit doulas from low-income communities, and long-term sustainable payer funding through Medicaid reimbursement.[7] In 2014, Minnesota and Oregon were the first and only states that mandated coverage of doula services through Medicaid. Today, 15 states have passed doula-related legislation.[8]

Developing legislation to determine appropriate reimbursement rates and to encourage uptake of these benefits by doulas has posed a challenge. Due to the nonclinical role of doulas, in providing emotional support, referrals to social supports, and comfort measures, Medicaid reimbursement can be complex. Additionally, understanding the role of a doula and its importance in reducing poor outcomes, especially in the Black and Indigenous communities, is a challenge for payers and hospital systems that are more familiar with clinical models and pathways. Traditionally, doulas are paid per birth, where the doula is paid a lump sum for all work related to birth. While some private, non-community-based doulas may provide most of their care during labor and delivery, community-based doula programs typically involve significantly more client contact. Engaging doulas in policymaking is crucial to ensuring that the diverse lived experiences of training, supporting families, and compensation are centered in development of legislation.

New Jersey's Medicaid office established a stakeholder group in 2019 to advise Medicaid on equitable policy development and implementation for doula care. New Jersey trained nearly 100 doulas in counties with high Black infant mortality rates following a series of successful doula pilot programs run by community-based organizations supported by state and local foundations. These initiatives enabled New Jersey to become one of the first states to include community doula care in its Medicaid coverage system.

To accelerate the legislation's success, HC One was selected to establish the statewide New Jersey Doula Learning Collaborative (DLC). HC One's experience with Medicaid fee-for-service reimbursement and managed care organizations will enhance the partnership, which will serve as an important learning opportunity for doulas and organizations around the state and nation. In addition to working with payers, the DLC will increase the number of trained community doulas, help doulas engage with multiple health systems, and process Medicaid reimbursement claims for their services. The DLC is part of First Lady Tammy Murphy's Nurture NJ Maternal and Infant Health Strategic Plan, released in January 2021. The plan's goal is to reduce New Jersey's maternal mortality by 50% over five years and to eliminate racial disparities in birth outcomes. It is a culmination of more than a year of in-person and virtual meetings with more than 100 critical stakeholders, including national public health experts, New Jersey state departments and agencies, health systems, physicians, doulas, community organizations, and mothers and families. In this project, HC One will elevate the voices of community-based doulas and those they serve to ensure that they are centered throughout the ambitious statewide project.

Not only will reimbursing doulas ensure that the profession is valued and sustainable, but also it is a cost-effective solution for state Medicaid programs to reduce the costs associated with risk of preterm birth and cesarean deliveries.[9] To ensure that birthing families from communities of color have access to culturally competent medical care, reimbursement for these services is essential. Making doula care accessible to low-income birthing people who need it most is an overdue nationwide innovation to save lives.[10]

LOOKING AHEAD: FUTURE INNOVATION AND RECOMMENDATIONS

Due to their high level of engagement and individualized care for birthing families, community-based doulas often are viewed as the solution to all maternal health and societal issues, ranging from substance abuse and homelessness to mental health. While community-based doulas frequently address these issues, utilizing doulas as an innovation without appropriate pay, integration, and respect for the profession is unjust. For too long, community-based doulas and organizations have relied on grants and payment from sliding scales, despite their services' significant impact on birth outcomes.

The impact of doula care results in better birth outcomes, but maternity care budgets usually have only limited inclusion of costs for doula support. Although both private insurance and Medicaid plans have begun including reimbursement for doula services, this is painfully limited across the nation, in contrast to the way interventions that are as effective in a clinical setting would be covered without a second thought. The intentional exclusion of doula and doula advocates by payer organizations and in policy development is limiting shifts in reimbursement, as is the tremendous influence of hospital and clinical provider advocates that drowns out doula voices. Doula care must be covered as a standard practice by all payers.

There is no one-size-fits-all model of doula support, as each birthing person, birth, and infant is unique. Restrictive policies around what is and is not covered in doula support should be relaxed within reason to include à la carte options for birthing people as well as additional support to address higher needs and social determinants of health. In addition, COVID-19 has been a catalyst for telehealth innovation, including virtual doula and lactation support. Flexible support models centered on birthing people should be embraced, including virtual prenatal and postpartum doula support.

There are many doula training programs across the nation—some general, some community-based—that emphasize support for underrepresented Black, Brown, and Indigenous communities, and many variations on these common trainings. The more general training like that offered by DONA International and the Childbirth and Postpartum Professional Association are more widely accepted by funders, payers, and programs than community-based doula training like HC One and other Black, Brown, or Indigenous-led programs. Community-based doula programs are designed to support communities and to resonate with the doula trainees and those they serve. Culturally reflective training is an important first step in a community-based doula's journey to offering culturally reflective support. Doula training should not be restricted to white-led training organizations.

Community-based doulas know how to support birthing people and know how to support their communities. Providing education on high blood pressure, healthy eating, and exercise, as well as addressing social determinants of health and other needs, are within the skills of these experienced community health workers. Doulas are community health workers, and partnering with them on community health education beyond perinatal health is a valuable opportunity for individuals and potential clinicians and medical students.

Birthing parents in the United States are struggling with complicated and restrictive health plans, limited parental leave policies, and the difficulty of accessing and affording childcare when they return to work. Employer-sponsored doula support like that at CVS Health, Microsoft, Pioneer Construction, and other for-profit companies should become standard.[11] The support of a doula through the perinatal period could be game changing, especially for Black, Brown, and Indigenous staff employed by large corporations.

Mentorship and supervision are crucial components of community-based doula care. Yet reimbursement rates often do not account for program operation costs, which include billing assistance, supervision, and peer mentorship for doulas. Community-based doula organizations and programs are needed to support the work of individual doulas. As these professionals interact with community members and encounter challenging circumstances, it is essential that community-based organizations can offer mentorship, debriefing, and links to services to support them. While private foundation and grant funding may help to sustain community-based organizations as they establish themselves, governmental and third-party funding will allow community doula organizations to stand independently and will ensure that doulas have the structures to thrive.

REFERENCES

1. Louis JM, Menard MK, Gee RE. Racial and ethnic disparities in maternal morbidity and mortality. *Obstet Gynecol*. 2015;125(3):690–694. doi:10.1097/AOG.0000000000000704.

2. Altman MR, Oseguera T, McLemore MR, Kantrowitz-Gordon I, Franck LS, Lyndon A. Information and power: women of color's experiences interacting with health care providers in pregnancy and birth. *Soc Sci Med.* 2019;238:112491. doi:10.1016/J.SOCSCIMED.2019.112491.

3. Gruber KJ, Cupito SH, Dobson CF. Impact of doulas on healthy birth outcomes. *J Perinat Educ.* 2013;22(1):49. doi:10.1891/1058-1243.22.1.49.

4. HealthConnect One. *The Perinatal Revolution.* Chicago, IL: HealthConnect One; 2014.

5. Bey A, Brill A, Porchia-Albert C, Gradilla M, Strauss N. *Advancing Birth Justice: Community-Based Doula Models as a Standard of Care for Ending Racial Disparities.* Ancient Song Doula Services, Village Birth International, Every Mother Counts; 2019. https://everymothercounts.org/wp-content/uploads/2019/03/Advancing-Birth-Justice-CBD-Models-as-Std-of-Care-3-25-19.pdf.

6. Carvalho K, Kheyfets A, Maleki P, et al. A systematic policy review of Black maternal health-related policies proposed federally and in Massachusetts: 2010–2020. *Front Public Health.* 2021;9:1526.

7. HealthConnect One. Sustainable funding for doula programs: a study. 2017. https://healthconnectone.org/publication/read-sustainable-funding-for-doula-programs-a-study/

8. National Health Law Program. Medicaid coverage for doula care: state implementation efforts. 2021. https://healthlaw.org/medicaid-coverage-for-doula-care-state-implementation-efforts/. Accessed February 12, 2022.

9. Kozhimannil KB, Hardeman RR, Alarid-Escudero F, Vogelsang CA, Blauer-Peterson C, Howell EA. Modeling the cost-effectiveness of doula care associated with reductions in preterm birth and cesarean delivery. *Birth.* 2016;43(1):20–27.

10. Strauss N, Sakala C, Corry MP. Overdue: Medicaid and private insurance coverage of doula care to strengthen maternal and infant health. *J Perinat Educ.* 2016;25(3):145–149.

11. CVS Health and Microsoft cover the cost of doulas for some employees. Will other companies—and private insurance—follow suit? *The Lily.* 2021. https://www.thelily.com/some-big-companies-are-starting-to-cover-the-cost-of-doulas-will-others-follow/. Accessed February 15, 2022.

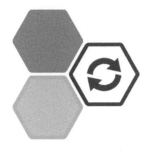

Chapter 36

From Grassroots to Telecommunication Innovation: Bridging the Gap in Perinatal Mental Health

CHRIS RAINES AND WENDY DAVIS

INTRODUCTION

Perinatal mood and anxiety disorders are the most common complications of pregnancy and the postpartum period.[1-2] Research has shown that up to one in seven birthing persons, and up to 10% of their partners, will experience a perinatal mood disorder.[3] With a range of affordable treatment options available, why are up to 15% of people diagnosed with a perinatal mood disorder not receiving treatment?[4] An additional 20% of perinatal mood disorders are not diagnosed, secondary to inadequate screening, inadequate education of providers, fragmentation of care, and other barriers.[5] This is most prevalent in Black, Indigenous, people of color (BIPOC) communities, where the rates of perinatal mood disorders can be two or three times greater than national averages.[6-7]

In addition to the mental health risks of missed, underdiagnosed, and untreated perinatal mental health disorders, there also comes a societal cost. Luca et al reported an average cost of $32,000 for the consequences of untreated perinatal mental health disorders per mother-child dyad in the United States, with an estimated total cost of $14.2 billion per year, including intergenerational consequences.[8]

To address these issues on a local, national, and global level, innovators have developed methods and means to engage patients, to reduce barriers, and to serve birthing people and their families with culturally sensitive care. A growing

Chris Raines and Wendy Davis, *From Grassroots to Telecommunication Innovation* In: *The Practical Playbook III*. Edited by: Dorothy Cilenti, Alisahah Jackson, Natalie D. Hernandez, Lindsey Yates, Sarah Verbiest, J. Lloyd Michener, and Brian C. Castrucci, Oxford University Press. © de Beaumont Foundation 2024. DOI: 10.1093/oso/9780197662984.003.0036

number of new platforms, initiatives, and organizations are focusing on serving the needs and closing the gaps in care and equity for pregnant and postpartum individuals. The innovation not only is technological but also includes newly formed efforts that revive the traditional and holistic strengths of communities, families, and collaboration.

As examples of telecommunications and community-led endeavors, this chapter highlights two organizations: Mahmee, a perinatal care management platform that empowers and facilitates connection between patients and providers, and Homeland Heart Birth & Wellness Collective, a community program in Nashville, Tennessee, that promotes optimal infant and maternal health in communities of color.

These two initiatives share a factor intrinsic to their strength and innovation: an intergenerational collaboration of mother and daughter, which highlights the importance of multigenerational mental wellness. In both cases, daughters saw their mothers as models of giving back and caring for the community and brought new skills to improve access and equity. Building on their support and collective skills, they made a difference in their community to improve perinatal mental health, and both have now expanded their model to help other communities. The generational aspect of these organizations exemplifies how important it is to have a strong and mentally healthy parental figure as a positive role model and thus how imperative it is for the well-being of families that perinatal mood disorders be recognized and treated.

MAHMEE

Mahmee's story begins with a mother and daughter. Linda M. Hanna, RNC, MSN/Ed, IBCLC, started her career as a registered labor and delivery nurse. She quickly made a name for herself as a staunch advocate for new mothers and began designing and scaling mother–baby care programs and lactation centers for large health systems, including Kaiser Permanente and Cedars-Sinai Medical Center. In 2010, she founded a first-of-its-kind mobile breastfeeding program, My Nursing Coach, in Los Angeles, providing community-based lactation care to a diverse patient population via a 25-foot-long RV. She and her staff often would drive 100 miles a day visiting patients in Los Angeles County.

Linda consulted with her daughter, Melissa Hanna, and expressed frustration about the lack of technology available to private-practice clinicians like herself. Recalling the electronic health record systems she used in hospital settings, Linda felt strongly that there had to be a better way for her to communicate and elevate clinical concerns to other members of her patients' care teams while working "outside of the building." She imagined giving patients the power to own their medical records and to easily share their information with maternity providers in the community, who often worked in disparate organizations.

Melissa understood the limited technology tools available to her mother. She saw enormous potential for technology to ease her mother's burden and to open new pathways for patients to receive education, to share information with their care team, and to participate more actively in their healthcare. After receiving her master's in business administration and her juris doctor, Melissa suggested to her mother that they team up to build a technology-driven solution that would remove the limitations Linda and her colleagues faced. Mahmee was born.

After incorporating Mahmee in 2014, they joined forces with seasoned technology leader Sunny Walia, who became a cofounder and chief technology officer in 2017. Melissa took on the role of chief executive officer and Linda stepped into the chief nursing officer position. Together, the trio set out to raise capital and to begin to design and build the digital infrastructure needed to connect patients and providers. During the multiyear design process, the team interviewed and analyzed data from over 1,000 patients, providers, and health system leaders.

By 2019, Mahmee had built an enterprise-level, HIPAA-compliant software solution and was offering a complete digital toolkit to community-based maternity providers to facilitate interconnectivity between them and their patients. Based on these early signs of progress, Mahmee closed a $3 million seed round with Serena Williams, Mark Cuban, Arlan Hamilton, and other investors to scale the platform nationwide. Mahmee empowered pregnant and postpartum individuals to create a unified, secure medical record accessible by multiple providers and organizations across a region to facilitate team-based care. This allows patients to track health vitals, to communicate with members of their care team, and to complete forms and screenings.

With its secure patient portal, Mahmee partnered with Cedars-Sinai Medical Center to administer its Childbirth Experience Survey, a two-part survey project funded by the Patient-Centered Outcomes Research Institute and administered to patients through the Mahmee platform. By the end of the project, the platform had facilitated collection of over 2,200 surveys across 16 hospital sites.

In 2020, Mahmee released more features for health professionals, providing tools to collaborate, to conduct secure video calls, to document interactions, to upload documents, to send educational materials, and to build customized forms for patients. By the end of that year, the platform had users in 35 states.

One of the earliest adopters of Mahmee's digital provider toolkit was Her Health First in Sacramento, California, an organization that offers education and support to Black women throughout pregnancy. Black Mothers United (BMU) collects and securely stores detailed data to document the support it provides to expectant mothers. When COVID-19 hit, BMU pregnancy coaches had no way to send forms to clients that they previously gave out in person. Mahmee provided a user-friendly, secure way to document and collect data. Screening clients for depression and anxiety became routine, and the ability to make referrals was simplified. Even reporting to funders was improved thanks to the platform's data export functionality, which was critical to Her Health First and BMU's achieving sustainability through partnerships with large institutions. BMU clients appreciated the platform, too; they valued having easy access to their own health information at any time and felt empowered by the educational resources they received. With Mahmee, they could easily message their care team and track updates to their care plan over time.

Also in 2020, Mahmee established its first regional partnership with the Los Angeles County Department of Health Services and its obstetric program, MAMA's Neighborhood, which is part of the Strong Start for Mothers and Newborns Initiative created by the US Department of Health and Human Services to decrease preterm birth and to improve outcomes. Mahmee provided HIPAA-compliant telehealth technology to increase accessibility of services and to better engage patients across the county. It also allowed MAMA's Neighborhood to host breastfeeding/chestfeeding classes and to provide education and emotional support to new and expectant parents, as well as to enable patients to sign up for classes by logging into their Mahmee patient dashboard. Using the technology, MAMA's Neighborhood could collect data on classes taken and provide patient feedback. Mahmee used the data to produce a guide with a free online library filled with hundreds of evidence-based articles and videos as class follow-up.

In 2021, Mahmee partnered with DC Health, the department of health for the nation's capital. The overarching goal of the Mahmee in DC program is to increase access to comprehensive maternal and infant healthcare for residents of the District by improving connectivity between prenatal care and labor and delivery options. Mahmee in DC created opportunities for organizations that provide a wide range of services, from mental healthcare to doula support to nutrition counseling, to list themselves in the Mahmee network and to increase their visibility to patients and providers.

Mahmee's technology targets three root problems that plague the maternal health industry: fragmentation, bias, and inaccessibility. Fragmentation and inaccessibility are addressed by the platform's comprehensive toolkit for providers who are likely to work outside of large health systems and hospitals and who lack access to secure electronic health records; the platform provides software that is uniquely beautiful and simple and has even been described as "fun" to use. Allied health professionals from nutritionists and therapists to doulas and pregnancy coaches use the platform daily to document the care they provide, to host secure virtual visits, and to participate in the expanded reimbursement landscape that is evolving to be more inclusive of professionals who are positioned to improve maternal health outcomes.

Mahmee's approach to tackling bias centers on mapping the maternity health landscape with a lens on health equity. Many of the organizations using the platform are grassroots organizations founded by individuals whose experiences motivated them to create a set of services to address the unmet needs of families in their communities. These organizations shaped Mahmee's understanding of how its product and technology need to evolve continuously to bridge gaps and smooth workflows for providers.

Melissa Hanna defines Mahmee as an integrated care delivery platform for maternal and infant health, but she is quick to underscore that Mahmee is so much more than a social network, an educational library, or a place to track health outcomes. "It can include all of those experiences, but it is really all about bringing multiple providers and organizations together in one place to coordinate and deliver care."

Looking to Mahmee's future, she says,

> I'm most interested in creating pathways to financial sustainability and economic power for community-based organizations and the professionals who work in them. Mahmee is moving this vision forward by forging partnerships with the players at both ends of the spectrum of the maternal health ecosystem and ultimately creating technologies and partnership models that allow for the efficient and equitable transfer of money and power in ways that keep patients centered and cared for by the individuals and organizations who share their lived experiences. (Melissa Hannah, Mahmee CEO, personal communication, January 2022.)

Organizations and providers can learn more about Mahmee at https://network.mahmee.com. New and expectant parents can learn about the program here: https://www.mahmee.com. Anyone can email the organization at hello@mahmee.com.

HOMELAND HEART BIRTH & WELLNESS COLLECTIVE

The formation of Homeland Heart Birth & Wellness Collective came about in response to the statistics on Black maternal and infant mortality. The rate of Black maternal death during and after childbirth is two times as high as the rate in the general population.[9] Kristin Mejia, a Black mother of two in Tennessee, found these statistics appalling and was moved to act. She founded Homeland Heart and incorporated the community-based organization as a nonprofit in 2020.

Mejia says she was compelled and inspired by her family's experience: "My mother was in medical school becoming an ER physician during my childhood. While she worked long hours and studied for board exams, my grandmother oversaw the care of myself and my older brother. Though still finding the time to be a mother . . . [my mother served] an entire city of underserved people at Martin Luther King Jr. Community Hospital in my hometown of Compton, California" (Kristin Mejia, personal communication, January 2022).

It is well documented that when people of color receive care from providers who share similar backgrounds, it yields better health outcomes,[10-11] and perinatal support is no exception. Mejia and her team believed in the importance of establishing community-based models of care in which family and community members play an integral role in the care team, ensuring an individual's well-being. Homeland Heart's mission is to promote and to protect maternal, perinatal, and infant health among families of color. "Corporate healthcare has to understand that there is a place for collaboration with community healthcare that can create positive outcomes beyond our wildest dreams," Mejia says.

As a doula herself, Mejia recognized the shortage of perinatal support in the local Black birthing community and developed community-based doula instruction to increase the number of trained doulas in her area. When denied funding from a local entity, she voiced her need to the community, and the community responded tenfold. This highlights the village-minded and reparations-based foundation on which Mejia birthed Homeland Heart as well as the way a community can come together to provide resources when they seem scarce and often earmarked for the more privileged.

A unique component of the Homeland Heart model is in the lengthened period of support that each family receives during the fourth trimester, the often-neglected 12-week postpartum period when women and families are left to figure it out for themselves. According to the Tennessee Maternal Mortality Review, 50% of maternal deaths occurred within one year postpartum, with an overwhelming majority of the deaths being from preventable causes.[12] Mejia reports, "Sometimes, it's not enough to help. Being able to relate to someone's situation is what makes a community-based doula such a vital member of the support team at any point in [a patient's] journey."

Homeland Heart partnered its community-based doula training with Nashville Strong Babies, a program supported by the local health department. The program gives patients access to free perinatal resources in seven ZIP Codes in the middle Tennessee region, which exhibits the state's highest maternal and infant mortality rates, and a majority of the deaths occur in Black families. As part of this partnership, Homeland Heart offers free prenatal and postpartum doula care as well as lactation support and resources for mothers and their families.

Homeland Heart also provides affordable perinatal care for families outside of these ZIP Codes by assigning each mother and family a birth team, which consists of a birth doula for prenatal and labor support, a postpartum doula, and lactation support. The families have access to an inclusive list of resources (both internally and in partnership with other local businesses and organizations), including childbirth education, a "community closet" full of donated items, prenatal and postnatal chiropractic care, and perinatal mental health support.

"We, as a society, so often remind birthing people that 'It takes a village' without reminding ourselves that we must actually be that village," Mejia says.

One of the organization's most innovative programs for addressing physical and mental health needs in the perinatal period is its Perinatal Health Community Garden. The goal of this project is to foster community involvement through a nurturing built environment in an underserved area, as well as to provide access to fresh produce and a multi-use space for community-building, education, and physical exercise. These services are a vital part of the health and well-being of families.

Particularly in the South, Black families are at high risk for developing health problems, such as diabetes and obesity, which can lead to adverse birth outcomes.[13] By building a positive environment directly in the communities that need it most, Homeland Heart is meeting mothers and families where they live and providing fertile ground for innovation and community engagement to address health disparities.

Taneisha Gillyard Cheairs, Homeland Heart's staff researcher and community garden coordinator, is passionate about the ways in which spaces not only support the health and well-being of the families who use them but also hold the potential for fostering the ancestral sense of community and village that somehow has been overlooked through the generations. Supporting mental and physical health for pregnant and postpartum families, Homeland Heart provides the bridge needed to begin to reduce maternal and infant mortality and morbidity in Black communities.

Part of future plans for Homeland Heart is developing ways to export its work to other communities. The infrastructure and knowledge learned can help other communities recognize the importance of community and support to reduce medical mistrust, racial bias, and stigma related to mental health and wellness. The organization also envisions establishing its own community-based birthing center/collaborative to serve as a one-stop shop for perinatal health, furthering the group's goal of creating an inclusive space that promotes optimal infant and maternal health in communities of color.

"We strive to be able to put ourselves out of business, ultimately," Meija says, "to live in a world where we aren't afraid for the lives of our daughters while we await the arrival of our granddaughters. The goal of Homeland Heart is to re-create the narrative of birth for the families we serve" (Kristin Mejia, personal communication, January 2022). Learn more about Homeland Heart at www.homelandheart.com.

MODELS OF COLLABORATION IN A COMPETITIVE WORLD

Collaboration in a competitive world helps everyone. One of the reasons Mahmee and Homeland Heart are featured in this chapter is to demonstrate their ability to collaborate with other groups working in the same space. This is an innovative model that takes effort, patience, and trust. By drawing on lived experience and engaging in authentic relationship-building, both groups have reduced barriers to care and increased trust for technology. These stories illustrate how getting back to the basics of grassroot efforts and meeting people where they are can be unique and innovative. The global pandemic has given new meaning to staying at home, having community, and living in safety.

By refocusing our thoughts to basic needs, organizations that can pivot and meet those needs are truly innovative. Wei et al[4] expressed it this way: "Collaboration among healthcare professionals is essential in creating a synergy to provide efficient, safe, and high-quality patient care. The culture of caring could be fostered through five processes: building caring relationships, developing an ownership mentality, providing constructive feedback, applying strengths-based practice, and acting as the first and last lines of defense."

The models of care discussed here address all these issues, as they create a supportive and collaborative environment and means for patient ownership that works to empower the people who need the care. Helping to support healthcare needs in a nurturing and equipped environment works to reduce stigma and to improve maternal mortality and morbidity. In our exploration of Mahmee, Homeland Heart, and the other innovative projects we interviewed through Postpartum Support International,[14] we were struck by this reality: If the United States, a country perceived as a leader in advanced technology—including maternity technology—has the worst record for maternal and infant mortality in the developed world, then it will be the innovations in collaboration and community involvement that make the difference. It will be the humanity behind the tech and outreach models that reduce barriers to wellness and provide equitable care for all families and communities.

It is also important to collaborate with established entities that focus on education, awareness, and legislation to ensure that help-seekers with perinatal mental health issues can find support and treatment that is evidence-based, affordable, and accessible. Postpartum Support International (PSI) was established over 35 years ago to support women and families during the stressful and vulnerable time of new parenthood. PSI founder Jane Honikman understood the need for community and established a support group for mothers and children in her living room in 1987. She also started the first PSI HelpLine using her own telephone. That resource continues today and is continuously improved technologically, allowing trained volunteers from all over the United States and 50 other countries to give help-seekers support, reassurance, and connection to resources in their own community.

PSI is a nonprofit organization dedicated to supporting pregnant, postpartum, and post-perinatal-loss individuals and their families. The group offers free support services for individuals and families struggling with perinatal mental health issues and offers evidence-based training for providers of all levels to recognize, screen, assess, and treat perinatal mental health disorders. PSI then provides the bridge to connect families with trained providers in their communities.

This connection is accomplished through the HelpLine and by offering more than 20 free, specialized groups per week that serve pregnancy, postpartum, grief and loss, NICU parents, military families, Black mothers, and LGTBQ+ individuals. PSI staffs its HelpLine with English- and Spanish-speaking volunteers who connect with more than 400 trained support volunteers in the United States and around the world. The online Perinatal Mental Health Provider Directory, managed by PSI, allows providers and help-seekers to find perinatal mental health specialists and support groups by search terms, including clinical specialty, language, and location.

Other support services offered by PSI include a facilitated Facebook group, weekly Chat with an Expert for mothers and monthly chat for fathers, and a novel peer mentor program created as a way for mothers who have recovered from perinatal mental health disorders to give back by matching them to pregnant and postpartum individuals who are struggling.

As part of PSI's vision, the organization has become a hub for other groups that work to raise awareness of perinatal mental health disorders and to collaborate for the common cause of keeping perinatal mental health at the table to improve policy and services. PSI developed a policy initiative called Mind the Gap to bring together like-minded organizations and government policymakers to activate improvements in US state and federal perinatal mental health policy. PSI's partners, including the Maternal Mental Health Leadership Alliance and 2020 Mom, have been instrumental in advancing support for legislation and policy initiatives, including the new National Maternal Mental Health Hotline specifically dedicated to maternal mental health.

Collaboration and innovation take a village. The programs highlighted here are just a sample of the local and national programs that use innovative methods to address perinatal mental health and maternal mortality rates across the country. Diversity, equity, and inclusion must be at the forefront of any program pushing for change going forward. Understanding and addressing cultural diversity and using innovation to increase access and concordance will help reduce stigma and save lives. The innovative community of perinatal mental health support is strongest when it works collaboratively, improving access and responsiveness for vulnerable pregnant and postpartum families so that they find the help they need, when and how they need it.

REFERENCES

1. American College of Obstetricians and Gynecologists. ACOG Committee Opinion No. 757: screening for perinatal depression. *Obstet Gynecol*. 2018;132(5):e208–e212.

2. Fawcett EJ, Fairbrother N, Cox ML, White IR, Fawcett JM. The prevalence of anxiety disorders during pregnancy and the postpartum period: a multivariate Bayesian meta-analysis. *J Clin Psychiatry*. 2019;80(4):18r12527.

3. Wisner KL, Sit DK, McShea MC, et al. Onset timing, thoughts of self-harm, and diagnoses in postpartum women with screen-positive depression findings. *JAMA Psychiatry*. 2013;70(5):490–498. doi:10.1001/jamapsychiatry.2013.87.

4. Wei H, Corbett RW, Ray J, Wei TL. A culture of caring: the essence of healthcare interprofessional collaboration. *J Interprof Care*. 2020;34(3):324–331. doi:10.1080/13561820.2019.1641476.

5. Cox EQ, Sowa NA, Meltzer-Brody SE, Gaynes BN. The perinatal depression treatment cascade: baby steps toward improving outcomes. *J Clin Psychiatry*. 2016;77(9):1189–1200. doi:10.4088/JCP.15r10174.

6. Sidebottom A, Vacquier M, LaRusso E, Erickson D, Hardeman R. Perinatal depression screening practices in a large health system: identifying current state and assessing opportunities to provide more equitable care. *Arch Womens Ment Health*. 2021;24(1):133–144. doi:10.1007/s00737-020-01035-x.

7. Harper MA, Espeland MA, Dugan E, Meyer R, Lane K, Williams S. Racial disparity in pregnancy-related mortality following a live birth outcome. *Ann Epidemiol*. 2004;14(4):274–279. http://www.annalsofepidemiology.org/article/S1047-2797(03)00128-5/abstract.

8. Luca DL, Margiotta C, Staatz C, Garlow E, Christensen A, Zivin K. Financial toll of untreated perinatal mood and anxiety disorders among 2017 births in the United States. *Am J Public Health*. 2020;110(6):888–896. doi:10.2105/AJPH.2020.305619.

9. Petersen EE, Davis NL, Goodman D, et al. Racial/ethnic disparities in pregnancy-related deaths—United States, 2007–2016. *MMWR*. 2019;68:762–765. doi:http://dx.doi.org/10.15585/mmwr.mm6835a3.

10. Alsan M, Garrick O, Graziani G. Does diversity matter for health? Experimental evidence from Oakland. *Am Econ Rev*. 2019;109(12):4071–4111. doi:10.1257/aer.20181446.

11. Foster VA, Harrison JM, Williams CR, et al. Reimagining perinatal mental health: an expansive vision for structural change. *Health Aff*. 2021;40(10):1592–1596. doi:10.1377/hlthaff.2021.00805.

12. Tennessee Department of Health, Division of Family Health and Wellness, Maternal Mortality Review Program. Tennessee maternal mortality annual report. https://www.tn.gov/content/dam/tn/health/program-areas/maternal-mortality/MMR_Annual_Report_2021.pdf. Published 2021. Updated March 25, 2021. Accessed February 1, 2022.

13. Noonan AS, Velasco-Mondragon HE, Wagner FA. Improving the health of African Americans in the USA: an overdue opportunity for social justice. *Public Health Rev*. 2016;37:12. https://doi.org/10.1186/s40985-016-0025-4.

14. Postpartum Support International. Community engagement grants. https://www.postpartum.net/about-psi/communitygrant/. Published 2021. Accessed February 1, 2022.

Chapter 37

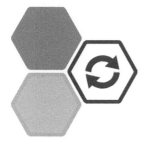

Using a Learning Community Model to Address Substance Misuse and Co-Occurring Mental Health Challenges among MCH Populations

SANAA AKBARALI, RAMYA DRONAMRAJU, KATRIN PATTERSON, ELLEN PLISKA, AND CHRISTINE MACKIE

INTRODUCTION

Recent trends suggest that behavioral health issues, including substance misuse, prenatal anxiety, and postpartum depression, continue to affect the well-being of women, infants, and families. Substance use, including use of illicit substances and misuse of prescribed medications, has increased year to year over the past decade.[1] In the United States, from 1999 to 2014, rates of opioid use disorder at delivery hospitalization more than quadrupled, and the incidence of neonatal abstinence syndrome (NAS) increased sevenfold.[2,3] Additionally, postpartum depression affects one in eight US women, and mental health conditions are one of the leading underlying causes of pregnancy-related deaths.[4,5] Given the complexity of this public health issue, effective provision of services requires close coordination among providers, health departments, and state and local agencies.[6]

The Association of State and Territorial Health Officials (ASTHO) is a non-profit organization committed to supporting the work of state and territorial health officials in each of the 50 states, Washington, DC, five US territories, and three freely associated states. State and territorial health officials (S/THOs) can

Sanaa Akbarali, Ramya Dronamraju, Katrin Patterson, Ellen Pliska, and Christine Mackie, *Using a Learning Community Model to Address Substance Misuse and Co-Occurring Mental Health Challenges among MCH Populations* In: *The Practical Playbook III*. Edited by: Dorothy Cilenti, Alisahah Jackson, Natalie D. Hernandez, Lindsey Yates, Sarah Verbiest, J. Lloyd Michener, and Brian C. Castrucci, Oxford University Press. © de Beaumont Foundation 2024. DOI: 10.1093/oso/9780197662984.003.0037

formulate and influence evidence-informed and evidence-based public health policy and ensure excellence in public health practice. As a membership organization, ASTHO primarily aims to develop strong and effective public health leaders; to improve public health through capacity-building, technical assistance, and thought leadership; and to advocate for resources and policies that improve the public's health and well-being.

Recognizing the importance of supportive policies and programs in facilitating this coordination, ASTHO leveraged a learning community model to support jurisdictions in advancing access to behavioral health services for pregnant and postpartum individuals and their families. ASTHO's Learning Community Model integrates several research-based implementation strategies, including organized meetings, centralized technical assistance, ongoing consultation from topical experts, dissemination of educational materials and resources, and networking opportunities to promote sharing of information and collaborative problem-solving. Through the Learning Community Model, ASTHO identifies technical assistance needs, develops resources and materials, and disseminates evidence-based and evidence-informed strategies. This chapter outlines critical areas in which participating states requested technical assistance, two learning communities in action, jurisdictional successes, and strategies health agencies can adapt in their own jurisdictions.

LEARNING COMMUNITIES IN ACTION

ASTHO's Learning Community Model has five standard components: (1) establishing cross-agency core teams, (2) developing action plans, (3) participating in virtual and in-person programming, (4) peer-to-peer sharing, and (5) technical assistance. Participating jurisdictions are selected through a request for applications process and actively engage in the learning community for at least 12 months. Learning communities that require a high level of agency commitment from their teams sometimes provide supplemental funding, staff support, or other paid components to selected agencies.

Opioid Use Disorder, Maternal Outcomes, and Neonatal Abstinence Syndrome Initiative Learning Community

In 2018, with funding from CDC's Division of Reproductive Health and the National Center for Birth Defects and Developmental Disabilities, ASTHO launched the Opioid Use Disorder, Maternal Outcomes, and Neonatal Abstinence Syndrome Initiative (OMNI) Learning Community. The purpose of the OMNI Learning Community was to support state policy implementation for identifying and treating pregnant and postpartum individuals experiencing opioid use disorder and strengthening systems of care for infants exposed to substances in utero. Over the course of the project, ASTHO engaged 15 state teams, each team comprising a health official or designee, Title

V/MCH director, substance use/mental health director, Medicaid provider champion, and perinatal quality collaborative representative. In Year 2 of the learning community, ASTHO received funding from the Health Resources and Services Administration's (HRSA) Bureau of Primary Health Care to encourage participation from state primary care associations, which provide comprehensive medical and behavioral health services in smaller communities. To guide team action plans and virtual/in-person programming, five key focus areas were identified, including: access to, and coordination of, quality services; provider awareness and training; data, monitoring, and evaluation; financing and coverage; and ethical, legal, and social considerations.[6] Stakeholder partnerships were classified as a cross-cutting strategy used to support implementation of activities in all focus areas.

In 2019, ASTHO and CDC launched the Local Enhancement Project, which provided a year-long, locally based field placement in five participating OMNI states. The objectives of the Local Enhancement Project were to bridge connections between state and local public health entities, to provide community-based support to jurisdictions heavily impacted by opioid use, and to identify opportunities to inform policy change. During the COVID-19 pandemic, field placements were invaluable to continuing and sustaining state activities, including provider engagement, partnerships, and care coordination.

Promoting Innovation in State and Territorial MCH Policymaking Learning Community

Funded through HRSA's Maternal and Child Health Bureau, the Promoting Innovation in State and Territorial MCH Policymaking (PRISM) Learning Community is a five-year (2018–2023) partnership between ASTHO and the Association of Maternal & Child Health Programs (AMCHP). PRISM is a learning community focused on building interagency state policymaking capacity to improve outcomes for women of reproductive age with mental health and substance use disorders (MH/SUD). Two state cohorts, totaling eight states and one territory, have participated in PRISM.

Participating teams focus their efforts on existing policies and strategies and, through a supported action-planning process, set objectives that are meant to be achievable within one to two years. Teams are encouraged to work on a singular policy or programmatic change within MH/SUD activities, with ASTHO and AMCHP providing ongoing support and technical assistance through resource development and distribution, virtual learning sessions, peer-to-peer networking, and other activities and products. The teams' goals reflect interventions and policies along the MH/SUD service continuum, including prevention, screening, treatment, and recovery. In the second cohort, teams continue to prioritize stakeholder engagement and collaboration and remain committed to interagency relationship-building even during the ongoing challenges of the pandemic. Team goals reflect strong interests in improving data-sharing, coordinating systems of care, and aligning with legislative and gubernatorial priorities around substance use and overdose prevention.

By the end of the first cohort, 33% of responding teams reached at least one of their originally identified implementation phases. One team held naloxone trainings for Title V nurses connected with their neonatal quality collaborative and supported the Medicaid flexibility expansions of telehealth for SUD treatment. Another completed a statewide gap analysis and began planning services exclusively for pregnant women with MH/SUD. All responding teams agreed they would sustain activities implemented during the PRISM Learning Community for three to six months after the end of their learning community engagement.

KEY TECHNICAL ASSISTANCE THEMES

Access to ongoing technical assistance provides meaningful capacity to health agencies and supports achievement of action plan goals. With support of federal and national partners, ASTHO provides a continuum of technical assistance, including on-demand technical assistance, trends analysis and research, and virtual/onsite site visits and expert consultation as part of the learning community model. Examples of technical assistance include connections to other jurisdictions and subject matter experts, policy scans, compilation of existing resources and tools, and site visits. As part of the learning communities described above, ASTHO identified three priority areas in which jurisdictions expressed the greatest need for tools and resources to support pregnant and postpartum individuals and their families experiencing SUD. These priority areas include expanding access to medication for opioid use disorder (MOUD), developing and implementing plans of safe care, and leveraging family-centered care strategies. These priority areas are briefly described below. For more detail, see the series of infographics ASTHO codeveloped with the CDC.[7]

Expanding Access to MOUD

MOUD is an evidence-based treatment protocol for people experiencing opioid use disorder. Methadone and buprenorphine are first-line therapy options for pregnant individuals, and they are administered in tandem with behavioral therapy and medical services.[8] While access to MOUD has been shown to improve patient outcomes, jurisdictions cited several barriers to access, including misconceptions among the public and medical community, associated stigma, reluctance among medical providers to prescribe MOUD, lack of consumer education about the benefits of MOUD, and geographic barriers to access. To address these obstacles, jurisdictions implemented several approaches to increase access to MOUD.

Internet-based learning networks, including Project ECHO and telemedicine programs, provide opportunities for consultation with experts in rural areas. States have also used the model to recruit physicians for buprenorphine waiver trainings and to deliver continuing medical education. Access to coordinated and quality care, including access to team-based care, is another successful strategy being used. The Ohio Maternal Opiate Medical Support (MOMS) project provides treatment to pregnant and postpartum individuals experiencing opioid use disorder during and after pregnancy through a Maternal Care Home model that leverages care coordination and wraparound services.[9] Finally, in recognition of financial and administrative barriers, state health agencies are working with their Medicaid agencies to ensure safe prescribing of opioids based on CDC guidelines.

Developing and Implementing Plans of Safe Care

A plan of safe care is a guide that assesses and directs services to ensure that pregnant individuals experiencing SUD and their infants are connected to appropriate medical and behavioral services upon discharge.[10] A plan of safe care focuses on the well-being of the family unit and is critical to improving health outcomes. Standard implementation of a plan of safe care can be challenging, and lack of clear reporting guidelines can cause confusion and diffusion of responsibility. To develop a comprehensive plan, states identified the importance of relationship-building and stakeholder engagement. The Florida OMNI team formed a new work group in partnership with the state's Department of Children and Families to develop and implement safe care plans statewide. Additional strategies include integrating the process of referrals and involvement of child welfare into plans of safe care and implementing standardized templates across hospital systems to reduce variability and to support equity.

Leveraging Family-Centered Care

Family-centered care focuses on parent–child relationships and provides holistic support to families experiencing SUD. This approach leverages clinical treatment, dyadic care to increase bonding activities (including skin-to-skin contact and breastfeeding), and community-based services. Several states are looking toward primary prevention methods and integrated care to improve health outcomes for pregnant and postpartum individuals and their families. One model of note is the Eat, Sleep, Console (ESC) model.[11] This model focuses on dyadic care and provides neonatal care through nonpharmacologic interventions. This approach has been shown to improve outcomes for families, including decreased length of hospital stay and reduced hospital costs. Additionally, integration of primary and behavioral health services is key to providing comprehensive, wraparound services. Pennsylvania's Centers of Excellence program uses a whole-person, family-centric approach to treat and care for families affected by SUD.[12] Additionally, the use of peer-recovery coaches and services has been critical to supporting this population. Peer-recovery specialists can support pregnant and postpartum individuals in reducing substance use and relapse rates, increasing treatment retention, ensuring greater housing stability, and decreasing criminal justice involvement.[13]

LEARNING COMMUNITY JURISDICTIONAL SUCCESSES

Below are examples of how learning community jurisdictions addressed the barriers described above and the impact of a learning community model on programmatic and policy uptake.

Rhode Island OMNI Team

Through the OMNI Learning Community, Rhode Island improved care coordination by emphasizing a multigenerational approach that prioritizes the mother–baby dyad to improve health outcomes. The Rhode Island team explored ways to support providers on how to identify and address bias and discrimination associated with MH/SUD. The state developed a Neonatal Abstinence Syndrome (NAS) Pilot Program using a two-generational approach to support the health and well-being of the entire family through care coordination and integration of medical services and home visiting for families of an infant diagnosed with NAS. In this program, each family was assigned an NAS liaison connecting them to a home-visiting program and, if needed, a peer-recovery specialist. Despite barriers caused by COVID-19, Rhode Island is committed to sustaining activities related to improving care coordination in the state, addressing stigma and bias in medical care, and increasing the number of pregnant individuals receiving screening for SUD.

Nevada PRISM Team

The Nevada PRISM team is capitalizing on progress toward removing barriers and increasing access to treatment for substance use and co-occurring disorders by addressing perinatal MH/SUD treatment needs. The team is well organized and is supported by a contractor that provides administrative and logistical structure. The state is building upon existing networks, such as its Perinatal Treatment Network, and expects to expand to, and intentionally include, maternal mental health. Newly developed state Screening, Brief Intervention, and Referral to Treatment (SBIRT) guides and trainings for identifying and treating general problematic substance use provided a starting point for the PRISM team to include specific screening for perinatal and postpartum mood and anxiety disorders.

Members of the PRISM team are themselves participants and subject matter experts on initiatives like the state Substance Use Response Working Group and the Advisory Committee for a Resilient Nevada, thereby strengthening the interdisciplinary and interdepartmental relationships of the team. The team occasionally hosts presentations where data and information are shared about the Patient-Centered Opioid Addiction Treatment alternative payment model for medication-assisted treatment (MAT) and the Pregnancy Risk Assessment Monitoring System (PRAMS), among others. The team cooperates with several work groups in the Nevada Perinatal Health Initiative and solicits feedback and expertise from a wide range of professionals, including medical providers, social workers, state staff representing divisions from the Department of Health and Human Services, staff from federally qualified health centers (FQHCs), and more. The team is committed to long-term progress and plans to formally codify memoranda of understanding (MOUs) among its various relationships as well as to develop a sustainability plan.

STRATEGIES FOR STATE HEALTH AGENCIES

In 2022, ASTHO's board of directors approved a new two-year strategic plan that reflects five priority areas in which health agencies have collective impact, influence, and authority.[14] The priority areas are health and racial equity, workforce development, sustainable infrastructure improvements, data modernization and interoperability, and evidence-based and promising public health practices. Within the five strategic priorities and based on learning community findings and technical assistance, ASTHO identified strategies health agencies can implement to improve health outcomes in their jurisdictions.

Health and Racial Equity

Grounding work in health and racial equity is critical to advancing care and treatment for pregnant and postpartum individuals experiencing substance use and their families. This includes implementing culturally competent systems and training; adapting healthcare delivery to meet a person's social, cultural, and linguistic needs; and using person-centered, nonstigmatizing language to reduce barriers to access. States and territories are encouraged to implement programs that center on health equity and support "whole-person" needs by examining and confronting systemic racism in provision of assessment, treatment, and recovery services. In addition, requiring cultural humility and implicit bias training for all staff involved in delivery of services was identified as an important strategy for addressing and eliminating race-based disparities.

Workforce Development

Improving care and increasing access to behavioral health services is a collaborative effort, and jurisdictions are encouraged to engage both traditional and nontraditional partners and systems. The partners include, but are not limited to, transportation, housing, information technology, education, and child welfare. As mentioned above, peer-recovery specialists are critical to this work and an especially important resource for pregnant individuals as a trusted source and messenger.

Sustainable Infrastructure Improvements

Critical to improving and expanding care and treatment is the ability to sustain funding, resources, and capacity to address substance use, even when resources are diverted to emergent and urgent public health issues. As part of the OMNI Learning Community, ASTHO launched a Local Enhancement project to bridge connections between state and local public health entities, to provide community-based support to jurisdictions heavily impacted by the opioid crisis, and to identify opportunities to inform programmatic and policy change. During the COVID-19 pandemic, field placements were invaluable for supporting continuous and sustained state opioid-related activities. These activities focused on provider awareness and trainings, stakeholder engagement, and access to, and coordination of, quality services.

Data Modernization and Interoperability

Supporting surveillance and data collection specifically related to NAS was identified as an important strategy to increasing care and treatment for infants and their families. In September 2021, ASTHO developed a report reviewing findings from the literature and current public health practices.[15] To inform the report, ASTHO conducted an environmental scan consisting of a literature, policy, and guidelines review and convened a series of focus groups with health agencies to identify and determine the consistency of key NAS data elements, case definitions, and standards in the field. The report outlines considerations for health agencies to include preliminary data elements that state health agencies are collecting and an overview of available NAS guidance and case definitions. (The report is available at: https://www.astho.org/globalassets/pdf/strengthening-health-agencies-nas-surve illance-through-consensus-driven-data-standards-practices.pdf.)

Evidence-Based and Promising Public Health Practices

Perhaps the most important strategy for improving care and access to treatment is implementation of evidence-based and promising public health practices, highlighted throughout this chapter. Expanding access to coordinated and quality care and treatment for pregnant and postpartum individuals, including MOUD, is an evidence-based treatment protocol for people experiencing opioid use disorder. Promoting dyadic care to ensure optimal health outcomes for birthing persons, infants, and their families is a key strategy in this effort. Developing services that emphasize the importance of family and relationships in treatment and recovery and adjusting programs to support the holistic needs of parenting people and families affected by substance use are also important strategies. Finally, collaboration with, and involvement of, multiple stakeholders is critical to success.

CONCLUSION

Substance misuse and co-occurring mental health challenges are multifaceted public health issues. Given their complexity and their exacerbation by the COVID-19 pandemic, it is imperative that health agencies work across sectors and communities to assess and improve existing policies and programs to increase access to comprehensive, person-centered services. ASTHO's learning community model provides a dedicated, supportive space for health agencies to work across sectors and jurisdictions to advance progress and to ensure optimal health outcomes for birthing persons, infants, children, and families.

Box 37.1 | Leveraging Short-Term Resources to Achieve Long-Term and Sustainable Perinatal Quality in Kentucky

Mary Beth Allen, Monica Clouse, Jordan Murphy, and Connie White

The Centers for Disease Control and Prevention (CDC) developed the Perinatal Quality Collaborative (PQC) framework to improve outcomes for mothers and babies.[1] PQCs are state or multistate organizations that engage cross-functional teams to apply evidence-based quality improvement (QI) in perinatal care settings.[i] The PQC model was created to reduce maternal and infant mortality, because the United States leads the developed high-income world in preventable perinatal deaths.[2,3] The sustainability of PQCs requires engagement of stakeholders and continuous access to funding and resources.[i]

In 2014, the PQC model was first applied in Kentucky with leadership from the Kentucky Perinatal Association. Priorities of the PQC focused on substance use disorder (SUD), the most consistent cause of maternal deaths in Kentucky. Also, the need for a PQC was well understood, because maternal and infant mortality rates in Kentucky are higher than the national average.[4,5] Despite strong engagement, a lack of dedicated funding resulted in the PQC's disbanding in 2016.

In 2018, Kentucky was selected to participate in the Association of State and Territorial Health Officials (ASTHO) Opioid Use Disorder, Maternal Outcomes, Neonatal Abstinence Syndrome Initiative (OMNI) Learning Community. Participation in OMNI established guidance and resources leading to the development of the Kentucky Perinatal Quality Collaborative (KyPQC) in 2019, which included an advisory committee and a temporarily designated ASTHO Health Policy Specialist Field Placement.

In 2019, the Kentucky Department for Public Health (KDPH) secured funding for the development of the KyPQC through CDC's Overdose to Action (OD2A) Grant under Strategy 7: Provider and Health Support System Activities. Combined support from ASTHO, the OMNI Learning Community, and CDC funding provided the foundational resources that led to the successful launch meeting of the KyPQC on October 22, 2019. Blended funding streams also supported necessary resources, including three full-time KyPQC Central Office positions dedicated to facilitating engagement, managing operations, disseminating education and communication, and reporting achievements to program sponsors. The KyPQC applied technology to expand infrastructure and engagement during the COVID-19 pandemic, leading to the current implementation of First Initiatives focused on SUD and neonatal abstinence syndrome (NAS).

In March 2021, Kentucky was accepted into the Alliance for Innovation on Maternal Health (AIM) program sponsored by the Health Resources and Services Administration (HRSA) and American College of Obstetricians and Gynecologists (ACOG). AIM develops packaged QI bundles targeting causes of maternal mortality in the United States[6] and provides training, data, and funding that supported the 2021 KyPQC Annual Meeting. In addition, AIM will provide resources to Kentucky facilities participating in QI. In September 2021, Kentucky was awarded a one-time supplemental grant from HRSA that will be used to improve AIM data reporting processes and provide Central Office staff with advanced QI training.

Box 37.1 | Continued

PQCs are proven models that result in measurable QI. However, sustainability remains a challenge because programs depend on continuous access to dedicated resources that often rely on short-term grant cycles. Advanced PQC management involves consistently identifying and appropriating new funding sources, which are critical in remaining a sustainable partner, collaborator, and leader in perinatal care.

References

1. Borders A, et al. *Developing and Sustaining Perinatal Quality Collaboratives: A Resource Guide for States*. https://www.cdc.gov/reproductivehealth/maternalinfanthealth/pdf/best-practices-for-developing-and-sustaining-perinatal-quality-collaboratives_tagged508.pdf. Published March 4, 2016.

2. *Maternal Mortality in the United States: A Primer*. Commonwealth Fund. https://www.commonwealthfund.org/publications/issue-brief-report/2020/dec/maternal-mortality-united-states-primer. Published December 16, 2020.

3. Organisation for Economic Co-operation and Development (OECD). *Infant Mortality Rates*. https://data.oecd.org/healthstat/infant-mortality-rates.htm#indicator-chart. Published 2021.

4. *Maternal Mortality and Maternity Care in the United States Compared to 10 Other Developed Countries*. Commonwealth Fund.

   https://www.commonwealthfund.org/publications/issue-briefs/2020/nov/maternal-mortality-maternity-care-us-compared-10-countries. Published November 18, 2020.

5. Centers for Disease Control and Prevention (CDC). *Reproductive Health: Infant Mortality*. https://www.cdc.gov/reproductivehealth/maternalinfanthealth/infantmortality.htm. Updated January 2, 2018.

6. Alliance for Innovation on Maternal Health. 2020. https://saferbirth.org.

REFERENCES

1. Substance Abuse and Mental Health Services Administration. 2017 National survey on drug use and health: detailed tables. https://www.samhsa.gov/data/report/2017-nsduh-detailed-tables. Published September 14, 2018. Accessed January 5, 2022.

2. Haight SC, Ko JY, Tong VT, Bohm MK, Callaghan WM. Opioid use disorder documented at delivery hospitalization—United Sates, 1999–2014. *MMWR*. 2018;67:845–849.

3. Patrick SW, Shumacher RE, Benneyworth BD, Krans EE, McAllister JM, Davis MM. Neonatal abstinence syndrome and associated care expenditures: United States, 2000–2009. *JAMA*. 2012;307:1934–1940.

4. Centers for Disease Control and Prevention. Vital signs: identifying maternal depression. https://www.cdc.gov/reproductivehealth/vital-signs/identifying-mater

nal-depression/VS-May-2020-Maternal-Depression_h.pdf. Published May 2020. Accessed January 5, 2022.

5. Petersen EE, Davis NL, Goodman D, et al. Vital signs: pregnancy-related deaths, United States, 2011–2015, and strategies for prevention, 13 states, 2013–2017. *MMWR.* 2019;68:423–429.

6. Kroelinger CD, Rice ME, Cox S, et al. State strategies to address opioid use disorder among pregnant and postpartum women and infants prenatally exposed to substances, including infants with neonatal abstinence syndrome. *MMWR.* 2019;68:777–783.

7. Supporting Pregnant and Postpartum Women with Opioid Use Disorder; An Infographic Series. https://www.astho.org/topic/population-health-prevention/ women-infant-family-health/supporting-pregnant-and-postpartum-women-with- opioid-use-disorder/. Published June 2022. Accessed June 30, 2022.

8. Centers for Disease Control and Prevention. Treatment before, during, and after pregnancy. https://www.cdc.gov/pregnancy/opioids/treatment.html#:~:text=Med ication%2DAssisted%20Treatment%20(MAT)%20During%20Pregnancy&text= SAMHSA%20and%20the%20ACOG%20recommend,behavioral%20therapy%20 and%20medical%20services. Published July 21, 2021. Accessed April 19, 2022.

9. Maternal Opiate Medical Support. MOMs care coordination. http://momsohio. org/sites/momsohio/files/2018-12/MOMS%20Decision%20Tree_F4_6-27-16.pdf. Accessed April 19, 2022.

10. National Center on Substance Abuse and Child Welfare. A planning guide: steps to support a comprehensive approach to plans of safe care. https://www.cffutures. org/files/fdc/A-Planning-Guide_-Steps-to-Support-a-Comprehensive-Approach- to-Plans-of-Safe-Care-3.21.18-final.pdf. Published March 2018. Accessed April 19, 2022.

11. Grossman MR, Lipshaw MJ, Osborn, RR, Berkwitt AK. A novel approach to assessing infants with neonatal abstinence syndrome. *Hosp Pediatr.* 2018;8(1):1–6.

12. Pennsylvania Department of Human Services. Centers of excellence. https://www. dhs.pa.gov/Services/Assistance/Pages/Centers-of-Excellence.aspx. Accessed April 2022.

13. Association of State and Territorial Health Officials. The role of peer support in federally qualified health centers. https://www.astho.org/globalassets/brief/the-role- of-peer-support-in-federally-qualified-health-centers.pdf. Published July 2020. Accessed April 2022.

14. Association of State and Territorial Health Officials. ASTHO's strategic plan. https:// www.astho.org/about/strategic-plan/. Published January 2022. Accessed April 2022.

15. Association of State and Territorial Health Officials. Strengthening health agencies' neonatal abstinence syndrome surveillance through consensus-driven data standards and practices. https://www.astho.org/globalassets/pdf/strengthening-hea lth-agencies-nas-surveillance-through-consensus-driven-data-standards-practices. pdf. Published September 2021. Accessed April 2022.

Chapter 38

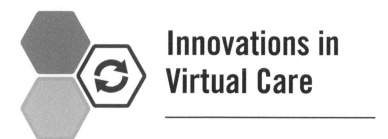

Innovations in Virtual Care

LESLIE DEROSSET, HALLE NEELEY, AND AUNCHALEE PALMQUIST

BACKGROUND: TELEMEDICINE AND TELEHEALTH

Telemedicine has been used since the 1950s to provide specialized healthcare to patients who could not otherwise access needed services.[1] However, it was not until the late 1980s and early 1990s that technological advancements allowed telemedicine to become more available to both patients and healthcare providers.[1] Between 2016 and 2019, telemedicine utilization in the United States doubled, from 14% to 28%.[2]

Telemedicine is defined as "the use of medical information exchange from one site to another via electronic communication to improve the patient's clinical health status," while telehealth is defined as "the use of electronic information and telecommunications to support long-distance clinical healthcare [and] health-related education."[3] For the purpose of this chapter, the terms *telemedicine* and *telehealth* are used interchangeably. Telemedicine and telehealth help patients and healthcare providers to communicate using electronic platforms that include audio and video that are either synchronous or asynchronous.[4] In 2019, approximately 28% of the US population used telehealth as their "go to" for healthcare access.[2] By April 2021, telehealth uptake was 38 times higher.[5]

Since its inception, telehealth has failed to address the structural inequities of access to healthcare.[6] Access to telemedicine, telehealth, and remote services is not equitable in the United States.[7-9] Telehealth is most challenging for people with low digital literacy, those who are non-English-speaking and need an interpreter, people living in rural areas (where broadband is insufficient or limited), and those without access to computers or devices (or who must share them with other family members). In addition, those who face barriers in access

Leslie deRosset, Halle Neeley, and Aunchalee Palmquist, *Innovations in Virtual Care* In: *The Practical Playbook III*. Edited by: Dorothy Cilenti, Alisahah Jackson, Natalie D. Hernandez, Lindsey Yates, Sarah Verbiest, J. Lloyd Michener, and Brian C. Castrucci, Oxford University Press. © de Beaumont Foundation 2024.
DOI: 10.1093/oso/9780197662984.003.0038

to education and/or undocumented populations have long had inequitable access to these services.[9-11]

In the United States, although approximately 90% of the population has regular access to the Internet, the remaining 10% are similar to those who are most unlikely to successfully access telehealth services: people who live in rural areas, have a high school education or less, and identify as a person of color.[10] Those with the greatest need for access to telemedicine and telehealth services are often the least likely to have it.

Prior to COVID-19, telemedicine in maternal care was seen as an option for addressing challenges in providing perinatal care either during natural disasters and/or due to geographic limitations of available providers. Telehealth was used to increase access to specialists, to provide additional support for high-risk perinatal patients, to reduce scheduling and transportation barriers, and to provide cost-savings opportunities.[12,13] For the average perinatal patient, however, telemedicine was not the primary option provided or utilized. Expanding uptake of perinatal care via telemedicine or telehealth services was challenging for a number of reasons, including access to broadband service, privacy and confidentiality, low levels of medical and health literacy among low-income patients and healthcare providers, addressing the needs of complex perinatal cases, and concerns about how patients use medical equipment, such as blood pressure cuffs and infant scales.[10,14]

Prior to COVID-19, telemedicine for infant, child, and adolescent healthcare was not routine. Services typically were used to overcome barriers to care, such as geographic location, the need for specialized services, or transportation challenges. However, neonatologists and school-based settings were early adopters of telemedicine.[15] Neonatologists used telemedicine to address geographic barriers in providing care to high-risk newborns who were unable to transfer to a NICU.[15] Prior to COVID-19, asthma prevention and care for children and adolescents in a school-based setting was used to improve quality of life measures, to bolster communication between patients and providers, and to more effectively manage chronic conditions.[16]

Telemedicine and telehealth expansion held great potential to deliver critical COVID-19-related healthcare and education to pregnant and postpartum populations facing barriers of transportation, childcare, access to healthcare, and so on.[4] However, the rapid expansion of, and reliance on, telemedicine, telehealth, and remote services during the pandemic paradoxically worsened preexisting health disparities among these populations.[17,18] Although telemedicine and telehealth did provide greater access for some during this period, there were significant challenges in reaching other populations. Working to overcome challenges and to ensure equitable access to healthcare provided great opportunities for innovation.

This chapter focuses on innovations in telemedicine, telehealth, and emerging forms of remote maternal and infant care services—largely in response to COVID-19—that hold potential for sustainable and equitable access to care beyond the pandemic. The pandemic also provided novel opportunities for healthcare policy innovation and creative solutions to rapidly fund community-based organizations that provide telehealth services. For example, rapid policy innovations provided health insurance reimbursement adjustments to meet the healthcare needs of diverse populations. Healthcare organizations, community-based organizations, and clinical care providers had to pivot quickly and learn how to provide online care to their patients and clients. While some solutions were introduced almost immediately, others required overcoming other emerging barriers, such as the 2020 fires in California. That state's record-setting wildfire season and resulting infrastructure challenges eliminated the possibility for needed healthcare virtual support. From these types of experiences, incredible innovative programs were developed and implemented in maternal and child health across the country.

INNOVATIONS IN VIRTUAL CARE

Mental Healthcare

As healthcare systems and community-based care providers pivoted to online learning and online healthcare, finding ways to ensure that children and parents continued to receive behavioral and mental health support was critical. For example, to meet the needs of its patients, a mental health clinic in upstate New York quickly transitioned care to online services. After six months and more than 43,000 services provided to more than 2,500 unique patients, the clinic found that although behavioral and mental health services were being delivered to both adults and children, service utilization and satisfaction were higher among adults.[19]

The Substance Abuse and Mental Health Services Agency (SAMHSA) released an evidence-based resource guide to help providers implement telehealth treatment for serious mental illness and substance use disorder (SUD).[20] In reviewing the research, SAMHSA found that both therapeutic and evidence-based treatments were comparable to in-person services (the data do not distinguish age). The natural experiment of COVID-19 provided opportunities in real time for mental and behavioral health services to compare virtual delivery methods with in-person treatments. This natural experiment has provided increased access to high-quality and equitable care, regardless of geographic and other barriers.[20]

Doulas, Childbirth Education, and Midwifery Care

Perinatal doulas provide care to women and gender-diverse childbearing populations during the prenatal and postpartum period. Doulas are "trained professionals who provide continuous physical, emotional, and informational support" to birthing persons before, during, and after childbirth.[21] Evidence demonstrates that doulas have a positive impact on the well-being of the entire family. COVID-19 caused hospitals and birthing centers to reduce the number of people who could be present during the birthing experience to zero or one family member only, and doula organizations quickly had to find new ways to support their clients to ensure a healthy birth experience. Healthy Mothers, Healthy Babies Coalition of Georgia,[22] for example, developed a Virtual Doula Toolkit. The online resource[23] ensured that doulas had access to the necessary training, technology, and policy-related information needed to support their clients.[14]

Bellies to Babies Foundation[24] in Atlanta is a small midwifery practice that assists the community with access to birth workers, doula training, and health-care services. Before COVID-19, the organization provided less than 25% of care in a virtual setting and primarily focused on in-home prenatal, birth, and postpartum care. In-person classes and training for doulas and birth assistants were also available. During the pandemic, virtual care doubled, and the practice transitioned in-person trainings to online platforms. The group offered in-person support to provide access to screening tools and assessments while also educating each participant on self-assessment under virtual supervision. To supplement childbirth preparation, the practice provided online resources and videos. These steps ultimately kept team members and families protected.

Before COVID-19, Accompany Doula Care[25] in Boston provided over 75% of perinatal care in person (including care during labor and delivery). Using funds from the Maternal Telehealth Access Project (MTAP), the organization invested in online training for its doulas, who in turn could provide online support to their clients. The online training consisted of a 90-minute presentation and brainstorming with all doulas on topics like fostering rapport and trust when providing care online, considerations for safeguarding personal health information while providing virtual care, and adapting instruction on topics like comfort measures to an online platform, among others. Accompany Doula Care also invested in the online platform Mahmee,[26] where doulas record client visit notes and schedule virtual visits directly on a client's phone through a HIPAA-compliant platform. As Accompany Doula Care began the transition from in-person to online services, the doulas and leadership experienced several challenges. The challenges included training leadership and doulas to use the electronic platform to capture visits with patients. (Doulas had various levels of experience with the Internet and using an electronic platform.) Regardless of the challenges, the organization reported positive outcomes among the patients they cared for over the last two years and demonstrated the clear value of doula care, even when delivered virtually, as evidenced by 96% satisfaction with doula care in 2021. Lessons learned from COVID-19 will guide the organization as it continues to train and educate its doulas to provide hybrid care.

Mandala Midwifery Care[27] in the Minnesota area delivered less than one-quarter of its care online prior to COVID-19, offering perinatal home care, in-person classes for clients, and in-person classes and training for doulas. Pivoting to online, Mandala Midwifery Care provided education and training videos to supplant childbirth education for clients and remote technology for listening to fetal heart tones, monitoring blood pressure, measuring fundal height, and measuring weight. The team reports that birth outcomes for patients receiving virtual care have been similar to outcomes for those receiving in-person care. Table 38.1 shows additional examples of how doula and midwifery organizations have transitioned to online care.

Maternal Health Organizations Provide Telemedicine

Mujeres Ayudando Madres (MAM)[28] in Puerto Rico is a grassroots organization that provides maternal–infant healthcare through a network of obstetricians, pediatricians, mental health support specialists, midwives, and doulas. Prior to COVID-19, MAM conducted its work in person, via community outreach and group education as well as labor and delivery assistance at home and in local hospitals. MAM provided free online perinatal education on its Facebook page. Despite the lack of dependable Internet and an efficient electric grid on the

Table 38.1	Examples of MTAP Grantees Providing Innovative, Virtual Support during COVID-19

Birth Matters (South Carolina) provided cell phones, breast pumps, and blood pressure cuffs for expectant mothers and used TikTok and Instagram Live to connect with families.

Community Birth Companion (Louisiana) hosted "grab and go" events and relied on social media and word of mouth to connect the community with resources.

Southeast Michigan IBCLCs of Color (Michigan) leveraged community relationships to gain access to loaner breast pumps and other supplies that otherwise would have gone unused.

New Familia Health Support Services (California) utilized funds to purchase tablets, electronic record systems, and equipment for doulas, lactation consultants, and mental health providers.

Raising Resilience (North Carolina) utilized funds to host remote groups that catered to new and existing mothers. Support groups focused on maternal mental health services.

Big Springs Medical Association (Missouri) directed funds to purchase and install telemedicine equipment in six of the 12 highest-need clinics that lacked OB services.

Chicago Family Health Center (Illinois) used funds to purchase and distribute telehealth supplies, including broadband access and telephone cards, to high-risk pregnant women in Chicago.

Children's National Medical Center (Washington, DC) utilized funds to provide NICU parents with free subscriptions to mindfulness apps and additional support resources (e.g., notebooks and increased broadband access). The organization established an app for screening for perinatal mood-associated disorders and provided referral and support services.

Great Lakes Intertribal Council (Wisconsin) utilized MTAP funding to train and support peer-to-peer educators from the 22 tribes in Wisconsin and surrounding areas. Trained educators conducted educational sessions and outreach in the areas of breastfeeding (education and lactation support) and management of chronic disease (diabetes and obesity).

island, MAM assisted thousands of people throughout the pandemic via virtual visits and support. To support telehealth visits, MAM outreach staff provided prenatal remote monitoring supplies and taught patients how to use them. Patients say they felt a level of empowerment, taking charge of their health virtually while also having MAM staff available online (telehealth, video, and/or telephone). MAM transitioned its in-person childbirth classes to online and maintained sufficient enrollment. In addition, even with the challenges of the pandemic, MAM continued to host bilingual midwifery students during their rotations, assisting them in attaining their degrees.[28] The switch to telemedicine was not without challenges. The inability to offer in-person hospital doula care because of COVID-19 restrictions may have contributed to an increase in cesarean delivery rates over the past two years in the patients seen by MAM staff. This, in turn, affected breastfeeding rates. The addition of a 24-hour hotline for virtual visits and emphasis on the collaborative care model with obstetric and pediatric providers are positive changes MAM hopes to maintain after the pandemic.

Mamatoto Village[29] in Washington, DC, has a mission to "create pathways for economic advancement [and] leadership and [to help] Black and Brown parents forge self-determination leading to person and community transformation." Before COVID, Mamatoto Village conducted less than 25% of its work via telehealth. The pandemic limited home visits, in-person education, and community outreach and forced the organization to limit labor support. Mamatoto Village instead introduced virtual support groups, community conversations, and childbirth classes. As of January 2022, up to 75% of its work remained virtual, and the organization was developing protocols for a hybrid strategy to fully engage with its community by mid-Spring 2022.

In Atlanta, Mamas and Tatas[30] provides private lactation consultations, prenatal breastfeeding classes, and a weekly virtual support group. During the height of the pandemic, Mamas and Tatas connected by Zoom with families as nearby as Savannah, Georgia, and as far away as Ghana. As most organizations transitioned to virtual meetings, Mamas and Tatas implemented interactive platforms like Kahoot to combat Zoom fatigue, and GroupMe, which gives families 24-7 access to a breastfeeding chat and community. Mamas and Tatas also developed a nutritionist partnership to provide nutritionist support to families with limited access to nutrition information.

In Queens, New York, the obstetrics and gynecology department at Jamaica Hospital Medical Center[31] pivoted its CenteringPregnancy prenatal program to virtual services in the early days of COVID-19. Like most hospitals across the country, the hospital had conducted perinatal care and education in person, and less than one-quarter of visits to the OB-GYN department were conducted online prior to the pandemic. New York was the epicenter of COVID-19 in early Spring 2020, and the department had to quickly figure out how to continue to provide quality and accessible care to its perinatal patients. With support

> **Box 38.1 | All virtual: A patient describes how a doula helped them navigate their labor and delivery options**
>
> "I could not have done this without [my doula]. I had no idea how many options were available to me during labor. [My doula] supported my husband as well. This was all done virtually! I didn't have a doula with my first two pregnancies, and I wish had."

from the larger medical center and a grant from MTAP, the OB-GYN department supplied patients with remote monitoring equipment and developed educational videos about their use. As the pandemic recedes, Jamaica Hospital Medical Center continues to see its virtual CenteringPregnancy offerings thrive.

Healthcare Providers and Telemedicine

Local, state, and national surveys of the use of telehealth for maternity care found common challenges to using telehealth during COVID-19. Improving patient access via patient navigators, assisting with smart technology, and increasing support for remote patient monitoring (e.g., blood pressure cuffs, glucometers) were identified as critical needs. The majority of healthcare providers in a national survey agreed that there is a need to expand maternal telemedicine. Telemedicine can work in a variety of settings, but it is critical that patients have access to, and familiarity with, digital technology to participate in virtual healthcare options.[12]

Project ECHO (Extension for Community Health Outcomes) was developed more than 20 years ago by Dr. Sanjeev Arora at the University of New Mexico Health Science Center to meet the healthcare needs of New Mexico residents.[32] Project ECHO is an online, video-conferencing medical education model that provides training and education, as well as advice and support, to primary care providers in rural and underserved areas. An evidence-based strategy that has been proven to improve the health of rural and underserved communities, the model was identified by Montana Obstetrics & Maternal Support (MOMS)[33] as a best practice to implement with Maternal Health Innovation funding, even before COVID-19.

The MOMS program, funded by a Health Resources and Services Administration Maternal and Child Health Bureau (HRSA-MCHB) five-year grant, is a collaboration among the Montana Department of Public Health and Human Services (DPHHS), Billings Clinic, and the University of Montana's Rural Institute. One of the largest and least populated states in the country, Montana has 56 counties, of which 46 are identified as frontier (six or fewer people per square mile), and all counties (except for one) are designated mental health provider shortage areas. With only 26 birthing hospitals in the state, Montana has distinct challenges to providing comprehensive maternal healthcare.[34] Billings Clinic implemented the MOMS Project ECHO series in June 2020 and provides twice-monthly educational clinics via Zoom. MOMS Project ECHO clinics attract groups of 35 to 50 participants per session, including students from nursing programs around the state and residents from the two Montana family medicine residency programs. ECHO is an excellent pathway for bringing new physicians and nurses into the maternal health discussion and connecting them with other maternal health provider teams across the state. According to the MOMS Web site, Project ECHO has created a virtual space for bringing together urban-based experts and rural providers. Providers share their expertise via mentoring, guidance, feedback, and didactic education.[33]

University Health Partners of Hawaii was home to the Midwifery Integrated Home Visitation Program (MI-Home),[35] located in Honolulu. (In December 2021, the midwifery program went on hiatus.) MI-Home provided in-home and street-based midwifery services to the community, then transitioned during the pandemic to seeing patients virtually. To continue to provide services to pregnant people, MI-Home purchased and mailed to clients' homes INVU by Nuvo monitors. The INVU devices provide remote maternal and fetal vitals monitoring for patients. INVU tracks maternal heart rate and blood pressure, the baby's heartbeat, and non-stress tests (as of November 2021); the provider receives the data remotely. The adoption of virtual care for pregnant persons and the remote monitoring devices allowed MI-Home to expand its services to neighbor islands, where care was already limited before COVID-19. Even with this innovative approach, barriers existed for patients without telephones, Wi-Fi, or cell service. Telemedicine care was also extremely difficult for patients with mental health disabilities.

COVID-19 and the shutdown of a majority of US public schools created opportunities to provide alternate school-based health services. To care for students and families who utilized a school-based health center (SBHC),

> **Box 38.2 | Available day or night: A patient describes how a doula helped them feel confident**
>
> "Whenever I had a question, whether it was at 1 a.m. or 4 p.m., [my doula] responded quickly— she was there when I needed her. She made me feel really confident and had an answer to every question I had. She wanted me to get the best care possible and was very sincere. The doula is a great support system for people who want it. I was very pleased and happy that [Doula name] and I connected so well. I felt so close to her even though we couldn't meet in person much due to COVID."

> **Box 38.3 | "Women drive change, families drive change."**
> **—Kiana Ayers, Mamas and Tatas**
>
> Village. Innovating. Perinatal. Support in Action. (V.I.P.S. in Action), Episode 5 https://www.youtube.com/watch?v=gcT2JkMq0V4

these programs switched to virtual care and expanded the types of services provided. During COVID-19, SBHCs provided more acute care, mental and behavioral healthcare, and even a collaboration to address pediatric obesity. The transition to telehealth for SBHCs was innovative, and data on outcomes suggest it has the potential to expand educational opportunities beyond the pandemic. Increasing options for telehealth in SBHCs may also increase coordinated care with primary care providers, thus decreasing some inequities.[36]

Telehealth Resources and Training Materials

Rapid expansion of training and resources to implement telehealth and to evaluate the success of programs and care is critical. The National Consortium of Telehealth Resource Centers (NCTRC)[37] was established in 2017 and supports 12 regional and two national telehealth resource centers (TRCs) in implementing telehealth programs for rural and underserved communities. NCTRC and local TRCs provide telehealth experts, technical assistance, no-cost resources, and support for organizations, practices, federally qualified health centers, rural health clinics, and rural communities. Throughout the pandemic, NCTRC expanded and ramped up its projects, technical assistance, and education. Policy analyses with the Center for Connected Health Policy (CCHP) and assessment of video platforms by the Telehealth Technology Assessment Resource Center (TTAC)[37] are two NCTRC projects that stand out and are discussed briefly below.

NCTRC and TRCs

NCTRC and the TRCs offer a wealth of easily accessible information. NCTRC's 2021 annual report highlighted individual TRC projects as well as national programs implemented by NCTRC. More information is available at https://telehealthresourcecenter.org/about-us/.

CCHP Training Materials

CCHP provided timely, user-friendly information on new state and federal policies.[37] The organization also developed a Medicaid series of webinars focused on educating telehealth users about important issues associated with Medicaid policies and implementation of virtual care for patients.[37]

TTAC Training Materials

TTAC "used a network emulator to do an assessment of the largest video platforms to determine how they handled spotty cell networks, low bandwidth, delays, packet loss, satellite interruptions, or extremely rural locations."[37] This assessment allowed those implementing telehealth services to make better, more informed decisions.[37]

The National Perinatal Association Expanded Its Courses to Attract New Audiences

The National Perinatal Association (NPA)[38] received funding to expand its online healthcare provider education. Courses on trauma-informed care for NICU and maternity care were adapted to address the multitude of needs that arose during COVID-19. The new courses attracted a more diverse audience than previous courses, in part due to marketing provided by the partners involved with MTAP. The most popular modularity for the course was a prerecorded, one-hour webinar. Even before the pandemic, NPA successfully provided online education; it now has an even larger, more diverse audience for its provider trainings.

Community-Centered Funding Models for Telehealth in Public Health Emergencies

Georgia breastfeeding support organization Reaching Our Sisters Everywhere (ROSE)[39] designed an equitable application process for CARES Act funds available through MTAP. The goal was to ensure that organizations with limited technology access, time, and resources (especially during the pandemic) could apply for funding to enhance telehealth access in their communities. ROSE created a mobile-friendly app using JotForm[40] and ensured that video applications could be accepted. Required paperwork was set up for electronic submission using DocuSign,[41] another mobile-friendly app, which eliminated the need for applicants to print, sign, and scan documents. ROSE offered MTAP awardees additional training opportunities, including a grant-writing workshop to promote organizational sustainability.

Evidence is mounting to support telehealth use, and hybrid models that employ both telehealth and in-person care are needed, even in high-risk obstetric scenarios.[42] A recent study in North Carolina found that 81% of providers surveyed would like to continue some type of hybrid care for their perinatal patients.[12] Perinatal telemedicine can help reduce barriers like transportation, child care, and lack of services for pregnant or postpartum people who work remotely or cannot get time off work.[43]

Many organizations that integrated telehealth into their practice in response to COVID-19 restrictions have discovered that these programs continue to fill a need. For example, the Carolina Global Breastfeeding Institute (CGBI)

> ## Box 38.4. | Perspectives from Doulas, Midwives, and Birthing People on Addressing Inequities in Telehealth*
>
> "The strongest interventions for telehealth are based on trust."
> "Understand that different communities will have different needs related to telehealth."
>
> "Trusted community-based organizations with experience [are needed] to provide support [and] will know how to overcome structural barriers within their communities and offer viable solutions."
>
> *Reaching Our Sisters Everywhere (ROSE) Maternal Telehealth Access Project (MTAP) Grantees.

launched a virtual version of its evidence-based prenatal breastfeeding education, *Ready, Set, Baby Live,* that meets the training needs of its clinical lactation students and provides free virtual facilitated prenatal breastfeeding education. *Ready, Set, Baby Live* was adapted to incorporate specific emerging guidance on best practices for breastfeeding in the context of COVID-19. This education was offered in English and Spanish at no cost to participants. CGBI continues to offer *Ready, Set, Baby Live,* and preliminary evaluation shows that the virtual platform makes completing the education a convenient alternative for many participants. It also provides a new opportunity for students enrolled in the CGBI clinical lactation training program to practice education competencies and to become familiar with using a virtual platform to offer lactation education.

Training Is Critical to Expanding Services to Ensure Equitable and High-Quality Care

Telehealth training is not only for patients and providers but also for healthcare systems.[37] The American Medical Association developed the AMA Telehealth Implementation Playbook [44], which can help healthcare systems understand the complexities of developing and implementing telehealth services as well as patient encounters.

Participants from community assessment listening sessions, as well as recent research, have identified numerous ways that community organizations and healthcare systems can meet the needs of underserved communities, thus improving access and equity of telehealth. The recommendations include:

- Ensure that digital literacy education is provided to all recipients of any telehealth intervention. [45]
- Promote and disseminate information about available telehealth in priority communities. [45]
- Consider the needs of the community and offer non-video-based and video-based telehealth appointments.[46]

- Fund community-based organizations based on their identified needs. [45]
- Design telehealth products and services with the end user in mind, especially vulnerable or priority populations. [47]
- Expand telehealth coverage, including policies and reimbursements. [47]
- Increase funding to federally qualified health centers, rural health clinics, and other organizations to implement and support telehealth services.[47]
- Integrate telehealth into value-based care.[47]

Several MTAP grantees[48] offered suggestions to help ensure that maternal and infant telehealth services meet emerging needs:

- Engage with people with lived experience in the development, implementation, and evaluation of services.
- Ensure that visual aids and resources are translated and adapted for communicating with special needs populations.
- Work to ensure that families in need can receive rapid referrals for governmental and philanthropic resources.
- Ensure that organizations and agencies have referrals to, and provision of, mental health services that provide culturally appropriate, respectful, and compassionate trauma-informed care.
- Ensure that birthing people have access to real-time, responsive health and birthing advocates, especially when support persons are not permitted to accompany birthing people.
- Develop "Know your rights" resources and referrals to virtual advocates on call.

CONCLUSION AND FUTURE STEPS

As this chapter is being written, COVID-19 has been in the world for over three years. More than 6 million people have died of the virus. Prior to COVID-19, most people worldwide accessed healthcare services in person. Since COVID-19, primary and secondary healthcare services, mental and behavioral health services, and specialty care have moved online. Community-based organizations focused on offering maternal and child health services, such as doulas,

> ### Box 38.5 | The future of telemedicine
>
> Future efforts in telemedicine should "focus on support for remote patient monitoring (e.g., blood pressure cuffs, glucometers) and improving patient access (e.g., using a patient navigator, assisting with smart technologies).

> **Box 38.6 | Mujeres Ayudando Mujeres (MAM) shared this experience of their client, a female, age 30**
>
> [Name] was a mother of two children who was pregnant with her third child. Due to COVID-19, her partner had lost his job, and the family was struggling to make ends meet, [so] the family had disconnected cable and Wi-Fi. MAM's Parent Coach had only been able to connect to the client via the phone but sensed that there were mental health issues taking place with the mother. The Parent Coach encouraged [the] mother to borrow an iPad so they could connect via video, which the mother was initially reluctant to do. When she finally agreed and connected via Zoom it was apparent that client had a flat affect and was deeply depressed. Her Parent Coach quickly connected her to a mental health agency that specializes in maternal mental health. The mother has begun therapy and will continue receiving services with the program until her baby is nine months old. Being able to connect with the mother via Zoom was essential in getting her the help that she needed.

lactation consultants, and child and adolescent health providers, have pivoted from in-person visits to learning how to use virtual platforms to meaningfully engage with their patients and clients.

Telehealth is not a perfect solution. Inequities and disparities regarding who has access to and is using virtual services continue to exist. According to the study Provider and Practice-Based Perceptions of Telehealth for Maternity Care During the COVID-19 Pandemic,[12] telehealth best lends itself to sessions that involve information-gathering and verbal interactions, such as patient education, genetic and preconception counseling, mental health visits, maternal–fetal medicine consults for single-issue management, follow-up visits, decision-making conversations, patient questions, postpartum visits, and centering groups.[12] These providers believe that telehealth use will become more common.

What can we expect over the next five or ten years? What is our responsibility as public health professionals to ensure equitable access, high-quality care, and services that are affordable via public, private, or self-pay? What are the skills and tools that our providers, doulas, health educators, policymakers, outreach workers, and the overall maternal and child health workforce need to learn, employ, and develop?

Answering these questions and ensuring that we listen to, and follow, the recommendations of those "on the ground" with clients and patients is critical to establishing equitable care that is accessible, of high quality, and medically appropriate. We must work with state and federal policymakers on reimbursement policies and legislation to expand what is working and to revise or adapt what is not. It is imperative to ensure that rural, frontier, and geographically isolated places have sufficient broadband by working with local and state partners and leaders, including local, state, and national businesses and corporations.

Even before the pandemic, states and jurisdictions like Hawaii, Alaska, American Samoa, and the Marshall Islands were expert at implementing telehealth. Working with those who came before us, who know how to provide virtual care and how to ensure a quality-improvement approach, is key. Telehealth is here to stay.

REFERENCES

1. Nestor M. A collaboration and history of communication technologies. *Dermatol Clin.* 2001;19(2):379–385. doi:10.1016/s0733-8635(05)70275-8.

2. American Medical Association. *Telehealth Implementation Playbook.* American Medical Association; 2020:128. https://www.ama-assn.org/system/files/2020-04/ama-telehealth-implementation-playbook.pdf.

3. Voran D. Telemedicine and beyond. *Mo Med.* 2015;112(2):129–135.

4. Wakefield A, Mather Conray J, McLafferty S, et al. *National Institutes of Health Pathways to Prevention Workshop: Improving Rural Health Through Telehealth-Guided Provider-to-Provider Communication.* National Institutes of Health; 2022:18. https://prevention.nih.gov/sites/default/files/documents/NIH-P2P-RuralHealthPanelReportDraft-FINAL-508.pdf.

5. Bestsennyy O, Gilbert G, Harris A, Rost J. Telehealth: a quarter-trillion-dollar post-COVID-19 reality. McKinsey & Company. https://www.mckinsey.com/industries/healthcare-systems-and-services/our-insights/telehealth-a-quarter-trillion-dollar-post-covid-19-reality. Published July 9, 2021. Accessed January 18, 2022.

6. Nouri S, Khoong EC, Lyles C, Karliner L. Addressing equity in telemedicine for chronic disease management during the Covid-19 pandemic. *NEJM Catalyst.* 2020;55(2):366–388. https://catalyst.nejm.org/doi/full/10.1056/CAT.20.0123. Published May 4, 2020. Accessed December 15, 2021.

7. Friedline T, Chen Z. Digital redlining and the fintech marketplace: evidence from US ZIP Codes. *J Consumer Aff.* 2021;55(2):336–338. doi:10.1111/joca.12297.

8. Dorsey E, Topol E. State of telehealth. *N Engl J Med.* 2016;375(2):154–161. doi:10.1056/NEJMra1601705.

9. Scott Kruse C, Karem P, Shifflett K, Vegi L, Ravi K, Brooks M. Evaluating barriers to adopting telemedicine worldwide: a systematic review. *J Telemed Telecare.* 2018;24(1):4–12. doi:10.1177/1357633X16674087.

10. Perrin A, Atske S. 7% of Americans don't use the Internet. Who are they? Pew Research Center. https://www.pewresearch.org/fact-tank/2021/04/02/7-of-americans-dont-use-the-internet-who-are-they/. Published April 2, 2021.

11. Artiga S, Hill L, Oregera K, Damico A. Health coverage by race and ethnicity, 2010–2019. https://www.kff.org/racial-equity-and-health-policy/issue-brief/health-coverage-by-race-and-ethnicity/. Published July 16, 2021. Accessed January 10, 2022.

12. Mallampati D, Talati A, Menard MK. *Provider and Practice-Based Perceptions of Telehealth for Maternity Care During the COVID-19 Pandemic.* University of North Carolina at Chapel Hill, Division of Maternal Fetal Medicine, Department of Obstetrics and Gynecology; 2020:29. https://maternalhealthlearning.org/wp-content/uploads/2020/12/Executive-Provider-Assessment_FINAL.pdf.

13. Lurie N, Carr BG. The role of telehealth in the medical response to disasters. *JAMA Intern Med.* 2018;178(6):745–746. doi:10.1001/jamainternmed.2018.1314.

14. Palmquist AEL, Griffin A, Chung S. *Community Assessment: Online Stories from the Field.* University of North Carolina at Chapel Hill; 2020:17. https://maternalhealthl earning.org/wp-content/uploads/2020/11/FINAL_ES_Online-Stories_10-13.pdf.

15. Culmer N, Smith T, Stager C, et al. Telemedicinal asthma education and health care outcomes for school-age children: a systematic review. *J Allergy Clin Immunol.* 2020;8(6):1908–1918. doi:10.1016/j.jaip.2020.02.005.

16. Maddox LJ, Albritton J, Morse J, Latendresse G, Meek P, Minton S. Implementation and outcomes of a telehealth neonatology program in a single healthcare system. *Front Pediatrics.* 2021;9:648536. doi:https://doi.org/10.3389/fped.2021.648536.

17. Ramsetty A, Adams C. Impact of the digital divide in the age of COVID-19. *J Am Med Inform Assoc.* 2020;27(7):1147–1148. doi:10.1093/jamia/ocaa078. Published online April 28, 2020.

18. Erchula C, Pichardo M, Bhradwaji M, et al. The expanding digital divide: digital health access inequities during the COVID-19 pandemic in New York City. *J Urban Health.* 2021;98(2):183–186. doi:10.1007/s11524-020-00508-9. Published online January 20, 2021.

19. Hoffnung G, Feigenbaum E, Schechter A, Guttman D, Zemon V, Schechter I. Children and telehealth in mental healthcare: what we have learned from COVID-19 and 40,000+ sessions. *Psychiatr Res Clin Pract.* 2021;3:105–113. doi:10.1176/appi.prcp.20200035.

20. Substance Abuse and Mental Health Services Administration (SAMHSA). *Telehealth for the Treatment of Serious Mental Illness and Substance Use Disorder.* National Mental Health and Substance Use Policy Laboratory; 2021:75. https://store.samhsa.gov/sites/default/files/SAMHSA_Digital_Download/PEP21-06-02-001.pdf.

21. DONA International. What is a doula? https://www.dona.org/what-is-a-doula/. Published 2022. Accessed January 18, 2022.

22. Healthy Mothers, Healthy Babies Coalition of Georgia. https://hmhbga.org/. Published January 27, 2022. Accessed January 27, 2022.

23. Healthy Mothers, Healthy Babies Coalition of Georgia. Virtual doula toolkit. https://hmhbga.org/wp-content/uploads/Virtual-Doula-Toolkit-2020-COVID-19-Respo nse-3.pdf. Published online March 2020.

24. Bellies to Babies Foundation. http://safematernityconference.org/. Published January 27, 2022. Accessed January 27, 2022.

25. Accompany Doula Care. https://www.accompanydoulacare.com. Published January 27, 2022. Accessed January 27, 2022.

26. Mahmee. https://www.mahmee.com/. Published January 27, 2022. Accessed January 27, 2022.

27. Mandala Midwifery Care. http://mandalamidwiferycare.com/. Published January 27, 2022. Accessed January 27, 2022.

28. Mujeres Ayudando Madres. http://mujeresayudandomadres.org/. Published January 27, 2022. Accessed January 27, 2022.

29. Mamatoto Village. https://www.mamatotovillage.org/. Published January 27, 2022. Accessed January 27, 2022.

30. Mamas and Tatas. https://mamasandtatas.com/. Published January 27, 2022. Accessed January 27, 2022.

31. Jamaica Hospital Medical Center. https://jamaicahospital.org/. Accessed April 28, 2022.

32. Agency for Healthcare Research and Quality. Project ECHO. https://www.ahrq.gov/patient-safety/resources/project-echo/index.html. Published September 2020. Accessed January 3, 2022.

33. Montana Obstetrics & Maternal Support (MOMS). https://www.mtmoms.org/about/. Published January 27, 2022. Accessed January 27, 2022.

34. Rural Health Information Hub (RHIhub). State guides. https://www.ruralhealthinfo.org/states/montana. Published January 7, 2022.

35. MI-HOME. https://mihomehawaii.org/. Published January 27, 2022. Accessed January 27, 2022.

36. Goddard A, Sullivan E, Fields P, Mackey S. The future of telehealth in school-based health centers: lessons from COVID-19. *J Pediatr Health Care*. 2021;35(3):304–309. doi:10.1016/j.pedhc.2020.11.008.

37. National Consortium of Telehealth Resource Centers. https://3f9znz109u3oybcpa3vow591-wpengine.netdna-ssl.com/wp-content/uploads/2021/02/NCTRC-White-Paper-FINAL.pdf. Published online 2020. Accessed December 2, 2021.

38. National Perinatal Association. https://www.nationalperinatal.org/. Accessed April 28, 2022.

39. Reaching Our Sisters Everywhere (ROSE). https://breastfeedingrose.org/. Published June 7, 2018. Accessed January 27, 2022.

40. Jotform. https://www.jotform.com/. Published January 27, 2022. Accessed January 27, 2022.

41. DocuSign. https://www.docusign.com/. Published January 27, 2022. Accessed January 27, 2022.

42. DeNicola N, Grossman D, Marko K, et al. Telehealth interventions to improve obstetric and gynecologic health outcomes: a systematic review. *Obstet Gynecol*. 2020;135(2):371–382. doi:10.1097/AOG.0000000000003646.

43. Aziz A, Zork N, Aubey JJ, et al. Telehealth for high-risk pregnancies in the setting of the COVID-19 pandemic. *Am J Perinatol*. 2020;37:800–808.

44. American Medical Association. Telehealth Implementation Playbook. https://www.ama-assn.org/system/files/ama-telehealth-playbook.pdf. Published 2022. Accessed September 12, 2023

45. Bugg K, Bugg W, Godbolt D, et al. Maternal Telehealth Access Project community assessment: listening sessions. https://maternalhealthlearning.org/wp-content/uploads/2020/11/Listening-Session-ES_10-14_FINAL.pdf. Published 2020.

46. Centers for Disease Control and Prevention. Using telehealth to expand access to essential health services during the COVID-19 pandemic. https://www.cdc.gov/coronavirus/2019-ncov/hcp/telehealth.html. Published 2020. Accessed January 27, 2022.

47. Madubuonwu J, Mehta P. How telehealth care be used to improve maternal and child health outcomes: a population approach. *Clin Obstet Gynecol*. 2021;64(2):398–406.

48. Palmquist AEL, Reddy J, Griffin A, et al. Maternal Telehealth Access Project community assessment: literature scan. University of North Carolina at Chapel Hill. https://maternalhealthlearning.org/wp-content/uploads/2020/11/MTAP-Lit-Scan-EXECUTIVE-SUMMARY.pdf. Published 2020.

Systems and Scalability

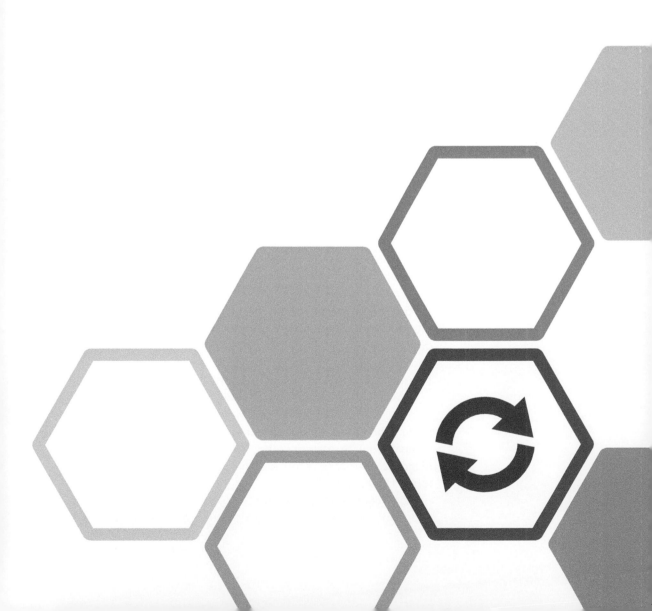

Breanna's Story

I'm nervous about the unknown, so I plan. I keep a notebook, jot down questions and ask them rapid-fire at each appointment. When the doctor and nurse start chatting about whether Pitocin or misoprostol would be more appropriate to start contractions, I jump in. I say I'm nervous about misoprostol because of what I've learned about possible side effects.

"Can we try Pitocin?"

"Sure," she says.

Half a day later, my dilation is stalled at five centimeters. The doctor is concerned about infection and fetal distress. She recommends a C-section and asks what we think. We agree. I'm an active part of choosing my care. The doctors treat me with dignity and respect.

Two weeks later, I wake in a room, not remembering how I got there. I'm wearing a hospital bracelet with the name of a doctor I don't know. My daughter was born on the 12th, but the bracelet says I was admitted on the 26th. I walk into the hallway. Tile floors, doors lining one side, dim safety lighting. It looks like a psych ward. I'm told to go back to my room. I am alone and scared.

The bathroom has a pull cord, and when I pull it, nursing staff appear asking what I need. I can't find the words to tell them, so they leave. Alone. Again, I pull the cord, and they come, but leave when there's no emergency. The third time, they tell me I need to stop, but what I need is for someone to tell me what's happening. Why I'm here.

I need to know I'm going to be okay. I shuffle up and down the hallway. Memories start coming. My nonstop talking, extreme insomnia, my Tasmanian Devil whirlwind of energy, starting five tasks without finishing any. My doctor saying postpartum mania. My trip to the emergency room. This place looks like a psych ward because it is.

My care team is led by a matter-of-fact psychiatrist. I make a joke and she doesn't smile. She talks to me like I'm a child. Nurses keep asking if I need to pump. How would I know? I've been lactating for two weeks, and I've been sedated for over a day as part of the intake process. The nurse stays in my room while I pump, and she freezes my milk. But I'm taking lithium, which is potentially dangerous for my baby. The psychiatrist didn't consider this or didn't care. She certainly never asked me.

In an outpatient program, another psychiatrist tells me what to do. When I ask what medications we will use, and are they compatible with breastfeeding, she adds anxiety to my list of diagnoses. She doesn't consider that at baseline I value being informed about my care.

I find a community psychiatrist who's willing to listen. She asks about my priorities. When I say I'm interested in switching meds so I can breastfeed, she says it's my body and those decisions are up to me. Someone is listening to me again, and that's all I wanted.

Source: Illinois Maternal Health Digital Storytelling Project. Breanna's Story. October 26, 2022. https://www.youtube.com/watch?v=tWajRPGUqGc

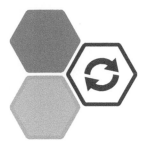

Chapter 39

Scaling Up and Sustaining Improvements in Maternal Health Equity

J. LLOYD MICHENER

Earlier sections of this *Playbook* demonstrated that maternal health equity in the United States falls short because of multiple factors, which combine and reinforce to disadvantage all birthing people, some much more than others. Each of the underlying issues has been the object of one or more related innovations, but these are rarely linked to other innovations or methods of sustaining effective change. Building and sustaining systems for maternal health equity requires the ability to track and weave together different programs and innovations, to realign funding streams and training models, and to advocate for needed changes, all centered on the leadership and guidance of engaged communities. There are no easy or quick fixes, nor one solution that works for all, but rather an opportunity to create enduring systems of maternal health for individuals and communities.

There are several key threads, or "plays," that need to be mastered to build sustained systems of maternal health equity. These are outlined in the US Department of Health and Human Services' *Action Plan to Improve Maternal Health in America* (https://aspe.hhs.gov/topics/public-health/hhs-initiative-improve-maternal-health#maternal-health; accessed July 27, 2022). This section of the *Practical Playbook* begins with a critical component of that plan: the services provided to states and communities. This opening chapter, by Michael Warren and colleagues at the Maternal and Child Health Bureau (MCHB) of the Health Resources and Services Administration, discusses examples of state-level innovations underway and provides advice about how to leverage MCHB-funded programs to improve local maternal health equity.

J. Lloyd Michener, *Scaling Up and Sustaining Improvements in Maternal Health Equity* In: *The Practical Playbook III*. Edited by: Dorothy Cilenti, Alisahah Jackson, Natalie D. Hernandez, Lindsey Yates, Sarah Verbiest, J. Lloyd Michener, and Brian C. Castrucci, Oxford University Press. © de Beaumont Foundation 2024.
DOI: 10.1093/oso/9780197662984.003.0039

Next, Jessica Smith and colleagues at the Georgia Health Policy Center review how Medicaid can help advance maternal health. Their chapter includes an overview of Medicaid's role in birthing services as well as some innovations being undertaken.

Academic health systems have long had major roles in maternal health, as providers of care, as sites of training, and as centers of research. Olufunmilayo Chinekezi and colleagues describe how academic health centers are embracing systems approaches to community health and health equity and are reassessing their roles and activities to advance maternal health equity.

Amy Mullenix and Kate Menard write in their chapter about the complex workforce required for maternal health equity, including clinical, community, and public health professionals. They also describe how that workforce varies across communities and provide examples of innovation in workforce training.

Julie Wood at the American Academy of Family Physicians next describes how a national physicians' organization advocates and provides training for maternal health, especially in rural communities. With so many closures of rural hospitals, finding solutions for, and advocating on behalf of, rural communities, and for and on behalf of birthing people, is an increasing priority for many medical groups.

Advocacy and policy change are at the root of innovation and are central to sustainability, and Anna Kheyfets and colleagues describe six focus areas for policy in improving maternal health equity, including improved data collection, expanded Medicaid, improved telehealth, and mandated cultural competency training.

States play a critical part in supporting and scaling innovation. The next chapter, about the role of state and territorial health offices in maternal health equity, by Ellen Pliska and colleagues, describes how states can test new models of maternal health, share lessons learned, and scale successful innovations (and their funding models) to other states.

In their chapter, Dana Smith and Stephanie Teleki describe the California Health Care Foundation's approach to innovation in maternal health equity across the state. The foundation is a strong example of what a state philanthropy can achieve as a thought leader, coalescing teams and finding multiple levers for driving change.

Adam Zolotor and team at the North Carolina Area Health Education Centers (NC AHECs) describe the core role state AHECs can play in developing a diverse workforce pipeline, supporting practices, and providing graduate and continuing education across diverse communities and practice settings, with a goal of healthier mothers and babies.

Innovation, policy, and sustainability can seem impersonal and removed from life "in the field," so in the final chapter, Lisa Harrison and Abi Kenney share their ground-level perspective as leaders of a small, rural health department that has been listening to its community and forming partnerships to support maternal health equity, as part of a larger goal of supporting health for all.

No community or state has all the "plays" described in this section. However, all have access to most, and all are part of learning collaboratives that link community, medical, public health, and academic groups in unique networks. These networks are creating new, sustainable models of care for birthing people, building on available resources and the ideas and passions of those who know that we can do better at supporting our mothers and babies. Please reach out to the authors and those whose stories are shared in these chapters as we work together to achieve maternal health equity.

Chapter 40

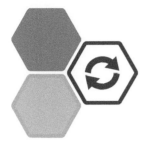

The Role of the Maternal and Child Health Bureau in Supporting States and Communities to Advance Maternal Health Equity

MICHAEL D. WARREN, KATHY K. BEST, ERIN PATTON, AND BELINDA PETTIFORD

ABOUT THE MATERNAL AND CHILD HEALTH BUREAU

The mission of the federal Maternal and Child Health Bureau (MCHB) is to improve the health and well-being of America's mothers, children, and families. The MCHB is part of the Health Resources and Services Administration (HRSA) of the US Department of Health and Human Services (HHS). MCHB partners with states, jurisdictions, tribes, communities, and a variety of organizations to advance improvements in maternal health and to reduce health disparities.

MCHB's efforts to improve maternal health have roots extending back more than a century. Julia Lathrop, the first chief of the Children's Bureau (predecessor of today's MCHB) wrote in 1916 "that maternal mortality is in great measure preventable, that no available figures show a decrease in the United States in recent years, and that certain other countries now exhibit more favorable rates."[1] In its earliest years, and in a time before consistent birth and death registration, MCHB staff partnered with states and communities to collect and report data on the causes and frequencies of maternal deaths.[2]

Over the last 106 years, the bureau's efforts to improve maternal health have evolved substantially. Major legislation—including the Sheppard-Towner Maternity and Infancy Act (1921) and Title V of the Social Security Act (1935)— laid the foundation for federal/state partnerships to improve maternal and child

Michael D. Warren, Kathy K. Best, Erin Patton, and Belinda Pettiford, *The Role of the Maternal and Child Health Bureau in Supporting States and Communities to Advance Maternal Health Equity* In: *The Practical Playbook III.* Edited by: Dorothy Cilenti, Alisahah Jackson, Natalie D. Hernandez, Lindsey Yates, Sarah Verbiest, J. Lloyd Michener, and Brian C. Castrucci, Oxford University Press. © de Beaumont Foundation 2024. DOI: 10.1093/oso/9780197662984.003.0040

health, yielding the framework for today's Title V Maternal and Child Health (MCH) Services Block Grants to states.[3] Projects specifically focused on maternal health have also emerged over the years. During World War II, MCHB directed the Emergency Maternity and Infant Care Program, which provided care during pregnancy, labor and delivery, and for six weeks postpartum to the wives and infants of service members.[4] The Healthy Start program was established in 1991 to address high rates of infant mortality, and it included a focus on comprehensive women's healthcare to improve perinatal outcomes.[5] The Patient Protection and Affordable Care Act (ACA), passed in 2010, authorized the Maternal, Infant, and Early Childhood Home Visiting (MIECHV) Program and also established requirements for insurance coverage of preventive services for women.[6] In the last five years, Congress has appropriated additional funds to support a variety of maternal health initiatives, including the State Maternal Health Innovation program, the Alliance for Innovation on Maternal Health (AIM), and the National Maternal Mental Health Hotline.

MCHB's programs have substantial reach across MCH populations, providing important support for advancing maternal health. MIECHV-funded home-visiting programs are implemented in one-third of all US counties and serve 140,000 parents and children per year.[7] Healthy Start serves approximately 70,000 pregnant women, infants, and postpartum women annually.[8] In addition to these programs that provide more direct services, some MCHB-funded programs support population/systems-level activities that extend their reach. The Title V MCH Services Block Grants reach 98% of infants, 93% of pregnant women, and 60% of all children, including those with special healthcare needs.[9] At the time of this writing, 44 states and the District of Columbia were implementing AIM in approximately 1,700 birthing facilities.[10] The preventive services guidelines for women and children set important standards for coverage of individuals covered by most insurance plans in the United States.

In 2021, MCHB released an updated strategic plan, which focused on four key goals: (1) ensuring access to high-quality and equitable health services to optimize health and well-being for all MCH populations, (2) achieving health equity for MCH populations, (3) strengthening public health capacity and workforce for MCH, and (4) maximizing impact through leadership, partnership, and stewardship.[11]

HOW MCHB SUPPORTS STATES AND COMMUNITIES TO ADVANCE MATERNAL HEALTH EQUITY

MCHB utilizes multiple approaches to advance maternal health equity in the United States. The Bureau provides funds directly to states and communities to support a variety of grant programs in response to the needs of MCH populations. MCHB supports national data infrastructure—through performance measures and a national survey—that states and communities can use to inform and evaluate programmatic efforts. MCHB also oversees development and implementation of preventive services guidelines that set insurance coverage standards for MCH populations. Finally, MCHB provides national leadership by convening relevant federal, state, and local partners; funding technical assistance; and leveraging resources across various programs.

At the state and community levels, grantees implement MCHB-funded programs in response to local data. Every five years, state* Title V programs conduct a comprehensive needs assessment to identify state-specific needs and priorities; the states then implement an action plan for the next five years to address priorities across MCH population domains (women/maternal, perinatal/infant, child, adolescent, children with special healthcare needs, cross-cutting/systems-building). The flexibility of the MCH Block Grant recognizes that the needs of MCH populations vary across states, and states assess their needs and priorities to tailor their approaches. In the most recent MCH Block Grant Application/ Annual Reports, states reported plans to fund a variety of maternal health activities, including providing patient navigation and health education (Alaska), supporting smoking cessation for pregnant women (Indiana), and promoting oral health in pregnant women (Puerto Rico).[12]

Similarly, MIECHV grantees are required by statute to use a needs assessment to identify communities at risk for poor maternal and child health outcomes. Grantees then develop plans to implement voluntary, evidence-based home-visiting programs in response to the identified needs. Among other activities, home visitors screen for postpartum depression and intimate partner violence and help new mothers with referrals for a postpartum visit. The Healthy Start program also funds community grants in areas with high rates of poor perinatal outcomes—specifically, those with infant mortality rates at least 1.5 times the national average. Once these target areas are identified, community organizations implement activities to improve women's health, to improve family health and wellness, and to promote systems change. Healthy Start grantees advance maternal health by conducting screening and referral for needed services, providing case management, assisting with needed resources (e.g., transportation and housing), and increasing access to health services (by hiring clinical providers or increasing the availability of doulas in communities).

The state Maternal Health Innovation (MHI) program provides funds for states to convene a maternal health task force, to identify maternal health needs from a variety of data sources (e.g., maternal mortality review committees, vital statistics, hospital discharge data), and to implement innovative strategies to improve outcomes. One such strategy might be to encourage birthing facilities to participate in AIM. The program provides safety bundles—collections

---

* The term *states* here refers to states, territories, and freely associated states, including the 50 states, District of Columbia, Puerto Rico, US Virgin Islands, Guam, American Samoa, Commonwealth of the Northern Mariana Islands, Republic of Palau, Federated States of Micronesia, and Republic of the Marshall Islands.

of evidence-based practices that have been shown to improve patient outcomes when performed collectively and reliably in a delivery setting. For example, a state MHI program might identify obstetrical hemorrhage as a key contributor to maternal mortality or morbidity. The state might then encourage implementation of the AIM obstetric hemorrhage bundle at birthing facilities throughout the state.

MCHB also supports key data infrastructure that can be used to guide state and community maternal health activities. The Title V National Performance Measures and National Outcome Measures, available at the national and state levels, can help states identify opportunities for intervention and measure the success of their efforts. States might, for instance, track improvements in maternal mortality and morbidity (outcome measures) alongside efforts to reduce low-risk cesarean deliveries or increase well-woman visits (performance measures). Each year, the National Survey of Children's Health provides national- and state-level estimates of health outcomes, access to health, and family, neighborhood, school, and social context. States can use estimates of chronic health conditions or preventive care utilization for adolescent females. MCHB also funds the State Systems Development Initiative (SSDI) program to ensure key MCH data capacity support for state Title V programs, enhancing state capacity to inform, monitor, and evaluate program efforts addressing MCH. Maryland, for example, has used SSDI funds to support a comprehensive Perinatal Periods of Risk analysis and the creation of census-tract-level risk maps to enhance local program design to improve preconception and maternal health.[13]

In addition to these grant programs, MCHB supports development of preventive services guidelines for infants, children, and adolescents (Bright Futures), and women (Women's Preventive Services Initiative). Under the ACA (§2713[a]), these preventive services must be covered with no cost-sharing.[6] Given the contribution of chronic disease to maternal morbidity and mortality, efforts to optimize health through preventive care are essential to ensuring that women are healthy before, during, and after pregnancy.

MCHB also supports national organizations and academic institutions that provide resources and technical assistance to promote improvements in maternal health. One such example is the Innovation Hub, created by the Association of Maternal and Child Health Programs (AMCHP).[14] This Web-based repository of effective practices from states and communities offers a variety of examples related to maternal health, ranging from preconception health programs to universal nurse home-visiting initiatives.

A key role for MCH programs is to convene relevant stakeholders. At the national level, MCHB led HRSA's global maternal mortality summit in 2018, bringing together various national and international stakeholders to provide recommendations for reducing maternal mortality.[15] MCHB convenes the Secretary's Advisory Committee on Infant and Maternal Mortality, which advises the Secretary of HHS on programs and policies to reduce infant and maternal mortality.[16] MCHB staff regularly engage with other federal agencies, including the Centers for Medicare & Medicaid Services and the Centers for Disease Control and Prevention (CDC) to explore opportunities for alignment and collaboration in improving maternal health. Similarly, state Title V programs regularly convene key MCH stakeholders—community-based organizations, clinical providers and professional organizations, insurance payers, and academic institutions, for example—to obtain input on programming, to develop strategies, and to explore opportunities for collaboration.

Through stakeholder engagement and partnership-building efforts, MCHB grantees frequently leverage various funding streams to achieve greater reach or impact. For example, Iowa's Title V program, through its local Title V maternal health agencies, partnered with HRSA-funded community health centers to increase the number of women served and to improve the quality of their visits.[17] Tennessee's Title V program utilized MCH Block Grant funds and administrative funds from the Special Supplemental Nutrition Program for Women, Infants, and Children (WIC) to support a 24-7 breastfeeding hotline.[18] As a final example, 11 states utilize MCH Block Grant funds to pay for the state portion (80%) of support for a CDC Maternal and Child Health Epidemiology Assignee, bringing vital MCH data capacity to state MCH programs. Grantees can engage their project officers, or MCHB-funded technical assistance providers, for suggestions or guidance about leveraging resources across programs.

"BRIGHT SPOTS"—PRACTICAL EXAMPLES OF STATES LEVERAGING MCHB-FUNDED PROGRAMS TO ADVANCE MATERNAL HEALTH EQUITY

Perhaps the best way to illustrate the ways that HRSA supports states and communities to advance maternal health is to share examples from states. These "bright spots" are two examples of many that may inspire partnerships in other states or communities.

North Carolina—Perinatal Health Equity Collective

In 2014, North Carolina's Title V program convened partners to develop a collaborative Perinatal Health Strategic Plan (PHSP) with a focus on infant mortality, maternal health, maternal mortality, and the overall health of individuals of reproductive age. As a result of North Carolina's efforts with the HRSA MCHB-funded Collaborative Improvement and Innovation Network to address infant mortality, the initial leadership team recognized the need for an "upstream" plan focused on equity and inclusive of social determinants of health. The collaborative selected as its framework the life-course approach, which "conceptualizes birth outcomes as the end product of not only the nine months of pregnancy but the entire life course of the mother before the pregnancy."[19] After receiving feedback from over 120 thought leaders and meetings with funders (e.g., foundations, legislative aides), the collaborative released a 12-point plan in 2016. The plan had three goals: to improve healthcare for women and men, to strengthen families and communities, and to address social and economic inequities. Within each goal are four points that support the goal, for a total of 12 points.[20] In 2021, Title V supported development of the Perinatal Health Equity Collective, an outgrowth of the PHSP planning team. The Collective was created to provide guidance and movement on the PHSP.

The strategic plan has been a blueprint for addressing perinatal health in North Carolina. Partners, including agencies, communities, and individuals with lived experience, are engaged in moving the PHSP forward. Entities turn to the plan when applying for funding opportunities or looking for ways to improve perinatal health in their communities. The Collective operates with five work groups: community and consumer engagement, data and evaluation, communications, policy, and maternal health.

More recently, the PHSP has been updated to utilize more inclusive language and to strengthen the focus on addressing social and economic inequities. This specific goal is inclusive of undoing racism, supporting working mothers and families, reducing poverty, and closing the education gap. Within the last year, several efforts have moved forward, including:

- Extending Medicaid for 12 months in the postpartum period
- Increasing access to contraception through pharmacy distribution
- Conducting a doula landscape analysis to determine the workforce
- Expanding Preconception Peer Education Programs to community colleges and 4-H organizations
- Completing CDC's Level of Care Assessment Tool (LOCATe) to continue discussions with hospitals about developing maternal levels of care

North Carolina's Title V program continues to enhance partnerships and implement efforts to address the state's ongoing inequities in infant and maternal outcomes. Title V's leadership has been instrumental in keeping these issues in the forefront, in engaging communities, and in centering individuals with lived experience in the work.

Illinois—Maternal Health Task Force

Illinois is leveraging two HRSA MCHB investments—the Title V MCH Services Block Grant and the State MHI program—to advance maternal health equity. The Illinois Title V MCH Services Block Grant program, administered by the Illinois Department of Public Health's Office of Women's Health and Family Services, collaborates with the University of Illinois at Chicago (UIC) on I PROMOTE-IL (Innovations to ImPROve Maternal OuTcomEs in Illinois). UIC was awarded this cooperative agreement in 2019 through HRSA MCHB's State MHI program. I PROMOTE-IL will assist Illinois in addressing disparities in maternal health and in improving maternal health outcomes, with a particular emphasis on preventing and reducing maternal mortality and severe maternal morbidity. A key component of I PROMOTE-IL is the Illinois Maternal Health Task Force, which addresses maternal health needs identified from a variety of data sources (e.g., maternal mortality review committees, vital statistics, hospital discharge data). The Title V director serves as co-chair of the task force.[21]

As a convener of key MCH stakeholders, Illinois Title V has connected the Illinois Maternal Health Task Force with the state's legislatively mandated Task Force on Infant and Maternal Mortality among African Americans to foster collaboration on addressing maternal mortality in Illinois with a focus on social determinants of health and health equity. As of September 2021, the Illinois Maternal Health Task Force included 86 members representing more than 60 organizations. The members include representatives from maternal mortality review committees, state government agencies, elected officials, local public health, the state perinatal quality collaborative and perinatal networks, clinical providers and organizations, nonprofits, and community-based organizations (A.C. Handler, personal communication, February 1, 2022). These partners initiated development of the Illinois Maternal Health Strategic Plan. The vision for the plan calls for "health equity for women, pregnant persons, and families in Illinois, across race, ethnicity, class, geography, immigration status, and ability, where all have what they need to be healthy and reach their full potential."[22] Co-leadership by Title V in this project has ensured that the task force is fully integrated into the state's existing maternal health infrastructure without duplication of effort. Title V has also leveraged this partnership to address gaps outside of Title V's efforts.

Partnership Opportunities during and after COVID-19

The COVID-19 pandemic has disrupted normal patterns of maternal healthcare and posed unique threats to MCH populations (such as the increased risk of intensive care admission, mechanical ventilation, and death for pregnant people with COVID-19 infection).[23] The flexibility of the Title V MCH Services Block Grant positions states to be nimble and to respond to emerging issues like the pandemic. State Title V programs have provided subject matter expertise, have expanded partnerships, have adapted existing programmatic approaches, and have leveraged new funding opportunities to meet MCH population needs during the pandemic.

COVID-19 prompted many state Title V programs to explore partnerships with other agencies, in some cases outside state and local health departments; New York's Title V Program provided staffing for the COVID-19 Maternity Task Force led by the governor's office. This group convened in early 2020 to develop recommendations for the COVID-19 response among MCH populations. Recommendations included centering birth equity, supporting birthing site choice, testing pregnant people for the virus, and promoting an increased understanding of the impact of COVID-19 on pregnancy and childbirth in New York.[24]

Title V programs also adapted existing initiatives as a way to support pregnant women during the pandemic. Nebraska's Pregnancy Risk Assessment Monitoring System added a COVID-19 supplement to the questionnaire to better understand the impacts of COVID on women during pregnancy. In addition, Nebraska's Title V program supported changes to the WIC program in how women received benefits during this time, supported by feedback from participants regarding their experiences.[25] During the pandemic, the New Jersey Department of Health began utilizing frontline workers, such as community health workers and doulas, to provide information and healthcare to local communities. In 2020, New Jersey's Title V program supported development of this workforce by establishing the Community Health Worker Institute, which was initiated in 2019 through a Department of Labor Apprenticeship award.[26]

Supplemental funding has augmented Title V pandemic response efforts. With funding from the Coronavirus Aid, Relief, and Economic Security (CARES) Act, HRSA's MCHB partnered with AMCHP to make grants to state programs to support telehealth efforts; these funds assisted states in providing prenatal care and home-visiting services through telehealth, improving access for pregnant women during this time. American Rescue Plan Act (ARPA) funds provide additional opportunities for partnership. MCHB has encouraged state Title V programs to explore ARPA funding and to consider partnership with agencies outside of health, such as education, transportation, and housing, to address pandemic-related needs of MCH populations.

PRACTICAL NEXT STEPS FOR LEVERAGING MCHB-FUNDED PROGRAMS TO ADVANCE MATERNAL HEALTH EQUITY

Entities interested in advancing maternal health equity should consider opportunities to engage MCHB-funded grantees in their states and communities. Community-based organizations might have programming that helps a state address its Title V needs and priorities. Individuals with lived experience can provide valuable input in the design, implementation, and evaluation of maternal health activities. Advocacy organizations may be able to push for policies that impact the root causes of poor maternal health outcomes.

Some potential next steps for organizations wishing to partner with MCHB-funded efforts include:

1. Explore the Title V Information System (TVIS). The TVIS website (mchb. tvisdata.hrsa.gov/) provides contact information for each state's Title V director, along with recent copies of each state's Title V MCH Services Block Grant Application/Report and Five-Year Needs Assessment.
2. Review your state's MCH priorities and action plan. Identify alignment between your goals and Title V activities and consider ways that your organization could help Title V achieve items in the action plan.

3. Engage in the Title V Needs Assessment. At a minimum, find out ways to offer input into the Needs Assessment (often there are opportunities for public comment or other stakeholder engagement). Consider partnering with Title V to facilitate engagement with particular segments of the MCH population or around specific topic areas.

4. Utilize MCHB data to help prioritize your efforts. The Title V National Performance and Outcome Measures (available at mchb.tvisdata.hrsa.gov/) show your state's performance in comparison to the rest of the nation and can help prioritize your efforts. The National Survey of Children's Health can yield information about the health of children and adolescents and can influence more "upstream" work to improve health outcomes across the life course.

5. In addition to Title V, consider whether other MCHB activities align with your efforts. You can find information on MCHB-funded projects in your state or community on the MCHB Website (data.hrsa.gov/topics/mchb/mchb-grants). Perhaps your organization could refer community members to MCHB-funded programs, or you may be able to offer training or other professional development opportunities for local program staff.

6. Look out for new funding opportunities. MCHB routinely posts grant opportunities at grants.gov/. Consider engaging other community partners to develop a proposal. Non-health partners, such as local housing authorities or social service agencies, can help you address social determinants of health that influence maternal health outcomes. To advance health equity, consider how to engage community members with lived experience to plan and implement the proposal. Also consider minority-serving institutions, which include historically Black colleges and universities, Hispanic-serving institutions, tribal colleges and universities, and institutions serving Asian Americans and Pacific Islanders.[27]

CONCLUSION

Julia Lathrop's description of maternal mortality in the United States in 1916, reported at the beginning of this chapter, unfortunately still rings true today. Persistently poor maternal health outcomes, including marked disparities, underscore the need for continued efforts to partner at all levels to improve outcomes. The MCHB supports multiple efforts at the state and community levels to advance maternal health equity. MCHB-funded programs and initiatives provide significant opportunities for partnership, for leveraging other federal, state, and local investments, and for aligning efforts.

REFERENCES

1. US Department of Labor, Children's Bureau. *Maternal Mortality from All Conditions Connected with Childbirth in the United States and Certain Other Countries*; 1917. Miscellaneous Series No. 6, Bureau Publication No. 19. http://

books.google.com/books?id=E4svaxqpNGkC&printsec=titlepage. Accessed February 13, 2022.

2. Virginia Commonwealth University VCU Libraries Social Welfare History Project. Children's Bureau: Part 1. 2018. https://socialwelfare.library.vcu.edu/programs/child-welfarechild-labor/childrens-bureau-part-i-2/. Accessed February 13, 2022.

3. Schmidt WM. The development of health services for mothers and children in the United States. *Am J Public Health.* 1973;63(5):419–427.

4. Eliot MM. Emergency maternity and infant care program for the wives and infants of men in the armed forces. *JAMA.* 1944;124(13):833–838.

5. Escarne JG, Atrash HK, de la Cruz DS, et al. Introduction to the Special Issue on Healthy Start. *Matern Child Health J.* 2017;21(Suppl 1):1–3.

6. Patient Protection and Affordable Care Act of 2010. Pub L No. 111–148, 124 Stat 119 (2010).

7. US Department of Health and Human Services, Health Resources and Services Administration, Maternal and Child Health Bureau. Program brief: maternal, infant, and early childhood home visiting program. https://mchb.hrsa.gov/sites/default/files/mchb/about-us/program-brief.pdf. Accessed February 13, 2022.

8. US Department of Health and Human Services. Fiscal year 2022 Health Resources and Services Administration justification of estimates for appropriations committees. https://www.hrsa.gov/sites/default/files/hrsa/about/budget/budget-justification-fy2022.pdf. Accessed February 16, 2022.

9. US Department of Health and Human Services, Health Resources and Services Administration, Maternal and Child Health Bureau. Title V information system. https://mchb.tvisdata.hrsa.gov/. Accessed February 13, 2022.

10. US Department of Health and Human Services, Health Resources and Services Administration, Maternal and Child Health Bureau. Alliance for Innovation on Maternal Health (AIM) and AIM-Community Care (AIM-CCI). https://mchb.hrsa.gov/programs-impact/programs/alliance-innovation-maternal-health-aim-aim-community-care-aim-cci. Accessed February 13, 2022.

11. US Department of Health and Human Services, Health Resources and Services Administration, Maternal and Child Health Bureau. Mission, vision, and work. https://mchb.hrsa.gov/about-us/mission-vision-work. Accessed February 13, 2022.

12. Health Resources and Services Administration, Maternal and Child Health Bureau. Maternal and Child Health Services Title V Block Grant FY2022 Application/FY2020 Annual Report (Alaska, Indiana, and Puerto Rico). https://mchb.tvisdata.hrsa.gov/Home/StateApplicationOrAnnualReport. Published 2021. Accessed February 14, 2022.

13. Health Resources and Services Administration, Maternal and Child Health Bureau. Maternal and Child Health Services Title V Block Grant, Maryland FY2022 Application/FY2020 Annual Report. https://mchb.tvisdata.hrsa.gov/Home/StateApplicationOrAnnualReport. Published 2021. Accessed February 17, 2022.

14. Association of Maternal and Child Health Programs. Innovation Hub. https://www.amchpinnovation.org/. Accessed February 17, 2022.

15. US Department of Health and Human Services, Health Resources and Services Administration. *HRSA Maternal Mortality Summit: Promising Global Practices to Improve Maternal Health Outcomes Technical Report.* https://www.hrsa.gov/sites/

default/files/hrsa/maternal-mortality/Maternal-Mortality-Technical-Report.pdf. Accessed February 13, 2022.

16. US Department of Health and Human Services, Health Resources and Services Administration, Maternal and Child Health Bureau. Secretary's Advisory Committee on Infant and Maternal Mortality. https://www.hrsa.gov/advisory-com mittees/infant-mortality/index.html. Accessed February 17, 2022.

17. Health Resources and Services Administration, Maternal and Child Health Bureau. Maternal and Child Health Services Title V Block Grant, Iowa FY2022 Application/ FY2020 Annual Report. https://mchb.tvisdata.hrsa.gov/Home/StateApplicationOrA nnualReport. Published 2021. Accessed February 14, 2022.

18. Health Resources and Services Administration, Maternal and Child Health Bureau. Maternal and Child Health Services Title V Block Grant, Tennessee FY2018 Application/FY2016 Annual Report. https://mchb.tvisdata.hrsa.gov/Home/StateAp plicationOrAnnualReport. Published 2017. Accessed February 14, 2022.

19. Lu MC, Kotelchuck M, Hogan V, et al. Closing the Black–white gap in birth outcomes: a life-course approach. *Ethn Dis*. 2010;20(1 suppl 2):62–76.

20. North Carolina Department of Health and Human Services. *North Carolina's Perinatal Health Strategic Plan 2016–2020*. 2021. https://whb.dph.ncdhhs.gov/docs/ PerinatalHealthStrategicPlan-WEB.pdf. Accessed February 13, 2022.

21. Health Resources and Services Administration, Maternal and Child Health Bureau. Maternal and Child Health Services Title V Block Grant, Illinois FY2022 Application/FY2020 Annual Report. https://mchb.tvisdata.hrsa.gov/Home/StateAp plicationOrAnnualReport. Published 2021. Accessed February 14, 2022.

22. I PROMOTE-IL. Illinois Maternal Health Strategic Plan 2020-2024, Version 1— February 2021. http://ipromoteil.org/wp-content/uploads/2021/03/IL-Maternal-Health-Strategic-Plan-V1_February-2021.pdf. Accessed February 13, 2022.

23. Zambrano LD, Ellington S, Strid P, et al. Update: characteristics of symptomatic women of reproductive age with laboratory-confirmed SARS-CoV-2 infection by pregnancy status—United States, January 22–October 3, 2020. *MMWR*. 2020;69:1641–1647.

24. Health Resources and Services Administration, Maternal and Child Health Bureau. Maternal and Child Health Services Title V Block Grant, New York FY2022 Application/FY2020 Annual Report. https://mchb.tvisdata.hrsa.gov/Home/StateAp plicationOrAnnualReport. Published 2021. Accessed February 14, 2022.

25. Health Resources and Services Administration, Maternal and Child Health Bureau. Maternal and Child Health Services Title V Block Grant, Nebraska FY2022 Application/FY2020 Annual Report. https://mchb.tvisdata.hrsa.gov/Home/StateAp plicationOrAnnualReport. Published 2021. Accessed February 14, 2022.

26. Health Resources and Services Administration, Maternal and Child Health Bureau. Maternal and Child Health Services Title V Block Grant, New Jersey FY2022 Application/FY2020 Annual Report. https://mchb.tvisdata.hrsa.gov/Home/StateAp plicationOrAnnualReport. Published 2021. Accessed February 14, 2022.

27. US Department of the Interior. Minority Serving Institutions Program. https://www. doi.gov/pmb/eeo/doi-minority-serving-institutions-program. Accessed February 4, 2022.

Chapter 41

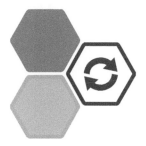

Driving Access, Health Equity, and Innovation in Maternal Healthcare through Medicaid

JESSICA C. SMITH, EMILY HEBERLEIN, ANGELA SNYDER, AND KAREN MINYARD

INTRODUCTION

The Medicaid program covers a large portion of births in the United States (43%). Medicaid pays for an even greater share of births for women in rural areas (50%), Black women (65.9%), and women under age 19 (77.5%).[1] In addition to covering deliveries, Medicaid is an important source of coverage for many women before and after giving birth. Approximately half of women who are uninsured when they become pregnant gain access to insurance coverage through Medicaid or the Children's Health Insurance Program (CHIP).[2] This coverage provides access to the full range of Medicaid benefits, allowing women to receive care in inpatient and outpatient settings, to fill prescriptions, and to receive services from healthcare providers from the time they become pregnant through at least 60 days after delivery. Coverage beyond 60 days varies by state and household income.

Medicaid is funded jointly by the federal government and state governments, and each state operates its own Medicaid program according to federal rules. Because each state is responsible for its Medicaid program, there are variations from state to state in who is covered, length of coverage, what services and provider types are covered, and quality improvement strategies. While this variation can lead to disparities in healthcare access and quality between states, it can also spur innovation, so that state programs can learn from one another and work with their communities to design the most appropriate care for the populations covered.

Jessica C. Smith, Emily Heberlein, Angela Snyder, and Karen Minyard, *Driving Access, Health Equity, and Innovation in Maternal Healthcare through Medicaid* In: *The Practical Playbook III*. Edited by: Dorothy Cilenti, Alisahah Jackson, Natalie D. Hernandez, Lindsey Yates, Sarah Verbiest, J. Lloyd Michener, and Brian C. Castrucci, Oxford University Press.
© de Beaumont Foundation 2024. DOI: 10.1093/oso/9780197662984.003.0041

Providing insurance coverage and minimizing coverage disruptions are important pieces of the policy puzzle to help reduce maternal morbidity and mortality. Because Medicaid covers so many pregnancies in the United States, finding ways to promote equitable access to quality healthcare through Medicaid is critical to improving maternal health for many low-income women, women in rural areas, and women of color.

MEDICAID BASICS

Variations in Medicaid

Since states run and partially fund their own Medicaid programs, political, ideological, and budgetary considerations influence Medicaid coverage and how care is paid for. Medicaid eligibility limits vary by state, with some states offering generous eligibility and others restricting coverage, and can depend on individuals' health status, age, or whether they are a parent. Disparities exist in who can be covered by Medicaid before, during, and after pregnancy. Medicaid eligibility is primarily tied to a household's income level as it relates to the federal poverty level (100% FPL). For example, in states that expanded Medicaid under the Affordable Care Act (ACA), any individual in a household earning less than 138% FPL qualifies for Medicaid. To illustrate the differences in Medicaid eligibility, different state and individual scenarios for coverage are detailed in Table 41.1.

Table 41.1 State Medicaid Coverage Variation				
State Medicaid Coverage Rules	**Covered Individual**	**Covered before Pregnancy**	**Covered during Pregnancy**	**Covered after Pregnancy**
State A: Expanded Medicaid and covers pregnant women in households earning up to 200% FPL	Childless adult	If income ≤ 138% FPL	If income ≤ 200% FPL	For 60 days if 138% < income ≤ 200% FPL Covered beyond 60 days if income ≤ 138% FPL
	Parent	If income ≤ 138% FPL	If income ≤ 200% FPL	For 60 days if 138% < income ≤ 200% FPL Covered beyond 60 days if income ≤ 138% FPL
State B: Did not expand Medicaid, covers pregnant women in households earning up to 200% FPL, and covers parents earning up to 35% FPL	Childless adult	Not covered	If income ≤ 200% FPL	For 60 days if 35% < income ≤ 200% FPL Covered beyond 60 days if income ≤ 35% FPL
	Parent	If income ≤ 35% FPL	If income ≤ 200% FPL	For 60 days if 35% < income ≤ 200% FPL Covered beyond 60 days if income ≤ 35% FPL

Income Limits and Eligibility Categories

In states that have not expanded Medicaid, able-bodied adults are not eligible for Medicaid coverage unless they are a parent earning less than their state's income eligibility limit for parents. This eligibility limit also varies significantly in states without Medicaid expansion, but it is below the 138% FPL minimum in all non-expansion states. This means that many childless adults in non-expansion states living below 138% of the poverty line may have no access to Medicaid coverage until they become pregnant. Similarly, whether an individual is eligible for Medicaid coverage during pregnancy, and how long coverage lasts after delivery, depends on the state of residence. All states are required to provide Medicaid coverage through 60 days postpartum for women living in households earning below 138% FPL, but eligibility limits beyond that minimum again vary significantly by state, with many states setting much higher income limits. States can decide to increase their income eligibility limits for pregnant women to ensure that more women and infants have access to free perinatal care.

Postpartum Coverage Limits

While many women gain access to Medicaid coverage during pregnancy, because states are required to cover women only through 60 days postpartum, more than half of the women experience a lapse in insurance coverage within six months of delivery.[2] In states that have not expanded Medicaid, a postpartum coverage gap exists for women living in households earning too much to qualify for Medicaid as low-income parents but earning too little to qualify for support to purchase a healthcare plan on the ACA insurance exchanges (under 100% FPL).[3] Even in states that have expanded Medicaid, mothers in households with incomes just above the expansion income limit (138% FPL) who are able to purchase private coverage on the ACA exchanges may find the out-of-pocket costs unaffordable and often have to change providers, leading to more care disruptions.[4]

Reimbursement Structure

Medicaid programs can use different reimbursement structures to pay for services: fee-for-service, managed care, or a combination of both. Under fee-for-service, state Medicaid programs act as an insurance company, setting payment rates and reimbursing providers for each service they provide. In managed care, states contract with a third-party company and pay a set rate per month for each Medicaid member assigned to the managed-care organization; this is referred to as a per member per month rate. The managed-care organization is then responsible for covering all members in its plan with this pool of money.

Around two-thirds of individuals on Medicaid are covered by a managed-care organization. Some states, like Tennessee, cover all their Medicaid population under managed care.[5] Other states, like Georgia, cover only select eligibility groups (e.g., pregnant women) under managed care. A smaller number of states use no managed care—covering all members under the fee-for-service structure.

The structure of managed care makes it a useful vehicle for providing non-medical services and supports or enhanced medical services while also providing a predictable level of spending for states. However, proper oversight of managed-care organizations is required to ensure that Medicaid enrollees receive the services they are entitled to.

INNOVATION IN MATERNAL AND CHILD HEALTH THROUGH MEDICAID

States have many opportunities to make changes to their Medicaid programs and to enhance services provided to their maternal and infant populations under existing Medicaid regulations. These changes might include providing eligibility to additional populations, covering optional benefits, or providing coverage through a managed-care delivery system. The most basic tool used to make the changes is a state plan amendment. In effect, the state alters its existing agreement with the federal government to administer its Medicaid program and collect federal matching funds that provide financial support to the program. Additionally, when states seek to innovate Medicaid beyond the rules of the standard federal program, tools like Section 1115 waivers are available to allow states to test and develop new programs and policies to best meet the state's unique needs. Because the waivers are seeking federal funds to demonstrate improvements in care or efficiencies, states need to implement rigorous evaluations and to show that the innovations are cost-neutral to the federal government; therefore, waivers come with more federal oversight and state administrative burden.

Expanding Eligibility

As mentioned above, states are required to provide Medicaid coverage for pregnant women with incomes at or below 138% of the FPL extending to 60 days postpartum. States also have expanded coverage to pregnant women through state plan amendments, waivers, and, in some cases, state-only-funded programs to improve maternal and infant outcomes. These enhancements have included presumptive eligibility, immigrant coverage, postpartum coverage extensions, and place-based coverage in response to environmental exposures.

Presumptive Eligibility

As of 2020, 31 states allowed women to obtain Medicaid-covered prenatal care via presumptive eligibility.[6] Certain qualified state partners, including public health, medical care, and/or social service providers, can screen women for income eligibility and temporarily enroll them in Medicaid, granting them immediate access to coverage. Presumptive eligibility ensures that providers are paid for any services they deliver during the eligibility period, even if the pregnant woman is not subsequently determined to be eligible.

Immigrant Coverage

Legal permanent residents of the United States entering after August 1996 typically must wait five years before they can receive full Medicaid benefits, but states can cover lawful residents during pregnancy before the five-year waiting period ends. States also have the option to provide coverage to other immigrants, but they may only use state funds to do so. As of 2020, 27 states provided coverage to immigrant pregnant women.[7]

Postpartum Coverage

When the 60-day Medicaid postpartum period expires, some postpartum women may qualify for Medicaid through another pathway; others may not. To address maternal health equity and decrease morbidity and mortality in the postpartum period, several states have extended coverage to all, or a targeted population of, pregnant women. In July 2021, Georgia implemented a Medicaid 1115 waiver that extends full Medicaid coverage from 60 to 180 days postpartum for all pregnant women. Beginning in April 2022, the American Rescue Plan Act of 2021 gives states the option to extend postpartum Medicaid coverage to 12 months via a five-year state plan amendment.[8]

Geographic Coverage

Using the 1115 waiver, Michigan provides full Medicaid coverage to pregnant women and children in Flint, Michigan, who were affected by that city's water crisis. Coverage is available to all income levels with no cost-sharing for those under 400% of the FPL.

Coverage for Different Services under Medicaid

In addition to variation in eligibility rules, states vary in their benefits and coverage policies that affect maternal health. While states must provide core inpatient and outpatient medical care under federal law, they have considerable flexibility in determining the scope for pregnancy-related support services and other nonhospital services.[9]

Midwifery Services and Birth Centers

States vary in coverage, licensing, and credentialing rules for Medicaid coverage of midwives and free-standing birth centers. Particularly suitable for women with low-risk pregnancies, midwifery-led care is an evidence-based maternity model that includes prenatal, intrapartum, and postpartum services, with a philosophy of shared decision-making and supporting "watchful waiting and nonintervention in normal processes." Different types of midwives have different training, certification, and scopes of practice. When care is needed beyond the midwifery scope, midwives may consult with physicians, manage care with physicians, or transfer the patient for medical management. Practices have developed varied staffing models for physicians and midwives. The number of midwife-attended births in the United States has steadily increased, with most births occurring in hospitals, including "alongside" birth centers housed on a hospital campus (98.5%).

Free-standing birth centers are physically separate from a hospital and comprise a small part of the US maternity care system. Between 2010 and 2020, the number of birth centers grew by 97%, to a total of 384. Strong evidence supports positive outcomes and increasing access to birth centers; these settings are much more common and well-integrated into healthcare systems in European countries. Medicaid reimbursement requires that birth centers be licensed, with regulations varying by state, and states that license birth centers must cover birth center deliveries under Medicaid. The Institute for Medicaid Innovation's 2020 report, "Improving Maternal Health Access, Coverage, and Outcomes in Medicaid," is a comprehensive guide to the midwifery-led model of care opportunities and policy landscape under Medicaid.[10]

Doula Care

A doula is a "trained professional who provides continuous physical, emotional and informational support to a mother before, during, and shortly after childbirth to help her achieve the healthiest, most satisfying experience possible."[11] Multiple research studies have demonstrated that pregnant women who receive doula services are more likely to have healthy birth outcomes and a more positive birth experience, and Medicaid-funded doula programs could experience a significant return on investment.[12] As of 2020, six states had state-level Medicaid doula reimbursement programs (Indiana, Oregon, Minnesota, Nebraska, Washington, and New Jersey) and New York was piloting a program in several counties; 13 state Title V Maternal and Child Health Block Grant programs also had long-standing doula services. In 2019, 13 state legislatures were considering Medicaid reimbursement for doula services.[12] Payment strategies include using Title V block grant funds for services for Medicaid-enrolled women and adding doula services as an optional pregnancy care benefit, where doulas work under the supervision of a Medicaid-enrolled provider (Minnesota) or enroll as Medicaid providers (Oregon). In Nebraska, one managed-care organization has selected doula services as a value-added service for pregnant females involved in the foster care system.

Group Prenatal Care

Group prenatal care models, usually serving women with low-risk pregnancies, integrate health assessment, health education, and peer support. Group sessions are facilitated by a healthcare provider and follow a curriculum; women with similar due dates participate in two-hour sessions every two to four weeks. Partners and support people are welcome to attend. CenteringPregnancy (Centering Healthcare Institute) is the most researched of these models and has approximately 350 sites across 40 states.[13] Women participating in group prenatal care are more likely to receive adequate care and to breastfeed; some evidence suggests that participants, particularly Black women, may experience better birth outcomes. Group prenatal care can be more costly and logistically challenging for providers to implement.

A handful of states (Maryland, Montana, New Jersey, Ohio, and South Carolina) lead in offering group prenatal care, providing enhanced Medicaid reimbursement, investing state funds to improve access (e.g., grants to support start-up or pilot programs), and reaching a greater proportion of pregnant women. States may also include group prenatal care in alternative payment method initiatives. Prior to COVID-19, only 10% of states had at least 5% of pregnant women access CenteringPregnancy, and the pandemic significantly curtailed this type of group care.[13]

Home-Visiting Services

Although they cover a range of models, home-visiting services generally tend to offer screening, case management, health education, parenting support, and other interventions to improve a combination of health outcomes, skills, and child development. Case management is a broad term for activities that link families to needed services and supports. Research has demonstrated a range of positive health and developmental effects and a return on investment for home visiting, depending on the program's focus (e.g., education, justice system involvement, healthcare costs, public assistance reliance).[14] The home-visiting workforce may include nurses, social workers, early childhood educators, lactation counselors, and others.

As of 2018, 20 states were using a variety of approaches under Medicaid to fund home visiting. Some initiatives are decades-old, state-level policies; others are pilots, localized, or more recently developed. Most commonly, states use the targeted case-management benefit under a Medicaid state plan amendment or finance home visiting as a demonstration or pilot program under a larger Medicaid waiver (e.g., Section 1115 or 1915b waiver). Some states use existing benefits. Blending/braiding with Title V funds is a strategy to expand capacity. Because most pregnant women are covered under Medicaid managed care, home-visiting services often are incorporated into state contracts with managed-care organizations.[14]

Community Health Workers

A community health worker (CHW) is a trusted community member or has a very close understanding of the community and uses these relationships to connect health and social services with the community, facilitating access and improving quality and cultural competence.[15] CHWs support women in following recommended care and health screenings, accessing child vaccinations, and improving nutrition. The Affordable Care Act officially recognized CHWs as an important resource for improving care and population health and reducing costs. States vary in training and certification standards for CHWs.

States have used Medicaid waivers to fund CHW programs and to reimburse for CHW services. Healthcare providers use waiver funds to pay CHWs to work with patients to enroll in Medicaid, to manage their health, to connect to community resources, and to navigate health services. Some states (including Massachusetts) use the designation "medically necessary early intervention" to allow Medicaid reimbursement to CHW-like providers directly through fee-for-service or within a managed-care contract structure.

Maternity Medical Homes

Maternity medical homes are enhanced models of prenatal care that track patients over time, coordinate services and supports, and aim to be more patient-centered, providing additional psychosocial support and health education.[16] These models are relatively new and vary in their implementation.[17] North Carolina's Pregnancy Medical Home initiative is one example, where Medicaid pays a primary care case-management organization a per member per month bundled payment. Other states, including Texas and Wisconsin, have implemented these models.

Optional Services

When states expand eligibility to additional populations, they can provide full Medicaid coverage, a limited package of services, or innovative benefits not currently available to beneficiaries. Home visiting, doula services, and models of care delivery like pregnancy medical homes and group prenatal care are described above. Additionally, states have added behavioral healthcare, substance use disorder services, and family planning to their Medicaid plans to improve the array of services available to women during pregnancy and their childbearing years. Although most states provide full Medicaid benefits to all pregnant women, five states (Arkansas, Idaho, New Mexico, North Carolina, and South Dakota) cover only pregnancy-related services.

Maternal Depression Screening

In 2016, the Centers for Medicare & Medicaid Services issued a bulletin clarifying that state Medicaid agencies may allow maternal depression screenings to be claimed as a service for the child as part of the well-child benefit, in effect expanding screenings to women who lose Medicaid coverage after 60 days postpartum.[18] For example, North Dakota Medicaid covers maternal depression screening as a separate service when performed in conjunction with a Health

Tracks (EPSDT) screening or any other pediatric visit. Providers are allowed to bill the child's Medicaid ID when using one of the standardized screening tools up to three times in the child's first year.

Substance Use Disorder (SUD) Services

Under a Section 1115 waiver, Massachusetts Medicaid managed-care organizations must provide acute treatment services, structured outpatient addiction programs, clinical support services, residential rehabilitation services, recovery coaches, and recovery-support navigators for people with SUDs. Pregnant women receive specialized services to ensure coordination between their obstetrical care, acute addiction treatment, and clinical support services. Structured outpatient addiction and residential rehabilitation programs may also include specialized services and staffing for pregnant women.[6]

Family Planning

Family planning services must be provided without cost-sharing to individuals of childbearing age who qualify for Medicaid. Many states also extend eligibility for family-planning-only services through waivers or under their state plan. Through these stand-alone benefit packages, 31 states have a payment policy specifically designed to encourage long-acting reversible contraception insertion immediately postpartum. Multiple studies have found that these programs prevent unintended pregnancies and abortions, thus improving women's health and saving money for federal and state governments.[19] The Healthy Texas Women program started in 2016 as a non-Medicaid-funded program and provides women's health and family planning services at no cost to eligible low-income Texas women.

IMPROVING QUALITY THROUGH VALUE-BASED PURCHASING

Because Medicaid covers many people, the program can drive quality improvement for specific populations, including pregnant women, by linking payments to quality metrics or other policies that can improve patient care. In 2016, changes to federal rules around managed care gave states and managed-care organizations greater flexibility to pilot value-based payment (VBP) programs, to cover a broader scope of services, including services that address social determinants of health, and to implement payment reforms. Money that is not spent by managed-care organizations on providing care or administering services to Medicaid members can be used for other purposes, such as investing in care-coordination services or providing value-added services (e.g., covering breast pumps and infant car seats to new mothers). More than half of states have managed-care quality initiatives in place that are tied to perinatal outcomes.[5]

Pay for Performance

As of 2020, the most popular VBP program was the pay-for-performance model.[20] In this model, financial incentives are used to increase the quality of care. Providers or health systems are given quality targets and are rewarded for meeting or exceeding the targets. For example, Medicaid could provide bonus payments to managed-care organizations that increase by 5% the number of Black women who have a prenatal care visit during their first trimester. Managed-care organizations can also develop and implement their own programs to meet the goals, such as offering OB-GYNs in their provider network $100 bonus payments for each delivering mother who attends a postpartum visit within six weeks of delivery.

Episode of Care

For perinatal services, Medicaid programs can utilize an episode-of-care approach to reimburse providers for bundles of services. This model essentially sets acceptable costs for providing a service or set of perinatal services. It is designed to control costs by rewarding providers who deliver services for less than the set acceptable cost and by penalizing providers who deliver services for more than the acceptable cost.

Medical Homes

As mentioned above, states can support a holistic approach to perinatal healthcare using the maternity medical home model. This model encourages care coordination across providers and services, in both clinical and behavioral care, as well as social supports.[20] Medical homes may be supported by offering financial incentives for activities like completing risk assessments or through the creation of other payment approaches, such as shared savings programs that encourage coordination across provider types and care settings.

CONCLUSION

Medicaid is an essential tool for building and sustaining maternal and child systems of care at the state and local levels. Mapping what populations and services are currently covered by state Medicaid programs to determine the current context and to identify gaps is one place stakeholders can begin a process of comprehensive system planning and improvement. Complementary steps in the planning process involve identifying other relevant funding streams, grants, and demonstration projects to test and fill the gaps, sometimes through additional blending and braiding of funds. Home-visiting programs are an example of how multiple federal and state funding streams, including Medicaid and the Maternal, Infant, and Early Childhood Home Visiting Program, can be successfully combined to target women and their families.

One place stakeholders can get data to inform system effectiveness and planning is the state maternal mortality review committee (MMRC). MMRCs are multidisciplinary teams that conduct comprehensive reviews of women's deaths during, or within a year of, pregnancy. The committees often include representatives from the maternal and child health practitioner community, public health and behavioral health professionals, and advocacy or community-based organizations. Reports from MMRCs can identify opportunities to address system shortcomings related to hospital protocols, payment mechanisms, and gaps in clinical and preventive services. Stakeholder engagement is crucial in driving system improvements, with each member playing a unique role in the policy change process.

This chapter describes the basics of the Medicaid program, how Medicaid funding can be leveraged for innovation, and how some states have used Medicaid to improve maternal and child outcomes in their unique contexts. While Medicaid plays an important role in covering many pregnant women and their children, variation in eligibility rules and covered services by state can make the program difficult to navigate for patients, providers, and community-based organizations. Like many policies, Medicaid policies in some states are more progressive than in others. Having a clear understanding of a state's Medicaid income eligibility rules, reimbursement structure, and scope of covered services is the first step in identifying who the program can cover now and who could benefit from more generous coverage requirements or policies.

REFERENCES

1. MACPAC. Medicaid's role in financing maternity care: fact sheet. 2020:16. https://www.macpac.gov/wp-content/uploads/2020/01/Medicaid%E2%80%99s-Role-in-Financing-Maternity-Care.pdf. Accessed November 19, 2021.

2. Daw JR, Hatfield LA, Swartz K, Sommers BD. Women in the United States experience high rates of coverage 'churn' in months before and after childbirth. *Health Aff*. 2017;36(4):598–606. doi:10.1377/hlthaff.2016.1241.

3. Garfield R, Damico A, Orgera K. *The Coverage Gap: Uninsured Poor Adults in States That Do Not Expand Medicaid*. National Library of Medicine Digital Collections. 2016. https://collections.nlm.nih.gov/catalog/nlm:nlmuid-101717244-pdf.

4. Ranji U, Gomez I, Salganicoff A. Expanding postpartum Medicaid coverage. https://www.kff.org/womens-health-policy/issue-brief/expanding-postpartum-medicaid-coverage/. Published 2020.

5. Hinton E, Rudowitz R, Stolyar L, Singer N. 10 Things to know about Medicaid managed care. https://www.kff.org/medicaid/issue-brief/10-things-to-know-about-medicaid-managed-care/. Published 2020.

6. Medicaid and Chip Payment and Access Commission. Inventory of state-level Medicaid policies, programs, and initiatives to improve maternity care and outcomes. https://www.macpac.gov/publication/inventory-of-state-level-medic

aid-policies-programs-and-initiatives-to-improve-maternity-care-and-outcomes/. Published 2020.

7. MACPAC. Report to Congress on Medicaid and CHIP. 2020:99–132. https://www. macpac.gov/wp-content/uploads/2020/06/Chapter-5-Medicaid%E2%80%99s-Role-in-Maternal-Health.pdf.

8. H.R.1319 - 117th Congress (2021-2022): American Rescue Plan Act of 2021, Congress (Yarmuth JA 2021). March 11, 2021. https://www.congress.gov/bill/117th-congress/house-bill/1319.

9. Gifford K, Walls J, Ranji U, Salganicoff A, Gomez I. Medicaid coverage of pregnancy and perinatal benefits: results from a state survey. 2017:38. https://www.kff.org/wom ens-health-policy/report/medicaid-coverage-of-pregnancy-and-perinatal-benefits-results-from-a-state-survey/. Accessed December 20, 2021.

10. Moore JE, George KE, Bakst C, Shea K. Improving maternal health access, coverage, and outcomes in Medicaid: a resource for state Medicaid agencies and Medicaid managed care organizations. https://www.medicaidinnovation.org/_images/cont ent/2020-IMI-Improving_Maternal_Health_Access_Coverage_and_Outcomes-Report.pdf. Published 2020.

11. DONA International. What is a doula? https://www.dona.org/what-is-a-doula/.

12. Platt T, Kaye N. Four state strategies to employ doulas to improve maternal health and birth outcomes in Medicaid. https://www.nashp.org/four-state-strategies-to-employ-doulas-to-improve-maternal-health-and-birth-outcomes-in-medicaid/. Published July 13, 2020. Accessed December 20, 2021.

13. Prenatal-to-3 State Policy Roadmap. Group Prenatal Care. https://pn3policy.org/pn-3-state-policy-roadmap-2021/us/group-prenatal-care/.

14. Johnson K. Medicaid financing for home visiting: the state of states' approaches. https://ccf.georgetown.edu/wp-content/uploads/2019/01/Medicaid-and-Home-Visiting.pdf. Published January 2019. Accessed December 20, 2021.

15. Association of State and Territorial Health Officials. Utilizing community health workers to improve access to care for maternal and child populations: four state approaches. Issue brief. Association of State and Territorial Health Officials. https://www.astho.org/Maternal-and-Child-Health/AIM-Access-CHW-Issue-Brief/. Published 2016. Accessed December 20, 2021.

16. Rakover J. The maternity medical home: the chassis for a more holistic model of pregnancy care? [Blog post]. Institute for Healthcare Improvement. http://www. ihi.org/communities/blogs/_layouts/15/ihi/community/blog/itemview.aspx?List= 7d1126ec-8f63-4a3b-9926-c44ea3036813&ID=222. Published 2016.

17. Hill I, Benatar S, Courtot B, Dubay L, Blavin F. *Strong Start for Mothers and Newborns Evaluation: Year 4 Annual Report*. Vol 1. *Cross-Cutting Findings*. Urban Institute. 2018:204. https://downloads.cms.gov/files/cmmi/strongstart-snhancedprenatalcaremodels_evalrptyr4v1.pdf. Accessed October 13, 2020.

18. U.S. Dept. of Health and Human Services Guidance Portal. Maternal Depression Screening and Treatment: A Critical Role for Medicaid in the Care of Mothers and Children. Published May 11, 2016. https://www.hhs.gov/guidance/document/mater nal-depression-screening-and-treatment-critical-role-medicaid-care-mothers-and

19. Walls J, Gifford K, Ranji U, Salganicoff A, Gomez I. Medicaid coverage of family planning benefits: results from a state survey. 2016:44. https://files.kff.org/attachment/Report-Medicaid-Coverage-of-Family-Planning-Benefits-Results-from-a-State-Survey.

20. MACPAC. Value-based payment for maternity care in Medicaid: findings from five states. 2021:16. https://www.macpac.gov/wp-content/uploads/2021/09/Value-Based-Payment-for-Maternity-Care-in-Medicaid-Findings-from-Five-States.pdf.

Chapter 42

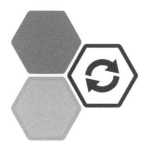

Role of Academic Health Systems in Improving and Sustaining Maternal Health

OLUFUNMILAYO MAKINDE CHINEKEZI, KAREY M. SUTTON,
CRISTA E. JOHNSON-AGBAKWU, AND YHENNEKO J. TAYLOR

Academic health systems have a moral responsibility to support and improve the health and well-being of the birthing people, children, families, and communities they serve. The maternal and child health crisis in the United States is well known; it also is widely acknowledged that maternal deaths are avoidable with proper tools and technology, human capital, and services. Research has shown that factors related to systems of care have contributed to over half of all pregnancy-related deaths and have affected rates of infant deaths.

CALL TO ACTION FOR MATERNAL AND CHILD HEALTH

The US Department of Health and Human Services (HHS) is working to ensure that the United States becomes one of the safest countries for women to give birth in and that mothers can expect a healthy life span for their infants. In its plan of action, HHS (https://health.gov/healthypeople/tools-action/browse-evidence-based-resources/healthy-women-healthy-pregnancies-healthy-futures-action-plan-improve-maternal-health-america) addresses challenges and the role of health systems. The challenges include racial and ethnic disparities in maternal health, rural disparities in access to care, health insurance coverage, practice patterns, payment misalignment, and data quality and timelines. The academic health system is a pivotal partner for the solutions outlined by HHS. Substantial work is needed on differences in quality of care and clinical practice and in improving healthcare access for birthing people who reside in maternity deserts. The academic health system advocates for more comprehensive

Olufunmilayo Makinde Chinekezi, Karey M. Sutton, Crista E. Johnson-Agbakwu, and Yhenneko J. Taylor, *Role of Academic Health Systems in Improving and Sustaining Maternal Health* In: *The Practical Playbook III*. Edited by: Dorothy Cilenti, Alisahah Jackson, Natalie D. Hernandez, Lindsey Yates, Sarah Verbiest, J. Lloyd Michener, and Brian C. Castrucci, Oxford University Press. © de Beaumont Foundation 2024. DOI: 10.1093/oso/9780197662984.003.0042

insurance coverage for birthing people, families, and communities. In addition, there is a need for solid data systems that can help identify areas of focus for new interventions to improve maternal and child health. Without meaningful partnerships with community members and community-based organizations, this work is challenging. Thus, centering the wisdom of birthing persons, family supports, and community-based organizations throughout the research and training models used by academic health systems is imperative for reducing maternal health and health inequities.

Building a Community Health System

An academic medical system is a complex organization that usually comprises a teaching hospital, an accredited medical school, and other health professions schools. It is documented that medical schools and teaching hospitals are working to address inequities in health and healthcare. One benefit of building the capacity at academic health systems is that this work will span the key mission areas of research, education, clinical care, and community collaborations to improve the health of all. A potential limiting factor is that work affecting the communities most in need often is siloed and uncoordinated. To address the immediate need for creating sustainable, efficient community health systems, the Association of American Medical Colleges (AAMC) embarked on a three-year initiative to develop resources for academic health centers to build capacity to create efficient community health systems. The AAMC is a not-for-profit association with a membership that includes 155 accredited US medical schools and 17 accredited Canadian medical schools; more than 400 teaching hospitals and health systems, including Department of Veterans Affairs medical centers; and more than 70 academic societies. Academic health systems were encouraged to build a systems approach to community health and health equity by:

1. Conducting an inventory of all community-partnered or relevant activity at their institution
2. Mapping how their community-relevant activity could be better coordinated across mission areas
3. Identifying critical pieces of their system to implement for the future
4. Identifying critical stakeholders needed for the success of their future system
5. Developing an evaluation plan that includes metrics salient to all key stakeholders, including community partners

These steps are integral to building a system for community health and health equity, scaling systems-change initiatives, and incorporating communication methods for sustainability. The goal is for academic health systems to achieve their ideal states, ultimately improving the health and well-being of birthing people, children, and the community.

Academic Health

Academic health systems play a critical role in advancing maternal health equity for Black, Indigenous, and People of Color (BIPOC) communities. Understanding and confronting the myriad challenges in addressing maternal morbidity and mortality necessitates a coordinated, multipronged approach that engages stakeholders both within and across academic institutions, as well as the very communities served by the academic health system(s). In 2021, the American Medical Association (AMA) published a strategic plan detailing a roadmap for action and accountability in embedding racial justice and advancing health equity. The AMA's five strategic approaches—(1) embed equity, (2) build alliances and share power, (3) ensure equity in innovation, (4) push upstream, and (5) foster truth, reconciliation, racial healing, and transformation—provide an important framework for academic health systems to advance maternal health equity.

Embed Equity

Embedding equity in practice, process, action, innovation, and organizational performance and outcomes necessitates an understanding of the interconnected nature of the social and political identities of minoritized communities. The interplay of factors like race, ethnicity, age, gender, sexuality, language, education, class, religion, culture, history, heritage, and migratory pathways was originally popularized by the late feminist writer bell hooks in the early 1980s. The idea became codified as *intersectionality* by Kimberlé Williams Crenshaw in 1989.[1] Intersectionality provides an analytical framework for understanding how overlapping and intersecting social and political identities may create interdependent systems of oppression, domination, discrimination, or privilege. Such factors manifest in the experiences of care for BIPOC women, mothers, and birthing people, whereby structural racism, cultural hegemony, and implicit bias collide to result in the pervasive "othering" of BIPOC bodies.[2]

Efforts to embed equity in advancing maternal health should include a focus on the care interactions experienced by BIPOC patients: Is verbal and nonverbal communication by the healthcare provider during patient care encounters conveyed in a nonstigmatizing, respectful, validating manner? Does this take place in a safe space and employ careful listening and linguistically inclusive care? Are patients empowered to ask questions and to seek a second opinion, as well as encouraged to bring along a peer advocate? Is health messaging tailored to BIPOC communities in a manner that is respectful, culturally congruent, and trauma-informed? Are there efforts to nurture and sustain trust with BIPOC communities that have historically been marginalized and disadvantaged? What efforts are being made to ensure the recruitment, inclusion, and retention of BIPOC participants in clinical trials and other forms of research? What structural changes are being put in place to recruit, retain, and promote a diverse healthcare workforce with greater representation of BIPOC faculty, learners, and staff? Is there mandatory, enduring, and iterative training across the health-care workforce in antiracism, implicit bias, and cultural competency?

While it is important to develop this infrastructure, it must also be accompanied by a mechanism to monitor and evaluate institutional cultural and structural change and quality improvement in the patient experience and maternal health outcomes over time. Recent years have brought increased attention to longitudinal quality-improvement initiatives that incorporate patient safety bundles and examine patient morbidity registries on maternal and perinatal health outcomes through such entities as the National Network of Perinatal Quality Collaboratives, the Centers for Disease Control and Prevention, and the Alliance for Innovation on Maternal Health (AIM). (A national, data-driven, maternal safety and quality-improvement initiative, AIM is funded by the American College of Obstetricians and Gynecologists and the Maternal and Child Health Bureau of the Health Resources Services Administration.)

Build Alliances and Share Power

Meaningful community engagement and embeddedness enables academic health systems to build alliances and share power. Such engagement must be firmly rooted in trust that is earned, nurtured, and sustained with historically marginalized populations. Systems changes to advance maternal health equity must center the voices of those with lived experiences of racism, bias, and discrimination. A critical first step is attending community meetings and participating in listening sessions to hear from those most affected by injustice. A next step is coalescing a community advisory board whereby academic health systems can leverage the community's expertise, knowledge, and lived experience by partnering with local champions who can help develop the programmatic, clinical, and research directions of the academic health system. Such alliances should share power and leadership, include BIPOC representation on both the academic health system and the community sides of the alliance, and be grounded in mutual respect, humility, and open, bidirectional dialogue. Attention should also be paid to ensuring appropriate remuneration (whether monetary or otherwise, as agreed on by the alliance) for the time, expertise, and effort of community partners. Such alliances should also ensure accountability and provide educational outreach and research engagement with hard-to-reach communities. Any research efforts should be grounded in the principles of community-based participatory research (CBPR), whereby the community remains centered throughout all phases of the research enterprise in driving the initial research idea, conceptual design, implementation strategy, interpretation of findings, and dissemination efforts. Critical discussions on data ownership, sustainability, benefits, and potential harms to the community (in the short and long term) must be addressed and revisited throughout the study. Building community capacity by integrating peer support/navigators and/or community health workers as vital members of the academic health system's workforce will advance maternal health equity through the roles these individuals play as reproductive and sexual health champions in their respective communities.

Ensure Equity in Innovation

Advancing data equity by improving measurement of maternal morbidity, mortality, and other maternal health indices has also received new attention. It is critically important that data are stratified by race and ethnicity and that they describe language, country of origin, and ethnocultural statistics. For instance, the racial category of Black/African American is an umbrella term that encompasses all people of African ancestry, including US-born Blacks, Africans, and Caribbean migrants, for which further disaggregation according to migratory pathway (e.g., voluntary immigrant, refugee, asylum-seeker, undocumented) is crucial. This has important implications for the "healthy migrant paradox," health status, health-seeking behavior, health services utilization, and access to care, not only at the time of arrival in the United States but generationally, considering the impacts of epigenetics and lifelong exposure to racism, discrimination, and microaggressions. Other considerations are the effects of chronic toxic stress and weathering on worsening maternal health inequities with increased length of residency in the country. Geospatial residential clustering of BIPOC people is another critically important consideration in measurement, given the pervasiveness of structural racism in the housing market that exacerbates maternal health inequities through historically redlined districts.[3] Validated instruments and assessment tools should achieve cross-cultural and linguistic equivalency, particularly when engaging with and/or examining maternal health equity and outcomes among BIPOC migrant populations with limited English proficiency. Precision population health is becoming widespread, with artificial intelligence (AI) and machine learning (ML) algorithms being applied to big data, such as electronic health records in academic health centers. Careful attention must be paid to AI/ML algorithms so that they do not perpetuate biases.

Push Upstream

To make substantive advances in maternal health equity, it is important to push upstream levers in considering social determinants of health (SDOH) that undergird the root cause of maternal health and healthcare inequities. Figure 42.1 shows the socio-ecological model of the impact of racism on the sexual and reproductive health of BIPOC women, mothers, and birthing people and outlines the multiple ways that racism manifests, whether internalized, personally mediated, or institutionalized. At the individual level, negative prior healthcare experiences, distrust of healthcare providers, and lack of quality care can manifest as avoidance and/or delay in care-seeking, with resultant adverse maternal health outcomes. This is exacerbated by internalized racism. At the interpersonal/family health level, a culture of mistrust, the school-to-prison pipeline of

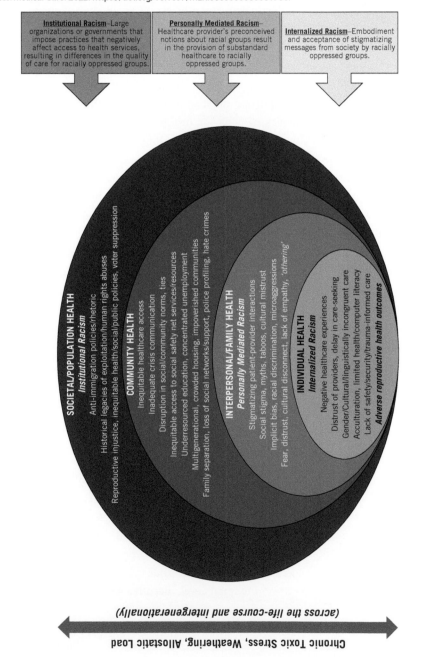

Figure 42.1 ▼

The socio-ecological model of the impact of racism on the sexual, gender, and reproductive health of BIPOC women, mothers, and birthing people, including migrant populations.

Source: Reprinted with Permission by Wolters Kluwer. Johnson-Agbakwu CE. The impact of racism and the sociopolitical climate on the birth outcomes of migrant women, mothers, and birthing people in the United States. *Medical Care*. 2022. https://doi.org/10.1097/MLR.0000000000001780.

mass incarceration, police brutality, exposure to various forms of violence (including domestic, interpersonal, and sexual violence), and adverse childhood experiences further compound inequities. At the community level, inequitable access to healthcare, residential segregation (and historic redlining), concentrated unemployment, impoverished communities, underresourced education, food deserts, environmental hazards, and crime—all of which are compounded by experiences of personally mediated racism—are at play. Finally, at the global level of society and population health, systemic, institutional racism manifests in voter-suppression efforts, the overturning of *Roe v Wade,* and inequitable health, social, and public policies that bear the vestiges of the historic, traumatic legacies of exploitation of BIPOC bodies (among them, Saartjie Baartman, medical experimentation, forced sterilizations, HeLa cells from Henrietta Lacks, and othering).[4] Across all these levels, both upstream and downstream, racism intersects with and influences a woman's lifelong experience of chronic toxic stress, weathering, and epigenetic memory. Ultimately, its impact manifests in adverse maternal health outcomes.

Foster Truth, Reconciliation, Racial Healing, and Transformation

Advancing maternal health equity requires truth, reconciliation, racial healing, and transformation. Silence and complicity are no longer options. We must foster cultural humility and cultural responsiveness and embrace empathy in our shared collective humanity. We must use our power, privilege, influence, and access to name, to acknowledge, and to dismantle systemic, social, and structural inequities that perpetuate disadvantage. We must not be afraid to step outside of our comfort zones in speaking truth to power when encountering instances of bias, prejudice, and microaggressions. We must advocate for our patients, those who are voiceless and disempowered and who possess the lived experience of bias and racism in healthcare. Patients must be enabled to seek care congruent with race, ethnicity, gender, culture and/or language as they desire, and we must normalize patients' self-advocacy in questioning providers' practices. In doing so, we will nurture safe, inclusive environments anchored in trust, empathy, dignity, and respect.

Training, Research, and Education in Health Systems: Implications for Maternal Health
Training

African Americans represent 13% of the US population yet comprise only 5.4% of the country's medical professionals, of which only 2.8% are African American women (0.8% of whom were full professors at US medical schools in 2020).[5] Over the course of nearly 50 years, representation of BIPOC health professionals has not advanced, while studies have cemented the advantages of racially concordant care. Given the underrepresentation of BIPOC health professionals in medicine, academic training institutions must prioritize recruitment, retention, and promotion of BIPOC faculty, who will become the mentors, role models, and care providers for BIPOC learners and patients. Nurturing and sustaining pipeline programs should be anchored in mentorship through longitudinal learning opportunities that also support financial incentivization models for the learners (scholarships, stipends, travel/housing support for elective clinical rotations, and so on). Workforce development must embed training on antiracism, implicit bias, and cultural competency that is rooted in a deep understanding of the historic legacies of slavery and the role of SDOH in the persistence of maternal health inequities. Antiracist frameworks should be operationalized at the individual, interpersonal, and institutional levels through iterative trainings across all administrative leaders, administrative staff, ancillary staff, clinical support staff, faculty, and learners. Such trainings should provide for self-reflection that allows the individual to challenge assumptions and biases; to consider cultural, racial, and gender power hierarchies; and to consider patient–provider interactions, both verbal and nonverbal. These trainings should also be easily accessible as online, enduring educational materials. Safe spaces should also be created that anonymize the reporting of instances of bias, discrimination, racism, and/or microaggressions by providers, staff, and patients without fear of repercussion, thereby cultivating a culture of inclusive excellence.[6]

Patient and Community Engagement Models

As the largest public safety net healthcare system in Arizona and the only public teaching hospital in the state, Valleywise Health (VH) serves a vital role in educating and training healthcare professionals and caring for diverse, medically underserved, and underrepresented communities. VH has a teaching hospital for learners from four area medical schools and trains residents from across critical primary care fields of medicine. In addition to the hospital system, VH has multiple behavioral health centers, comprehensive health centers, and community health centers, such as the Refugee Women's Health Clinic (RWHC), which was founded in 2008 and is anchored in eliminating health disparities and structural barriers to care. Cultural competency training in refugee women's health, including sexual health and maternity care, is offered to provider staff as well as students, residents, and fellows in training across the health and social science professions. In the 14 years since its inception, the RWHC has expanded to include refugee pediatrics and family medicine clinics and serves over 16,000 patients from more than 60 countries using a novel cultural health navigator (CHN) model to enhance health literacy, to mitigate the digital divide, to address SDOH, and to empower refugees to navigate complex healthcare ecosystems. The robust team of multilingual and bicultural CHNs streamlines patient navigation and care coordination in the health system and across the refugee community, stakeholders, and partners. Through this model, the RWHC has cultivated trusted relationships with, and improved health outcomes among, some of the most marginalized, vulnerable, underserved, underrepresented, and hard-to-access populations in Arizona, including newly arrived refugees from sub-Saharan Africa, Southeast Asia, and the Middle East. Through its Refugee Women's Health Community Advisory Coalition, VH has nurtured long-standing community partnerships through a consortium of refugee community stakeholders that represent the patient populations served. These voices directly inform the clinical, programmatic, and research directions of refugee health services.

Examples of Community-Based Participatory Research Training Models

Multiple national programs train healthcare professionals from across all fields of medicine and public health to advance health equity, policy, and population health. The programs listed have a long track record of success in building critical skills in community-based participatory research.

- National Clinician Scholars Program (nationalcsp.org)
- RWJF Culture of Health Leaders–Robert Wood Johnson Foundation
- Commonwealth Fund Fellowship in Minority Health Policy–Harvard University
- Duke Margolis Center for Health Policy

At RWHC, a multilingual staff includes refugee women who themselves serve as CHNs and, as certified medical interpreters, speak up to 18 languages fluently and facilitate an integrated team-based approach to healthcare delivery. These CHNs possess a shared, lived experience of forced displacement and are embedded in the fabric of their respective communities. They facilitate an integrated team-based model of healthcare delivery that involves intensive care coordination, community outreach and education, and intensive case management that engenders trust and empowers women toward enhanced health literacy and self-efficacy in navigating the healthcare system. This facilitates their journey to economic self-sufficiency, health, and wellness for themselves, their children, and their families.

The RWHC is the first clinic of its kind in Arizona to pilot a value-based model of maternity care with a major Medicaid health plan (Mercy Care). CHNs are the cornerstone of this initiative, whereby they assist refugee women in securing access to care, trust-building, navigating the healthcare system, scheduling interpretation services, obtaining behavioral health screenings and other referrals, enhancing health literacy, complying with medical visits, organizing transportation, accessing community outreach and education, and minimizing loss to follow-up. Preliminary analyses of obstetrical outcomes among refugee women insured by Mercy Care demonstrate improved maternal and perinatal outcomes and quality of care, as well as cost savings along such key quality indicators as emergency room use, hospital readmission rates, birth weight, and early initiation of prenatal care. These findings provide clear justification for scaling up value-based healthcare delivery models that integrate CHNs as part of the critical healthcare workforce to advance health equity for vulnerable and marginalized communities across the state and nation.

Advancing Institutional Advocacy

Over the last decade, there has been an increase in proposed policies, both at the national and state level, that address racial disparities in maternal health.[7] Although few of these proposals have become law, recently introduced legislation, such as the federal Momnibus act, offers a promising outlook for eliminating persistent gaps in health outcomes for birthing persons. Given the wealth of learning and engagement opportunities that exist in academic health systems, the systems are both uniquely and favorably positioned to influence policies that promote maternal health equity.

Academic health systems can support federal and regional efforts by creating and/or joining existing coalitions that address critical aspects of maternal health, some of which are:

- Extended Medicaid coverage and innovative payment models
- Mandated evaluation of hospital quality-improvement efforts
- Development of mechanisms for capturing and reporting patient experience data—particularly pertaining to respectful care—given the role that bias and discrimination play in exacerbating disparities[8]

Policy development, proposals, support, and implementation must be informed by institutions as well as the communities they serve. Ensuring that community voices are represented across the spectrum of pregnancy and childbirth is a critical component of institutional advocacy. Maternal health is a cornerstone of community health; in addition to seeking out, amplifying, and centering the voices of birthing persons, advocates must also account for the perspectives of families and community members. Academic health systems must be trustworthy pillars of their communities to effectively inform and advocate for policy. Furthermore, they need to be accessible, meaning there should be bidirectional communication between the broader service population that works for both parties. Partnering with community members to develop, execute, and evaluate maternal health equity initiatives is not enough. When there are opportunities to influence policy—such as federal requests for information or public comment—health systems should ensure that communities not only participate but also affirm awareness, applicability, and usefulness.

Another realm of expertise that academic health systems can engage in service of maternal health equity is multisector partnerships. Various sectors of society—including transportation, education, housing, and criminal justice—are directly connected to SDOH. Alliances between academic health systems and these sectors can enhance advocacy for policies that promote maternal health and strengthen related policy proposals. These alliances capture a broader range of expertise and insights about the many factors outside of clinical care that affect maternal health outcomes. For example, if a hospital learns that many of its pregnant patients walk to a bus stop to catch a bus to their doctor's visit but there are few sidewalks in the neighborhood, the hospital can enlist the local department of public works to address the safety issue.

The suggestions below are a few practical steps academic health systems can take to leverage multisector partnerships for advocacy on matters that affect maternal health equity.

- Review the latest Community Health Needs Assessment to identify potential policy needs/priorities both within and beyond the healthcare sector.
- Take inventory of existing hospital partnerships with organizations in different sectors.
- Develop strategies to enhance or diversify partnerships, particularly with governmental agencies, such as local or state departments of health, education, transportation, and housing and community development.

Institutional advocacy is an investment of time, energy, and financial/human resources. Academic health systems will be unable to optimize their role in the maternal health policy space without buy-in from health system leadership. Entities in an academic health system that already are involved in advocacy efforts will need to make the case for scaling up those efforts with support from outcomes data, hospital partners, and relevant projections, such as cost–benefit analyses and health impact assessments (formal critiques of proposed or existing policies to determine how they may harm or promote health). If an academic health system is truly committed to maternal health equity and health equity at large, C-suite leadership must actively support infrastructure that enables robust advocacy for structural and systems-level changes that protect the health of all pregnant and birthing persons.

Ensuring Sustainability

Like any other aspect of healthcare, optimal health for birthing persons, mothers, and babies requires a mindset of continuous improvement. Promising interventions must be implemented with an eye toward sustainability and with a focus on evaluation to monitor gaps in care and to ensure that target outcomes are achieved. While resources and cost are central to many discussions about sustainability, other critical factors include partner buy-in, adaptability, and long-term outcomes. Engaging partners, designing adaptable interventions, and measuring long-term outcomes are important elements in efforts to improve maternal health.

The importance of partner engagement has become more apparent to researchers and public health practitioners over the last several decades. Still, while the terms *community engagement, community-based participatory research*, and *patient-centered research* are now familiar, not many people do these things well or at all. True sustainability cannot be achieved without designing interventions that consider the perspectives and the unique circumstances of the subjects of the intervention as well as the intended implementers of the intervention. Hospital administrators, doctors, midwives, and other members of the care team as well as birthing persons, mothers, fathers, and other family members are important partners in maternal health. Outside the health system, organizations that touch women anywhere along their perinatal care journey should be considered, including home-visiting programs, doulas, and organizations focused on social needs like housing, food, and transportation. Partner engagement must be intentional and rooted in mutual trust. The Principles of Trustworthiness developed by the AAMC is a suite of tools and resources that academic medical centers and their partners can use to build relationships based on trust. Partner groups can take the form of community advisory boards, and they often begin with a core group who then identify additional relevant partners. The trustworthiness principles emphasize valuing the knowledge that diverse partners bring to the table as well as meaningful and long-term engagement with the issues at hand. In the case of maternal health, proposed interventions should consider the cumulative experiences that contribute to maternal health before, during, and after pregnancy and allow adequate time to understand and incorporate stakeholder-driven solutions.

Adaptability is another key element for designing sustainable interventions to improve maternal health. In this context, adaptability refers to tailoring an intervention to the local context while still achieving the desired outcomes. Because of their local knowledge, partners can play an important role in adaptability. This and similar roles allow partners to actively participate in designing an intervention and enhance trust. Adaptability considers the resources required to implement an intervention and alternatives that could be used to achieve similar results. One must consider diverse settings where interventions may be implemented as well as diverse circumstances in which participants may find themselves. Importantly, one must consider how to ensure that interventions endure beyond a brief trial period or limited funding opportunity. Academic medical centers are uniquely positioned to function in this capacity, given their traditional community focus. Pilot programs are useful for assessing adaptability of interventions in addition to providing results that can be used to advocate for further funding and investment. For example, Nurse–Family Partnership is an evidence-based program with benefits that include higher patient satisfaction and reduced infant mortality. Implementing this type of program across an entire health system may be costly. However, piloting the program with a few practices can provide useful information for adapting the program workflow and securing funding for program expansion. Pilot programs can easily be implemented as part of ongoing quality improvement initiatives. Technological interventions like health apps may also provide opportunities for academic–private partnerships to test novel technologies that address barriers to optimal maternal health.

Plans for data collection and evaluation should accompany any program implementation and are necessary for ensuring sustainability. Partners should agree on outcomes that matter both in the short term and in the long term. Identifying key measures using standard definitions allows results to be tracked over time and compared with peer groups. The Alliance for Innovation on Maternal Health has identified several care bundles and associated outcome measures that can be adopted and tracked in various settings. These include obstetric hemorrhage, severe hypertension in pregnancy, and primary cesarean delivery. Other relevant metrics for partners include program participation and patient satisfaction. Logic models that provide a visual representation of program activities and outcomes are a useful tool for outlining activities and reasonable outcomes that proceed from those activities. Data sources for evaluation may include existing quality-improvement dashboards or dedicated databases for tracking maternal health outcomes. Community Health Needs Assessments are another source of data to identify community trends that affect maternal health. Partnering with trained evaluators will ensure that data are analyzed objectively and that conclusions about program outcomes can be adequately supported by program data.

REFERENCES

1. Crenshaw K. Demarginalizing the intersection of race and sex: a Black feminist critique of antidiscrimination doctrine, feminist theory and antiracist politics. *U Chi Legal F*. 1989;1:Article 8.

2. Johnson-Agbakwu CE, Manin E. Sculptors of African women's bodies: forces reshaping the embodiment of female genital cutting in the West. *Arch Sex Behav*. 2020;50(5):1949–1957. https://doi.org/10.1007/s10508-020-01710-1.

3. Hollenbach SJ, Thornburg LL, Glantz JC, Hill E. Associations between historically redlined districts and racial disparities in current obstetric outcomes. *JAMA Network Open*. 2021;4(9):e2126707. doi:10.1001/jamanetworkopen.2021.26707.

4. Washington HA. *Medical Apartheid: The Dark History of Medical Experimentation on Black Americans from Colonial Times to the Present*. New York: Doubleday Books; 2006.

5. Bajaj SS, Tu L, Stanford FC. Superhuman, but never enough: Black women in medicine. *Lancet*. 2021;398(10309):1398–1399. https://doi.org/10.1016/S0140-6736(21)02217-0.

6. Johnson-Agbakwu C, Ali N, Oxford, C, Wingo S, Manin E, Coonrod D. COVID-19: racism, COVID-19 and health inequity in the US: a call to action. *J Racial Ethnic Health Dispar*. 2020;9(1):52–58. https://doi.org/10.1007/s40615-020-00928-y.

7. Carvalho K, Kheyfets A, Maleki P, et al. A systematic policy review of Black maternal health-related policies proposed federally and in Massachusetts: 2010–2020. *Front Public Health*. 2021;9:664659. doi:10.3389/fpubh.2021.664659.

8. Crear-Perry J, Hernandez-Cancio S. Saving the lives of moms and babies: addressing racism and socioeconomic influences. National Partnership for Women and Families and National Birth Equity Collaborative. https://www.nationalpartnership.org/our-work/resources/health-care/saving-the-lives-of-moms-and.pdf. Published August 2021.

Chapter 43

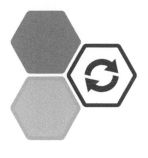

Building a Maternal Health Workforce to Advance Equity, Partnerships, and Healthy Communities

AMY J. MULLENIX AND M. KATHRYN MENARD

INTRODUCTION

Maternal healthcare clinicians provide services for individuals before, during, and after pregnancy. Public health professionals are charged with a broader agenda to promote an environment in which "all people can achieve their full potential for health and well-being across the lifespan."[1] Medical and public health workforces, together with community partners, comprise a national maternal health workforce, striving to produce healthy and equitable outcomes for maternal populations.

While maternal health professionals across the country share a common commitment to improving outcomes and decreasing disparities, the insufficient number of professionals in the field is a challenge. A second key challenge is the lack of racial and ethnic diversity in the workforce. Finally, the uneven distribution of providers across geographic regions makes it difficult to ensure underserved communities can access high-quality services. However, the COVID-19 pandemic demonstrated that workforce deployment does not have to be static. Careful attention to appropriate workforce recruitment, development, deployment, and retention can lead to robust support for maternal health populations. Strategic partnerships with community professionals can enhance systems and care.

This chapter touches on critical workforce systems and skills needed to ensure that equity remains centered in workforce initiatives. It is recognized that a myriad of clinical, community, and public health professionals contribute

Amy J. Mullenix and M. Kathryn Menard, *Building a Maternal Health Workforce to Advance Equity, Partnerships, and Healthy Communities* In: *The Practical Playbook III*. Edited by: Dorothy Cilenti, Alisahah Jackson, Natalie D. Hernandez, Lindsey Yates, Sarah Verbiest, J. Lloyd Michener, and Brian C. Castrucci, Oxford University Press.
© de Beaumont Foundation 2024. DOI: 10.1093/oso/9780197662984.003.0043

to maternal health outcomes. In addition, other professionals, such as social workers, behavioral and mental health professionals, lactation consultants, dietitians, and many others, support the health of women and birthing people throughout the life course. The focus of this chapter is prenatal care providers, nurses, doulas, and maternal and child health (MCH) public health professionals in local and state health departments. The chapter also offers ideas about how effective partnership with community-based organizations and community health workers (CHWs) can bolster equity and the workforce itself.

Four primary mandates related to maternal workforce development thread throughout the practical strategies in this chapter: recruit and grow diverse talent, ensure the maternal health workforce is adequately prepared, collaborate across disciplines and integrate community voices, and continue innovating in service delivery.

CURRENT STATE OF THE WORKFORCE

Clinical Workforce

Geographic Distribution and Maternity Deserts

High-quality maternity care requires the development, distribution, and retention of a diverse, culturally responsive workforce that can meet the ever-changing needs of the birthing population. The 2020 March of Dimes report "Nowhere to Go: Maternity Care Deserts Across the U.S." describes maternity care deserts as counties in the United States in which access to maternal healthcare services is limited or absent.[2] Key points include that 8% of births nationwide occur in counties with limited or no maternity hospitals and obstetric care providers. The geographic distribution of maternity care hospitals and birth centers reflects the provider distribution, leaving women and birthing people in rural counties with less access to both providers and birthing facilities. The maldistribution of resources can contribute to inequities in pregnancy outcomes. According to the Centers for Disease Control and Prevention (CDC) Pregnancy Related Mortality Ratio (PRMR) data from 2011 to 2016, large metro counties had the lowest PRMR (14.8/100,000 live births) and rural counties had the highest (24.1).[3]

In the United States, most babies are born in a hospital (98.4%) with the birth attended by a physician.[2] Approximately 1 in 10 births are attended by a certified nurse midwife (CNM) (9.4%) or other type of midwife (0.8%). Births to American Indian/Alaska Native people are more likely to be attended by a CNM (19.7%), compared to 11.2% for non-Hispanic whites, 9.4% for Hispanic births, 8.4% among Black births, and 8.0% of births to Asian/Pacific Islander people. There has been an intentional effort to incorporate CNMs into the Indian Health Service, as historical American Indian values and practices align with midwifery care.

Access to subspecialty care for high-risk pregnancies and conditions is particularly challenging for people living in rural counties. Maternal–fetal medicine specialists and medical subspecialists tend to reside and work near subspeciality care facilities, and nearly all maternal, neonatal, and critical care units are concentrated in urban areas, some only blocks from one another. While most women of reproductive age live within 50 miles of a critical care facility, there are substantial differences across the United States.[4]

Supply and Demand Projections

In addition to examining the current geographic distribution of maternal healthcare providers, projections for the future overall supply and demand of the workforce can inform workforce strategies. While the assessment was not specific to maternal health, in June 2021, the Association of American Medical Colleges (AAMC) released an assessment of the capacity of the nation's future physician workforce to meet expected demands projected to 2034. Considering an estimated population growth of 10.6%, with a 42.4% growth in the number of people over 65, two in five currently active physicians will be of traditional retirement age (65 or older) within the next decade. The estimated shortage of primary care physicians is expected to be between 17,800 and 48,000. The shortage across nonprimary specialties is projected to be between 21,000 and 77,100.[5]

Appreciating the gender-specific needs of the birthing population, the National Center for Health Workforce Analysis (NCHWA) monitors trends. In March of 2021, the NCHWA released a report of projections for 2018 to 2030.[6] The report compares 2018 supply to projected supply and demand in 2030 for obstetrician/gynecologists (OB-GYNs), CNMs, certified midwives (CMs), nurse practitioners (NPs), and physician assistants (PAs) specialized in women's health and describes the role of family medicine in delivery of women's gender-specific care, assuming similar use patterns. In this analysis, considering the projected age distribution in 2030, the demand for women's health services is projected to increase by 4%.

- Based on current utilization patterns, demand for OB-GYNs is projected to exceed supply by 5,170 Full-Time Employees (FTEs) (expected decrease in FTEs by 7% due to retirement trends, work hours, and relatively fixed number of training programs). This estimate is inclusive of all OB-GYNs, including those who do not practice obstetrics.
- The number of CNM/CMs is expected to grow by 3,120 (32%) based on current level of annual new entrants. Applying current utilization patterns, supply will exceed demand by 2,690 FTEs.
- The women's health NP supply is projected to grow by 89% and PA supply by 56%. If utilization patterns are unchanged, supply for women's health NPs and PAs will exceed demand by 9,750 FTEs.

The adequacy of supply in number and type of provider varies by region. The Northeast currently has, and is projected to continue to have, an OB-GYN supply that exceeds demand, while the West, South, and Midwest are projected to have deficits. OB-GYN supply in metropolitan counties is currently sufficient to meet demand (106%), but by 2030 is projected to decline to 95% in metropolitan counties and 51% in rural areas, perpetuating challenges for rural residents. Nonmetropolitan counties have about twice as many CNM/CMs and four times as many PAs as metropolitan areas. The relative representation of nonphysician women's health providers is projected to increase significantly over time.[6] These providers are well suited to provide services related to uncomplicated pregnancy and childbirth. The declining OB-GYN supply may require a shift in these physicians' practices, increasing their focus on high-risk pregnancies, management of complex gynecological conditions, and surgical procedures.

Family medicine physicians have a prominent role in delivery of women's health services, particularly in rural areas. While primary care physicians may provide gender-specific services, such as birth control, cancer screening, and management of chronic conditions during pregnancy, family physicians are uniquely trained to provide obstetric care, with a skill set that overlaps those of OB-GYNs and CNM/CMs. Given their broad skill set, family medicine physicians are especially well suited to provide prenatal care and to attend births in sparsely populated settings because they can attend to the totality of the family's needs. When considering whether to provide obstetric care or not, family physicians can strategically collaborate with other maternal health professionals in a given community to build a well-coordinated maternal health system. With telehealth now a prominent feature of medical care, intentional collaboration among family physicians, OB-GYNs, midwives, doulas, and CHWs can produce effective systems of care.

Workforce Diversity

The AAMC maintains statistics on the diversity of the practicing physician workforce and medical applicants. They define "underrepresented in medicine" as racial and ethnic populations underrepresented in the medical profession relative to their numbers in the general population. While 2020 US census data indicates that 18.5% of the population identifies as Black,[7] in a 2018 AAMC survey, only 5.8% of active physicians and 8.4% of medical school applicants identified as Black.[8] In 2020, 1.3% of the US population identified as American Indian/Alaska Native.[7] Only 0.3% of active physicians and 0.2% of medical school applicants identified as American Indian/Alaska Native.[8] Workforce diversity statistics specific to women's health physicians and advanced practice providers are not abundant, but the AAMC Minority Physicians Database for 2014 indicated that OB-GYNs had the highest proportion of underrepresented minority (URM) physicians, 11.1% Black and 6.7% Hispanic.[9] URM OB-GYNs were more likely than whites or Asians to practice in areas with high poverty levels or in federally funded underserved areas.

Nurses (RNs), certified medical assistants (CMAs) and certified nursing assistants (CNAs) can play a key role in diversifying the workforce to reflect the communities they serve. Every two years, the National Council of State Boards of Nursing and the National Forum of State Nursing Workforce Centers conduct a survey of a sample of the entire US RN workforce.[10] In the 2020 survey, nearly 81% reported being white/Caucasian, 7.2% Asian, 6.7% Black/African American, and 0.5% American Indian/Alaska Native, while 5.6% reported Hispanic or Latinx ethnicity. National workforce data on CMAs and CNAs are not readily available.[10]

The active presence of community maternal health professionals, such as CHWs and doulas, is likely to advance equity for several reasons: The professionals are often members of the local community and reflect its values. They are culturally fluent and trusted by the community. They often serve as effective liaisons between community groups and more traditional clinical and public health workforces. They are often more racially and ethnically diverse than traditional maternal health professionals, and they increase the overall number of maternal health providers in a given community.

CHWs are known by many names, including promotoras, tribal community health representatives, community health advocates, outreach counselors, and navigators. CHWs were formally recognized in the Affordable Care Act as a resource for achieving the law's "triple aim" of improving care, improving population health, and reducing healthcare costs. In 2010, the Bureau of Labor Statistics implemented a national occupational code for CHWs that states that CHWs "assist individuals and communities to adopt healthy behaviors" through outreach, information and resource sharing, data collection, and provision of services, such as first aid or health screenings. Since that time, many states have begun credentialing and building payment structures to formally add CHWs to the health workforce. This is a key area of collaboration between health systems and public health, because public health can often support the policy changes required to build this workforce.

A doula is a nonclinical professional birth assistant who provides physical, emotional, and informational support to a mother during pregnancy, childbirth, and the postpartum period. Doulas often provide guidance and support around pregnancy health, continuous labor support, and guidance on breastfeeding and newborn care. Attention to physical comfort measures, emotional reassurance, and facilitation of effective communication with the hospital staff are among the services provided by a doula. Studies indicate that birthing people who receive continuous labor support are less likely to have medical intervention during delivery and are more likely to have a satisfying birth experience.[11]

There is a growing appreciation that increased access to doula care in low-income and underresourced communities can reduce the impact of social determinants of health by mitigating barriers like reduced health literacy and language and cultural barriers. In many areas of the United States, access to care by a doula is limited. While there is no reliable estimate of the number of doulas in the United States, a centralized online registry had over 10,000 registered doulas in 2020. Services are often not covered by insurance, which financially limits the growth of the culturally diverse workforce and leaves those who may benefit most without this support.

In addition to the maternity care professionals mentioned above, other providers who serve this population play a critical role in bolstering the maternal health workforce: mental health professionals, social workers, dietitians, WIC professionals, and many others contribute to the constellation of professionals who support maternal health populations.

MCH public health professionals are responsible for a wide range of programs, from prenatal care services in local health departments to oversight for state maternal mortality review committees. These public health professionals sometimes serve as a bridge between traditional clinical systems and local communities, a role that is necessary and unlikely to be filled by others, especially on regional or state levels. The public health workforce is severely understaffed. A 2021 analysis of public health workforce needs found that state and local government public health departments need an 80% increase in their workforce (80,000 additional full-time employees) to provide an adequate infrastructure and a minimum set of public health services to the nation. This includes 6,500 MCH professionals.[12] In addition to the sheer number of new professionals required, the field also continues to deepen its focus on addressing inequities in outcomes and partnership with local communities, requiring a workforce with nuanced skills in systems integration and community collaboration.

PRACTICAL STRATEGIES TO ENHANCE WORKFORCE CAPACITY AND CENTER EQUITY

Due to persistent inequities in maternal health outcomes, local, state, and federal agencies have responded by promulgating policies and allocating resources that support maternal health interventions. These welcome resources have presented opportunities for innovation and expansion of the maternal health workforce. The practical strategies described here represent just a fraction of the innovation possible in workforce development to support maternal health. Above all, the field as a whole must act with intention and alignment to build, rebuild, and support a maternal health workforce that is responsive to the needs of families across the country.

The practical strategies in this section cover a broad range of approaches and highlight workforce strategies that are most likely to address geographic and racial/ethnic inequities. As described elsewhere in this book, the reason for focus in these areas is that maternal health inequities are most pronounced in rural areas and among communities of color. While the individual programs described below can address the challenges described earlier in the chapter, for recruitment and retention of maternal health professionals in high-need areas, a strategic approach that includes multiple programs or strategies is likely to be more sustainable and effective.[13]

It has long been recognized that increasing the diversity of the workforce can have significant implications for improving healthcare delivery. Diversity in the workforce can increase access to care among minority and socioeconomically disadvantaged populations, improve adherence in healthcare with better opportunity for having a race-concordant provider, increase trust in the healthcare delivery system, and improve leadership and advocacy for programs for underserved populations.

The pipeline and professional education strategies described below are organized into the following areas:

- Youth programs: Programs that expose young people to maternal health career opportunities
- Undergraduate programs: Incentives and support programs for undergraduate students who want to pursue maternal health careers
- Graduate/residency programs: Incentives and support programs for graduate and residency programs in maternal health workforce.

Youth Programs

Programs that expose young people to the plethora of public health and medical career opportunities have been well documented and have served to build a pipeline of incoming potential students. (The Area Health Education Program discussed in Chapter 48 is an excellent example.)

> ### Box 43.1 | Medical Schools Building Their Own Pipelines
>
> In some cases, medical schools have chosen to build their own pipeline programs in an effort to increase their diversity and local representation. Tufts University School of Medicine's pipeline program has followed its mission of "growing a workforce equipped with the knowledge and skill needed to address the range of health challenges facing an increasingly diverse population and their communities" for over a decade. The Tufts program has supported Pipeline Programs for minority students interested in medicine and biomedical sciences. The program begins by identifying youth in middle and high school with an early interest, then offering informative courses and support that follow the students through college. Currently, over half of the medical student body identifies as nonwhite (https://medicine.tufts.edu/administration/multicultural-affairs).

Undergraduate Programs

There are several types of programs and incentives that can nurture undergraduate students who are interested in maternal health careers. Academic institutions have traditionally supported interest in health professions via their pre-professional student associations. Undergraduate learning communities can be an effective strategy for encouraging underrepresented minority students. In particular, identifying and supporting interested undergraduates who grew up in rural areas are especially important because a rural background is a strong predictor of future rural practice for physicians.

Many opportunities already exist that can be used to intentionally build the maternal health pipeline in underserved areas (Table 43.1). These strategies generally apply to both clinical and public health professionals. To grow both workforces, educational institutions and funders like HRSA can strategically focus on recruiting underrepresented individuals as a way to increase diversity in the workforce and to build more communities in which the maternal health workforce looks like the population it serves. Beginning in 2022, the Public Health AmeriCorps added a $400 million dollar investment, over five years, to

---

Box 43.2 | Leverage the Reproductive Justice Movement

In recent years, the reproductive justice movement has taken flight on college campuses across the country. Designing learning communities among students interested in reproductive justice and more traditional pre-med students on campuses can open additional opportunities to ground students' interest in health inequities early in their careers, while simultaneously exposing students interested in reproductive justice to the plethora of career opportunities that exist in clinical, community, or public health practice.

Box 43.3 | Build the Doula Workforce through Credentialing

Increasing training, support, and capacity development for doulas, particularly from racially, ethnically, culturally, geographically, and socioeconomically diverse communities, may prove to be an important strategy to improve birth outcomes and reduce maternal morbidity and mortality among women of color in the United States. Many states have moved to credential doulas as a first step toward reimbursement of their services through insurance. This has followed a similar pattern as the credentialing of community health workers, which may provide lessons for doula certification.

Table 43.1	Funding Opportunities for Maternal Health Workforce Development and Diversifying the Workforce	
Program	Description	Additional Information
For Students and Professionals		
Title V MCH Internship Program	Provides future MCH professionals (graduate and undergraduate students) with experience working in state and jurisdictional Title V agencies, with mentorship and guidance from Title V agency preceptors.	https://mchwdc.unc.edu/ Funder: HRSA's Maternal Child Health Bureau
National Health Service Corps	Supports primary care physicians and other healthcare professionals who have dedicated themselves to working in underserved, rural, and Tribal areas located in health professional shortage areas. Offer scholarships and loan repayment.	https://nhsc.hrsa.gov/
Public Health Americorps	Develops a new generation of public health leaders who are ready to respond to the public health needs of the nation by providing public health service in communities. AmeriCorps members serve primarily in state, local, Tribal, and territorial public health departments or in service to public health departments.	https://americorps.gov/ funding-opportunity/ fy-2022-americorps-state-national-public-health-americorps
Health Career Connections (HCC)	Provides opportunities to students of color and organizations hosting interns to help increase diversity in healthcare professions. HCC is a national nonprofit that inspires and empowers undergraduate students, recent graduates, and HCC alumni, particularly those from under-represented or disadvantaged backgrounds, to choose and successfully pursue authentic healthcare and public health careers.	https://www. healthcareers.org
Diverse Executives Leading in Public Health (DELPH)	Increases and strengthens participants' visibility and exposure in public health systems, access to key networks, and leadership development opportunities. Program participants are selected from experienced public health professionals who self-identify from an underrepresented group, including people of color, people with disabilities, women, and LGBTQ+ individuals.	https://www.astho.org/ topic/leadership-and-workforce-development/ delph/

(continued)

Table 43.1 Continued

Program	Description	Additional Information
For Educational Institutions, States, and Organizations		
Nursing Workforce Diversity Program	Increases nursing education opportunities for people from disadvantaged backgrounds.	https://www.hrsa.gov/grants/find-funding/HRSA-21-020
Teaching Health Center Graduate Medical Education (THCGME) Program	Supports residency training for future primary care physicians and dentists in community-based ambulatory care settings in rural and underserved areas.	https://bhw.hrsa.gov/funding/apply-grant/teaching-health-center-graduate-medical-education
Area Health Education Centers (AHEC)	Develops and enhances education and training networks in communities, academic institutions, and community-based organizations. In turn, these networks seek to increase diversity among health professionals, broaden the distribution of the health workforce, enhance healthcare quality, and improve healthcare delivery to rural and underserved areas and populations.	https://www.hrsa.gov/grants/find-funding/HRSA-22-053
Community Health Worker and Paraprofessional Training Program (CHWPTP)	Trains community health workers and paraprofessionals to provide public health emergency response and to address the public health needs of underserved communities.	https://www.hrsa.gov/grants/find-funding/HRSA-22-124
State Loan Repayment Program	Provides cost-sharing grants to states and territories, allowing them to operate their own loan-repayment programs. Programs must repay loans to primary medical, mental/behavioral, and dental healthcare clinicians. These clinicians must be working in Health Professional Shortage Areas (HPSAs) (https://bhw.hrsa.gov/workforce-shortage-areas/shortage-designation#hpsas).	https://nhsc.hrsa.gov/loan-repayment/state-loan-repayment-program

enable the recruitment, training, and development of a new generation of public health leaders who are ready to respond to the public health needs of the nation by providing public health service in communities. AmeriCorps members serve primarily in state, local, Tribal, and territorial public health departments or in service to public health departments.

Graduate/Residency Programs

Medical schools also have a role to play through their selection and scholarship processes. To address the projected shortage of obstetricians in rural and other underserved areas, providing advanced training for those interested in rural health is an essential strategy for growing the rural health workforce. It is well recognized that physicians who receive some of their training in underserved settings are more likely to practice in those settings.[14] Medical schools and other training programs (such as public health and midwifery programs) can partner with local public health and healthcare systems to provide training opportunities in underserved areas.

Beyond medical school, residency programs often attempt to attract the most academically accomplished medical students. This goal must not supersede the need to train a diverse workforce who will meet the needs of the population. Residency selection should target recruitment of health professionals with ties to, and experience with, the populations served.[15]

Residency program curricula can expose clinical trainees to healthcare delivery in high-need areas through rotations and curricular content tailored to the specific needs of the maternal health populations served. Ample evidence suggests that physicians trained in community-based settings are more likely to practice in those same settings, such as health centers, when they complete their training.[16] Training programs based in urban settings have also successfully included rural experience in their curricula. A number of Rural Immersion programs have been highlighted by the AAMC and can serve as models. The AAMC also has a new Center for Health Equity with a strong maternal health component.

Lifelong Learning and Equity

One clear goal of workforce development initiatives should be that all students and current maternal health practitioners demonstrate a nuanced understanding of maternal health inequities, with particular emphasis on disparate outcomes in communities of color and rural areas. Many workforce development initiatives across the training spectrum have added basic historical information about the origins of racial inequities and the movement of services away from rural areas over time to help learners understand why inequities are present at the individual patient level.

Training Programs Addressing Equity

The Institute of Medicine's 2003 report on unequal treatment described unacceptable variation in the quality of healthcare services provided to individuals of different racial and ethnic backgrounds.[17] A key recommendation was the need to "increase healthcare providers' awareness of disparities" and to

Box 43.4 | Family Medicine Residency Rural Track

The University of North Carolina's family medicine residency has a rural track that includes a longitudinal continuity clinic in a rural federally qualified clinic. In addition, the program includes experience working in a family medicine–directed rural maternity hospital. Trainees experience what it is like to practice obstetrics without obstetricians on site, in consultation with a tertiary care center. This training has the potential to provide them with the confidence needed to include obstetrics as part of their rural setting practice after residency. (Chapter 44 includes extensive information about how family medicine as a discipline can contribute to a robust maternal health workforce.)

Box 43.5 | Financial Incentives

Financial incentives to work in underserved areas should not be overlooked as a critical strategy for building the maternal health workforce. Table 43.1 offers examples of several programs that offer financial incentives for maternal health professionals who choose to work in an underserved area in return for educational financial aid. Undergraduate and medical schools can also actively promote resources that help students finance their educations. For example, the Association of American Medical Colleges (AAMC) offers resources on how to finance medical education (https://students-residents.aamc.org/applying-medi cal-school/pay-medical-school-through-service) through the completion of service requirements.

"integrate cross-cultural education into the training of all current and future health professionals." The report emphasized that lecture series were not sufficient, and that longitudinal curricula should be implemented, beginning in the preclinical years and carried through the clinical years, allowing points for active reflection. The AAMC has collated resources for health professionals and makes them available on their Anti-racism in Medicine Collection within MedEdPORTAL, which provides educators with practice-based, peer-reviewed resources to teach antiracist knowledge and clinical skills, elevates the educational scholarship of antiracist curricula, and aims to convene a community of collaborators dedicated to the elimination of racism in medical education.

Teaching about Racism

There are also examples of public health programs strengthening content related to racism, cultural competence, and rural health inequities. One course developed at the University of North Carolina at Greensboro teaches graduate-level public health students to name structural racism in their professional practice, to understand how it operates, and to collaborate for action. Key elements of the curriculum include use of the book *The Color of Law* as a means to understand racism as a structure, use of the Harvard Case Teaching Method, incorporation of local community health and nonprofit organizations' voices into the course, and engagement with minority-owned nonprofits to allow for practice applying the knowledge and skills learned in the course.[18]

Opportunities for synergy exist between clinical and public health training programs with mutual interest in maternal health. For example, clinical training programs can improve understanding of maternal health inequities by partnering with schools of public health to add population health data analysis skills to their curricula.

Professional Equity Education

In addition to clinical training programs, professional organizations are also playing an important role in promoting an awareness of, and providing strategies to undo, racism. In August of 2020, a consortium of professional organizations engaged in obstetrics and gynecology education and practice released a joint statement, "Obstetrics and Gynecology: Collective Action Addressing Racism," which professes their sustained commitment to guiding their organizations and their membership through needed change.[19] One example is that for the 2021 Maintenance of Certification exam (taken by every American Board of Obstetrics and Gynecology-certified obstetrician and gynecologist in the country), all clinicians were required to view a one-hour video training about implicit bias. Similarly, in the public health realm, a plethora of equity resources are available to current practitioners through the American Public Health Association.

There are current initiatives in many states across the country to fund and disseminate implicit bias training for practicing maternal health professionals via the Maternal Health Innovation grants sponsored by the Maternal and Child Health Bureau, the March of Dimes, and other organizations.

People with Lived Experience as Teachers

For current practitioners, one often-overlooked resource is local community organizations. These groups can be the "lead teachers" about what maternal health equity looks like in a given location. In some places, geographic access will be the dominant concern. In other communities, disparate outcomes by race will be the leading challenge named by community members. These concerns often surface in the periodic community health needs assessments performed by healthcare and public health systems but can be brought to life in authentic partnerships with local community-based organizations, who can teach maternal health professionals about their reality and how they think practitioners can support improvements. Many local community-based organizations have deep knowledge of their communities and passion to improve them, but they often lack the capacity (or knowledge about) funding opportunities that are frequently accessed by local health systems. By joining forces, traditional workforce programs and local community-based organizations can improve their individual efforts to advance the workforce capacity of maternal health professionals.

In addition to local groups, maternal health professionals charged with workforce capacity-building can also reach out to national organizations to make connections. One example is MoMMA's Voices. This national coalition of patient organizations and individuals is the first-ever maternal health patient-advocacy coalition. Their goal is to amplify the voices of those

Box 43.6 | The EMBRACe Model

EMBRACe (Equity for Moms and Babies Realized Across Chatham) is a community coalition based in rural Chatham County, North Carolina. It is an effective model for engaging community members in improving maternal health and healthcare through system and service alignment. EMBRACe is led by community members and includes representation from Chatham Hospital, the UNC Family Medicine Department, the Chatham County Health Department, the Chatham County Department of Social Services, and Piedmont Health Services, the local federally qualified health center.[i] The group is facilitated by members with commitment, knowledge, and experience in work to advance health equity by engaging communities and building equitable partnerships and processes. Initially funded through the Robert Wood Johnson Foundation, this outcomes-focused initiative launched out of an ongoing effort to work collaboratively across sectors to address root causes of the county's most pressing health disparities. With funding, the group was able to complete a mixed-methods equity assessment. A popular and ongoing activity that is regularly scheduled is group "story circles." These are facilitated conversations with coalition members, using prompts selected by community representatives. The realities that are revealed in these honest conversations help to shape training and patient-informed changes needed at the public health and clinical service levels.

Reference

i. The Public Health National Center for Innovations. Cross-sector Innovation Initiative Profile: Chatham County Public Health Department (NC). https://phnci.org/uploads/resource-files/CSII-Profile-Chatham-County-Public-Health-Department.pdf. Accessed June 2022.

who have experienced pregnancy and childbirth complications or loss, especially those who have been historically marginalized, and to ensure they are equipped and activated as partners with providers and researchers to improve maternal health outcomes. Family Voices also has local affiliates in every state that can connect people with lived experience to workforce development initiatives.

STRATEGIC SKILLS FOR MATERNAL HEALTH PROFESSIONALS

It is not sufficient to understand history and have knowledge about maternal health outcomes. Ensuring that the workforce is equipped with the strategic skills needed to make change is the next critical step to actually tackling and advancing equity. Particularly for public health professionals charged with improving or supporting the health of entire maternal health populations, strategic skills can boost the workforce's capacity to make change. Many of these skills are also essential for clinical health professionals to thrive in systems-change initiatives related to maternal health. Several iterations of critical "strategic skills" have been described over the past two decades in the public health literature, with the most recent version holding a laser-sharp vision for skills that are most critical to advancing equity.[20]

In 2021, the de Beaumont Foundation published a report titled "Adapting and Aligning Public Health Strategic Skills".[20] The report provides definitions for each of nine strategic skills. They are:

1. Effective Communication
2. Data-Based Decision Making
3. Justice, Equity, Diversity and Inclusion
4. Resource Management
5. Change Management
6. Systems and Strategic Thinking
7. Community Engagement
8. Cross-Sectoral Partnerships
9. Policy Engagement

Strategic skills trainings should engage the maternal health workforce in creative ways, and bringing many types of maternal health professionals together to learn together can advance several goals at once. Training opportunities can be used as trust-building activities that lead to further collaboration between community organizations and public and clinical healthcare groups in local communities. People with lived experience from local community organizations can provide context and wisdom about how these skills can improve their communities.

RETAINING AND SUPPORTING THE EXISTING WORKFORCE

Collaboration as a Retention Strategy

Given the insufficient numbers of maternal health clinicians in many communities, retaining and supporting the current maternal health workforce is a critical strategy. Several studies have concurred that the "community culture" of the local community, defined as "open, helpful and supportive of healthcare professionals," is essential in attracting and retaining healthcare professionals.[21] To translate this into a concrete strategy, employers should highlight the friendliness of local people, the relationships between professionals and the hospital, and the ability of community groups and other healthcare professionals to collaborate. In essence, offering ongoing opportunities for maternal health providers to collaborate within the community can help retain them in local health systems.

One workforce implication of this finding is that many groups in a given local community—beyond the employer—should collaborate to recruit and retain the maternal health workforce in their community. This can be a key role for community members who are already engaged in, and committed to, improving maternal health outcomes in their own community. Collaborations between hospital systems and local public health and community organizations can produce authentic and thriving maternal health workforces, even in small, rural communities. The strategic skills described above can be jointly learned and applied across all types of maternal health providers to advance equity and to improve outcomes. Other maternal health training opportunities might also be undertaken across silos in a local community, further building knowledge, trust, and skills. While on the surface community engagement may not seem like an obvious recruitment/retention strategy for clinical professionals, many factors contribute to their satisfaction, and collaboration across silos is likely to have additional benefits to the community as well as increasing the chances that providers will stay in a given area.

Another strategy to support and retain the existing workforce is to offer and to fund ongoing professional development that helps professionals of all types feel connected to their peers in other locations and to stay abreast of emerging trends in maternal health. All clinical and public health professionals have professional membership organizations that offer annual conferences and training. HRSA and their funded partners offer many opportunities for professionals to participate in maternal health webinars and other continuing education activities. State agencies often offer learning opportunities via their state perinatal quality collaboratives. The Maternal Health Learning and Innovation Center (MHLIC) offers free resources related to maternal health topics and a free national annual symposium.

Reimagining Service Delivery

Another approach to workforce retention is to reimagine how some services are provided entirely. Many examples exist; the three described here are perinatal regionalization, telehealth, and an emerging community model.

Perinatal Regionalization

Perinatal regionalization provides a formal infrastructure for the provision of risk-appropriate maternal care, similar to systems established for neonatal care. To standardize system integration, resources and capabilities of birthing facilities are categorized as basic (Level I), specialty (Level II), subspecialty (Level III), and regional perinatal health centers (Level IV). The higher-level facilities support the Level I and II hospitals through outreach education and quality improvement and receive patients in need of advanced resources in transfer. A shared understanding of the capacity and resources available in the facilities in the region and a system for seamless communication and referral can help ensure that pregnant and postpartum individuals are cared for by the provider type and facility that best meets their needs.

Telehealth

Telehealth educational programs, such as Project ECHO, and direct patient care through telemedicine can increase access to subspecialty consultation. Telehealth has emerged as a powerful means of supporting providers and their patients residing in rural or otherwise underserved areas. Policy changes enacted in response to the COVID-19 pandemic enabled rapid expansion of telemedicine in most states. In the past, growth in telehealth has been limited by high start-up cost, limited Internet access in rural areas, inconsistent reimbursement requirements across different insurance plans, and state-to-state variation of professional licensing regulations. Many of these barriers were overcome out of necessity during the COVID-19 pandemic, illustrating a clear path to continued provision of this important service.

Pregnancy Care ECHO

Pregnancy Care ECHO, based at the University of Utah, leverages technology-enabled collaborative learning to help address specialty-care health concerns in the primary care setting. The premise is to bring knowledge to the rural community rather than requiring rural community members to travel long distances to receive subspecialty care. Specialist teams comprised of several disciplines conduct weekly or biweekly sessions with community providers via videoconference. The

---

Box 43.8 | High-Risk Pregnancy Care via Telehealth

The University of Arkansas for Medical Sciences (UAMS) was a pioneer in design and implementation of telehealth. Formerly referred to as ANGELS, the UAMS High-Risk Pregnancy Program now links clinicians and patients from across the state with UAMS, where most of the state's high-risk and specialty maternal health providers are located.[i] Providers and patients around the state can access real-time telehealth consultation with a variety of specialists. The program also develops and disseminates guidelines for obstetric best practice and facilitates referrals to the medical center through a patient/provider call center.

Reference

i. Institute for Digital Health & Innovation, University of Arkansas for Medical Sciences. High-Risk Pregnancy Program. https://idhi.uams.edu/high-risk-pregnancy-program/#:~:text=The%20High%2DRisk%20Pregnancy%20Program%20mission%20is%20to%20ensure%20that,a%2024%2F7%20call%20center. Accessed June 2022.

Box 43.9 | Maternal Health Services via Telehealth

One example of a local adaptation of the UAMS concept is Vidant hospital in Greeneville, North Carolina, which serves as the regional perinatal center for 29 counties in eastern North Carolina. In July of 2020, they launched a telemedicine program whereby experts can remotely treat high-risk patients in collaboration with local obstetricians. The program, MOTHeRS (Maternal Outreach through Telehealth for Rural Sites), not only addresses medical and obstetric complications of pregnancy, but also screens for social factors, such as food insecurity and mental health concerns, and provides support and services as needed.

The Vidant regional perinatal center also provides support to their referring hospitals through training and simulations. In small rural hospitals with 300 to 400 deliveries annually, obstetric emergencies like eclampsia and severe postpartum hemorrhage are infrequent events. To ensure that the staff are prepared for the infrequent event, the regional perinatal center providers travel to the community hospital to assist with simulations and drills in emergencies like hemorrhage, eclampsia, and shoulder dystocia.

provider groups together discuss specialized healthcare topics, and community providers present patient cases to determine the best treatment options. This case-based learning has improved patient health outcomes and provider confidence.

The collaboration and partnership strategies described above can also lead to innovative service-delivery systems in which community engagement is the essential ingredient of the innovation. In this emerging model, local strengths serve as the starting point for strategic planning efforts, which then build wraparound services, including maternal health services, in each community based on the community's partnership and input. A recent National Academy of Medicine commentary describes a new conceptual model to support assessment of health equity in transformed or transforming systems via community engagement.[22]

These practical strategies for building and maintaining a diverse and strategically skilled workforce, along with innovative service-delivery approaches, can advance equity in maternal health outcomes. With continued collaboration and commitment, the maternal health workforce can build on and accelerate broader societal efforts to ensure equity for all maternal health populations.

SUMMARY/CONCLUSION

This chapter provides an overview of the current state of the maternal health workforce and projections for the workforce of the future, as well as practical strategies, strategic skills, and innovative service delivery. The essential takeaways are shown in Figure 43.1.

Figure 43.1 ▼
Key strategies for developing the maternal health workforce.

Recruit and grow diverse talent
Grow, with intention, the diversity of the workforce to advance equity
Recruit diverse talent by starting early and providing incentives to achieve the desired outcome of a geographically and racially diverse workforce.
Ensure the maternal health workforce is adequately prepared
Actively support, elevate, and integrate the breadth of the maternal health workforce, leveraging their diverse expertise to more effectively provide holistic care for families.
Ensure that the public health workforce has the strategic skills necessary to support systems integration and cross-sector collaboration and then serves in the role of convener and bridge to advance health equity.
Ensure that maternal health professionals access ongoing personal development opportunities to advance their equity practice, including learning from and with community members and organizations.
Collaborate across disciplines and integrate community voices
Be strategic, particularly in underresourced communities, about how the maternal health workforce collaborates to best meet the needs of the community served.
Leverage collaboration in support of rural communities to advance adequate distribution of the maternal health workforce.
Continue innovating in service delivery
Reimagine services by applying innovative technology and community perspectives to expand access to risk-appropriate care and services.

REFERENCES

1. US Department of Health and Human Services, Office of Disease Prevention and Health Promotion. *Healthy People 2030*. https://health.gov/healthypeople. Accessed June 15, 2022.

2. March of Dimes. Nowhere to go: maternity care deserts across the U.S. https://www.marchofdimes.org/research/maternity-care-deserts-report.aspx. Published 2020. Accessed June 15, 2022.

3. Centers for Disease Control and Prevention. Pregnancy Mortality Surveillance System. https://www.cdc.gov/reproductivehealth/maternal-mortality/pregnancy-mortality-surveillance-system.htm#urban-rural. Accessed July 4, 2022.

4. Brantley MD, Davis NL, Goodman DA, Callaghan WM, Barfield W. Perinatal regionalization: a geospatial view of perinatal critical care, United States, 2010–2013. *Am J Obstet Gynecol*. 2017;216(2):185.e1. https://doi.org/10.1016/j.ajog.2016.10.011.

5. IHS Markit Ltd. *The Complexities of Physician Supply and Demand: Projections From 2019 to 2034*. Washington, DC: AAMC; 2021.

6. US Department of Health and Human Services, Health Resources and Services Administration, National Center for Health Workforce Analysis. *Projections of Supply and Demand for Women's Health Service Providers: 2018–2030*. Rockville, MD: Health Resources and Services Administration & US Department of Health and Human Services; 2021.

7. US Census Bureau. Improved race and ethnicity measures reveal U.S. population is much more multiracial. https://www.census.gov/library/stories/2021/08/improved-race-ethnicity-measures-reveal-united-states-population-much-more-multiracial.html#:~:text=The%20largest%20Multiracial%20combinations%20in,Other%20Race%20(1%20million). Published 2020. Accessed July 4, 2022.

8. Association of American Medical Colleges. Diversity in medicine: facts and figures 2019. https://www.aamc.org/data-reports/workforce/report/diversity-medicine-facts-and-figures-2019. Accessed July 4, 2022.

9. Rayburn WF, Xierali IM, Castillo-Page L, Nivet M. Racial and ethnic differences between obstetrician–gynecologists and other adult medical specialists. *Obstet Gynecol*. 2016;127(1):148–152.

10. Smiley RA, Ruttinger C, Oliveira CM, et al. The 2020 national nursing workforce survey. *J Nurs Reg*. 2021;12(1):S1–S96.

11. Gruber KJ, Cupito SH, Dobson CF. Impact of doulas on healthy birth outcomes. *J Perinat Educ*. 2013;22(1):49–58. doi:10.1891/1058-1243.22.1.49.

12. de Beaumont Foundation. Staffing up: workforce levels needed to provide basic public health services for all Americans. Research brief. October 2021. https://debeaumont.org/wp-content/uploads/2021/10/Staffing-Up-FINAL.pdf.

13. Rural Policy Research Institute. Health Panel report: access to rural health care—a literature review and new synthesis. 2014. https://rupri.org/2014/08/10/access-to-rural-health-care-literature-review-and-new-synthesis/.

14. McWillistrem-Evenson A. Informing rural primary care workforce policy: what does the evidence tell us? 2011. https://www.ruralhealthinfo.org/assets/1145-4634/informing-rural-primary-care-workforce-policy.pdf.

15. Martinsen K. Goodman M. Case study: state innovations in training In: Michener JL, Castrucci BC, Bradley DW, et al, eds. *The Practical Playbook II: Building Multisector Partnerships That Work*. New York, NY: Oxford University Press; 2019.

16. Talib Z, Jewers MM, Strasser JH, et al. Primary care residents in teaching health centers: their intentions to practice in underserved settings after residency training. *Acad Med*. 2018;93(1):98–103. https://pubmed.ncbi.nlm.nih.gov/28834845/.

17. Institute of Medicine, Committee on Understanding and Eliminating Racial and Ethnic Disparities in Health Care. *Unequal Treatment: Confronting Racial and Ethnic Disparities in Health Care*. Smedley BD, Stith AY, Nelson AR, eds. Washington, DC: National Academies Press; 2003.

18. Rosario C, Al Amin S, Parker C. [Un]forgetting history: preparing public health professionals to address structural racism. *J Public Health Manag Pract*. 2022;28(suppl 1):S74–S81. doi:10.1097/PHH.0000000000001432.

19. American College of Obstetricians and Gynecologists. Joint statement: collective action addressing racism. https://www.acog.org/news/news-articles/2020/08/joint-statement-obstetrics-and-gynecology-collective-action-addressing-racism#:~:text=Within%20the%20specialty%20of%20obstetrics,free%20from%20racism%20and%20bias. Published 2020.

20. de Beaumont Foundation. Adapting and aligning public health strategic skills. March 2021. https://debeaumont.org/strategic-skills.

21. MacDowell M, Glasser M, Fitts M, Nielsen K, Hunsaker M. A national view of rural health workforce issues in the USA. *Rural Remote Health*. 2010;10(3):1531.

22. National Academy of Medicine, Organizing Committee for Assessing Meaningful Community Engagement in Health & Health Care Programs & Policies. Assessing meaningful community engagement: a conceptual model to advance health equity through transformed systems for health. https://nam.edu/assessing-meaningful-community-engagement-a-conceptual-model-to-advance-health-equity-through-transformed-systems-for-health/. Published February 14, 2021. Accessed June 15, 2022.

Chapter 44

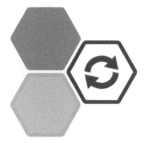

The Role of the Family Physician in Pregnancy Care: Striving for Birth Equity and Reducing Maternal Morbidity and Mortality

JULIE K. WOOD

Approximately 700 people die from pregnancy-related complications annually in the United States.[1] Among the maternal deaths for which timing is known, 31.3% occur during pregnancy, 16.9% occur the day of delivery, 18.6% occur one to six days postpartum, 21.4% occur one week to 42 days postpartum, and 11.7% occur 43 days to one year postpartum.[1] Data from 13 state maternal mortality review committees from 2013 to 2017 indicated that more than 60% of pregnancy-related deaths were preventable.[1] Many other individuals suffer pregnancy-related complications that do not result in death but place their health at significant risk. The leading causes of pregnancy-related morbidity and mortality include hemorrhage, infection, cardiovascular conditions, preeclampsia and eclampsia, and embolism.[1,2]

In 2018, the maternal mortality rate in the United States was 17.4 deaths per 100,000 live births, more than double the rate of every other country in the developed world.[2] The rate is significantly higher for pregnant people age 40 and older (81.9 per 100,000 live births) and people of color. At 37.1 deaths per 100,000 live births, the maternal mortality rate for non-Hispanic Black people in the United States is more than double that of non-Hispanic white people (14.7) and more than three times the rate for Hispanic people (11.8). These reported rates notably exclude maternal deaths that occur more than 42 days postpartum, which represent 11.7% of all maternal deaths, according to the Centers for Disease Control and Prevention.[2]

Many of the disparities that exist in maternal morbidity and mortality are exacerbated by other social determinants of health. Closure of rural hospitals

Julie K. Wood, *The Role of the Family Physician in Pregnancy Care* In: *The Practical Playbook III*. Edited by: Dorothy Cilenti, Alisahah Jackson, Natalie D. Hernandez, Lindsey Yates, Sarah Verbiest, J. Lloyd Michener, and Brian C. Castrucci, Oxford University Press. © de Beaumont Foundation 2024. DOI: 10.1093/oso/9780197662984.003.0044

and obstetrics programs has led to rapidly decreasing access to prenatal and perinatal services for pregnant people living in rural communities—a threat that, unfortunately, continues to grow. Gaps in insurance coverage and availability of affordable care for people with low incomes also increase the risk of morbidity and mortality, particularly during the postpartum period.

According to the Accreditation Council for Graduate Medical Education (ACGME),

> Nearly one-third of U.S. women who are pregnant report having received care from a family physician in the previous year. Family physicians regularly provide prenatal care, labor and delivery care, and postpartum care as well as primary care before and after pregnancy to people who are among those most vulnerable to maternal morbidity and mortality, including Medicaid beneficiaries, people of color, low-income families, and rural residents. Therefore, family physicians have a unique role and opportunity to support improvements in maternal health.[3]

FAMILY MEDICINE EDUCATION AND TRAINING

All family physician residents in an accredited family medicine residency program receive core training in maternity care. Specifically, "residents must demonstrate competence in their ability to provide maternity care, including distinguishing abnormal and normal pregnancies, caring for common medical problems arising from pregnancy or coexisting with pregnancy, performing a spontaneous vaginal delivery, and demonstrating basic skills in managing obstetrical emergencies." Some residencies and/or maternity care fellowships offer additional training in high-risk maternity care and may include surgical maternity care.[4]

At the time of this writing, ACGME is anticipated to update requirements for family medicine residency programs that will affect pregnancy care training for family physicians. A core minimum required training experience is expected to continue for all family medicine residents to establish comprehensiveness of care and competency as a family physician. In addition, for those family physicians planning to incorporate comprehensive pregnancy care into their practice, additional training, curriculum, and continuity requirements are expected.

At a summit held to re-envision family medicine education and consider changes to the family medicine residency training guidelines overall, a written commentary by Barr regarding maternity care training stated that:

> Maternity care continues to be a defining and essential feature of our specialty. No other specialty cares for the mother–baby dyad throughout the perinatal period and no other specialty routinely provides comprehensive primary care for women. If our society and the healthcare system want to

address the inequities in health outcomes, particularly for rural and BIPOC [Black, Indigenous, and people of color] women, we must embrace this challenge and train the next generations of family physicians to provide this care.[4]

Beyond training, maternity care provided by family physicians is not a one-size-fits-all approach and varies widely by state. Levels of care depend on the individual needs of the patient and the availability of services in the community. Family physicians have historically provided maternity care, especially in rural and underserved populations. Family physicians provide delivery services and, in some rural areas, may provide 100% of maternity care. In fact, approximately 26% of family physicians working in rural communities in 2020 delivered babies as part of their scope of practice, more than three times the number of their urban counterparts.

AMERICAN ACADEMY OF FAMILY PHYSICIANS TASK FORCE ON MATERNAL MORBIDITY AND MORTALITY

Understanding family physicians' potential to improve pregnancy-related health outcomes, the American Academy of Family Physicians (AAFP) convened a Task Force on Maternal Morbidity and Mortality based on action taken by the AAFP's policymaking body, the AAFP Congress of Delegates. This task force brought together multiple stakeholders both to inform the Academy's efforts to decrease maternal morbidity and mortality as well as to determine areas of potential collaboration.

Participating organizations included the AAFP (representing 133,500 family physicians, residents, and medical students), American College of Obstetricians and Gynecologists (ACOG), National Rural Health Association, American College of Nurse Midwives, American Hospital Association, Society of Teachers of Family Medicine, and Association of Departments of Family Medicine, who met to address the following objectives:

- To evaluate evidence-based methods to decrease maternal morbidity and mortality
- To review methods to increase recognition of implicit bias and reduce disparities in maternal morbidity and mortality
- To develop strategies to improve resident education and support practicing family physicians in providing maternity care
- To address the growing loss of rural obstetric services across the nation

Recommendations from the task force were presented to the AAFP's board of directors and to the AAFP Congress of Delegates in 2019. These recommendations shaped the AAFP's actions and policies around maternal morbidity and mortality and resulted in a position paper describing the findings and recommendations, "Striving for Birth Equity: Family Medicine's Role in Overcoming Disparities in Maternal Morbidity and Mortality."[5]

The paper's Call to Action (see Box 44.1) outlines what actions family physicians, educators, and policymakers can take.

Box 44.1 | Call to Action from the American Academy of Family Physicians Position Paper "Striving For Birth Equity: Family Medicine's Role in Overcoming Disparities in Maternal Morbidity and Mortality"

Family physicians have a vested interest in policies and practices that advance the health of their patients and their communities. Several structural and institutional barriers to achieving better outcomes and equity in maternal morbidity and mortality exist, and solutions must be actionable and supported by broad-based policy changes. As medical experts and trusted members of their communities, family physicians can serve as effective agents in facilitating and advocating for change.

Actions Family Physicians Can Take

- Learn about the effects of implicit bias and develop an action plan for addressing personal biases
- Work in a rural community to provide obstetrical services or partner with other clinicians providing obstetrical services in rural communities
- Identify and encourage continuing medical education and other training opportunities on topics like patient safety bundles, implicit bias, and health/birth equity
- Participate in a local maternal health review committee
- Advocate for policies to increase birth equity within their practice and the hospital system, including the standardization of mandatory data collection and reporting
- Advocate for Medicaid expansion, payment parity and postpartum coverage to increase access to care for patients across their reproductive life course

Actions Educators Can Take

- Learn about the effects of implicit bias and develop an action plan for addressing personal biases
- Develop best-practice guides to help family physicians retrain and gain privileges to provide obstetric care[5]
- Support family medicine preceptorship programs for medical students and advocate for funding to expand opportunities into rural communities
- Advocate for the funding of additional graduate medical education opportunities for family physicians and obstetricians to train in rural communities[6]

> **Box 44.1 | Continued**
>
> *Actions Policymakers Can Take*
> - Learn about the effects of implicit bias and develop an action plan for addressing personal biases
> - Advocate to expand Medicaid coverage and to extend coverage of mothers to one year postpartum and to provide adequate reimbursement for obstetric services
> - Advocate for the expansion of current loan-repayment programs or incentives, including the National Health Service Corps and the federal Public Service Loan Forgiveness Program, to obstetric care providers, such as family physicians, OB-GYNs, certified nurse-midwives, labor and delivery nurses, and community health centers
> - Advocate to allow rural obstetric care providers, and potentially rural hospitals, to be eligible for Federal Tort Claims Act medical malpractice liability protection

EVIDENCE-BASED METHODS TO DECREASE MORBIDITY AND MORTALITY

The AAFP supports dissemination, participation, and use of evidence-based tools, such as the Alliance for Innovation on Maternal Health (AIM) maternity safety bundles, and regularly collaborates with ACOG and other key stakeholders to further this program. AAFP is a partner of the AIM Community Care Initiative (AIM CCI), which focuses on opportunities to prevent maternal morbidity and mortality by making available to community partners, women, and families education and safety bundles for the nonhospital setting. Family physicians are well positioned to inform the AIM CCI initiative, which is built on an equity framework, and to assist with implementation in their communities. In addition, the AAFP calls for standardization of data collection and reporting on maternal mortality and encourages family physician participation and perspectives on maternal mortality review committees, as their unique experience of continuing care for mothers, babies, and families provides invaluable perspective.

BARRIERS TO, AND ACTIONS FOR ACHIEVING, EQUITY IN MATERNAL MORBIDITY AND MORTALITY

The AAFP recognizes that the root causes of racial and ethnic disparities in maternal morbidity and mortality are institutional racism, implicit bias, and social inequities, and it has declared racism a public health crisis. One of the first actions after the task force completed its work was to implement "Striving for Birth Equity," a policy that states:

The AAFP recognizes that significant disparities exist in the rates of maternal morbidity and mortality, with higher rates occurring among Black women, women who have a low income, and women living in rural areas. According to data from the Centers for Disease Control and Prevention's Pregnancy Mortality Surveillance System (PMSS), between 2007 and 2016, the maternal mortality rate for Black women was 40.8 deaths per 100,000 live births. This is more than three times the rate for white women, which was 12.7 deaths per 100,000 live births.

The AAFP also recognizes that the root causes of racial and ethnic disparities in maternal morbidity and mortality are institutional racism in the healthcare and social service delivery system and social and economic inequities. Family physicians are well positioned to address these root causes as they are trained to provide comprehensive care, including prenatal, perinatal, and postpartum care for women in the communities in which they live.

The AAFP defines birth equity as the assurance of the conditions of optimal births for all people with a willingness to address racial and social inequalities in a sustained effort. The AAFP recommends educating physicians about inequities in maternal morbidity and mortality and supports strategies that integrate birth equity into the delivery of family-centered maternity care.[6]

IMPLICIT BIAS TRAINING

The AAFP and its Center for Diversity and Health Equity support physician education and development by creating and disseminating health-equity-focused education and practice tools that are based on evidence and align with accepted educational standards. In 2020, the AAFP released its *Implicit Bias Training Guide* (https://www.aafp.org/dam/AAFP/documents/patient_care/health_equity/implicit-bias-training-participant-guide.pdfrlink?) for use by members and other healthcare professionals. The training has also been expanded to AAFP state chapters to facilitate dissemination and implementation of training across the country. The primary goal of this training is to promote awareness of implicit bias among all members of the healthcare team and to provide resources for mitigating the negative effects of implicit bias on patient care.

Training activities include self-assessments, application of skills to case-study examples, small-group discussions, and development of an implementation plan. The training format incorporates both online modules and in-person activities. Learning objectives of the training include:

- To increase self-awareness by reflecting on the results of the implicit bias self-assessment
- To demonstrate conscious mitigation strategies to overcome implicit bias

- To apply implicit bias reduction skills to case-study examples
- To understand the effect of implicit bias on real-life patients

HEALTH EQUITY EDUCATION FOR FAMILY PHYSICIANS

In 2021, the AAFP partnered with the American Board of Family Medicine to implement "Health Equity: Leading the Change," a series of modules focused on health effects of disparities and solutions family physicians can use in vulnerable populations. These modules provide continuing medical education to assist with maintaining board certification.

The AAFP Center for Diversity and Health Equity continues to provide information to physicians and practices via the EveryONE Project Toolkit to address social needs, including practice tools, and the Neighborhood Navigator, to help patients locate resources in their communities.

There also are needs and opportunities to increase diversity in the pregnancy care workforce, and particularly among family physicians, who often provide care to vulnerable populations. A 2021 study by Eden et al determined that family physicians of color were less likely to include pregnancy care in their practices. The authors concluded, "A diverse and racially/ethnically representative maternity care workforce, including family physicians, may help to ameliorate disparities in maternal and birth outcomes. Enhanced efforts to diversify the family physician care workforce should be implemented."[7] This is vital information to consider as the new ACGME maternity care training guidelines are finalized.

RURAL DISPARITIES AND OPPORTUNITIES

Current trends in hospital and obstetric unit closures will widen rural health disparities. There have been 135 rural hospital closures in the last 10 years, with an additional 453 facilities that are vulnerable and could close. Of the rural hospitals that remain, 54% do not offer maternity care. Access to OB services is disappearing at the rate of 24 rural hospitals each year. "Significant service deserts are emerging—not just in areas where a hospital has closed"[8]; a rural hospital may stay open, but close its OB unit. Distance to maternity care has a direct impact on outcomes for both pregnant women and newborns.[8] In 2021, Deutchman et al studied the impact of family physicians delivering in rural communities and their absence, noting that "many patients would have to drive an average of 86 miles round-trip to access care if those FPs were to stop delivering." Further, they concluded that family physicians are essential providers of maternity care in the rural United States. Family medicine residency programs should ensure that trainees who intend to practice in rural locations have adequate maternity care training to maintain and expand access to maternity care for rural patients and their families.[9]

EDUCATION ON RECOGNITION AND TREATMENT OF OBSTETRIC EMERGENCIES

The AAFP and ACOG both offer courses to provide education and to build skills focused on recognizing obstetric emergencies. These evidence-based, interprofessional, and multidisciplinary programs train medical staff and first responders through a blend of didactic learning and simulated obstetric emergencies, with a focus on team-based care.

Advanced Life Support in Obstetrics (ALSO®) is an AAFP program that equips the entire maternity care team with skills to effectively manage obstetric emergencies. This comprehensive course encourages a standardized team-based approach among physicians, residents, nurse-midwives, registered nurses, and other members of the maternity care team to improve patient safety and maternal outcomes.

Basic Life Support in Obstetrics (BLSO®) is designed to improve management of normal deliveries, as well as obstetric emergencies, by standardizing the skills of first responders, emergency personnel, and maternity care providers. AAFP's BLSO curriculum is directed at prehospital care providers; first responders and emergency personnel; and medical, nursing, and physician assistant students.

Emergencies in Clinical Obstetrics is an ACOG course that trains healthcare professionals at all levels to work together during obstetric emergencies.

OB READY

The AAFP believes it is vital to increase maternity care readiness for practice teams, first responders, hospitals, communities, and maternity care professionals so that they are "OB Ready." Low-resource hospitals and communities where physicians no longer provide obstetric services need adequate funding and the ability to connect with appropriate healthcare resources to become OB Ready by building competencies in basic and advanced obstetric care.

In addition to training, rural medical professionals and first responders need access to necessary supplies and equipment during obstetric emergencies. This includes basic or prepackaged delivery kits, postpartum hemorrhage kits, and medications for both deliveries and/or common complications. The AAFP is eager to collaborate with public and private stakeholders on ways to further develop and implement the OB Ready concept to better support communities in need.

The AAFP also encourages funding of the implementation and validation of a scalable demonstration OB Ready pilot project to integrate training, supplies, and communication plans with community input and a sustainability plan. It is imperative to concurrently address the upstream issues that create the lack of services while assisting the communities that are struggling with this dire impact.[10]

CONCLUSION

The factors driving the high rates of maternal morbidity and mortality in the United States are complex and highly relevant to the practice of family medicine. Limited access to quality prenatal and postpartum care, which is caused by workforce shortages and closures of rural hospitals and obstetrics programs and is exacerbated by social determinants of health, creates disparities that family physicians are uniquely positioned to address. The AAFP is committed to working with stakeholders across the continuum of healthcare to implement evidence-based strategies aimed at achieving equity in maternal morbidity and mortality. Through continued engagement, learning, and a willingness to confront implicit biases, family physicians can continue to serve as leaders to overcome this critically important public health challenge.

REFERENCES

1. Petersen EE, Davis NL, Goodman D, et al. Vital signs: pregnancy-related deaths, United States, 2011–2015, and strategies for prevention, 13 states, 2013–2017. *MMWR*. 2019;68(18):423–429.

2. Hoyert DL, Miniño AM. Maternal mortality in the United States: changes in coding, publication, and data release, 2018. *Natl Vital Stat Rep*. 2020;69(2):1–18.

3. ACGME. ACGME Program Requirements for Graduate Medical Education in Family Medicine. Accreditation Council for Graduate Medical Education. 2020.

4. Barr WB. Women deserve comprehensive primary care: the case for maternity care training in family medicine. *Fam Med*. 2021;53(7):524–527. https://doi.org/10.22454/FamMed.2021.451637.

5. American Academy of Family Physicians. Striving for birth equity: family medicine's role in overcoming disparities in maternal morbidity and mortality. https://www.aafp.org/about/policies/all/birth-equity-pos-paper.html. Accessed February 9, 2022.

6. American Academy of Family Physicians. Striving for birth equity policy. https://www.aafp.org/about/policies/all/striving-for-birth-equity.html. Accessed February 9, 2022.

7. Eden AR, Taylor MK, Morgan ZJ, Barreto T. Racial and ethnic diversity of family physicians delivering maternity care. *J Racial Ethnic Health Dispar*. 2022;9(4):1145–1151. https://www.chartis.com/insights/crises-collide-covid-19-pandemic-and-stability-rural-health-safety-net.

8. Chartis Center for Rural Health. Crises collide: Covid-19 and the stability of the rural health safety net. https://www.iowawatch.org/wp-content/uploads/2021/02/Chartis-Rural_Crises-Collide-Rural-Health-Safety-Net-Report-Feb-2021-1.pdf. Published 2021. Accessed February 9, 2022.

9. Deutchman M, Macaluso F, Bray E, et al. The impact of family physicians in rural maternity care. *Birth*. 2022;49(2):220–232. https://doi.org/10.1111/birt.12591.

10. Centers for Medicare & Medicaid serivces. Improving access to maternal health care in rural communities. Issue brief. 2019. https://www.cms.gov/About-CMS/Agency-Information/OMH/equity-initiatives/rural-health/09032019-Maternal-Health-Care-in-Rural-Communities.pdf. Accessed February 9, 2022.

Chapter 45

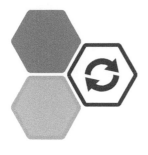

Employing Policy and Advocacy for Sustainable Reduction of Maternal Mortality and Maternal Health Inequities

ANNA KHEYFETS, MARIA GABRIELA RUIZ, KERI CARVALHO, CANDACE STEWART, AND NDIDIAMAKA AMUTAH-ONUKAGHA

BACKGROUND

The Black maternal health crisis has been a consistent focus of the media for the past few years, but sustained progress will be required to eliminate the Black–white racial disparity gap.[1,2] While there are very many new publications, policy proposals in state and national legislatures,[1,3-5] and media attention across the country on this topic, there still is much work to be done for years to come to address structural factors, including structural racism, that cannot be changed within the confines of a single generation. Racism is a significant contributor to poor health outcomes and acts as an obstacle to health equity by affecting birthing individuals both interpersonally and systemically. Systemic racism includes a combination of structures, policies, and norms built into the American healthcare system that contribute to the health disparities that adversely affect birthing people of color.[6,7] Social determinants of health directly correlate to an individual's health outcomes, and these inequities persist throughout the life course.[8] Disparities have been exacerbated by COVID-19 by way of policy changes and barriers to care during the pandemic as well as increased stress for birthing people.[9,10] Black birthing people are two to three times as likely as their white counterparts to die as a result of delivery or pregnancy-related complications.[11] These differences are not due to biology or sociodemographic factors, but can be attributed to the weathering, psychosocial stress, and inequities in healthcare that persist because of systemic racism.

Anna Kheyfets, Maria Gabriela Ruiz, Keri Carvalho, Candace Stewart, and Ndidiamaka Amutah-Onukagha, *Employing Policy and Advocacy for Sustainable Reduction of Maternal Mortality and Maternal Health Inequities* In: *The Practical Playbook III*. Edited by: Dorothy Cilenti, Alisahah Jackson, Natalie D. Hernandez, Lindsey Yates, Sarah Verbiest, J. Lloyd Michener, and Brian C. Castrucci, Oxford University Press. © de Beaumont Foundation 2024. DOI: 10.1093/oso/9780197662984.003.0045

Although the obstacles to equitable maternal healthcare are embedded in the systems that make up American society, there are numerous evidence-based solutions that can be implemented to improve the status quo for Black maternal care and to promote a more equitable health space. The way to achieve systemic change is to modify and implement more advantageous policies. Increasing access to doula care, implementing standardized data collection on maternal and infant deaths, promoting cultural competence, expanding virtual programming, and diversifying the healthcare workforce are policy efforts that can have significant effects on maternal health equity.

POLICY CHANGES TO IMPROVE MATERNAL HEALTH

As part of the effort to reduce racial disparities in maternal morbidity and mortality, the authors put forth a set of six policy recommendations to engender systematic and sustainable health equity improvements.

Invest in Doula Care to Improve Maternal Health Outcomes

Access to, and increased use of, doula care can play a key role in improving maternal health outcomes among Black women. Studies have shown that births assisted by doulas were twice as likely to avoid complications and that mothers were significantly more likely to breastfeed.[12] The Giving Voice to Mothers study found a statistically significant difference in mistreatment reports by race, including reports of "being ignored."[13] Community-based approaches to maternal healthcare help empower birthing individuals by connecting them with local perinatal companions who guide birthing individuals and partners through the entire birthing process.[14] Doulas help mitigate poor maternal outcomes by addressing barriers to care, discrimination, and other social determinants of health.[15] Through the use of doulas, women in marginalized communities can access trusted and empowering resources, including not only support during and after pregnancy but also health literacy, social support, and culturally competent providers.[16]

Doulas offer support in five key areas: agency, personal security, respect, knowledge, and connectedness.[15] They provide clients with a sense of agency and knowledge through empowerment, advocacy, and informational support, and they promote open communication between patient and healthcare provider. Doulas impart the assurance of personal security and connectedness through social and emotional support as well as community-building and being a personal champion.[15] They provide clients with a sense of respect through cultural competence and, in cases where doulas originate from the same community, shared experience.

An important aspect of increasing access to doula care includes insurance reimbursement for doula and other support services, including those provided by midwives, lactation consultants, and community health workers. These reimbursements are essential to ensuring access to respectful, culturally competent care for women of color.[17] Research has shown that covering doula services can reduce costs for state Medicaid programs, because doula care has been found to reduce the risk of preterm birth, cesarean delivery, and their associated costs.[5] Doula care can be made more available to women of color with new policies that allow for service reimbursement via expanded Medicaid and private insurance coverage, as well as accessible doula training programs in communities of color.

Implement a Standardized Data-Collection System on Maternal and Infant Deaths in All States to Enhance Readiness

The Centers for Disease Control and Prevention (CDC) reports that approximately 60% of pregnancy-related deaths between 2011 and 2015 were preventable, highlighting the importance of targeted interventions and improved data-collection methods.[18] Previous research found that relying solely on obstetric codes to identify maternal deaths was insufficient and resulted in inaccurate maternal mortality ratios.[19] In 2018, in response to underreporting of pregnancy-related deaths, the United States adopted a pregnancy checkbox on death certificates.[20] This checkbox gave researchers the ability to classify pregnancy-related deaths more accurately, although concerns regarding quality of the data persisted, and precise reasons for pregnancy-related deaths, especially deaths incidental to pregnancy, cannot be fully determined through use of the checkbox or other improvements in computerized data-collection methods.[20] Poor data collection and monitoring of maternal health issues nationally are contributing to a lack of progress in reducing national maternal mortality rates and the racial disparities that persist.[21]

Data collection needs to be further standardized, including expanding analysis of maternal deaths to include those that were associated with, but not related to, pregnancy. Over 20% of pregnancy and postpartum deaths in this country are attributed to drug-related causes, suicide, or homicide. These deaths often are not included in measures of maternal mortality but are disproportionately prevalent among pregnant and postpartum groups.[22] Data should also be stratified by race and ethnicity to accurately determine the causes behind maternal death and the respective disparities.

While disparities in rates of maternal mortality and morbidity between Black and white women have been identified in the literature, the causes of these gaps are not entirely understood.[3,4] Disparities persist after controlling for socioeconomic factors, insurance, and neighborhood factors.[5,23] Systematic data collection to analyze the impact of structural and interpersonal racism on health outcomes of Black people is lacking, despite recent evidence suggesting racism as a cause of these disparities.[24,25] There is need for a validated measure and the collection of data on experiences of racism, specifically structural racism, across the life course to fully grasp its effects on outcomes like maternal mortality and morbidity.[26]

Establishment of the CDC's "Review to Action" Maternal Mortality Review Information Application (MMRIA) program was one step in improving data collection around maternal deaths.[27] The Preventing Maternal Deaths Act of 2018 sought to address Black maternal health by identifying disparities through improved data collection, including establishment of maternal mortality review committees (MMRC) across the country to systematically document maternal mortalities using the MMRIA program, including deaths that resulted directly from pregnancy and those where the decedent was pregnant or postpartum but the death itself was not caused by the pregnancy.[28] The MMRIA seeks to standardize reporting and analysis of maternal deaths nationally, to identify specific contributing factors, to assess preventability, and to determine recommendations for preventing future maternal deaths. In 2020, a CDC working group added three contributing factors—interpersonal racism, structural racism, and discrimination— to the MMRIA, as well as recommendations for MMRC members to use when these factors were identified as contributing to a maternal death.[7] Future work should assist in identifying racism and discrimination from medical documents in the MMRC process. With systematic analysis of the impact of these factors and identification of the physiological and social causes of maternal deaths, clear ties can be made to evidence-based recommendations that can prevent future mortality. Identifying the causes of the disparities and the maternal deaths themselves through improved data collection would allow specific quality-improvement projects to address factors like structural racism and interpersonal racism. Lack of clear and systematic data can stall progress, especially among those resistant to acknowledging the effects of discrimination in adverse maternal outcomes.

Increase Access to Maternal Health Resources by Expanding Medicaid to One Year Postpartum

Medicaid provides coverage for pregnant women in over 40% of births in the United States.[29] This coverage is mandated to extend to at least 60 days postpartum. However, nearly one-third of maternal mortalities occur between one week and one year postpartum.[18] Furthermore, a retrospective cohort study from a large national commercial claims database found that almost 24% of postpartum women had a problem visit, a visit with a physician other than a scheduled physical or follow-up, compared with 19.7% of age-matched nonpostpartum women; in addition, emergency department visits were more likely among postpartum women.[30] These disparities in healthcare utilization persist beyond 60 days postpartum,[30] suggesting the need for expansion of Medicaid coverage to one year postpartum.[31] Doing so would give mothers access to critical care they might not otherwise receive. In states where new mothers receive Medicaid coverage only through 60 days postpartum, low-income women lose access to affordable maternal health resources.[32] A New York study demonstrated that expanding Medicaid coverage from 60 days to one year postpartum significantly decreased severe maternal morbidity in low-income women.[31] The year after birth is critical for both mother and child: it has been shown that more than 70% of complications, some of which prove fatal, occur during this period.[18]

One tactic for reducing maternal and infant mortality is for the Centers for Medicare & Medicaid Services' Center for Medicare & Medicaid Innovation's aim to develop additional quality-based alternative payment models, which would improve the quality of clinical care for pregnant women and new mothers.[33] Increasing access to coverage through Medicaid would give mothers from rural areas and minority women more resources for preventing maternal mortality. States can apply for a waiver to extend postpartum coverage, but only the federal government can alter the length of postpartum coverage. The American Rescue Plan Act of 2021 established a new state option to extend Medicaid and CHIP (Children's Health Insurance Program) coverage for pregnant women from 60 days to one year after the baby's birth.[34] Currently, 25 states have either implemented a waiver expanding Medicaid coverage to one year postpartum or have announced a plan for implementation.[35] Organizations, including the American College of Obstetricians and Gynecologists (ACOG), are advocating to extend Medicaid coverage nationwide to at least one year postpartum.[36]

Expand Virtual Healthcare Options and Coverage

With the onset of the COVID-19 pandemic, healthcare providers, including perinatal service providers, have increasingly relied on telehealth, or remote care through telecommunications, to reach patients.[37] Given the increased need for telehealth, there have been substantial healthcare policy revisions. Before the pandemic, only 19 state Medicaid programs covered telehealth services, with some reimbursing at a lower rate than for in-person care.[38] As of 2020, all 50 states included coverage for telehealth services in their Medicaid programs.[39] Telehealth is associated with improved maternal outcomes because of better access to specialized care for mothers as well as more frequent prenatal check-ins, particularly among mothers who are otherwise unable to access care.[40] Lack of access to adequate and timely care in maternal health disproportionately affects those in rural areas who experience physical barriers, which may compound other factors that influence access to care.[41] This is especially true in maternal mental health, which has been an issue of particular importance with the emergence of COVID-19. Telehealth fulfills the need to overcome barriers like physical access and points to a solution to the health gap faced by many women, even beyond the pandemic.[42]

Although significant improvements have been made during the pandemic to enhance implementation of virtual health services, there still are problems to be addressed. Notably, evidence suggests that low-income communities, communities of color, and rural communities disproportionately lack telehealth access because of Internet inaccessibility.[43,44] Maternal mortality and severe morbidity are increasing in rural areas due to the challenges patients face that require specific attention, particularly in increasing healthcare access.[45] The urban–rural disparities in maternal mortality and morbidity are associated with the place-based risk inherent in a medically isolated location and are compounded by racial disparities associated with comorbidities, such as hypertension, that disproportionately affect Black and Hispanic mothers.[46]

While telehealth services became more available during the pandemic, telehealth and teletherapy must also be integrated into future care. For example, patients identified with high-risk pregnancies in rural areas where high-risk OB services are not readily accessible can consult virtually with a maternal–fetal medicine specialist. Patients with mental health risks or who report significant psychosocial stressors can schedule telehealth visits with a mental health professional in the immediate area. In addition, while lack of Internet access can be difficult to address, patients should always have the option to obtain virtual care in private spaces.

Incorporate Cultural Competence Training in Health Practice at All Levels to Ensure That Providers Administer Culturally Appropriate Care

Cultural competence training can teach more effective communication, treatment, and advocacy for patients. Cultural competence is defined as the policies, attitudes, and behaviors within a system that enable professionals to work more effectively in cross-cultural settings.[47] Although they are similar, cultural competence should not be confused with cultural congruence, which is the state of effective communication between provider and patient developed through a mutual understanding of the patient's culture that can result in a higher quality of care.[48] Community-based, culturally congruent care has been shown to improve outcomes.[49] A study from 2020 demonstrated that infants who were treated by racially congruent doctors had more positive outcomes, particularly among Black newborns.[50] Not many studies have been conducted to analyze the impact of racial congruence on patient outcomes, and although no significance was found in the improvement of maternal health outcomes in the same conditions, more research needs to be done on culturally congruent care.

Increasing diversity and cultural competence among healthcare practitioners, particularly in women's health, will decrease the biases that can impede delivery and quality of care.[51] Implicit bias can be defined as a set of group-based behaviors that are influenced by indicators of another's social group.[52] Implicit biases are propagated in medical training by standardized exam questions that test students on stereotypically associated disease processes.[53] Implicit bias can be addressed and culturally competent care can be increased by spotlighting the role of the misrepresentation of race in medical school training.[54] These biases are ingrained in students' training and persist as they administer care unless they are given tools to unpack and address the behaviors.[51,55] The responsibility to confront structural racism in medicine lies with medical educators, because they can teach antiracist practices to inform the care future physicians deliver as well as the culture surrounding physicians of color. By recognizing the socialization of race and its distinction from disease processes and genetics, schools can improve cultural competency and help decrease institutional racism among the next generation of physicians. This will increase conversations about structural racism and the patient experience.

Increase Diversity of Medical Professionals

Although there are higher rates of Black and Hispanic OB-GYN professionals than in other categories of medicine (e.g., surgical training),[56,57] Black individuals account for only 5% of medical professionals in the United States overall.[58] Research demonstrates that racial representation in medical settings can significantly mitigate perceptions of racial bias, enhance perceptions of cultural competence, and improve patient outcomes.[57,59] In addition, the experience of medical students can be improved by increasing admission of students underrepresented in the field.[60] As in other educational settings, increased diversity leads to greater satisfaction in educational experiences, an increased sense of community, and heightened cultural awareness.[61] Lack of diversity in the OB-GYN workforce has been found to contribute to poor maternal health outcomes and increased incidence of mistreatment.[49] Increasing diversity in the workforce, training about implicit bias, and other support services will increase access to trusted, culturally competent maternal care services and thus improve outcomes.[62]

EXAMPLES OF SUCCESSFUL POLICY AND PROGRAM IMPLEMENTATION

This section provides examples of successful policies and programs that address disparate maternal health outcomes. By evaluating disparities at the patient, provider, and system levels, policies can be implemented to successfully address the many aspects of health inequity.[8] While over 30 bills were introduced nationally between 2010 and 2020 to address this issue, only two were signed into law.[17] With the support of an array of medical organizations, progress is being made in policy implementation that addresses maternal outcome disparity. The American Rescue Plan Act of 2021 has allowed and incentivized states to expand Medicaid and CHIP coverage for pregnant women up to a year postpartum—although only half of US states have undertaken or indicated plans to implement this expansion.[35] Signed into law in 2021, the Protecting Moms Who Served Act is part of the Black Maternal Health Momnibus Act of 2021, a combination of 12 comprehensive bills introduced by Congresswoman Lauren Underwood, Congresswoman Alma Adams, Senator Cory Booker, and members of the Black Maternal Health Caucus to address the Black maternal health crisis.[63-65] Portions of several other bills from the Momnibus Act have also been included in the proposed Build Back Better Act.[66]

The role of implicit bias among physicians in causing lower quality of care is well documented.[55,67] To address the impact of implicit bias and to improve cultural competency, California passed Assembly Bill 241 in 2021, making California the first state to mandate implicit bias training for physicians, nurses, and physician assistants.[68] The requirement was implemented January 1, 2022, and the impact of this bill on quality of care and health disparities is to be seen.

One federal program that yielded improved maternal health outcomes is the Alliance for Innovation on Maternal Health (AIM). In 2014, the US Department of Health and Human Services funded ACOG to develop AIM to help improve quality and safety of maternal care.[69] Through AIM safety toolkits, state and hospital partners have improved maternal outcomes and decreased maternal morbidity in four states.[70] AIM also developed a conceptual safety bundle to reduce peripartum racial and ethnic disparities, and the bundle is being adapted and implemented in several states, including California, Massachusetts, and Illinois, through their state perinatal quality collaboratives.[71-73]

Quality improvement efforts have been made through various state perinatal quality collaboratives (PQCs), which were made possible by federally funded initiatives, including the Maternal, Infant, and Early Childhood Home Visiting (MIECHV) Program and AIM.[74] Due to recent policy changes and funding opportunities, the number of state maternal care quality collaboratives has substantially increased. According to the CDC, there are 40 states with available PQCs and 10 states with PQC development in progress.[75,76] The California Maternal Quality Care Collaborative (CMQCC) is a locally and federally funded organization designed to end preventable maternal morbidity and mortality. It works in partnership with many public and private agencies, groups, and health systems.[77] Through the use of PQCs and an updated surveillance system (the Maternal Data Center), CMQCC has decreased maternal mortality by 50%.[78]

Several state programs have implemented components from the aforementioned suggested policies. The Postpartum Visit (PPV) Quality Improvement Project in Massachusetts is a Medicaid-driven initiative established to improve postpartum outcomes through the Text4Baby mobile application.[77] The Text4Baby app allows expectant parents to receive information that complements provider resources via text message and relevant articles.[79] Participants in Text4Baby were found to have an 82% increase in health knowledge, 63% increase in appointment attendance, and 65% increase in agency when using the app.[79] A state policy introduced in Minnesota (hard-stop early elective delivery) was enacted to minimize unnecessary pregnancy inductions and thus their associated costs.[77] Keeping medically unnecessary procedures to a minimum can reduce overall costs to states and health systems by thousands of dollars.[80]

The Tampa Bay Doula Program in Florida trains multilingual women in the community to provide doula services in local dialects. The program is also supported by social services to provide more holistic care, including housing stability and nutrition needs.[77] Participation in this program has lessened the need for urgent medical intervention and has increased the duration of breastfeeding.

THE NEXT GENERATION OF HEALTHCARE PROVIDERS

To achieve the ideal of a more equitable future in healthcare, a multipronged approach that addresses the issues of structural racism in the US medical system must be employed. This can be achieved through several strategies, including promotion of diversification of the workforce as well as implementing cultural competence policies in healthcare settings. Physicians are becoming increasingly important advocates for their patients, and thus must be representative of the populations they serve. In addition, increasing awareness of one's own implicit biases is a key component to the future of healthcare.[81,82] Cultural competence requires continuous learning and is only one part of the puzzle. Self-awareness and addressing the biases that inevitably exist in all of us must be practiced in conjunction with the lifetime of learning that comes with cultural competence.

According to the Association of American Medical Colleges, white students still make up the majority of medical students, at almost 50% of all students enrolled, while Black medical students account for about 8%.[83] This is important, given that many studies have demonstrated the benefits of having patient–doctor racial or ethnic concordance for positive patient outcomes.[50,84] A significant barrier to health equity is the lack of trust among many communities of color that results from systemic racism, medical assault, and the unfavorable sociopolitical contexts that permeate the nation's history.[85] Diversifying the field means introducing a greater number of medical, nursing, and physician assistant students of color so that the healthcare space reflects the population it serves. Representation is key for numerous reasons, particularly because it helps practitioners wage the battle against implicit biases, navigate the structural racism that persists in the medical field, improve trust among patients, and nurture the advocacy that can be necessary in patient care.[86]

These future implications are of particular importance in maternal care, where significant racial disparities persist and result in extremely poor patient outcomes. The above strategies for improving the next generation of healthcare providers are evidence-based measures that are essential for improving maternal health outcomes in the United States. Diversification of the maternal healthcare workforce is a crucial strategy for combating current stark disparities, particularly regarding Black maternal health outcomes. Not only do Black mothers experience less mortality and morbidity with Black doctors, but also having a more diverse workforce improves the overall cultural competence of the healthcare space.[57,59] Physician–patient relationships are important components of the success of maternal health because mutual trust is required to ensure the safety of Black birthing people.[87]

Mentorship is instrumental in bringing about a diverse workforce. An example of the role of mentorship in the field of healthcare, specifically in maternal and child health, is MOTHER Lab.[88] Housed in the Tufts University School of Medicine, MOTHER Lab has the specific goals of training and mentoring maternal health scholars of color and white allies and providing a research and training space to ensure that maternal health scholars are supported as they prepare to go into their respective fields to dismantle systemic racism. Labs like these provide a framework for developing advocacy, research, and leadership skills among future providers and public health scholars with an emphasis on growing diversity in the next generation.

The future of maternal healthcare providers is a diverse workforce with an awareness not only of their internalized biases but also of the social determinants that affect patients' health. They are culturally competent and ready to advocate for the well-being of their patients. Improving maternal care is not a one-size-fits-all approach; it requires a multipronged effort to tackle the root causes at play. The strategies to improve Black maternal health outcomes discussed here are essential for the future of the field.

THE ROLE OF ADVOCACY AMONG HEALTHCARE PROVIDERS

There is a growing role for advocacy among healthcare professionals. Advocacy can be accomplished through a variety of mechanisms to push for important legislation to be passed and implemented. There has been a significant increase in proposed legislation to address maternal health disparities over the last decade, and staying abreast of proposed state and national legislation relevant to the Black maternal health crisis is the first step in advocacy.[17] Healthcare professionals can write and present testimony in support of such legislation and contact their local and federal representatives to push for support. Writing op-eds in local papers, magazines, and online to share knowledge and personal experiences about how policy can improve outcomes will help garner more widespread support for these efforts.

REFERENCES

1. Villarosa L. Why America's Black mothers and babies are in a life-or-death crisis. *New York Times*. April 11, 2018. https://www.nytimes.com/2018/04/11/magazine/black-mothers-babies-death-maternal-mortality.html. Accessed January 15, 2022.

2. Martin N. Lost mothers. ProPublica. 2017. https://www.propublica.org/series/lost-mothers. Accessed January 15, 2022.

3. Chinn JJ, Eisenberg E, Artis Dickerson S, et al. Maternal mortality in the United States: research gaps, opportunities, and priorities. *Am J Obstet Gynecol.* 2020;223(4):486–492.e6. doi:10.1016/j.ajog.2020.07.021.

4. Creanga AA, Bateman BT, Kuklina EV, Callaghan WM. Racial and ethnic disparities in severe maternal morbidity: a multistate analysis, 2008–2010. *Am J Obstet Gynecol.* 2014;210(5):435.e1–435.e8. doi:10.1016/j.ajog.2013.11.039.

5. Howell EA, Egorova NN, Janevic T, et al. Race and ethnicity, medical insurance, and within-hospital severe maternal morbidity disparities. *Obstet Gynecol.* 2020;135(2):285–293. doi:10.1097/AOG.0000000000003667.

6. Jones CP. Systems of power, axes of inequity. *Med Care.* 2014;52(10):5.

7. Hardeman RR, Kheyfets A, Mantha AB, et al. Developing tools to report racism in maternal health for the CDC Maternal Mortality Review Information Application (MMRIA): findings from the MMRIA Racism & Discrimination Working Group. *Matern Child Health J.* Published online January 4, 2022;26(4):661–669. doi:10.1007/s10995-021-03284-3.

8. Yearby R. Structural racism and health disparities: reconfiguring the social determinants of health framework to include the root cause. *J Law Med Ethics.* 2020;48(3):518–526. doi:10.1177/1073110520958876.

9. Carvalho K, Kheyfets A, Lawrence B, et al. Examining the role of psychosocial influences on Black maternal health during the COVID-19 pandemic. *Matern Child Health J.* Published online August 21, 2021;26(4):764–769. doi:10.1007/s10995-021-03181-9.

10. Lemke MK, Brown KK. Syndemic perspectives to guide Black maternal health research and prevention during the COVID-19 pandemic. *Matern Child Health J.* 2020;24(9):1093–1098. doi:10.1007/s10995-020-02983-7.

11. Hoyert DL Maternal mortality rates in the United States, 2021. NCHS Health E-Stats. 2023. doi: https://dx.doi.org/10.15620/cdc:124678.

12. Gruber KJ, Cupito SH, Dobson CF. Impact of doulas on healthy birth outcomes. *J Perinat Educ.* 2013;22(1):49–58. doi:10.1891/1058-1243.22.1.49.

13. GVtM-US Steering Council, Vedam S, Stoll K, et al. The Giving Voice to Mothers study: inequity and mistreatment during pregnancy and childbirth in the United States. *Reprod Health.* 2019;16(1):77. doi:10.1186/s12978-019-0729-2.

14. Declercq E, Zephyrin L. Maternal mortality in the United States: a primer. Commonwealth Fund. Published online 2020:14: https://www.commonwealthfund.org/publications/issue-brief-report/2020/dec/maternal-mortality-united-states-primer.

15. Kozhimannil KB, Vogelsang CA, Hardeman RR, Prasad S. Disrupting the pathways of social determinants of health: doula support during pregnancy and childbirth. *J Am Board Fam Med.* 2016;29(3):308–317. doi:10.3122/jabfm.2016.03.150300.

16. DeAngelis T. In search of cultural competence. *Monit Psychol.* 2015;46(3):64. https://www.apa.org/monitor/2015/03/cultural-competence. Accessed January 18, 2022.

17. Carvalho K, Kheyfets A, Maleki P, et al. A systematic policy review of Black maternal health-related policies proposed federally and in Massachusetts: 2010–2020. *Front Public Health.* 2021;9:664659. doi:10.3389/fpubh.2021.664659.

18. Petersen EE, Davis NL, Goodman D, et al. Vital signs: pregnancy-related deaths, United States, 2011–2015, and strategies for prevention, 13 states, 2013–2017. *MMWR*. 2019;68(18):423–429. doi:10.15585/mmwr.mm6818e1.

19. Baeva S, Saxton DL, Ruggiero K, et al. Identifying maternal deaths in Texas using an enhanced method, 2012. *Obstet Gynecol*. 2018;131(5):762–769. doi:10.1097/AOG.0000000000002565.

20. Hoyert DL, Minino AM. *Maternal Mortality in the United States: Changes in Coding, Publication, and Data Release, 2018*. Washington, DC: US Department of Health and Human Services; 2020:18.

21. Nichols CR, Cohen AK. Preventing maternal mortality in the United States: lessons from California and policy recommendations. *J Public Health Policy*. 2021;42(1):127–144. doi:10.1057/s41271-020-00264-9.

22. Margerison CE, Roberts MH, Gemmill A, Goldman-Mellor S. Pregnancy-associated deaths due to drugs, suicide, and homicide in the United States, 2010–2019. *Obstet Gynecol*. 2022;139(2):172–180. doi:10.1097/AOG.0000000000004649.

23. Janevic T, Zeitlin J, Egorova N, Hebert PL, Balbierz A, Howell EA. Neighborhood racial and economic polarization, hospital of delivery, and severe maternal morbidity: an examination of whether racial and economic neighborhood polarization is associated with severe maternal morbidity rates and whether the delivery hospital partially explains the association. *Health Aff*. 2020;39(5):768–776. doi:10.1377/hlthaff.2019.00735.

24. Liu SY, Fiorentini C, Bailey Z, Huynh M, McVeigh K, Kaplan D. Structural racism and severe maternal morbidity in New York State. *Clin Med Insights Womens Health*. 2019;12:1179562X1985477. doi:10.1177/1179562X19854778.

25. Davis DA. Obstetric racism: the racial politics of pregnancy, labor, and birthing. *Med Anthropol*. 2019;38(7):560–573. doi:10.1080/01459740.2018.1549389.

26. Szanton SL, LaFave SE, Thorpe RJ. Structural racial discrimination and structural resilience: measurement precedes change. *J Gerontol Ser A*. Published online December 23, 2021. doi:10.1093/gerona/glab344.

27. Review to Action. Report from nine maternal mortality review committees. 2018:1–76. http://reviewtoaction.org/2018_Report_from_MMRCs. Accessed January 15, 2022.

28. Kaiser Family Foundation (KFF). Analysis of federal bills to strengthen maternal health care. *Womens Health Policy*. https://www.kff.org/womens-health-policy/fact-sheet/analysis-of-federal-bills-to-strengthen-maternal-health-care/. Published December 21, 2020.

29. Medicaid and CHIP Payment and Access Commission (MACPAC). *Medicaid's Role in Financing Maternity Care*. MACPAC; 2020:1–16. https://www.macpac.gov/wp-content/uploads/2020/01/Medicaid%E2%80%99s-Role-in-Financing-Maternity-Care.pdf.

30. Steenland MW, Kozhimannil KB, Werner EF, Daw JR. Health care use by commercially insured postpartum and nonpostpartum women in the United States. *Obstet Gynecol*. 2021;137(5):782–790. doi:10.1097/AOG.0000000000004359.

31. Guglielminotti J, Landau R, Li G. The 2014 New York State Medicaid expansion and severe maternal morbidity during delivery hospitalizations. *Anesth Analg*. 2021;133(2):340–348. doi:10.1213/ANE.0000000000005371.

32. Perleoni A. House Energy and Commerce Subcommittee discusses maternal mortality. Association of American Medical Colleges (AAMC); 2019. https://www.aamc.org/advocacy-policy/washington-highlights/house-energy-and-commerce-subcommittee-discusses-maternal-mortality. Accessed January 18, 2022.

33. Perleoni A. AAMC responds to Senate Committee request for information on maternal health. Association of American Medical Colleges (AAMC); 2020. https://www.aamc.org/advocacy-policy/washington-highlights/aamc-responds-senate-committee-request-information-maternal-health.

34. Ranji U, Salganicoff A, Gomez I. Postpartum coverage extension in the American Rescue Plan Act of 2021. Kaiser Family Foundation (KFF); 2021. https://www.kff.org/policy-watch/postpartum-coverage-extension-in-the-american-rescue-plan-act-of-2021/.

35. Kaiser Family Foundation (KFF). Medicaid postpartum coverage extension tracker. https://www.kff.org/medicaid/issue-brief/medicaid-postpartum-coverage-extension-tracker/. Published January 13, 2022.

36. American College of Obstetricians and Gynecologists (ACOG). Extend postpartum Medicaid coverage. ACOG; 2022. https://www.acog.org/advocacy/policy-priorities/extend-postpartum-medicaid-coverage.

37. Hill I, Burroughs E. Maternal telehealth has expanded dramatically during the COVID-19 pandemic: equity concerns and promising approaches. Urban Institute; 2020:10. https://www.urban.org/research/publication/maternal-telehealth-has-expanded-dramatically-during-covid-19-pandemic. Accessed January 30, 2022.

38. Center for Connected Health Policy (CCHP). State telehealth laws & reimbursement policies: a comprehensive scan of the 50 states & the District of Columbia. The National Telehealth Policy Resource Center; 2020:466. https://cdn.cchpca.org/files/2020-05/CCHP_%2050_STATE_REPORT_SPRING_2020_FINAL.pdf. Accessed January 27, 2022.

39. Augenstein J, Marks JD, Andrade M. Executive summary: tracking telehealth changes state-by-state in response to COVID-19. Manatt on Health; 2022. https://www.manatt.com/insights/newsletters/covid-19-update/executive-summary-tracking-telehealth-changes-stat. Accessed January 30, 2022.

40. Ahn R, Gonzalez GP, Anderson B, Vladutiu CJ, Fowler ER, Manning L. Initiatives to reduce maternal mortality and severe maternal morbidity in the United States: a narrative review. *Ann Intern Med*. 2020;173(11 suppl):S3–S10. doi:10.7326/M19-3258.

41. Madubuonwu J, Mehta P. How telehealth can be used to improve maternal and child health outcomes: a population approach. *Clin Obstet Gynecol*. 2021;64(2):398–406. doi:10.1097/GRF.0000000000000610.

42. Guille C, Johnson E, Douglas E, et al. A pilot study examining access to and satisfaction with maternal mental health and substance use disorder treatment via telemedicine. *Telemed Rep*. 2022;3(1):24–29. doi:10.1089/tmr.2021.0041.

43. Chunara R, Zhao Y, Chen J, et al. Telemedicine and health care disparities: a cohort study in a large health care system in New York City during COVID-19. *J Am Med Inform Assoc*. 2021;28(1):33–41. doi:10.1093/jamia/ocaa217.

44. Weber E, Miller SJ, Astha V, Janevic T, Benn E. Characteristics of telehealth users in NYC for COVID-related care during the coronavirus pandemic. *J Am Med Inform Assoc*. 2020;27(12):1949–1954. doi:10.1093/jamia/ocaa216.

45. Kozhimannil KB, Interrante JD, Henning-Smith C, Admon LK. Rural–urban differences in severe maternal morbidity and mortality in the US, 2007–15. *Health Aff*. 2019;38(12):2077–2085. doi:10.1377/hlthaff.2019.00805.

46. Cameron NA, Molsberry R, Pierce JB, et al. Pre-pregnancy hypertension among women in rural and urban areas of the United States. *J Am Coll Cardiol*. 2020;76(22):2611–2619. doi:10.1016/j.jacc.2020.09.601.

47. Cross TL, Bazron BJ, Dennis KW, Isaacs MR. Towards a culturally competent system of care: a monograph on effective services for minority children who are severely emotionally disturbed. National Institute of Mental Health; 1989:88. https://www.ojp.gov/ncjrs/virtual-library/abstracts/towards-culturally-competent-system-care-monograph-effective. Accessed January 18, 2022.

48. Marion L, Douglas M, Lavin MA, et al. Implementing the new ANA Standard 8: culturally congruent practice. *Online J Issues Nurs*. 2017;22(1). doi:10.3912/OJIN.Vol22No01PPT20.

49. Zephyrin L, Seervai S, Lewis C, Katon JG. Community-based models to improve maternal health outcomes and promote health equity. Commonwealth Fund. doi:10.26099/6s6k-5330. Published online March 3, 2021.

50. Greenwood BN, Hardeman RR, Huang L, Sojourner A. Physician–patient racial concordance and disparities in birthing mortality for newborns. *Proc Natl Acad Sci*. 2020;117(35):21194–21200. doi:10.1073/pnas.1913405117.

51. Chapman EN, Kaatz A, Carnes M. Physicians and implicit bias: how doctors may unwittingly perpetuate health care disparities. *J Gen Intern Med*. 2013;28(11):1504–1510. doi:10.1007/s11606-013-2441-1.

52. De Houwer J. Implicit bias is behavior: a functional-cognitive perspective on implicit bias. *Perspect Psychol Sci*. 2019;14(5):835–840. doi:10.1177/1745691619855638.

53. Ripp K, Braun L. Race/ethnicity in medical education: an analysis of a question bank for Step 1 of the United States Medical Licensing Examination. *Teach Learn Med*. 2017;29(2):115–122. doi:10.1080/10401334.2016.1268056.

54. Amutah C, Greenidge K, Mante A, et al. Misrepresenting race—the role of medical schools in propagating physician bias. *N Engl J Med*. 2021;384(9):872–878. doi:10.1056/NEJMms2025768.

55. FitzGerald C, Hurst S. Implicit bias in health care professionals: a systematic review. *BMC Med Ethics*. 2017;18(1):19. doi:10.1186/s12910-017-0179-8.

56. López CL, Wilson MD, Hou MY, Chen MJ. Racial and ethnic diversity among obstetrics and gynecology, surgical, and nonsurgical residents in the US from 2014 to 2019. *JAMA Netw Open*. 2021;4(5):e219219. doi:10.1001/jamanetworkopen.2021.9219.

57. Nair L, Adetayo OA. Cultural competence and ethnic diversity in health care. *Plast Reconstr Surg Glob Open*. 2019;7(5):e2219. doi:10.1097/GOX.0000000000002219.

58. Association of American Medical Colleges (AAMC). Figure 20: percentage of physicians by sex and race/ethnicity. Association of American Medical Colleges (AAMC); 2019. https://www.aamc.org/data-reports/workforce/interactive-data/figure-20-percentage-physicians-sex-and-race/ethnicity-2018.

59. Green TL, Zapata JY, Brown HW, Hagiwara N. Rethinking bias to achieve maternal health equity: changing organizations, not just individuals. *Obstet Gynecol*. 2021;137(5):935–940. doi:10.1097/AOG.0000000000004363.

60. Nieblas-Bedolla E, Christophers B, Nkinsi NT, Schumann PD, Stein E. Changing how race is portrayed in medical education: recommendations from medical students. *Acad Med*. 2020;95(12):1802–1806. doi:10.1097/ACM.0000000000003496.

61. Milem JF. The educational benefits of diversity: evidence from multiple sectors. In: Chang MJ, Witt D, Jones J, Hakuta K, eds. *Compelling Interest: Examining the Evidence on Racial Dynamics in Colleges and Universities*; Redwood City: Stanford University Press 2003. https://search.ebscohost.com/login.aspx?direct=true&scope=site&db=nlebk&db=nlabk&AN=1433726.

62. Ona FF, Amutah-Onukagha NN, Asemamaw R, Schlaff AL. Struggles and tensions in antiracism education in medical school: lessons learned. *Acad Med*. 2020;95(12S):S163–S168. doi:10.1097/ACM.0000000000003696.

63. Black Maternal Health Momnibus Act of 2021. https://www.congress.gov/bill/117th-congress/senate-bill/346/amendments.

64. Underwood L, Adams A, Booker C. Black Maternal Health Caucus. Black Maternal Health Momnibus. https://blackmaternalhealthcaucus-underwood.house.gov/Momnibus.

65. Underwood L. President Biden signs first bill in Underwood's historic "Momnibus" legislation into law. https://underwood.house.gov/media/press-releases/president-biden-signs-first-bill-underwood-s-historic-momnibus-legislation-law. Published November 30, 2021.

66. Taylor J, Bernstein A. Tracking progress of the Black maternal health Momnibus. The Century Foundation; 2022. https://tcf.org/content/data/black-maternal-health-momnibus-tracker/. Accessed January 24, 2021.

67. Hall WJ, Chapman MV, Lee KM, et al. Implicit racial/ethnic bias among health care professionals and its influence on health care outcomes: a systematic review. *Am J Public Health*. 2015;105(12):e60–e76. doi:10.2105/AJPH.2015.302903.

68. Kamlager-Dove S. Implicit bias: continuing education; requirements. 2019. https://leginfo.legislature.ca.gov/faces/billTextClient.xhtml?bill_id=201920200AB241.

69. American College of Obstetricians and Gynecologists (ACOG). Alliance for Innovation on Maternal Health (AIM). 2020. https://www.acog.org/practice-management/patient-safety-and-quality/partnerships/alliance-for-innovation-on-maternal-health-aim.

70. American College of Obstetricians and Gynecologists (ACOG). AIM program awarded millions to expand efforts to reduce maternal mortality and morbidity. https://www.acog.org/news/news-releases/2018/08/aim-program-awarded-millions-to-expand-efforts-to-reduce-maternal-mortality-and-morbidity. Published August 1, 2018.

71. Howell EA, Brown H, Brumley J, et al. Reduction of peripartum racial and ethnic disparities: a conceptual framework and maternal safety consensus bundle. *Obstet Gynecol*. 2018;131(5):770–782. doi:10.1097/AOG.0000000000002475.

72. Illinois Perinatal Quality Collaborative (ILPQC). Birth equity. 2019. https://ilpqc.org/birthequity/.

73. California Maternal Quality Care Collaborative (CMQCC). Birth equity. https://www.cmqcc.org/content/birth-equity.

74. US Commission on Civil Rights, Cantu N, Llamon CE, et al. *Racial disparities in maternal health*. US Commission on Civil Rights; 2021:1–405. https://www.usccr.gov/reports/2021/racial-disparities-maternal-health.

75. King PAL, Henderson ZT, Borders AEB. Advances in maternal fetal medicine: perinatal quality collaboratives working together to improve maternal outcomes. *Clin Perinatol.* 2020;47(4):779–797. doi:10.1016/j.clp.2020.08.009.

76. Centers for Disease Control and Prevention (CDC). State perinatal quality collaboratives. https://www.cdc.gov/reproductivehealth/maternalinfanthealth/pqc-states.html. Accessed January 18, 2022.

77. Association of Maternal & Child Health Programs (AMCHP). *Health for Every Mother: A Maternal Health Resource and Planning Guide for States.* AMCHP; 2015:1–120. http://www.amchp.org/programsandtopics/womens-health/Focus%20Areas/MaternalHealth/Pages/default.aspx. Accessed January 15, 2022.

78. Main EK. Reducing maternal mortality and severe maternal morbidity through state-based quality improvement initiatives. *Clin Obstet Gynecol.* 2018;61(2):319–331. doi:10.1097/GRF.0000000000000361.

79. MassHealth. Text4baby program & home visiting in Massachusetts: harnessing the power of mobile for maternal & child health in the U.S. Massachusetts Department of Health & Social Services; 2015:48. https://www.mass.gov/service-details/text4baby.

80. Main E, Morton C, Hopkins D, Giuliani G, Melsop K, Gould J. Cesarean deliveries, outcomes, and opportunities for change in California: toward a public agenda for maternity care safety and quality. California Maternal Quality Care Collaborative (CMQCC); 2011:86. https://www.cmqcc.org/research/cmqcc-publications/archived-2013-2006-publications. Accessed January 18, 2022.

81. FitzPatrick ME, Badu-Boateng C, Huntley C, Morgan C. 'Attorneys of the poor': training physicians to tackle health inequalities. *Future Healthcare J.* 2021;8(1):12–18. doi:10.7861/fhj.2020-0242.

82. Zestcott CA, Blair IV, Stone J. Examining the presence, consequences, and reduction of implicit bias in health care: a narrative review. *Group Process Intergroup Relat.* 2016;19(4):528–542. doi:10.1177/1368430216642029.

83. Association of American Medical Colleges (AAMC). 2021 FACTS: enrollment, graduates, and MD-PhD data. AAMC; 2022. https://www.aamc.org/data-reports/students-residents/interactive-data/2021-facts-enrollment-graduates-and-md-phd-data. Accessed January 15, 2022.

84. Nicolau B, Marcenes W. How will a life course framework be used to tackle wider social determinants of health? *Community Dent Oral Epidemiol.* 2012;40:33–38. doi:10.1111/j.1600-0528.2012.00717.x.

85. Alsan M, Garrick O, Graziani GC. Does diversity matter for health? Experimental evidence from Oakland. Am Econ Rev. 2019;109(12):4071–4111.

8:6. Paez KA, Allen JK, Carson KA, Cooper LA. Provider and clinic cultural competence in a primary care setting. *Soc Sci Med.* 2008;66(5):1204–1216. doi:10.1016/j.socscimed.2007.11.027.

87. Haley J, Benatar S. Improving patient and provider experiences to advance maternal health equity. Urban Institute. 2020. https://www.urban.org/research/publication/improving-patient-and-provider-experiences-advance-maternal-health-equity.

88. Maternal Outcomes for Translational Health Equity Research (M.O.T.H.E.R.) Lab. https://motherlab.org. Published January 2022. Accessed January 29, 2022.

Chapter 46

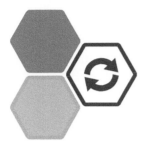

Sustainability and Finance: The Role of State and Territorial Health Agencies

ELLEN PLISKA, BRITTA CEDERGREN, KRISTIN SULLIVAN, MELISSA TOUMA, KARL ENSIGN, SOWMYA KURUGANTI, DEBORAH BACKMAN, ALEX WHEATLEY, HEATHER PANGELINAN, MARIJANE CAREY, SHANNON VANCE, AND SANAA AKBARALI

THE ASSOCIATION OF STATE AND TERRITORIAL HEALTH OFFICIALS

The Association of State and Territorial Health Officials (ASTHO) is the only national nonprofit organization representing public health agencies across the United States, its island jurisdictions, and the District of Columbia. ASTHO has built a network of 59 current and 230 alumni state and territorial health leaders who share expertise, preserve historical knowledge, and grow the skills and capacity of the over 100,000 people in the public health workforce that they represent.

ASTHO's mission is to support, equip, and advocate for state and territorial health officials in their work of advancing the public's health and well-being. For 80 years, ASTHO has supported its members, their staff, and others in the fields of community health and prevention, social and behavioral health, infectious disease, emergency response, equity and diversity initiatives, population health and data informatics, public health policy, and more. ASTHO continues to build state and territorial public health capacity to improve collecting and utilizing public health data, to expand access to care and treatment, and to create new preparedness frameworks to respond to crises. By providing state and territorial health officials with guidance and support, ASTHO empowers leaders as they craft more holistic preventive policies and lead in service delivery aimed at addressing the root causes of inequities and improving health outcomes.[1]

ASTHO operates under six core values: leadership, integrity, collaboration, respect, diversity and inclusion, and responsiveness. ASTHO's 2022–2024

Ellen Pliska, Britta Cedergren, Kristin Sullivan, Melissa Touma, Karl Ensign, Sowmya Kuruganti, Deborah Backman, Alex Wheatley, Heather Pangelinan, Marijane Carey, Shannon Vance, and Sanaa Akbarali, *Sustainability and Finance* In: *The Practical Playbook III*. Edited by: Dorothy Cilenti, Alisahah Jackson, Natalie D. Hernandez, Lindsey Yates, Sarah Verbiest, J. Lloyd Michener, and Brian C. Castrucci, Oxford University Press. © de Beaumont Foundation 2024.
DOI: 10.1093/oso/9780197662984.003.0046

Strategic Plan[2] reflects the organization's pathway to addressing the primary needs and demands of state and territorial health agencies and their staff through the following strategic priorities:

- Health and racial equity: ASTHO prioritizes implementing policies and programs that advance health and racial equity to achieve optimal health for all.
- Workforce development: ASTHO cultivates a workforce that is engaged at all levels, is well resourced, is well trained, and is connected to the communities it serves.
- Sustainable infrastructure improvements: ASTHO identifies and sustains sufficient, predictable, flexible capabilities, resources, and authorities to effectively protect and promote the health of their communities.
- Data modernization and interoperability: ASTHO builds an enterprise-level data infrastructure in which public health data systems are interoperable, secure, and supported by a well-trained workforce.
- Evidence-based and promising public health practices: ASTHO implements equitable evidence-based public health policies and programs in their jurisdictions that are achieving tangible improvement in public health outcomes across all programs and populations.

FUNDING FOR SUSTAINABILITY

Rates of maternal mortality and morbidity from pregnancy-related complications in the United States have increased steadily since the 1990s, resulting in a rate almost double that of other economically developed nations.[3] Black and American Indian/Alaska Native women die at a rate that is nearly three to four times higher than the rate for their white counterparts, and nearly two-thirds of all maternal deaths are preventable.[4]

Historically, the federal government has delegated the role of supporting the health and well-being of mothers and children to the states and territories. Since 1935, the federal government shifted funding streams, allocating federal Title V of the Social Security Act (funded by the Health Resource and Services Administration's Maternal and Child Health Bureau) to states and territories to manage. Over the last century, other federal agencies that have allocated dollars to states and territories with provisions to support maternal and infant health include the Department of Health and Human Services, CDC, and the Centers for Medicare & Medicaid Services.

Unfortunately, even with the growing national conversation on the health and wellness of mothers and the increasing need to address the factors contributing to mortality and morbidity, funding and scalability of programming lag. Appropriately funding and sustaining programming for interventions aimed at improving maternal health are vital. Cuts in federal spending on social programs over the decades have left state and territorial health agencies challenged by insufficient resources. What dollars are allocated are often siloed into specific programs or initiatives that can lack flexibility in meeting the most pressing public health needs due to historical contexts and challenges.[5] Finance reform is a top priority for foundational change as noted by over 50% of executive-level health leaders across the country citing the need for further training on budget and financial management.[5,6]

Often, funding streams do not perfectly align with public health needs. This requires health leaders to identify financing strategies that creatively combine multiple funding sources to support a public health initiative.[7] Realigning funding streams through the practices of blending, braiding, and layering have been common practices in international development for decades to fund and sustain initiatives. Those practices are now receiving attention domestically in public health as a way of addressing growing funding gaps, sustaining programming, and even mobilizing partners. Definitions of blending, braiding, and layering are:

- Blending is the merging of two or more funding sources into one award to fund a specific part of a program or initiative. With blending, each individual award loses its award-specific identity and spending is not necessarily allocated and tracked by individual funding source. Blending often increases efficiency and economies of scale, but specific grant requirements generally preclude this approach. Blending may require specific waiver authority.[8,9]
- Braiding is the coordination of two or more funding sources to support an activity while each individual award maintains its identity and meets reporting and tracking requirements. Very clear and concise cost-allocation methods are required in braiding to ensure that there is no duplicate funding of service and that each funding source is charged appropriately by partners or stakeholders.[8-10]
- Layering may be used when one source of funding cannot comprehensively cover an activity, project, or initiative. Instead of replacing the inadequate funding source, other sources are used to supplement and better meet the comprehensive needs of the activity.[10]

At its most basic level, funding by blending, braiding, or layering takes constant communication by leadership to staff, combined with diligent accounting and clear reporting structures. Truly successful blending, braiding, or layering takes creativity, dedication, and vision by leaders who empower their organizations by asking the question, "What if?" To answer this question, ASTHO hosted a pilot program with Colorado, Washington, and Rhode Island, providing leadership development and technical support to conduct programs aimed at using braided and layered funds to build the foundational capabilities needed to address the social determinants of health.[11]

Box 46.1 | ASTHO Braiding and Layering Pilot: Rhode Island's Health Equity Zone Project

In 2020, ASTHO reported on a pilot focused on braiding and layering funding through addressing the social determinants of health and building foundational capabilities.[i] Although dramatic examples of innovation were found, multiple challenges were also identified at both the state and federal levels. To help address the challenges, ASTHO provided leadership development, assembled existing resources, and provided technical support. Rhode Island, a participating state, built the Health Equity Zone Initiative through a braided funding model. This model, funded by the Rhode Island Department of Health, provides flexible funding to community-led initiatives to address the socioeconomic and environmental conditions driving disparities and to improve health outcomes, including addressing the health and well-being of mothers and children. Since the Health Equity Zone Initiative's inception, the state has invested more than $10.4 million to create sustainable change to support the health of Rhode Islanders and to reduce disparities.[ii] Similar strategies can be used to broaden the impact and reach of public health improvement initiatives and create policy and system changes that contribute to better maternal health outcomes.

ASTHO emphasizes the importance of constant leadership attention to address siloed funding, at both the state and federal level, which often hinders the true potential of programs and their impact.[i] Further steps to overcoming these silos include:

- Assessing and prioritizing how innovation will be targeted to make change and coming to clear and explicit agreement on the priorities.
- Identifying methods for allocating funding and reporting across multiple cost centers.
- Managing the process with dedicated staffing.
- Supporting ongoing learning and improvement.
- Documenting and communicating value.

Successfully braiding and layering funds requires adequate planning, leadership engagement, needs assessments, and stakeholder collaboration. The critical first step is engaging leadership by clearly framing the health issue to be addressed. Assessments of all stakeholders should be conducted, specifically those who would be involved in either the provision of funds or the execution of services. Project plans and budgets should be developed to identify relevant funding streams, cost-allocation processes, standards for translating work plans and budgets into practice, and monitoring and accountability mechanisms. Evaluation of results will communicate value to funders and policymakers. Communication and collaboration are necessary to openly address and resolve challenges and barriers during implementation.

Box 46.1 | Continued

References

i. Ensign K, Kain JC. Braiding and layering funding: doing more with what we have. *J Public Health Manage Pract.* 2020;26(2):187–191. https://journals.lww.com/jphmp/fulltext/2020/03000/braiding_and_layering_funding__doing_more_with.15.aspx. Accessed February 1, 2022.
ii. Rhode Island's Health Equity Zone (HEZ) Initiative. https://health.ri.gov/programs/detail.php?pgm_id=1108. Accessed February 1, 2022.

ASTHO DEVELOPS PUBLIC HEALTH LEADERS AND SUPPORTS ROBUST HEALTH AGENCIES

At all levels of health agencies, ASTHO provides leadership coaching, meeting facilitation, peer-to-peer connections, tools, and resources. At the highest levels, ASTHO helps leaders to employ strategies and practices to find and partner with others, to identify and connect over commonalities, and to reimagine structures and to innovate strategies to solve complex problems and begin the transformation of public health systems.[12] ASTHO facilitates training for state leaders on direction, alignment, and commitment across organizations, addressing the boundaries that prevent achieving a higher vision or goal.[13] ASTHO's Executive Leadership Forums bring together CFOs, senior deputies, legislative liaisons, public health lawyers, and others to enhance executive leader collaboration, communication, and management, and to discuss cutting-edge leadership practices to help meet the significant challenges and changes they face. Since 2000, ASTHO's Leadership Institute has equipped and empowered over 125 health officials with the tools necessary to help expand their influence on decisions affecting the health of the populations of their states and territories, and nationally.[14]

ASTHO responds to its members by providing direct training and peer-to-peer engagement opportunities for health officials, their deputies, agency chief financial officers, and other health agency leaders. Health leaders use these ASTHO Peer Networks as opportunities to connect, strategize, and share best practices on navigating federal funding initiatives, as well as building and sustaining flexible funding mechanisms. Previous financing trainings, pilots, and capacity-building activities for health agencies led by ASTHO have focused on reallocation of funds, spend-down processes, successfully innovating the alignment of funding streams to meet health needs, standardizing practices related to the translation of workplans into budgets, and meeting compliance through reporting requirements.[11] An analysis of the impact of ASTHO's capacity-building activities demonstrated that 95% of respondents found the activities valuable to their work, and 79% of respondents indicated they would apply information learned from ASTHO activities in their public health practice. ASTHO's Peer Network model provides a forum for sharing best practices between executive-level public health leaders through in-person and virtual events, skill-building workshops, discussion boards, and mentoring.[15] An internal survey of ASTHO's Peer Network showed that 95% of evaluation respondents indicated that they found their peer network to be valuable for their work.

HOW ASTHO DELIVERS: BEST PRACTICES IN SUPPORTING ENTIRE HEALTH AGENCIES

ASTHO's Learning Community model provides direct technical assistance and peer to peer engagement to state and territorial health programs through both funded and unfunded projects specific to different topic areas (see Section V, "Innovations"). Examples of how ASTHO has applied the Learning Community model to support states and territories as they increase capacity and build tools for sustainability in their agencies' maternal health programs include:

- In 2022, ASTHO kicked off a four-state learning community aimed at adopting or improving risk-appropriate and coordinated plans of care to ensure equitable access to obstetric services for all pregnant and postpartum people. Authority to designate levels of maternal and neonatal care is within the influence and authority of state health officials and their agencies. State health officials provide oversight of public health policy implementation, including coordination of policy and reimbursement for risk-appropriate care services. ASTHO builds the capacity of state and territorial health agencies by disseminating best practices for working with their medical partners to ensure that pregnant women and infants at high risk of complications receive equitable care at a birth facility that is best prepared to meet their health needs.
- ASTHO identified that improving access to regular well-woman care, including preconception and interconception care, and access to family planning services is a priority evidence-based health practice. From 2014 to 2018, ASTHO convened a learning community of 28 states to tackle issues surrounding access to contraceptive services, including securing Medicaid reimbursement for long-acting reversible contraceptive methods, such as intrauterine devices. In 2022, ASTHO convened a second learning community of six states dedicated to identifying and implementing creative, promising practices for addressing equitable access to contraception through telehealth services, securing and sustaining funding, and workforce improvements.

Box 46.2 | ASTHO's Breastfeeding Learning Community

A STHO's Breastfeeding Learning Community (BLC) builds sustainability of breastfeeding initiatives in 16 states funded by the Centers for Disease Control and Prevention's (CDC) State Physical Activity and Nutrition (SPAN) program through capacity-building, technical assistance, and sub-awards. The 2020–2021 ASTHO BLC State Innovations to Advance Breastfeeding and Health Equity grants provided funding to 10 total state health agencies and not-for-profit state and local organizations to collaborate with partners in implementing innovative cross-sector strategies to advance breastfeeding equity. Multisector partners have included local health agencies, community-based health and social services organizations, business networks, state and local breastfeeding and obesity prevention coalitions, healthcare organizations, and hospital associations. The Innovation grants have enabled participating states to implement structures that foster sustainability of their projects. The structures included new breastfeeding coalitions and workgroups, leveraging other funding opportunities, and establishing new hospital systems and procedures geared at providing long-term lactation care services and support in communities:

- A hospital-based Innovation grantee developed a clinic for new parents providing lactation support and other healthcare services to socioeconomically marginalized families, and it established a billing system for lactation support services.
- One state integrated components of their Innovation grant project into their Title V Maternal and Child Health Block Grant, WIC, and SPAN work.
- Two states formed coalitions and workgroups consisting of Black, Indigenous, and People of Color (BIPOC) lactation support providers and advocates who are focused on improving breastfeeding supports and services for Black and Hispanic/Latinx families.

The 2021–2022 BLC Sustaining Breastfeeding Innovations Through Policies and Programs initiative provides states that participated in the Innovations grant program with additional funding and support to work with multisector partners to sustain, enhance, or replicate their Innovations projects. In addition to programmatic efforts to sustain their Innovations projects, ASTHO trained participants to engage with policy processes in their state, resulting in policy-level action-learning deliverables to support programmatic efforts.

- Pennsylvania and Illinois are establishing programs to train and support BIPOC individuals or persons who have a lower income status in becoming professional lactation support providers. These states concurrently worked on policy initiatives related to Medicaid reimbursement for professional lactation care services.
- Washington implemented wraparound prenatal, intrapartum, and postpartum services for families while exploring Medicaid reimbursement for doula services, including lactation services.

Box 46.2 | Continued

- Utah is providing employers of women with low wages with funds to improve on-site workplace lactation accommodations, while also working with employers to establish new, or to improve existing, lactation accommodation policies.

By supporting states and multisector partners in addressing both programmatic and policy-level breastfeeding barriers, the Sustaining Breastfeeding Innovations initiative enables states to implement breastfeeding equity programs as well as establish organizational and public policy structures that will help maintain the programs for years to come.

Box 46.3 | ASTHO's Pregnancy Risk Assessment Monitoring System Learning Community

The Pregnancy Risk Assessment Monitoring System (PRAMS) survey was launched by CDC in 1987, collecting data from new mothers on their experiences before, during, and shortly after pregnancy. ASTHO's Linking PRAMS and Clinical Outcomes Data Multi-Jurisdiction Learning Community, launched in 2021, provides capacity-building support and technical assistance to 12 states as they link their PRAMS data set with outcomes-based data sets like hospital discharge and home visiting to help inform future clinical quality improvement and patient-centered outcomes research priorities. The PRAMS Learning Community builds capacity for state health agencies by laying the groundwork for future data-driven funding requests, programmatic initiatives, and leadership decisions to support maternal health.

The PRAMS Learning Community works with Alaska, Georgia, Massachusetts, Montana, Nebraska, New Mexico, Rhode Island, South Dakota, Tennessee, Texas, Virginia, and Washington, all states seeking to link their PRAMS data sets to different maternal and child health-related data sets to inform their state programs and policies. For example, the Nebraska, Rhode Island, Tennessee, and Texas teams focused heavily on leveraging their linked data sets to inform reducing severe maternal morbidity (SMM).

- The Nebraska, Rhode Island, and Tennessee Departments of Health linked PRAMS with their respective statewide hospital discharge data. By strengthening the amount of race, ethnicity & language (REAL) data that are accessible, the Nebraska team is hoping to be able to surveille SMM and other maternal outcomes more properly. Rhode Island, as part of their Title V strategic plan, is seeking to use their linked data set to inform programming and priorities from the PRAMS steering committee, including their "MomsPRN" program, which provides psychiatric teleconsultation services to reduce pregnancy-related depression. Tennessee is also linking an additional birth statistical file, to analyze the burden of SMM and to enhance recommendations about the burden of maternal health issues, specifically hypertensive disorders and mental health.

Box 46.3 | Continued

- The Texas Department of Health and Human Services linked their PRAMS data set to the Texas Health Care Information Collection research file to answer whether patient–provider conversations before and during pregnancy can reduce SMM and identify specifically what type of SMM is most affected by inadequate access to prenatal care.

ASTHO engaged each state team throughout the learning community to develop detailed action plans, including goals, strategies, and activities states would need to take to successfully link their PRAMS and clinical outcomes data sets. ASTHO worked with many of the state teams to process map their data-linkage protocols to streamline systems and to identify barriers and areas for improvement. Direct capacity-building and guidance to states included connecting teams with federal, nonprofit, academic, and other state health agency experts to solve direct linkage problems. Examples include identifying training materials for a variety of linkage software and providing guidance on Medicaid ICD-10 injury codes.

Additionally, ASTHO conducted a five-part webinar series in the spring of 2022 where expert panelists discussed common challenges in data linkage, the importance of partnerships in executing data-use agreements, navigating legal barriers with data-sharing, and ensuring data quality and equity in data linkage.

ASTHO's policy statements[16] reflect the official position of ASTHO and strategically align members around best practices on public health issues. Public health priorities and policies can vastly differ across the country. ASTHO members are the face and voice of state and territorial public health and are often called on by federal and state lawmakers and national organizations to provide input on developing public health policy. To support their leadership, ASTHO generates policy statements to be used by state and territorial health officials to develop and defend policy decisions to Congress, their own legislatures, and the public on a variety of topics backed by evidence-based findings. To ensure ownership of policies and consensus, 35 out of 59 active ASTHO members must vote to even begin crafting a statement. Policy statements provide a basis for ASTHO to speak on behalf of its members, to back national policy, to respond to federal comment periods, and to develop op-eds and other publicly facing actions.

In 2021, ASTHO's members and Board approved the Maternal Mortality and Morbidity (MMM) Policy Statement.[17] The MMM Policy Statement includes recommendations to promote health equity in all policies to reduce racial disparities in birth outcomes, to promote patient-centered care, to promote quality improvement and development of data infrastructure, to address issues around state policy and funding, and to expand workforce development opportunities to improve access to care. By approving the MMM policy statement,

ASTHO's members affirmed through one of the statement's recommendations that leveraging federal and state dollars through flexible funding mechanisms is vital to improving and sustaining programs that promote maternal health and reduce disparities.[18]

SUCCESS STORIES FROM STATE AND TERRITORIAL HEALTH OFFICIALS AND THEIR AGENCIES

ASTHO's 80 years of success are directly attributable to the organization's mindset of listening to its members, proactively addressing emerging public health issues, reacting quickly to urgent public health crises, and sustaining support for ongoing public health priorities that demand system-level change. The following are examples of how ASTHO has responded to health agencies and partners as part of the organization's commitment to improving the health of the nation.

Box 46.4 | Commonwealth of the Northern Mariana Islands

Heather Pangelinan

The Commonwealth of the Northern Mariana Islands (CNMI), located over 5,800 miles from the coast of California, is a United States territory with a population of approximately 57,500.[i] The territory's department of health, known as the Commonwealth Healthcare Corporation (CHCC), oversees both public health programming and acute care services, including administration of the territory's public hospital. In a recent restructure, CHCC leadership strengthened cross-cutting connections to improve outcomes in their family planning program.

The CHCC family planning program maintains integrated funding, staffing, data collection, and referral structures across its clinical care and public health programming. These integrated structures have facilitated the cross-cutting connections that underlie the territory's efficient and effective maternal and child health (MCH) care today.

As in other health systems in the Pacific, many CNMI public health programs are located at the local public hospital. This "one-stop shop" structure facilitates connections across programs as well as proximal relationships among complementary clinical and public health staff.

Funding for MCH staffing further reinforces these connections. CHCC blends local and federal Title X funds to ensure that public health and clinical staff and services are coordinated. Physicians, midlevel providers, and clinical care staff are funded through federal grants, Medicaid dollars, and local revenue generated by clinics offering family planning services. Contraceptive supplies are covered by Title X, with contraceptives purchased at a discount from the federal 340B pharmacy program. Collectively, these funding and staffing structures create a sustainable revenue cycle that supports many clients across Saipan, the territory's most populous island.

Box 46.4 | Continued

Cross-cutting referral structures also ensure coordinated care. At the CHCC Women's Clinic, patients seeking pregnancy testing are seen through family planning, and pregnant clients are immediately connected with prenatal care and other public health programs on site, including OB-GYN, tobacco cessation, and home-visiting support. This "warm handoff" between providers results in continuity of care services and support and takes the burden off patients as they are seamlessly enrolled in prenatal or other care.

Even MCH data structures were built to be collaborative. When the CNMI began plans for transitioning into an updated electronic health record system, the family planning program worked closely with the IT department during development and implementation to ensure that critical data elements were embedded in the system, streamlining collection of key programmatic indicators (e.g., household size) in clinical settings. Structures like these ensure that public health staff work with their clinical partners to improve family planning access and utilization, strengthen communication with referral partners, and perform quality improvement.

Reference

i. Population, total—Northern Mariana Islands. World Bank. 2022. https://data.worldbank.org/indicator/SP.POP.TOTL?locations=MP. Accessed February 9, 2022.

Box 46.5 | Connecticut's State Health Improvement Plan and MCH Coalition

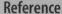

Marijane Carey

In Connecticut, braiding federal, state, and private grants supported the infrastructure of the State Health Improvement Coalition and its efforts to align partners around a common agenda for improving the state's health and ensuring that all people can attain their highest potential for health.[i] Acting as the backbone agency, the Connecticut Department of Public Health (CT DPH) convened a coalition of more than 100 stakeholders, led by a 30-member advisory council representing a diverse group of statewide partners representing health advocacy groups, including philanthropies, the Maternal and Child Health (MCH) Coalition, March of Dimes, housing enforcement, transportation, academia, healthcare access, tribal and local health, and organizations representing chronic and infectious disease. Coalition members identified a public health policy agenda, which was refined by the advisory council and grounded in evidence to target upstream factors and achieve the broadest impact on health. Braided funds were utilized to support CT DPH staffing in organizing and convening stakeholders to build the common agenda and establish a performance management system to monitor health-improvement outcomes.

Engaging cross-sector partners and coalitions, such as the MCH Coalition, through the State Health Improvement Plan (SHIP) structure helped expand the reach of advocacy efforts for paid family and medical leave, a policy designed to offer financial relief during times of significant life events. This resource offers financial security that can be used for basic needs, child care, and other specific needs of the household, and as a result it can improve health outcomes. Because Black, Latina, and Native women are often the primary earners in their families, paid leave helps to alleviate the financial and caregiver burdens experienced when the ability to work is compromised.[ii] Paid family medical leave may also have beneficial effects in terms of lowering prenatal and postpartum stress and may improve maternal mental and physical health.[iii] With advocacy led by the CT Women's Education and Legal Fund and supported by the MCH Coalition and SHIP structure, along with a number of advocates, Connecticut's Paid Family and Medical Leave program (Public Act 19-25) is among the country's most expansive[iv] and will help address health, racial, and gender inequities experienced by new mothers and babies.[v]

References

i. Connecticut Department of Public Health. Healthy Connecticut 2020. 2014. https://portal.ct.gov/-/media/Departments-and-Agencies/DPH/dph/state_health_planning/SHA-SHIP/hct2020/hct2020statehlthimpv032514pdf.pdf. Accessed January 27, 2022.

ii. Sanclemente D. Paid leave is a win for Connecticut workers, families, caregivers, and advancing racial justice. *CT Mirror*. January 10, 2022. https://ctmirror.org/2022/01/10/paid-leave-is-a-win-for-connecticut-workers-families-caregivers-and-advancing-racial-justice/. Accessed January 28, 2022.

iii. Jou J, Kozhimannil KB, Abraham JM, et al. Paid maternity leave in the United States: associations with maternal and infant health. *Maternal Child Health J*. 2018;22:216–225. https://doi.org/10.1007/s10995-017-2393-x.

iv. Connecticut Paid Leave. About the Paid Leave Authority. https://ctpaidleave.org/s/about-us?language=en_US. Accessed January 19, 2022.

v. Rossin-Slater M, Uniat L. Paid family leave policies and population health. *Health Aff*. March 28, 2019. https://www.healthaffairs.org/do/10.1377/hpb20190301.484936/full/. Accessed January 25, 2022.

FROM THOUGHT TO ACTION: ASTHO'S MATERNAL MORBIDITY AND MORTALITY TECHNICAL PACKAGE

In 2021, ASTHO began developing a series of technical packages, which prioritize the most high-impact strategies that ASTHO can take to support health leaders and their agencies. As of August 2022, packages have been developed in maternal health, chronic disease, social and behavioral health, and COVID-19 health equity. These packages guide the direction of funding requests and provide direct capacity-building and technical assistance activities. Due to the diverse nature of public health, no two ASTHO technical packages have been developed the same way, but they all serve to do the same thing—to provide direction and to identify long and short-term priority interventions.

The recommendations from the MMM Policy Statement formed the basis of the MMM technical package. ASTHO weighed MMM technical package recommendations against a theoretical functional model developed by ASTHO, depicting health agency leadership responsibilities (e.g., workforce development, promoting equity, establishing and advocating for policies that improve health) and cross-cutting factors necessary for achieving and sustaining those responsibilities (e.g., securing and sustaining funding; investing in strong data-collection, data-analysis, and data-sharing methods; and engaging and collaborating with partners). All areas must be rigorously evaluated.

ASTHO cross-walked the selected responsibilities with the ASTHO Strategic Plan. Promoting sustainability, financing, and scalability became core components of the technical package, including quality improvement and data infrastructure, state policy and funding, and workforce development.[19] The final MMM technical package includes recommendations that can only be achieved by developing and scaling-up flexible policies and mechanisms that leverage federal, state, and local funding to address and sustain initiatives. The priority recommendations include:

- Support agency leaders and their organizations as they creatively leverage, blend, braid, and layer federal funding streams, including the Title V Maternal and Child Health Services Block Grant, Title X Family Planning Program, and more, to increase reach and to sustain programming.
- Support or establish mechanisms for doula and community health worker reimbursement.
- Adopt risk-appropriate and coordinated plans of care to ensure equitable access to obstetric services for all pregnant and postpartum people.
- Promote the use of, and reimbursement for, evidence-based screening tools for mental health and/or substance use disorders, as well as intimate partner violence.

CONCLUSION

ASTHO is working to promote a shift in culture, skills in change management, active leadership engagement, and commitment to change and diverse partnerships, using data, funding, and staff to their maximum advantage. State and territorial health agencies have a unique role as both the recipients of funding and deliverers of essential public health services to innovate, sustain, and blend funding at the state, territorial, and community levels to help all mothers survive and thrive. The current political, social, and economic climate, changed forever by COVID-19, is the perfect opportunity to fundamentally reform operations in funding streams and data systems and to promote the culture change needed to best achieve health equity. The nation's health and wellness rely on the actions of its leaders. State and territorial health officials set the tone and direction of their organizations as they achieve their commitment to protect population health.[20] ASTHO is committed to advancing health equity and to achieving optimal health for our nation's mothers by equipping leaders with the tools they need to create change and the conditions in which families can survive and thrive.[21,22]

REFERENCES

1. Perrotte BM, Noorestani A. Going beyond public health 3.0: how flexible funding streams can help to break down silos, change systems, and advance health equity in local communities. *Am J Public Health.* 2021;111(S3):S189–S192.

2. Association of State and Territorial Health Agencies (ASTHO). Strategic plan. https://www.astho.org/about/strategic-plan/. 2022. Accessed August 5, 2022.

3. The Commonwealth Fund. Maternal mortality and maternity care in the United States compared to 10 other developed countries. November 18, 2020. https://www.commonwealthfund.org/publications/issuebriefs/2020/nov/maternal-mortality-maternity-care-us-compared-10-countries.

4. Petersen EE, Davis N, Goodman D, et al. Racial/ethnic disparities in pregnancy-related deaths—United States, 2007–2016. *MMWR.* 2019;68(35):762–765. https://www.cdc.gov/mmwr/volumes/68/wr/mm6835a3.htm?s_cid=mm6835a3_w. Accessed February 1, 2022.

5. DeSalvo K, Levi J, Hoagland B, Parekh A. Developing a financing system to support public health infrastructure. *Public Health Leadersh Forum.* https://www.resolve.ngo/docs/developing-a-financing-system-to-support-foundational-public-health-capabilities-final-draft-10.2.pdf. Published October 2018. Accessed February 1, 2022.

6. de Beaumont Foundation. Public Health WINS: 2021 findings. https://debeaumont.org/phwins/2021-findings/. Published August 2022. Accessed August 10, 2022.

7. Greater than the sum of its parts: blended finance roadmap for global health. USAID. https://www.usaid.gov/sites/default/files/documents/1864/Blended-Finance-Roadmap-508.pdf. Accessed February 1, 2022.

8. US Department of Health and Human Services, Administration for Children and Families. Online resource: https://childcareta.acf.hhs.gov/systemsbuilding/systems-guides/financing-strategically/maximizing-impact-public-funding/.

9. Association of Government Accountants (AGA), Intergovernmental Partnership, Collaboration Series. Blended and braided funding: a guide for policy makers and practitioners. December 2014. https://www.agacgfm.org/AGA/Intergovernmental/documents/BlendedandBraidedFunding.pdf.

10. Association of State and Territorial Health Agencies (ASTHO). Braiding and layering funding for adverse childhood experiences prevention. July 2021. https://

www.astho.org/ASTHOReports/Braiding-and-Layering-Funding-for-ACEs-Pre
vention/08-05-21/#:~:text=Braiding%20and%20layering%20refers%20to,a%20com
mon%20set%20of%20goals.

11. Ensign K, Kain JC. Braiding and layering funding: doing more with what we have. *J Public Health Manage Pract*. 2020;26(2):187–191. https://journals.lww.com/jphmp/ Fulltext/2020/03000/Braiding_and_Layering_Funding__Doing_More_With.15. aspx. Accessed 8-10-2022.

12. Fick-Cooper L, Williams A, Moffatt S, Baker E, Edward L. Boundary spanning leadership: promising practices for public health. J Public Health Manage Pract. 2019;25(3): 288–290. https://journals.lww.com/jphmp/Fulltext/2019/05000/Boundary_Spanning_ Leadership__Promising_Practices.12.aspx. Accessed February 1, 2022.

13. Center for Creative Leadership. Boundary spanning leadership. https://www.ccl.org/ leadership-solutions/leadership-topics/boundary-spanning/. Accessed February 1, 2022.

14. Association of State and Territorial Health Officials (ASTHO). Leadership institute. https://www.astho.org/members/ali/. Accessed August 8, 2022.

15. Association of State and Territorial Health Officials (ASTHO). Peer networks. https://www.astho.org/members/peer-networks/. Accessed August 11, 2022.

16. Association of State and Territorial Health Officials (ASTHO). Policy statements. https://www.astho.org/advocacy/policy-statements/. Accessed August 9, 2022.

17. Association of State and Territorial Health Officials (ASTHO). Maternal mortality and morbidity policy statement. https://www.astho.org/globalassets/pdf/policy-sta tements/maternal-mortality-and-morbidity.pdf. Accessed August 5, 2022.

18. https://astho.org/About/Policy-and-Position-Statements/Maternal-Mortality-and- Morbidity/. Accessed August 5, 2022.

19. Cedergren B, Pliska E, Mackie C. Supporting success: ASTHO's strategies for reducing maternal mortality and morbidity. *J Public Health Manage Pract*. 2022;28(3):317–320. doi:10.1097/PHH.0000000000001533.

20. 10 Essential Public Health Services. 2020. https://www.cdc.gov/publichealthgate way/publichealthservices/essentialhealthservices.html. Accessed August 5, 2022.

21. Association of State and Territorial Health Officials (ASTHO). About us. https:// www.astho.org/About/. Accessed January 4, 2021.

22. DeSalvo KB, Wang YC, Harris A, Aurebach J, Koo D, O'Carroll P. Public Health 3.0: a call to action for public health to meet the challenges of the 21st century. *Prev Chronic Dis*. 2017;14:170017.

Chapter 47

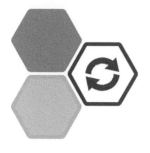

How State-Based Foundations Can Leverage Collaboration to Improve Maternal Health: A Case Study from California

DANA G. SMITH AND STEPHANIE S. TELEKI

From 1999 to 2006, the maternal mortality rate in California rose from 7.7 deaths per 100,000 births to 16.9 deaths, mirroring an upward trend in the United States (see Figure 47.1).[1] Shocked by these numbers, public and private stakeholders in the state joined forces to launch dozens of projects to improve maternal outcomes. Thanks to these efforts, over the next 10 years, the California maternal mortality rate dropped by more than 50%, to 5.9 deaths per 100,000 births in 2016,[1] one of the lowest rates in the country.[1] The US average continued to rise during that time, to 21.8 deaths per 100,000 births.[1]

California's initiative was launched in 2006 by the California Department of Public Health (CDPH) and was led by public health officer Connie Mitchell, MD, MPH. The work to improve maternal health began as a publicly funded effort, supported by federal Title V money, but as the project evolved, private funding became essential for growing and sustaining the work. State-based philanthropies came to play an especially important role, serving not only as funders but also as facilitators and thought leaders.

A significant state-based supporter of maternal health is the California Health Care Foundation (CHCF), which launched its maternal health portfolio in 2010. CHCF works to advance the health of Californians by supporting initiatives aimed at improving healthcare systems, particularly those serving the state's Medicaid population. The foundation has a funding budget of $40 million annually, with approximately $2 million dedicated to maternal health—a relatively modest sum in the face of the challenges—so it must be strategic about what it funds, with an emphasis on spread and scale.

Dana G. Smith and Stephanie S. Teleki, *How State-Based Foundations Can Leverage Collaboration to Improve Maternal Health* In: *The Practical Playbook III.* Edited by: Dorothy Cilenti, Alisahah Jackson, Natalie D. Hernandez, Lindsey Yates, Sarah Verbiest, J. Lloyd Michener, and Brian C. Castrucci, Oxford University Press. © de Beaumont Foundation 2024.
DOI: 10.1093/oso/9780197662984.003.0047

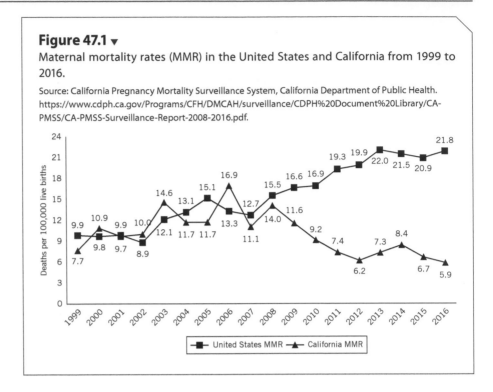

Figure 47.1 ▼

Maternal mortality rates (MMR) in the United States and California from 1999 to 2016.

Source: California Pregnancy Mortality Surveillance System, California Department of Public Health. https://www.cdph.ca.gov/Programs/CFH/DMCAH/surveillance/CDPH%20Document%20Library/CA-PMSS/CA-PMSS-Surveillance-Report-2008-2016.pdf.

CHCF's strategy is to "pull," or fund, multiple "levers" to bring about change: how care is delivered, how it's paid for, data and transparency, patient and community engagement, and public policy (see Figure 47.2). The tactic stems from the reality that major healthcare challenges are never solved by a single approach; instead, they must be addressed by pulling multiple levers. Along

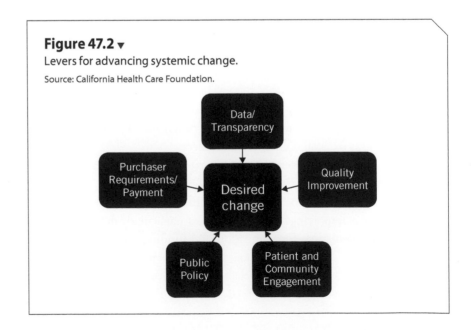

Figure 47.2 ▼

Levers for advancing systemic change.

Source: California Health Care Foundation.

these lines, CHCF frequently collaborates with other philanthropies for thought partnership and to make funding dollars go farther. Perhaps most importantly, CHCF views its role not just as a funder but as a partner to grantees and other stakeholders in the state. The organization believes that the perspective and connections foundations provide are often as vital, if not more so, as the financial investment itself.

When it comes to lowering maternal morbidity and mortality, this mindset is essential. The problem is too large for any one organization to solve on its own, and it is too complex to have a single solution. Collaboration around the levers, bringing together the right organizations and drawing on the strengths of each (in data analytics or community engagement or clinical interventions, for example), is what led to progress on tackling poor maternal outcomes in California.

This chapter uses CHCF's contributions in addressing California's maternal morbidity and mortality rates as a case study for how state-based philanthropies can help move the needle on complicated health issues not just by writing a check but by being conveners and thought leaders. CHCF's approach is not the only way, but it is one example of a strategy that has had success.

CESAREAN DELIVERIES

The clearest example of CHCF's multilever collaborative strategy is its five-year effort to reduce cesarean delivery rates for low-risk (nulliparous, term, singleton, vertex) births in California.

Cesarean deliveries (C-sections) can be lifesaving interventions when applied appropriately. However, rates of unnecessary procedures have skyrocketed over the past two decades and they now account for one-third of US births, including 26% of low-risk births.[2,3] C-sections increase the risk of hemorrhage, infection, and blood clots during and after delivery.[2] People who deliver via C-section are 90% more likely to have another one for a subsequent birth, and the cumulative impact of multiple C-sections dramatically raises a person's risk for maternal mortality.[2]

Despite a general acknowledgment in healthcare that C-section overuse is problematic, past efforts to reduce the prevalence have been met with resistance and ultimately have failed. In 2015, CHCF launched a five-year statewide effort to reduce California's C-section rates for low-risk births from 26.0% to the Healthy People 2020 target of 23.9%. The initiative focused on pulling four key levers and involved collaboration with multiple stakeholders across public and private sectors. This time, the effort was successful. By 2019, California had reduced its C-section rate from 26.0% to 22.8%.[4] The national rate remained steady at 26.0% during this time.

Quality-Improvement Lever

CHCF's first grant recipient for its C-section effort was the California Maternal Quality Care Collaborative (CMQCC), a quality-improvement organization based at Stanford University that focuses on data-driven delivery-system interventions.

CMQCC was founded in 2006 with support from CDPH to help address the rise in maternal mortality across the state. Under the direction of Elliott Main, MD, a maternal–fetal medicine specialist, CMQCC's initiatives to reduce some of the leading causes of maternal mortality—including hemorrhage, pre-eclampsia, and deep-vein thrombosis—had succeeded in improving obstetric care throughout the state.

CHCF funded CMQCC to develop a similar approach to tackle overuse of C-sections. The intervention included the Toolkit to Support Vaginal Birth and Reduce Primary Cesareans, a comprehensive "how to" manual for hospitals comprising evidence-based tools, algorithms, and guidelines.[5] CMQCC also launched a hospital-based quality-improvement learning collaborative consisting of small peer groups of physicians and nurses who met monthly to share their efforts, challenges, and progress. Each group was supported by a physician and nurse mentor pair who conducted site visits and provided hospitals with individualized support. By the end of the initiative, 91 of California's 238 delivery hospitals had participated in the learning collaborative.[4]

Data and Transparency Lever

Supporting the quality-improvement toolkit and learning collaborative was the CMQCC Maternal Data Center. The center—which was launched with funding from CDPH and the Centers for Disease Control and Prevention and then expanded with support from CHCF—provided hospitals with details on the number of C-sections performed each month as well as which physician ordered them and the reason for each procedure. This information told hospitals where they stood, how much they had to improve, and where to focus their efforts.

The data CMQCC needed to conduct these analyses was available in birth certificates and discharge diagnosis files, but the information had to be obtained fast and frequently enough to make it useful. Thanks to the partnership with CDPH, Dr. Main had the state send CMQCC a monthly feed of all California birth certificates. Next, he persuaded hospitals to directly provide CMQCC with their discharge diagnosis files rather than having to wait for the state to share them. This narrowed the time gap from 12 months to two months—a critical step that made the data more timely and thus more actionable. The key was making the request to hospitals as low-burden as possible—no extra processing needed, just share the data in the same format required by the state. Hospitals representing 95% of births in California now voluntarily contribute to the Maternal Data Center.

In return, the hospitals received valuable information about what was driving their cesarean deliveries. Were rates high because too many patients were induced? Were physicians intervening too early for slow labors? Was fetal distress being diagnosed too commonly? Once a cause was determined, the toolkit and learning collaborative showed the hospitals and physicians how to address the issue.

Comparing each hospital to its peers was another valuable set of data provided by CMQCC. This was important not only to the hospitals but also for consumers seeking to make informed decisions about where they received care. CHCF supported several projects to publish top-line information from the Maternal Data Center. First, each hospital's C-section rates were made publicly available by Cal Hospital Compare, a consumer-facing Web site that features performance information on all California hospitals. CHCF also funded a collaboration with Yelp to publish the maternity metrics on hospitals' Yelp pages alongside consumer ratings. Finally, CHCF and CMQCC worked with the California Health and Human Services Agency to release an annual honor roll recognizing hospitals that met the C-section target rate of 23.9%.

Purchaser and Payment Lever

Another important step was to get healthcare purchasers involved in the effort. Money drives behavior, so aligning payment with desired outcomes was critical. In 2015, CHCF convened Smart Care California, a group of the state's largest purchasers, including Covered California, the state's health insurance marketplace; Medi-Cal, California's Medicaid program; CalPERS, the public retirement system; and the Purchaser Business Group on Health (PBGH), a coalition of self-insured purchasers representing public and private employers. The goal was to bring these stakeholders together to focus on a few key issues where they could improve patient care by working together. One of the first causes the group elected to take up was limiting medically unnecessary C-sections.

The C-section problem had already emerged onto PBGH's radar when its board members flagged that they were seeing higher costs and poorer outcomes in maternity care. In 2014, PBGH launched a pilot project to lower C-section rates in three Southern California hospitals by changing the payment model.[6] C-sections cost nearly 50% more than vaginal births, so hospitals have a financial incentive to perform the surgery.[7] With a blended case rate, reimbursement is the same amount regardless of delivery method. A flat rate means payers spend a little more on vaginal births but a lot less on C-sections. On the provider side, increased reimbursement for low-risk births makes up for the lost revenue from the formerly more expensive C-sections. By realigning the payment system to support the desired outcome, the intervention reduced C-section rates by 20% in just six months.[6]

Inspired by PBGH's success, Smart Care California published a menu of payment options that insurance plans on the Covered California marketplace were required to choose from, with a blended case rate being the preferred option. Covered California also started holding plans accountable for the target

C-section rate of 23.9%—not as an average, but for each hospital included in the plan. If a hospital didn't work to reach that goal, it could be excluded from the plans offered on the marketplace. As a result, insurers pressured hospitals to lower their C-section rates using the CMQCC toolkit and quality-improvement collaborative.

At the end of 18 months, not every hospital had reached the 23.9% goal, but all either lowered their C-section rate or, if they couldn't lower the rate, stopped doing deliveries altogether. When the program started, the worst-performing hospital in California had a C-section rate exceeding 70%; by 2020, the highest rate was just over 40%.

Patient Engagement Lever

On the payer side of the equation, insurance plans were on board with Smart Care California's push to lower rates of unnecessary C-sections, but they were concerned about how the effort would be perceived by their members. When insurers change options for consumers, like limiting elective C-sections, it's often seen as the plans' taking away a benefit to save money rather than to improve care. To counter that impression, payers requested that a patient education component be added to the statewide effort, to inform consumers about why vaginal birth is preferable for low-risk pregnancies.

From these conversations, CHCF worked with CMQCC and *Consumer Reports* to produce the "My Birth Matters" campaign, comprising pamphlets and short videos to educate patients on the overuse of C-sections.[8] Content was approved by the American College of Obstetricians and Gynecologists and other stakeholders, and today the materials are distributed to women in doctor's offices, hospitals, and clinics.

By the end of the five-year initiative, messaging about reducing California's C-section rate was everywhere. Every major stakeholder was on board, including purchasers, payers, and providers. As a result of this cross-sector collaboration, the effort was a resounding success: from 2015 to 2019, the low-risk C-section rate in California dropped from 26.0% to 22.8% (see Figure 47.3).[4]

PERINATAL MENTAL HEALTH

In 2017, CHCF expanded its maternal health portfolio with a new initiative focused on improving perinatal mental health, which encompasses prenatal and postpartum depression, anxiety, bipolar disorder, and psychosis. Perinatal mental health issues are the number one complication of pregnancy and childbirth, with 63% of those screened reporting depressive symptoms.[9] In 2017, however, there was little knowledge about, or resources dedicated to, the issue. Consequently, the project required a substantial initial investment in data to lay the foundation and track changes over time. CHCF would later go on to pull other levers, but setting the stage with data was the first priority.

Figure 47.3 ▾
Cesarean delivery rates for low-risk births in California and the United States from 2014 to 2019. Abbreviation: NTSV, nulliparous, term, singleton, vertex.

Source: Rosenstein MG, Chang S, Sakowski C, et al. Hospital quality improvement interventions, statewide policy initiatives, and rates of cesarean delivery for nulliparous, term, singleton, vertex births in California. *JAMA.* 2021;325(16):1631–1639. doi:10.1001/jama.2021.3816.

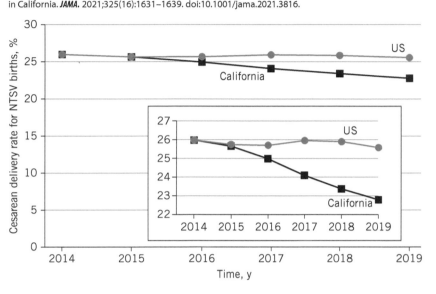

To start, reliable and valid measures to assess the problem were needed. These measures are typically developed by federal organizations and then disseminated to the states, so to have an impact in California, CHCF had to effect change at the national level. Because CHCF is not a national funder, it partnered with other state-based philanthropies to pool knowledge and funding to get the work done.

What Gets Measured Gets Counted

Despite the prevalence of perinatal mental health issues, providers rarely screen for them, and when they do, 75% of the time patients are not referred to appropriate care.[10] To increase accountability, CHCF and the ZOMA Foundation, a Colorado-based philanthropy, funded the National Committee for Quality Assurance to develop two Healthcare Effectiveness Data and Information Set (HEDIS) measures for perinatal mental health.

HEDIS measures are required by Medicare, Medicaid, and other national healthcare systems to evaluate payers and providers. If a measure is included in the HEDIS data set, then insurers and providers can be held accountable for that aspect of care. At the time, perinatal mental health had been overlooked, so CHCF and ZOMA funded the work to establish measures focused on screening and treatment for prenatal and postpartum mental health.

Ordinarily, development of HEDIS measures is funded by national organizations, so this interstate, interfunder collaboration was essential—not only to make an impact at a national level but also because the cost of the project would have been prohibitively expensive for either philanthropy to undertake alone.

The new measures require providers to collect information about whether depression screens were administered prenatally and postpartum, if there was follow-up for positive screens, and if there was treatment to remission. The measures were included in the 2020 HEDIS data set, and they could be made mandatory by 2024.

The Cost of Perinatal Mental Health

Another necessary metric was to determine just how big a problem perinatal mental health is, not only in terms of its human impact but also its financial cost. When people hear about a problem in healthcare, their first question is often, "What will it cost to fix?"—followed quickly by a litany of reasons why paying for the issue is not possible. Instead of funding a project about how much it would cost to screen and treat perinatal mental health, CHCF, ZOMA, and Perigee Fund, a national maternal and infant mental health funder based in Washington State, teamed up to turn the question on its head. They cofunded an analysis to show how much it costs not to treat the problem, highlighting the fact that money was already being spent on the issue—just not in effective ways.

The three organizations awarded a grant to Mathematica to create a model to generate estimates about the cost of untreated perinatal mental health issues. The model included medical costs and the economic toll of absenteeism, as well as costs associated with commonly linked developmental delays for the infant. The model revealed that perinatal mental health disorders cost the US $14.2 billion in a given year.[11] It also generated numbers for the funders' three home states to incentivize local governments and healthcare organizations to invest in the issue.

Building the model to run the numbers for just one state would have been extremely expensive, not to mention a wasted resource. By each foundation paying for a piece of it, the project became fiscally feasible for the three foundations, and the model is now available for other states to use to develop their own estimates.

Although there is still more data work to do, CHCF's perinatal mental health portfolio is now moving on to focus on additional levers, such as delivery-system interventions, payment, and policy change.

BIRTH EQUITY

For other issues related to maternal health, the data have long been clear: Regardless of the condition or measure, when it comes to maternal morbidity and mortality, Black birthing people have the worst outcomes. For example,

Figure 47.4 ▼

Black–white disparity in California maternal mortality ratio.

Source: California Pregnancy Mortality Surveillance System, California Department of Public Health. https://www.cdph.ca.gov/Programs/CFH/DMCAH/surveillance/CDPH%20Document%20Library/CA-PMSS/CA-PMSS-Surveillance-Report-2008-2016.pdf.

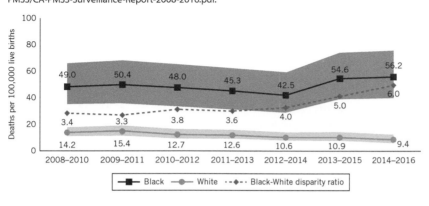

while the California maternal mortality rate has declined overall, the disparity between Black and white birthing people has grown. In 2008, the Black maternal mortality rate in the state was 3.5 times higher than the white maternal mortality rate; by 2016, it was six times higher (Figure 47.4).[†] Beyond the most extreme metric of mortality, the healthcare system fails Black birthing people in innumerable ways, including, but not limited to, higher cesarean delivery rates and lack of support for perinatal mental health issues.[12]

Supporting Community-Based Organizations

To try to start addressing the unacceptable birth-related inequities experienced by the Black population, CHCF first attempted to repeat the successful model used in the C-section initiative by funding CMQCC to develop and run a clinical quality-improvement collaborative focused on equity, which was to include antibias training and community engagement. The grant budget reflected this scope: Half was allocated to support CMQCC staff to do the quality-improvement work with hospital labor and delivery units and half was allocated to consultants to engage community to develop both a survey tool to elicit patient feedback and an antibias training for maternity care providers.

However, the structure (university-based) and leadership of the project proved problematic and ultimately required significant changes. Many lessons were learned in the process; some key ones are shared here. First, university-based efforts can struggle with community-centered competencies and relationships. Second, all those involved (especially white staff)

[†] As of this writing, 2016 is the most recent year that state data are available for California.

would have benefited from deep diversity, equity, and inclusion training before beginning the work. Third, to get to the root of birth inequities perpetuated by the healthcare system, racism (not just bias) must be named and tackled directly. Fourth, birth equity work necessitates a diverse set of skills not likely found in a single organization; therefore, collaboration and trust across teams are paramount. The work moves at the speed of trust, so significant time and support (facilitators and conflict mediators as needed) must be built in from the start to foster trust and resolve issues that arise within and across teams.

As a result of these lessons, CHCF pivoted to invest more deeply in Black-led initiatives to address birth equity, working with Black leaders at universities and think tanks and with Black-led community-based organizations (CBOs). Black-led projects now make up approximately 80% of CHCF's birth equity grantees. Central to CHCF's approach is an ongoing commitment to cultural humility that emphasizes self-evaluation and critique to address power imbalances (in this case between funders and grantees).

CHCF also convened a birth equity advisory group comprised of Black female healthcare and public health leaders. The advisory group provides CHCF with guidance and feedback on how to position its funding to make the greatest impact, as well as how it can collaborate as a true ally. The advisory group is one important way CHCF stays in touch with the community.

Partnering with community organizations is essential because these groups are the most knowledgeable about a problem and the best poised to deploy solutions. For example, in response to COVID-19, CHCF provided funding to Frontline Doulas, a CBO that established a hotline at the start of the pandemic to connect Black birthing people with virtual doula support when in-person care wasn't possible. CHCF's goal is to bring these types of solutions to scale by providing financial resources, raising awareness around them, and connecting them to the rest of the healthcare system to ensure uptake and sustainability. CHCF now tackles birth equity by pulling several levers—including data, public policy, and delivery-system interventions—but community engagement is always at the center.

Supporting Changes in Policy

With a problem as intractable as birth inequities, some interventions must come at the policy level to mandate change. CHCF does not lobby, but it often looks for ways to help support policy changes once they're passed.

One such change—the recently passed California Senate Bill 65 (California Momnibus bill)—aims to increase Black birthing people's access to doulas and midwives, particularly midwives of color, who can provide culturally congruent care. Continuous birthing support from doulas and midwives is linked to fewer pregnancy complications and unnecessary interventions,[13] which disproportionately affect Black birthing people. To support implementation of this bill,

CHCF, in partnership with the Yellowchair Foundation, is funding a mentoring program for midwives of color enrolled in California's two nurse-midwifery schools. The goal is to support new nurse-midwives through the multiyear training program and the launch of their careers.

Another bill aimed at reducing Black birth inequity is Senate Bill 464, the Dignity in Pregnancy and Childbirth Act, which, among other things, attempts to address implicit bias and racism in maternal care. To support this bill's goal, CHCF partnered with Black Women for Wellness, a CBO that cosponsored the bill, and Diversity Science, which specializes in developing diversity, equity, and inclusion educational tools, to develop an online module about implicit bias and racism in maternity care. The module is free for anyone to download and meets the training requirements stipulated in the law. While any organization serious about addressing systemic racism would need to do additional staff engagement at a deeper level, these tools help healthcare providers begin their journey to address implicit bias and racism.

CHCF's work to advance birth equity is just beginning. By supporting and collaborating with community organizations that know both the challenges and potential solutions, and by continuing to pull on multiple levers at opportune moments, CHCF hopes to contribute to progress in maternal health outcomes in California, especially in communities experiencing the greatest disparities.

REFERENCES

1. *CA-PMSS Surveillance Report: Pregnancy-Related Deaths in California, 2008–2016*. Sacramento, CA: California Department of Public Health, Maternal, Child and Adolescent Health Division; 2021. https://www.cdph.ca.gov/Programs/CFH/DMCAH/surveillance/CDPH%20Document%20Library/CA-PMSS/CA-PMSS-Surveillance-Report-2008-2016.pdf.

2. Teleki S. Working toward happier birthdays: an effort in California to lower C-section rates. *Health Affairs Blog*. 2015. doi:10.1377/hblog20151103.051561.

3. Main EK, Morton CH, Melsop K, et al. Creating a public agenda for maternity safety and quality in cesarean delivery. *Obstet Gynecol*. 2012;120(5):1194–1198. doi:10.1097/AOG.0b013e31826fc13d.

4. Rosenstein MG, Chang S, Sakowski C, et al. Hospital quality improvement interventions, statewide policy initiatives, and rates of cesarean delivery for nulliparous, term, singleton, vertex births in California. *JAMA*. 2021;325(16):1631–1639. doi:10.1001/jama.2021.3816.

5. Smith H, Peterson N, Lagrew D, et al. *Toolkit to Support Vaginal Birth and Reduce Primary Cesareans: A Quality Improvement Toolkit*. Stanford, CA: California Maternal Quality Care Collaborative; 2016.

6. *Case Study: Maternity Payment and Care Redesign Pilot*. San Francisco, CA: Pacific Business Group on Health; 2015. https://www.pbgh.org/wp-content/uploads/2020/12/TMC_Case_Study_Oct_2015.pdf.

7. Teleki S. Birthing a movement to reduce unnecessary C-sections: an update from California. *Health Affairs Blog*. 2017. doi:10.1377/hblog20171031.709216.

8. Pérez S, Peter D, Luca L. *"My Birth Matters" Research and Development: Creating Communications to Educate Low-Risk, First-Time Mothers About C-Sections.* Yonkers, NY: Consumer Reports; 2018. https://www.chcf.org/wp-content/uploads/2018/06/MyBirthMattersResearchDevelopment.pdf.

9. Declercq ER, Sakala C, Corry MP, et al. *Listening to Mothers II: Report of the Second National U.S. Survey of Women's Childbearing Experiences.* New York, NY: Childbirth Connection; 2006. https://www.nationalpartnership.org/our-work/resources/health-care/maternity/listening-to-mothers-ii-2006.pdf.

10. Byatt N, Levin LL, Ziedonis D, et al. Enhancing participation in depression care in outpatient perinatal care settings: a systematic review. *Obstet Gynecol.* 2015;126(5):1048–1058. doi:10.1097/AOG.0000000000001067.

11. Luca DL, Garlow N, Staatz C, et al. *Societal Costs of Untreated Perinatal Mood and Anxiety Disorders in the United States.* Cambridge, MA: Mathematica Policy Research; 2019. https://mathematica.org/publications/societal-costs-of-untreated-perinatal-mood-and-anxiety-disorders-in-the-united-states.

12. *Listening to Black Mothers in California.* Washington, DC: National Partners for Women and Families; 2018. https://www.nationalpartnership.org/our-work/resources/health-care/maternity/listening-to-black-mothers-in-california.pdf.

13. Bohren MA, Hofmeyr G, Sakala C, et al. Continuous support for women during childbirth. *Cochrane Database Syst Rev.* 2017;7:CD003766. doi:10.1002/14651858.CD003766.pub6.

Chapter 48

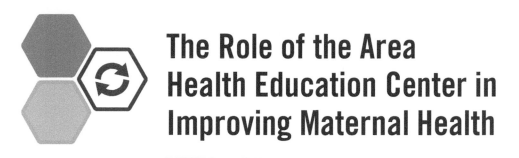

The Role of the Area Health Education Center in Improving Maternal Health

ADAM J. ZOLOTOR, JILL M. FORCINA, TARA OWENS SHULER, AND HUGH H. TILSON, JR.

INTRODUCTION

This chapter describes the current and potential roles of the North Carolina Area Health Education Center (NC AHEC) program in the recruitment, training, and retention of an available, accessible, appropriate, acceptable, and quality maternal health professional workforce. The NC AHEC program's vision is a state where every individual in North Carolina is healthy and supported by an appropriate and well-trained health workforce that reflects the communities it serves. The program's mission is to provide and support educational activities and services with a focus on primary care in rural communities and those with less access to resources to recruit, train, and retain the workforce needed to create a healthy North Carolina.

The NC AHEC program evolved from national and state concerns with the supply, distribution, retention, and quality of health professionals. In 1970, a report from the Carnegie Commission recommended the development of a nationwide system of Area Health Education Centers. Legislation and federal support since the early 1970s made the implementation of AHEC programs possible in many states, including North Carolina.

This national focus coincided with a growing effort in North Carolina to establish statewide community training for health professionals and to reverse a trend toward shortages and uneven distribution of primary care physicians in the state's rural areas. The North Carolina AHEC program began in 1972 under a federal AHEC contract with the University of North Carolina at Chapel Hill School of Medicine. In 1974, the North Carolina General Assembly approved and funded a plan to create a statewide network of nine AHEC regions. The plan

Adam J. Zolotor, Jill M. Forcina, Tara Owens Shuler, and Hugh H. Tilson, Jr., *The Role of the Area Health Education Center in Improving Maternal Health* In: *The Practical Playbook III*. Edited by: Dorothy Cilenti, Alisahah Jackson, Natalie D. Hernandez, Lindsey Yates, Sarah Verbiest, J. Lloyd Michener, and Brian C. Castrucci, Oxford University Press. © de Beaumont Foundation 2024. DOI: 10.1093/oso/9780197662984.003.0048

called for the establishment of 300 new primary care medical residency slots and the regular rotation of students to off-campus sites. The General Assembly provided funds to build or renovate AHEC educational facilities in the nine regions and to develop the proposed program components.

By 1975, all nine AHECs were operational and still operate today in all 100 North Carolina counties under the coordination of the NC AHEC Program Office in Chapel Hill. The program's work is organized through six service lines: Health Careers, Student Services, Graduate Medical Education, Continuing Professional Development, Practice Support, and Library Services.

- *Health Careers:* Emphasizing underrepresented minorities, rural communities, and economically/educationally disadvantaged populations, AHECs identify gaps in the educational pipeline and work to foster interest in healthcare careers. AHECs help students interested in health occupations to find enrichment activities and education programs before high school graduation so they can learn about health professions and job requirements. To address the need for a more diverse cadre of healthcare professionals, in 2018, NC AHEC launched the NC AHEC Scholars Program. With an emphasis on underrepresented minorities, rural areas, and first-generation college students, the NC AHEC Scholars Program provides a defined set of clinical didactic and community-based training activities in rural and/or underserved areas for health professions students.
- *Student Services:* Community-based student rotations are important parts of any health science student's education, and NC AHEC supports a variety of learning experiences, particularly at locations in rural and underserved areas. Health sciences students receive part of their training away from academic centers—in community hospitals, physicians' offices, rural health centers, public health departments, mental health centers, and other health-related settings. AHECs arrange short-term housing so students can complete their community rotations. AHECs also help facilitate community placement and problem-solve logistical issues.
- *Graduate Medical Education:* Supporting graduate medical education (also known as residency) is at the core of NC AHEC's mission. The program provides stipends at teaching hospitals across the state, and it helps support—and in some areas of the state, operate—the residency programs necessary for primary and community care, such as family medicine, pediatrics, internal medicine, general surgery, psychiatry, and obstetrics and gynecology. AHEC residents are more likely to stay in North Carolina than non-AHEC residents, which helps address the trend toward shortages and the uneven distribution of primary care physicians in the state's rural areas.[1]

- *Continuing Professional Development:* Continuing professional development (CPD) programs are important resources that provide healthcare professionals with the training and continuing education they need to meet state licensure and specialty certification and to stay abreast of new research, emerging technologies, and the latest innovations and advancements in their fields. CPD programs are often taught by health professions faculty from the state's health sciences academic centers, bringing university expertise into North Carolina communities.
- *Practice Support:* Clinical practices need to position themselves for new payment models, incentive programs, and other healthcare reforms, while focusing on patient-centered care. Nearly 50 practice-support coaches are trained to work with practices to transform the way in which care is delivered. To date, the team of coaches have helped more than 6,000 providers at 1,400 practices move toward promoting interoperability (formerly meaningful use) of their electronic health records; nearly 600 practices with Medicaid transformation education and issue resolution; over 500 practices with improving office systems for better care; and more than 300 practices with achieving patient-centered medical home recognition.
- *Library Services:* Libraries are a core part of the health education and support that AHEC provides to North Carolina's health professionals. Each of the nine AHEC locations has its own library, complete with a librarian staff prepared to meet the unique needs of the healthcare providers in their counties. In addition to this support, the AHEC Digital Library ensures that all providers in the state have high-quality health information at their fingertips.

All NC AHEC programs and services include cross-cutting emphasis on diversity, equity, and inclusion as well as interprofessional education and practice.

HEALTH WORKFORCE

The health and well-being of North Carolina's mothers and infants is like the "canary in the coal mine" and gives insight into the health of generations to come. Healthy pregnant persons are more likely to give birth to healthy infants and are less likely to face negative health outcomes themselves. Unfortunately, in North Carolina, access to maternal health providers remains a challenge.

According to the NC Rural Center, 80 of the 100 NC counties are considered rural and have an average population density of 250 people or fewer per square mile.[2] In 2017, 35 counties in North Carolina had no delivering physicians, certified nurse midwives (CNM), or delivery facilities, creating enormous barriers for women seeking maternal health services.[3] Compared to women living in urban areas, women living in rural areas experience higher rates of delayed prenatal care initiation. In North Carolina, approximately 68% of women receive prenatal care in the first trimester.[4] It is even more challenging to locate a maternal–fetal medicine (MFM) specialist. In North Carolina, most MFM specialists are geographically concentrated, which can be problematic for high-risk mothers and mothers in rural areas. In 2017, only 17 out of 100 counties had an MFM specialist.[3]

The total number of physicians providing obstetric deliveries slightly increased in North Carolina, from 928 in 2000 to 1,016 in 2017.[3] However, when compared to the total physician workforce in North Carolina over the same time, the percentage of obstetric providers making up the physician workforce declined, from 5.8% to 4.2%. Between 2000 and 2012, the number of family medicine physicians providing obstetric care declined, and then it began to increase. Unfortunately, the majority of family medicine providers who provide obstetric care live in metropolitan counties that have a family medicine residency program. From 1984 to 2017, the number of CNMs has steadily increased. Based on a 2017 Sheps presentation, CNMs reported primary practice locations in 57 counties.

In addition to the challenges of geographic distribution of healthcare providers, North Carolina is also challenged with the underrepresentation of historically minoritized persons in the healthcare workforce. Healthcare providers who identify as racial or ethnic minorities are more likely to provide care to lower-income, minority, and uninsured populations.[5] Minority health professionals play a critical role in efforts to reduce the disproportionate burden of diseases, including COVID-19, among communities of color.[6] For example, Black babies cared for by Black doctors have a significantly lower mortality rate than Black babies cared for by white doctors.[7] By building a more diverse health workforce, the United States would improve access and improve outcomes in underserved communities and for high-need populations.

Preparation of an interprofessional, diverse pipeline of maternal health professionals is an essential step in securing the future of maternal outcomes in the United States.[8,9] Studies show that outcomes improve with racially concordant, team-based care with a broad array of skills and specialties.[10,11] In a 2018 brief, 13% of North Carolina's obstetric delivery providers identified as Black or African American, compared to 21% of North Carolina's population identifying as Black or African-American. Three percent of North Carolina's obstetric providers identified as Hispanic or Latino, compared to 10% of North Carolina's population identifying as Hispanic or Latino.[12]

Recognizing that people from Black and Brown communities are underrepresented in the obstetric provider workforce, the NC AHEC program, inclusive of regional AHECs, is committed to offering CPD activities that promote understanding of dominant narratives that affect care and outcomes. Trainings specifically designed for maternal providers, newborn providers, and other health professionals are offered on implicit bias, impacts of structural racism, and cultural humility.

PRACTICE SUPPORT

The NC AHEC practice support service line is core to the way the AHEC program reaches across the state to support the system of care for women and families. To be successful working in community-based settings, health professionals must be able to enter a high-quality practice environment where they are supported by the latest information on management, billing, quality, and technology. Small, independent, and rural practices and health centers may have less access to such expertise than larger, urban, and health-system-connected practices. These practices and their patients may benefit from identifying and achieving high-value goals, electronic health record optimization, practice efficiency, and enhanced revenue.[13,14]

With nearly 50 practice coaches working in every county to support over 1,000 practices, AHEC practice coaches are a critical component of quality primary care in North Carolina. Practice coaches have historically worked with many FM providers, federally qualified community health centers, rural health centers, and county health departments. In those settings, coaches impact quality and access for women getting prenatal care across much of North Carolina's safety net. Practice coaches have worked with fewer obstetric practices, but that is quickly changing. In concert with NC Medicaid, practice coaches will work with obstetricians and family physicians to ensure providers of maternity services have up-to-date information on presumptive eligibility for Medicaid and the recent legislative extension of postpartum Medicaid. Practice coaches can also help practices with workflow, electronic health records, and billing optimization, as well as education on billing policies for telehealth and group prenatal care.

As Medicaid implements new quality metrics, including access to first trimester prenatal care, and goals around health equity for entry into first trimester prenatal care (initiation of prenatal care in the first trimester), practice coaches will develop data tools and workflows to improve rates of early prenatal care and address this inequity. AHEC practice coaches have used similar tools to improve quality of cardiovascular disease preventive care for all populations and especially Black patients.[15]

AHEC practice coaches assist in the deployment of important quality-improvement clinical trials, including a current trial with primary care providers who screen for and address unhealthy alcohol use—a program with 20 practices statewide that could have important consequences for decreasing alcohol consumption during pregnancy. Practice support is in the planning stages of a new project to measure the impact of doulas and a data dashboard on improving maternal and infant health and directly addressing health inequity. Twenty obstetric practices will be recruited and randomized into three intervention groups: no intervention, deployment of doulas at the practice level in combination with a data dashboard, and doulas, data dashboard, and practice workflow optimization. Studies like this build the evidence base for clinical interventions that address practice quality and health equity, and they also serve as a foundation for ongoing deployment of successful interventions.

CONTINUAL PROFESSIONAL DEVELOPMENT

In the rapidly evolving field of maternal health, maternal health professionals need access to quality, evidence-based, and up-to-date continuing professional development (CPD) opportunities to ensure the delivery of appropriate high-quality care. CPD is defined as "all educational programs that aim to enhance health professionals' practice and improve patient outcomes."[16] Because the breadth and depth of CPD vary across modalities, contexts, and audiences, it is difficult to demonstrate the direct effect that it has on patient outcomes; however, there is evidence that the majority of workshops, conferences, lectures, simulations, and even e-learning that target higher-level learning objectives are effective in achieving the desired results of behavior change and outcomes management.[16] According to the World Health Organization, the quantity of healthcare workers is only one component of the healthcare workforce that affects health outcomes.[17] Other essential components are the availability, accessibility, acceptability, and quality of health workers. The NC AHEC program strives to support the maternal health workforce through CPD opportunities that build the knowledge and expertise needed to meet the needs of the population; that target healthcare workers in rural and underserved areas of North Carolina; that integrate a diversity, equity, and inclusion framework; and that extend beyond knowledge gain to address behavior change and maternal health expertise.

CPD should be enjoyable and relevant to the learner. Once a learner is engaged, higher learning objectives, such as knowledge gain, can be achieved. Regional AHECs have impressive breadth and depth of CPD offerings. Regional AHECs provided at least 18 maternity-related programs to approximately 1,200 health practitioners in 2021 alone. Offerings on fetal monitoring and on substance use served an important role in 2021 regional CPD; historically, perennial offerings cover breastfeeding and high-risk maternity care. Many of the offerings are successful because of strong regional and state partnerships, such as South East AHEC's partnership with the North Carolina Lactation Consultant Association (NCLCA) and the Association of Women's Health, Obstetric and Neonatal Nursing (AWHONN).

Because coordination of care and team-based collaboration are key to achieving optimal outcomes in maternal health, NC AHEC CPD often incorporates interprofessional education as a means of optimizing efficiency and effectiveness of achieving learning objectives.[18] Eastern AHEC supports

ECU Health's Regional Intermediate Fetal Heart Monitoring and provides AWHONN training in fetal heart monitoring education, preparing learners to approach patient care utilizing standardized terminologies and interpretation tools from the National Institute of Child Health and Human Development. In partnership with their regional health system, Eastern AHEC also supports ECU Health's Regional In Situ Obstetric and Neonatal Emergency Drills, a program that engages teams at individual facilities to participate in quarterly on-site simulations. These low-fidelity simulations offer learners an opportunity to manage high-risk, low-frequency, obstetric emergencies with their own resources. Effective simulation debriefings uncover system barriers that inhibit safe care and transform them to positively affect maternal and neonatal outcomes.

Accessibility: Targeting Rural and Underserved Communities

To ensure quality maternal healthcare is accessible to the people of North Carolina, maternal healthcare providers in rural parts of the state must have access to CPD opportunities. Project ECHO (Extension for Community Health Outcomes) is an evidence-based tool both for reaching rural maternal healthcare workers and for extending specialty maternal care to the maternal health patient population in those areas. Project ECHO was developed to "ensure the right knowledge exists at the right place and time."[19] The ECHO platform is a team-support model that is based on two-way learning across a virtual community, using real-life case study presentations and consultations, discussions, and support through a formalized structure of assessment, planning, implementation, and evaluation. ECHO has been used to bridge the specialty gap that often exists in rural communities, by connecting local healthcare workers with experts, who are often located in large, urban centers. The NC AHEC program was involved in approximately 40 ECHOs in 2020 alone as a platform for both region-based education and regional communication on current topics. In maternal health, regional AHEC ECHOs have primarily focused on perinatal substance use disorder. At Eastern AHEC, the Perinatal ECHO, which has been in production for over a year, connects rural providers with the perinatal center in the region. Additionally, the Regional Tele-education via Perinatal ECHO is a monthly tele-education session in which regional obstetric providers present high-risk obstetric cases to subject-matter experts. Perinatal ECHO topics have included resource availability (e.g., mental health, dental care in pregnancy) and rapidly changing clinical recommendations (e.g., COVID-19 treatment and screening).

Acceptability: Diversity, Equity, and Inclusion

Diversity, equity, and inclusion (DEI) are key components in acceptable maternal healthcare. Regional AHECs have made significant efforts to expand DEI opportunities for the North Carolina healthcare workforce. In January 2022, the

NC AHEC Program launched a 12-module DEI curriculum. The curriculum focuses on implementing DEI strategies that are proven to improve patient care. The curriculum content is intended to articulate how DEI plays a heightened and essential role in today's healthcare environment; to educate clinical providers and nonclinical staff on fundamental concepts, such as cultural humility, structural racism, and other relevant content, to assist providers and staff to increase their knowledge and to adopt equitable practices; to integrate DEI values and core principles into the patient care environment; and to build core competency and shared language across staff. In addition, some regional AHECs embed DEI training directly in maternal health CPD offerings. For example, Eastern AHEC supports ECU Health's Regional Advanced Life Support in Obstetrics (ALSO), which directly integrates implicit bias training and awareness of the effects of structural racism. Eastern AHEC houses a region of counties to cover for the WIC Lactation program for the eastern part of the state, which includes conferences and training for healthcare providers in their support of low-income, pregnant, breastfeeding, and postpartum women, infants, and children. A little farther west, Southern Regional AHEC also partnered with the March of Dimes to provide CPD to healthcare professionals. The focus of these educational activities was preconception and interconception health. The goal was to decrease preterm birth rates, to decrease infant and maternal mortality, and to improve health equity.

Quality: Changing Behaviors and Outcomes

Multimodal CPD offerings are generally more effective in causing practice changes that can ultimately result in improved outcomes.[16] Several NC AHEC centers implement approaches that integrate multimodal learning, with didactic and clinical components, asynchronous and synchronous learning, and/or application of knowledge into deliverables. For 22 years, Northwest AHEC has coordinated the NC Lactation Educator Training Program. This biannual event involves six webinar days and two clinical days for nurses, dietitians, physicians, students, and others interested in counseling/educating breastfeeding families. Often, regional centers accomplish a multipronged approach to CPD offerings in maternal health by partnering with their regional healthcare partners. For example, Eastern AHEC supports their regional healthcare system in delivering large, multipronged training and education programs in maternal health. The Regional Advanced Life Support in Obstetrics (ALSO) prepares ALSO providers within the regional facilities and will generate in-house expertise to enhance maternal outcomes.

GRADUATE MEDICAL EDUCATION

AHEC was, in no small part, created to support enhanced investment in community-based education of primary care physicians. AHEC invests in, and supports, primary care specialties (family medicine, general internal medicine, general pediatrics, and OB-GYN) as well as the high-need physician specialties of psychiatry and general surgery. Advanced practice providers (nurse practitioners, physicians' assistants, and CNMs) comprise an increasingly valuable portion of North Carolina's primary care workforce but have historically received less focus and funding through AHEC.

Before the development of AHEC, most graduate medical education (also known as residency) took place in North Carolina's three medical schools: the University of North Carolina at Chapel Hill, Duke University, and Wake Forest University, resulting in two unintended consequences. It created urban centers with disproportionately high healthcare resources. In addition, most residency graduates practice within 100 miles of their residency, further contributing to the uneven distribution of providers.[20] Community-based education has emerged as one of the most important strategies for deploying physicians across the state. North Carolina now hosts residency programs in 26 communities throughout the state. AHEC supports residency programs in nearly all of these communities, including hosting residency programs in four communities. In a recent report by the National Academy of Science, Engineering, and Medicine, "Implementing High-Quality Primary Care," the training of primary care teams where people live and work was cited as one of the most important ways to improve access to primary care that is connected to community.[21]

NC AHEC has supported decentralized primary care graduate medical education for nearly 50 years. The clinical sites provide maternal care across the state, train the future workforce to provide that care, and are more likely to retain physicians close to the site of training.[1] Most of the 26 communities that host residency programs include family medicine residencies (23 residencies). Family medicine residency programs provide prenatal and hospital-based maternity care as part of a comprehensive program of training, and many graduates continue to provide maternity care; in addition, preconception care and chronic disease management are essential for a healthy pregnancy. North Carolina is home to eight OB-GYN training programs and one obstetric fellowship for family physicians. Several of these training programs are operated by a regional AHEC or are closely affiliated with an AHEC. Because of the close relationship between clinical services and training programs, faculty in one AHEC (Mountain AHEC) provide obstetric services to 90% of pregnant women with Medicaid in the most populous county in Western North Carolina. Regional obstetric services have become even more important in recent years, with the closure of six rural birthing units in Western North Carolina. Last, with an ever-increasing appreciation of the role of perinatal mood disorders in maternal health, it is important to recognize the AHEC-supported training in psychiatry. North Carolina is currently home to eight psychiatry residency programs similarly distributed across the state and supported by AHEC.

Having robust clinical and educational enterprises engaged in the care of women and children supports a number of care innovations to provide local high-quality care and to train learners in new models of care. Regional AHECs and their affiliated residency sites offer CenteringPregnancy® (Mountain AHEC, South East AHEC), services for pregnant women with substance use disorders (Mountain AHEC and South East AHEC), a community-based doula program for women of color (Mountain AHEC), and integrated behavioral healthcare. In addition, the distributive training infrastructure facilitates participation in multicenter quality-improvement initiatives through the implicit network to bring high-quality maternity care across the state.

CONCLUSIONS

By supporting the healthcare workforce along the entire learning continuum, the NC AHEC works toward a state where every individual is healthy and supported by an appropriate and well-trained health workforce that reflects the communities it serves. Pipeline/pathway programs reinforce the systems needed for maternal health by recruiting health professions students from a diverse background to build a more racially and ethnically diverse workforce. Training students and residents from rural communities and in rural communities is a well-recognized strategy to improve the distribution of health professionals. Supporting professionals in practice through practice support, library services, and CPD improves the quality of care and develops the needed skills of an effective health workforce to remain in NC communities taking care of pregnant persons.

REFERENCES

1. Spero J, Tilson H. Outcomes of NC medical school graduates: how many stay in practice in NC, in primary care, and in high needs areas? https://www.northcarol ina.edu/wp-content/uploads/reports-and-documents/academic-affairs/outcomes-of-nc-medical-school-graduates-2020.pdf. Publsihed 2020. Accessed February 2, 2022.

2. Rural-North-Carolina-at-a-Glance.pdf. 2021. https://www.ncruralcenter.org/wp-content/uploads/2021/03/Rural-North-Carolina-at-a-Glance.pdf. Accessed February 1, 2022.

3. Walker K, Fraher E, Spero J, Galloway E. Access to obstetric and prenatal care providers in North Carolina. Presented May 2, 2019, to North Carolina Institute of Medicine. https://nciom.org/wp-content/uploads/2018/12/ObstetricCareSlidesf orIOM_1-May-2019_COB-Fraher.pdf. Accessed February 2, 2022.

4. Risk factors and characteristics for 2019 North Carolina live births: overall, all mothers. North Carolina State Center for Health Statistics. 2021. https://schs.dph.ncdhhs.gov/schs/births/matched/2019/2019-Births-Overall.html. Accessed February 1, 2022.

5. Wilbur K, Snyder C, Essary AC, Reddy S, Will KK, Saxon M. Developing workforce diversity in the health professions: a social justice perspective. *Health Prof Educ*. 2020;6(2):222–229. doi:10.1016/j.hpe.2020.01.002.

6. Salsberg E, Richwine C, Westergaard S, et al. Estimation and comparison of current and future racial/ethnic representation in the US health care workforce. *JAMA Netw Open*. 2021;4(3):e213789. doi:10.1001/jamanetworkopen.2021.3789.

7. Greenwood BN, Hardeman RR, Huang L, Sojourner A. Physician–patient racial concordance and disparities in birthing mortality for newborns. *Proc Natl Acad Sci*. 2020;117(35):21194–21200. doi:10.1073/pnas.1913405117.

8. National Advisory Council on Nurse Education and Practice. Achieving health equity through nursing workforce diversity: Eleventh Report to the Secretary of Health and Human Services and the Congress. https://www.hrsa.gov/sites/defa ult/files/hrsa/advisory-committees/nursing/reports/2013-eleventhreport.pdf. Published 2013. Accessed February 2, 2022.

9. Homer CSE, Friberg IK, Dias MAB, et al. The projected effect of scaling up midwifery. *Lancet*. 2014;384(9948):1146–1157. doi:10.1016/ S0140-6736(14)60790-X.

10. Davis MB, Walsh MN. Cardio-obstetrics. *Circ Cardiovasc Qual Outcomes*. 2019;12(2):e005417. doi:10.1161/CIRCOUTCOMES.118.005417.

11. Laurie C. Zephyrin, Shanoor Seervai, Corinne Lewis, Jodie G. Katon. Community-based models to improve maternal health outcomes and promote health equity. 2021. https://www.commonwealthfund.org/publications/issue-briefs/2021/mar/ community-models-improve-maternal-outcomes-equity.

12. Julie Spero. NC health workforce—how diverse is NC's obstetric delivery workforce? 2020. https://nchealthworkforce.unc.edu/blog/obstetric_provider_race/. Accessed February 1, 2022.

13. Michaels L, Anastas T, Waddell EN, Fagnan L, Dorr DA. A randomized trial of high-value change using practice facilitation. *J Am Board Fam Med*. 2017;30(5):572–582. doi:10.3122/jabfm.2017.05.170013.

14. Phillips RL, Cohen DJ, Kaufman A, Dickinson WP, Cykert S. Facilitating practice transformation in frontline health care. *Ann Fam Med*. 2019;17(suppl 1):S2–S5. doi:10.1370/afm.2439.

15. Cykert S, Keyserling TC, Pignone M, et al. A controlled trial of dissemination and implementation of a cardiovascular risk reduction strategy in small primary care practices. *Health Serv Res*. 2020;55(6):944–953. doi:10.1111/1475-6773.13571.

16. Samuel A, Cervero RM, Durning SJ, Maggio LA. Effect of continuing professional development on health professionals' performance and patient outcomes: a scoping review of knowledge syntheses. *Acad Med J Assoc Am Med Coll*. 2021;96(6):913–923. doi:10.1097/ACM.0000000000003899.

17. Global Health Workforce Alliance. What do we mean by availability, accessibility, acceptability and quality (AAAQ) of the health workforce? Geneva, Switzerland: World Health Organization; 2022. https://www.who.int/workforcealliance/media/ qa/04/en/. Accessed January, 21, 2022.

18. Institute of Medicine (US) Committee on Planning a Continuing Health Professional Education Institute. *Envisioning a Better System of Continuing*

Professional Development. Washington, DC: National Academies Press; 2010. https://www.ncbi.nlm.nih.gov/books/NBK219797/. Accessed February 2, 2022.

19. University of New Mexico Health Sciences. About ECHO: We empower communities to tackle challenges in education, health care and more. https://hsc.unm.edu/echo/about-us/. Accessed February 2, 2022.

20. Fagan EB, Finnegan SC, Bazemore A, Gibbons C, Petterson S. Migration after family medicine residency: 56% of graduates practice within 100 miles of training. *Am Fam Physician*. 2013;88(10):704.

21. National Academies of Science, Engineering, and Medicine. *Implementing High-Quality Primary Care: Rebuilding the Foundation of Health Care*. Washington, DC: National Academies Press; 2021.

Chapter 49

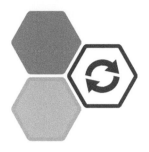

The Role of Local Health Departments in Women's Health and the Opportunity to Improve Rural Maternal Health Outcomes

LISA MACON HARRISON AND ABIGAIL KENNEY

Local health departments (LHDs) play a key role as essential community providers and healthcare access points across the rural–urban landscape in the United States. Granville Vance Public Health (GVPH) offers a critical access point for the provision of services to pregnant women in a rural two-county public health district in North Carolina. As a district, GVPH is a pseudo-independent public health entity in North Carolina serving two adjacent rural counties located just north and northeast of the triangle cities of Raleigh, Durham, and Chapel Hill. GVPH serves a combined population of approximately 100,000 and offers full-scale prevention, public health, and primary care services to the community. As a governmental entity, GVPH receives approximately 40% of its program-related funds from local, state, and federal sources combined. Funds from other sources are also necessary to support the workforce and the delivery of local public health in rural North Carolina. Both counties benefit from the cost-saving and the efficiency of shared leadership across one district health department.

Access to care can be especially challenging in rural and medically underserved areas, where transportation systems are not as robust as in suburban and urban areas and there are a limited number of obstetric (OB-GYN) providers. LHDs and rural areas are able to provide prenatal care using family physicians with additional training, including training in vaginal delivery and cesarean delivery. Advanced practice providers, such as certified nurse midwives, nurse practitioners, and physician assistants, also help to reduce the strain and provide prenatal care.[1] According to the University of North Carolina's Health

Lisa Macon Harrison and Abigail Kenney, *The Role of Local Health Departments in Women's Health and the Opportunity to Improve Rural Maternal Health Outcomes* In: *The Practical Playbook III*. Edited by: Dorothy Cilenti, Alisahah Jackson, Natalie D. Hernandez, Lindsey Yates, Sarah Verbiest, J. Lloyd Michener, and Brian C. Castrucci, Oxford University Press.
© de Beaumont Foundation 2024. DOI: 10.1093/oso/9780197662984.003.0049

Professional Supply data, as of October 31, 2019, approximately 25 counties in North Carolina do not have an active licensed physician with a primary area of OB-GYN practice, not including residents in training and employees of the federal government.[2] This is illustrated in Figure 49.1. It is difficult to accurately assess counties across the nation that do not have an OB-GYN provider in the jurisdiction, but using data from the 2010 Census, the American Congress of Obstetricians was able to identify that approximately half of the counties in the United States do not have an OB-GYN physician practicing in the county.[3] In an Issue Brief by the Centers for Medicare & Medicaid Services, a figure is presented that shows maternity care deserts in the United States.[4] This figure illustrates that urban counties have an average of 35 OB-GYNs per 1,000 residents, while rural counties suffer the most from physician shortages and there are less than two OB-GYNs per 1,000 residents.[4] Even more concerning, as we look through a health equity lens, counties with higher populations of Blacks, Hispanics, and those with lower median incomes were most at risk of not having

Figure 49.1 ▾

Physician with a primary area of practice in obstetrics and gynecology, general, per 10,000 population by county, North Carolina, 2019. Notes: Data include active, licensed physicians in practice in North Carolina as of October 31 of each year. Physician data are derived from the North Carolina Medical Board. Population census data and estimates are downloaded from the North Carolina Office of State Budget and Management via NC LINC and are based on US Census data.

Source: North Carolina Health Professions Data System, Program on Health Workforce Research and Policy, Cecil G. Sheps Center for Health Services Research, University of North Carolina at Chapel Hill. Created April 18, 2023, at https://nchealthworkforce.unc.edu/interactive/supply/.

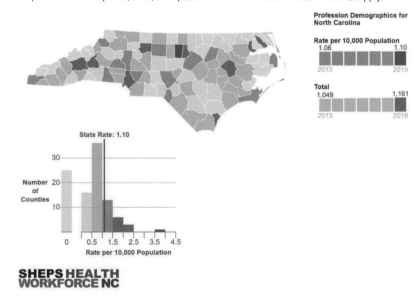

hospital obstetric services.[4] This is especially alarming, as there are known racial and ethnicity disparities when it comes to maternal mortality, with a threefold increased risk in mortality in non-Hispanic Black women compared to non-Hispanic white women.[5] Even when primary care physicians may be available to provide delivery in rural areas, there remains a high need for prenatal care and specialty care for high-risk individuals in maternity care deserts.

Often, LHDs fill the growing gap and address this inequity by becoming pregnancy care medical homes in rural counties that have few resources and OB-GYNs. One of the best ways to begin to address this problem is to focus on women's health through the life span, not just during pregnancy, but before and after pregnancy as well.[4] These services include family planning (FP), routine exams, mental health, substance use screening and treatment, and oral health.[4] Regardless of whether the agency provides full-scale primary care, the opportunity to connect a patient to all the services needed to be healthy is available at this critical entry point. LHDs also regularly connect individuals with services at the community level, where determinants of health, including housing security, nutrition security, transportation, and childcare referrals, can be addressed. In rural and medically underserved areas in particular, FP, maternal health, and child health, if offered together, can contribute to improved health outcomes for individuals and families, especially when mental health services and care management are available in the same location for ease of access.

Where there is investment in maternal health, even in counties with high poverty rates, there are improved birth outcomes.[6] LHDs can connect different sources of funding (local, state, federal, grant, and foundation funds) to comprise scalable, sustainable multidisciplinary teams that make a substantive impact on perinatal outcomes. In addition to offering FP, maternal health, and child health as clinic services, LHDs can address infant mortality through evidence-based public health interventions, education, and community connections.[7] One example of combining these approaches is CenteringPregnancy.[8] CenteringPregnancy is a model of prenatal care that combines peer support with health education and healthcare delivery.[9] In addition to reducing poor birth outcomes, prenatal care links patients to FP and child health services and is correlated with a decrease in maternal and infant deaths.[6] Preconceptual care, along with early, continuous prenatal care that all patients can access, has a direct impact on health outcomes. CenteringPregnancy is offered at GVPH and opportunities to connect to other services for pregnant women are offered in both individual patient care clinic settings and CenteringPregnancy sessions. These services offered include access to doula services (covered by Medicaid if eligible) and referrals in house for mental health and substance use treatment services, as well as care management for addressing housing security, nutrition needs, transportation, and childcare. Whole-person care delivered through coordinated care teams has arrived at GVPH and in other LHDs out of both necessity and community engagement. By bringing together a multidisciplinary team, a combination of funding sources, and creative approaches informed by evidence, LHDs can provide equitable, high-quality, coordinated care for women regardless of their insurance source.

THE IMPACT OF HEALTH DEPARTMENTS IN WOMEN'S HEALTH

LHDs make an impact by providing necessary and basic health services that promote health and prevent disease at all levels of the socio-ecologic model. Preconceptual care begins with FP services. As an LHD, FP is provided for all patients of reproductive age requesting services regardless of their immigration status. This is a crucial service to assess and identify risk factors that may affect health and pregnancy outcomes such as obesity, age, substance use, birth intervals, and family history.[10] Also, FP provides necessary preventative services such as pap smears, vaccination assessment and counseling, as well as mental health screening, substance use screening, and sexually transmitted disease (STD) screening and treatment. Referrals are made to other specialties as needed, based on the findings of the visit. Whether internally or through partnerships in the community, LHDs assist patients with accessing other sources of care such as primary care and behavioral health.[5]

Assessing patients' needs and medical conditions, and providing referrals when necessary, helps patients navigate the healthcare system by linking them to a broader range of services.[5] Further, FP services are available to those with or without health insurance. Women of all ages may seek a confidential space in the FP clinic at the LHD, including teenagers. Fees are assessed on a sliding scale basis based on a patient's household size and income, but care will not be refused if an individual is unable to provide that information. Birth control options such as long-acting reversible contraception, injectable contraception, and condoms are available on the same day of the visit, if appropriate. Other methods such as contraceptive pills and emergency contraception are provided through the LHD's stock at the local pharmacy. If it is determined that a patient meets criteria for those contraceptives, a prescription will be sent by the provider to be filled at the pharmacy using the LHD stock. These birth control options are purchased via the 340B drug pricing program. For uninsured patients, this ensures that patients have access to affordable contraception billed to them based on the percentage of pay that was assessed based on their household size and income. One main goal of the FP clinic is to help prevent unwanted pregnancies, but it also provides preconceptual and basic fertility counseling for those interested in becoming pregnant.[5]

Providing preconceptual and early, continuous prenatal care reduces poor outcomes such as low birthweight, preterm delivery, and infant mortality.[11]

The World Health Organization (WHO) stresses that early intervention reduces preventable mortality.[12] The three key components of preventable mortality that the LHD provides are availability, accessibility, and affordability.[12] For example, appointments are made available, and flexibility is provided as needed to meet the needs of the community. Care is accessible, and patients are not turned away for any FP, maternal or child health care services, regardless of the ability to pay. Women can receive an initial obstetric (OB) assessment within two weeks of a positive pregnancy test, or notification of the need to establish care. This initial assessment includes history-taking, a physical, counseling, education, laboratory testing, immunizations, and additional radiology orders as needed. This allows risk factors to be minimized with early identification and patients to be linked with higher levels of care for patients identified to be high-risk. In North Carolina, the above-mentioned initial OB as well as the return OB visit in the LHD is guided by the Agreement Addendum (AA) published by the NC Department of Health and Human Services Women's Health Branch. The AA is evidence-based and updated annually.[13] The AA is accessible via the North Carolina Department of Health and Human Services Women's Health Branch Web site and encompasses all aspects of health for the pregnant patient and allows for a complete and thorough assessment following best practices of care.[13]

FUNDING WOMEN'S HEALTH IN A HEALTH DEPARTMENT SETTING

Providing necessary care to women in rural areas through the LHD depends on a complex government agency budget with multiple sources of revenue and associated reporting requirements. Sources of funding to do the work of LHDs comes from local, state, and federal government levels in combination, some fee-for-service reimbursement, per-member-per-month Medicaid (PMPM) payments, as well as private foundation grants. In rural areas, where the revenues to the local county government from property taxes are smaller than in urban areas, there is often a need to supplement government sources of funding with nongovernment sources. The average cost for patient visits is something most clinics measure and work on for improving value, but value to whom? Value means that both cost and quality are considered, and for agencies whose mission it is to provide care as part of the safety net, value of services is measured by satisfaction with the services and health outcomes. Agencies focused on quality improvement, like GVPH, conduct optimal performance projects and institute quality-improvement councils to continually evaluate and improve patient flow and efficiency, to regularly monitor patient and staff satisfaction, and to work across a multidisciplinary team to ensure elements of the value of services provided are present.

Grants help fund quality-improvement initiatives and, at times, spur innovation. At GVPH, approximately 11 of 90 staff members across the agency are 100% grant-funded to do the work of health promotion, integrated care, quality improvement, and behavioral health services. For clinic services particularly, sources of funding can also include fees charged to patients and insurance companies, including Medicaid and Medicare. Often, the sources of funding for a program and its staff do not always cover the annual costs of the program and additional funding sources from grants and direct payments to draw down the federal share of Medicaid reimbursement round out the budget at the end of the year for Medicaid services provided and costs incurred. The mission is the focus; however, business practices are important to monitor and continually improve.

Public health has long existed to prevent disease, to promote health, and to serve the public based on priority health needs of the community identified in community health assessments. Many LHDs are focused on quality improvement, are trained to offer high-quality care to individuals and communities, and are used to working with partners to help fill any gaps in services that may be needed for patients. Figure 49.2 illustrates the funding or revenue sources for the maternal health program at GVPH. Each local health department will have some variation of these funding sources, because there are different levels of local, state, federal, and grant funding available in each county. The snapshot in Figure 49.2 is from GVPH for fiscal year 2020–2021 for maternal health only.

SYSTEMS IN PLACE TO PROVIDE HIGH-QUALITY CARE

For a small, rural LHD, providing equitable access to high-quality care is a priority. Providing prenatal care includes a multidisciplinary team that works closely together to promote positive birth outcomes and to ensure that patients

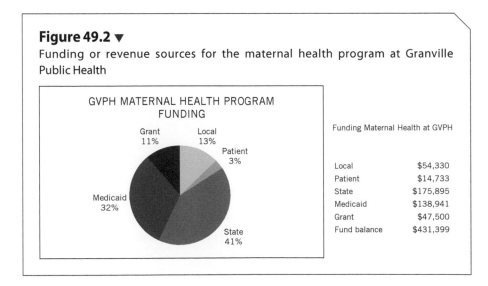

Figure 49.2 ▼
Funding or revenue sources for the maternal health program at Granville Public Health

have everything they need for a healthy pregnancy. In addition, at GVPH, a rural academic health department (AHD) model exists to augment quality, to connect innovation with evidence, and to address funding sustainability for different programs. These connections help GVPH to continue to grow as a LHD by connecting to innovators and grant opportunities. A unique long-standing partnership between GVPH and the University of North Carolina at Chapel Hill through the NC Institute for Public Health was started in 2013 to leverage the resources for patients and to elevate the practice of public health locally. This model provides real-time community relationships, and real-time testing for researchers interested in generating evidence based in rural public health practice. It also connects local public health practitioners to expertise in grant writing and management, evaluation, epidemiology, and health equity research. In 2017, the Duke University School of Nursing became another formal academic health department partner to GVPH. These relationships, as well as thinking strategically in the face of Medicaid transformation, have helped GVPH move along the AHD continuum toward comprehensive collaboration. GVPH intentionally takes on work that is consistent with GVPH's values and the community's priorities, includes collaborations with relevant stakeholders, and maximizes limited resources (including staff time to engage in efforts to seek grant funding). GVPH's unique "embedded researcher" structure allows for greater exchange of knowledge (empirical from research and experiential from practice), more nuanced understanding of contextual factors, and enhanced engagement between researchers, community members, and LHD staff. The AHD model depends on a researcher who has a mind for research, a heart for community, and an affinity for rural areas (even when those are not the places where a research project can get the largest numbers of participants). This partnership has allowed for practice support to increase capacity to address community needs by aligning strategic needs of the communities with the research and quality-improvement work of students and faculty. Further, this partnership allows for the amplification and dissemination of the innovative work of public health nursing and other innovative multidisciplinary collaborations that occur at GVPH and is another way health equity is addressed by bringing urban innovation to rural communities. For maternal health improvements at GVPH, the AHD model contributed to the grants the GVPH team wrote and received over the last decade for CenteringPregnancy, the doula program, and integrated care before those approaches became more commonly funded through state channels and Medicaid.

AN EXAMPLE OF GVPH'S USE OF A MULTIDISCIPLINARY TEAM THROUGHOUT A PATIENT'S PREGNANCY

A single pregnant patient arrives at GVPH for a return OB visit. This patient may see several different providers from multiple disciplines on the collaborative care team. After checking in, the patient is greeted by a management support professional. At this step, the management support professional helps the patient identify if she is eligible for Medicaid or emergency Medicaid, while taking care to help her fill out necessary forms and paperwork. Next, she is brought to an exam room by a registered nurse (RN) who has additional training in maternal health. At this point, vital signs are obtained, and an interview is completed. After this step, all paperwork and questionnaires are reviewed with the RN and healthcare provider. A prenatal check-up is then completed. CenteringPregnancy is offered to all patients in both English and Spanish. On some visits, the patient may participate in a scheduled CenteringPregnancy group session with other pregnant patients. Research has shown that CenteringPregnancy benefits low-income, teen, and racial/ethnic minority patients.[9] This is yet another example of LHDs' gap-filling capabilities to ensure equity in healthcare availability.

If risk factors are identified, wraparound services are available based on patient need. In addition, if requested by the provider, the patient can be linked with an OB care manager. The OB care manager may meet the patient at the visit or meet virtually on a telephone call. The care manager follows the patient during the pregnancy and continuously assesses the patient's needs and for any new risk factors that need to be addressed by either the OB care manager, provider, or both. The OB care manager may contact and collaborate with the RN or provider as needed.

While the dental office is not in the same building, a dental clinic is available to patients through GVPH. All pregnant patients are encouraged to visit the dentist for routine dental care and are provided a referral. On the other hand, the Special Supplemental Nutrition Program for Women, Infants, and Children (WIC) is housed at the LHD, and patients are linked to WIC at their initial visit. Through WIC, patients have access to supplemental foods, nutritional counseling, breastfeeding support, and a breastfeeding peer counselor.[14] Finally, behavioral health support is available for patients from a clinical mental health counselor if initial intake or formal assessment of the patient determines that is a needed service. Patients needing additional support through counseling may utilize this resource and see the counselor on the same day, if needed.

The maternal health team is invested in the care of patients and the importance of prenatal visits. If an appointment is missed, the RN contacts the patient to see if a new appointment can be scheduled. If the patient cannot be contacted, a reminder letter is sent in the mail regarding the missed appointment. Care does not stop after delivery. For example, postpartum visits are scheduled prior to delivery to ensure the patient does not fall through the gap in the transition between prenatal and postpartum care. WIC is available as needed to support breastfeeding, to provide breast pumps, and to aid in obtaining formula. A child health appointment can be made for the newborn to establish care, and the RN makes a postpartum home visit within the first few weeks after birth. This visit provides key postpartum and newborn education,

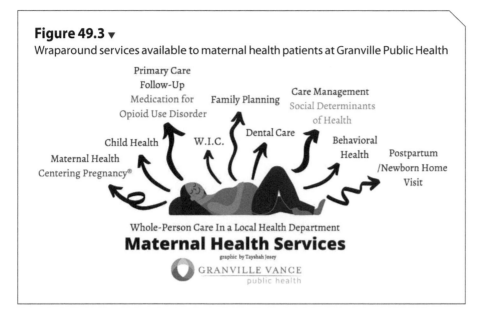

Figure 49.3 ▼

Wraparound services available to maternal health patients at Granville Public Health

Primary Care Follow-Up
Medication for Opioid Use Disorder
Family Planning
Care Management
Social Determinants of Health
Child Health
W.I.C.
Dental Care
Behavioral Health
Maternal Health Centering Pregnancy®
Postpartum /Newborn Home Visit

Whole-Person Care In a Local Health Department

Maternal Health Services

graphic by Tayshah Josey

GRANVILLE VANCE
public health

counseling, and assessment in the comfort of the patient's home. In conclusion, the LHD can provide thorough and comprehensive preconception to postpartum and FP care. This care is evidence-based, high quality, and delivered in a collaborative approach for community members. Figure 49.3 illustrates the different programs—the wraparound services—available to any maternal health patient who seeks care at GVPH.

THE FUTURE OF WOMEN'S HEALTH IN THE HEALTH DEPARTMENT SETTING

The future of maternal health in LHDs should include equitable access to all the services women, infants, and children need to achieve the best health outcomes. LHDs aim to address common gaps and challenges in access to care and can offer whole-person care and patient-centered approaches to care with multidisciplinary teams working together in the agency and across partners in the community. Partners are not just medical, behavioral, and healthcare-oriented partners, but also partners in housing, food security and nutrition, economic development, education, and transportation. LHDs can address maternal and infant mortality by ensuring access to value-based care for the individual while simultaneously paying close attention to the social determinants of health and systems change in a community. Value-based care in public health means ensuring the quality and affordability of community supports along with integrated care teams that, together, contribute to family health outcomes. By offering multiple services with easy access for women through a well-trained, diverse workforce, LHDs play a critical role in improving maternal and infant health outcomes and protecting and promoting health for everyone across the rural–urban continuum.

ACKNOWLEDGMENTS

The authors express their gratitude for the time and expertise contributed by the following colleagues as additional reviewers of this work: Tayshah Josey, BS, MedServe Fellow, Granville Vance Public Health; Shauna Guthrie, MD, MPH, FAAFP, Medical Director, Granville Vance Public Health; Leigh Anne Fowler, RN, Nursing Director, Granville Vance Public Health; and Devon Noonan, PhD, MPH, FNP-BC, Associate Professor, Duke School of Nursing.

REFERENCES

1. Deutchman M, Macaluso F, Bray E, et al. The impact of family physicians in rural maternity care. *Birth*. 2022;49(2):220–232. doi:10.1111/birt.12591.

2. Sheps Health Workforce NC. North Carolina health professional supply data. https://nchealthworkforce.unc.edu/interactive/supply/. Accessed March 11, 2022.

3. Rayburn WF, Klagholz JC, Murray-Krezan C, Dowell LE, Strunk AL. Distribution of American Congress of Obstetricians and Gynecologists fellows and junior fellows in practice in the United States. *Obstet Gynecol*. 2012;119(5):1017–1022. doi: 10.1097/AOG.0b013e31824cfe50.

4. Centers for Medicare & Medicaid Services. Improving access to maternal health care in rural communities. https://www.cms.gov/About-CMS/Agency-Information/OMH/equity-initiatives/rural-health/09032019-Maternal-Health-Care-in-Rural-Communities.pdf. Published June 2019. Accessed April 1, 2022.

5. Gavin L, Moskosky S, Carter M, et al; Centers for Disease Control and Prevention (CDC). Providing quality family planning services: recommendations of CDC and the U.S. Office of Population Affairs. *MMWR*. 2014;63(RR-04):1–54.

6. Bekemeier B, Yang Y, Dunbar MD, Pantazis A, Grembowski DE. Targeted health department expenditures benefit birth outcomes at the county level. *Am J Prev Med*. 2014;46(6):569–577. doi:10.1016/j.amepre.2014.01.023.

7. Mays GP, Smith SA. Evidence links increases in public health spending to declines in preventable deaths. *Health Aff*. 2011;30(8):1585–1593. doi:10.1377/hlthaff.2011.0196.

8. Centering Healthcare. CenteringPregnancy. https://www.centeringhealthcare.org/what-we-do/centering-pregnancy. Accessed March 11, 2022.

9. Liu R, Chao MT, Jostad-Laswell A, Duncan LG. Does CenteringPregnancy group prenatal care affect the birth experience of underserved women? A mixed methods analysis. *J Immigr Minor Health*. 2017;19(2):415–422. doi:10.1007/s10903-016-0371-9.

10. Brown W, Ahmed S, Roche N, Sonneveldt E, Darmstadt GL. Impact of family planning programs in reducing high-risk births due to younger and older maternal age, short birth intervals, and high parity. *Semin Perinatol*. 2015;39(5):338–344. doi:10.1053/j.semperi.2015.06.006.

11. Howell EA. Reducing disparities in severe maternal morbidity and mortality. *Clin Obstet Gynecol*. 2018;61(2):387–399. doi:10.1097/GRF.0000000000000349.

12. Owusu PA, Sarkodie SA, Pedersen PA. Relationship between mortality and health care expenditure: sustainable assessment of health care system. *PLOS One*. 2021;16(2):e0247413. doi:10.1371/journal.pone.0247413.

13. North Carolina Department of Health and Human Services, Women's Health Branch. Agreement addenda, audit tools and budget forms. https://wicws.dph.ncd hhs.gov/provpart/agreement-addenda.htm. Updated November 1, 2021. Accessed January 22, 2022.

14. Bersak T, Sonchak L. The impact of WIC on infant immunizations and health care utilization. *Health Serv Res*. 2018;53(suppl 1):2952–2969. doi:10.1111/1475-6773.12810.

Conclusion

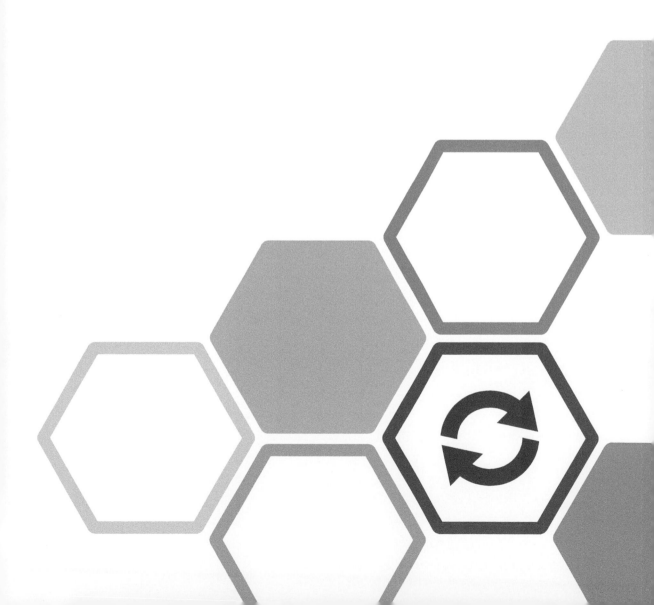

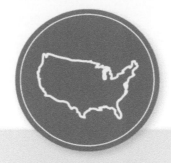

We have a long way to go, but we also have wonderful examples upon which to continue the journey forward.

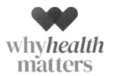

Source: Why Health Matters and Imaginari

Chapter 50

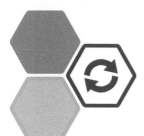

The Journey Forward

DOROTHY CILENTI, ALISAHAH JACKSON, NATALIE D. HERNANDEZ,
LINDSEY YATES, SARAH VERBIEST, AND J. LLOYD MICHENER

Throughout, *The Practical Playbook III* offers insight into, and awareness of, the many challenges to improving maternal health in the United States, as well as details about the organizations and partnerships at the community, state, and federal level that are aligning resources to ensure women and birthing people have optimal chances for a healthy pregnancy, birth, and delivery. Woven throughout the chapters are stories and examples of the disproportionate burden of maternal morbidity and mortality for Black and other racialized people, and those traumatized by historical abuses and present-day discrimination, racism, and stigma. While this book was being written, the current administration released the White House Blueprint for Addressing the Maternal Health Crisis (https://www.whitehouse.gov/wp-content/uploads/2022/06/Maternal-Health-Blueprint.pdf). The vision is to make the United States the best country to deliver a baby. So how does a practical playbook for improving maternal health help achieve this vision?

Previous Practical Playbooks have underscored that health can be achieved by working together, and *The Practical Playbook III* asserts the same. But the focus on maternal health is unique: we recognize that without healthy women and birthing people, the health of our families and communities is affected across the life span. We cannot delay implementation of efforts to prevent the nearly 1,000 maternal deaths each year, lest we lose our most important resource, our mothers and birthing people. The contributions of the many authors of this book describe ways to save mothers by centering equity in our practice, building partnerships and coalitions that share power with people with lived experience, decolonizing data to drive action at the state and local levels, piloting and expanding innovations that cross the many sectors that affect health and well-being, and leveraging backbone organizations, anchor institutions, financing,

Dorothy Cilenti, Alisahah Jackson, Natalie D. Hernandez, Lindsey Yates, Sarah Verbiest, and J. Lloyd Michener, *The Journey Forward* In: *The Practical Playbook III*. Edited by: Dorothy Cilenti, Alisahah Jackson, Natalie D. Hernandez, Lindsey Yates, Sarah Verbiest, J. Lloyd Michener, and Brian C. Castrucci, Oxford University Press.

and policy to scale and sustain what we know works. As we tackle complex, systemic, interconnected problems that are resulting in deepening and disparate health outcomes, there is an urgent need for new mindsets, approaches, and voices to move the field toward change. We hope that this Practical Playbook drives some important, and likely uncomfortable, conversations about the state of maternal health in this country. By having these conversations, we mobilize individuals, organizations, and communities to continue to demand change.

We began organizing and writing this book during the global pandemic. The contributors remained committed to sharing their stories and lessons learned, despite facing incredible challenges. We thank them for their contribution. We have been deeply enriched by their knowledge and willingness to work with us during unprecedented times.

We reached out to many people we believed had insight and perspectives to share about maternal health. Unfortunately, a number of them were unable to contribute at that time. As a result, there were several perspectives that we were unable to include in this version of the book. Among some of these are the perspectives of stakeholders people and partners who care for birthing people from the following populations: those living with disabilities, those living with mental illness, those suffering from intimate partner violence, and those who deliver in birthing centers or other nonclinical settings.

We are committed to learning from and sharing the best practices from people with those experiences. The partners spearheading this book, including the Maternal Health Learning and Innovation Center, are learning organizations. As part of our commitment to this work, we will continue to invest resources in collecting and disseminating stories from the field. This is just the beginning of what works for the field of maternal health. As this work moves forward, there will be new and exciting developments that can be scaled.

We hope this book will assist the wide range of partners working to improve maternal health so that they may support thriving, diverse communities in which women, birthing people, and children are valued and supported. We have a long way to go, but we also have wonderful examples upon which to continue the journey forward.

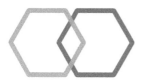

Index

For the benefit of digital users, indexed terms that span two pages (e.g., 52–53) may, on occasion, appear on only one of those pages.

Tables, figures, and boxes are indicated by *t, f,* and *b* following the page number

A

AAFP. *See* American Academy of Family Physicians

AAIMM Prevention Initiative. *See* African American Infant and Maternal Mortality Prevention Initiative

AAMC. *See* Association of American Medical Colleges

AAP (American Academy of Pediatrics), 96–97

academic centers, role in advancing maternal health
  academic medical centers and community benefits, 21–22, 22*f*
  community, 25–27
  general discussion, 32–33
  individuals, 22–23
  organizations, 23–25
  overview, 19–20, 20*f*, 21*f*
  policy and advocacy, 28–29
  relationships, 23
  society and scholarship, 29–32, 30*b*, 31*b*

academic health department (AHD) model, GVPH, 584–85

academic health systems
  advancing institutional advocacy, 486–87
  AMA strategic approaches to advance maternal health equity, 479–83, 482*f*
  community-based participatory research training models, 485–86
  community health systems, building, 478
  ensuring sustainability, 487–89
  and HHS call to action, 477–78
  overview, 448, 477
  patient and community engagement models, 484–85

  training in, 483–84, 485–86

academic medical centers (AMCs), 21–22, 22*f*

access
  to healthcare, and women's health, 364
  to healthcare, NC AHEC focus on, 573
  to healthcare, reproductive justice-focused approach to, 196
  to medication for opioid use disorder, expanding, 418–19
  to safe drinking water, 253–54
  for vulnerable populations at CommonSpirit Health, 60*b*, 63*b*, 64*b*

Accompany Doula Care, 430

accountability in postpartum care, 387

Accreditation Council for Graduate Medical Education (ACGME), 514

ACIMM (Secretary's Advisory Committee on Infant and Maternal Mortality), 11*t*

ACOG. *See* American College of Obstetricians and Gynecologists

action, intentional, by AAIMM Prevention Initiative, 182–83

action groups, IMPACT Collaborative, 156–57

adaptability, and sustainability of academic health systems, 488–89

Advanced Life Support in Obstetrics (ALSO®) program, AAFP, 520

advocacy
  advancing institutional, 486–87
  doula-supported, 398–99
  importance to success of IMPACT Collaborative, 161
  role among healthcare providers, 531–32
  in socioecological model for role of academic centers, 21*f*, 28–29

African American Infant and Maternal Mortality (AAIMM) Prevention Initiative
  activities born of intentional values, 169–72
  Black women/people up front and leading, 172–76, 176*b*
  fighting inequity while fostering equity, 173*f*, 177
  intentional values overview, 172
  lessons of intentionality, 181–83
  no blame game, 178–80, 179*b*
  overview, 75, 165–66
  as public-private-community partnership, 166*f*, 166–69, 167*f*, 168*f*, 169*f*
  racism as root cause, 172, 173*f*, 174*t*
  theory of causality, 169*f*, 169
  we are all pieces of the puzzle, 180–81, 181*b*
African American maternal health outcomes. *See* Black maternal health outcomes
AHD (academic health department) model, GVPH, 584–85
AHECs (Area Health Education Centers), 448, 499*t*, 567. *See also* North Carolina Area Health Education Center
AI/AN women. *See* American Indian/Alaska Native women; equity; Indigenous communities; racial MCH disparities; racism; structural racism
AIM. *See* Alliance for Innovation on Maternal Health
AIM CCI. *See* Alliance for Innovation on Maternal Health Community Care Initiative
AL (allostatic load) theory, 311–12
Alaska Native women. See American Indian/Alaska Native women; equity; Indigenous communities; racial MCH disparities; racism; structural racism
Alberti, P. M., 21–22
Alcade, Gabriela, 205
aligning across sectors, 78–79, 79*f*. *See also* maternal health zones of transformation model
Alliance for Innovation on Maternal Health (AIM), 11*t*
  enhancing workforce competency and outcomes, 506*b*

long-term outcomes, tracking, 489
MCHB support to advance maternal health equity, 451–52, 453–54
overview, 480, 530
patient safety bundles, 227–28
and Perinatal Quality Collaboratives, 283–84, 423*b*
postpartum discharge transition bundle, 381–82
Alliance for Innovation on Maternal Health Community Care Initiative (AIM CCI), 11*t*
  family physicians and, 517
  general discussion, 137–38
  holistic care models, 355
  lessons learned, 137
  New Orleans case study, 134–36
  overview, 74, 133–34
alliances, building to advance maternal health equity, 480–81. *See also* collaboration
allostatic load (AL) theory, 311–12
ALSO® (Advanced Life Support in Obstetrics) program, AAFP, 520
alternative dental workforce models, 95
AMA (American Medical Association), 479–83, 482*f*
AMCHP (Association of Maternal and Child Health Programs), 417–18, 454
AMCs (academic medical centers), 21–22, 22*f*
American Academy of Family Physicians (AAFP)
  education on obstetric emergencies, 520
  evidence-based methods to decrease morbidity and mortality, 517
  health equity education, 519
  implicit bias training, 518–19
  OB Ready concept, 520
  "Striving for Birth Equity" policy, 517–18
  Task Force on Maternal Morbidity and Mortality, 515–16, 516*b*
American Academy of Pediatrics (AAP), 96–97
American Board of Family Medicine, 519
American College of Obstetricians and Gynecologists (ACOG)
  Committee Opinion Number 736, 381
  Committee Opinion Number 832, 247
  informed consent, 357

innovations to postpartum practice, 381–82

maternal environmental health concerns, 250–51, 255

obstetric emergencies, education on, 520

patient-centered contraceptive counseling guidance, 356

Women's Preventive Services Initiative, 371

American Indian/Alaska Native (AI/AN) women. *See also* equity; Indigenous communities; racial MCH disparities; racism; structural racism

disparities in maternal and child health for, 297

forced sterilization of, 292*b*

midwifery care for, 492

American Medical Association (AMA), 479–83, 482*f*

American Public Health Association (APHA), 97

American Rescue Plan Act (ARPA), 458, 467, 527, 529–30

AmeriCorps, 498–500, 499*t*

Amnesty International, 227

analysis

in culturally responsive evaluation, 337, 338*b*

New Jersey MHI Program focus on, 114*b*

anchor institution programs, 26

antenatal screening, 48

Anti-racism in Medicine Collection (MedEdPORTAL), 501–2

anti-racist initiatives. *See also* African American Infant and Maternal Mortality Prevention Initiative; equity

in academic centers, 23–25, 29

decolonizing maternal health research, 289–98, 292*b*

reproductive justice as, 194–95

reproductive justice in incarcerated populations, 237–44

AN women. *See* American Indian/Alaska Native women; equity; Indigenous communities; racial MCH disparities; racism; structural racism

anxiety disorders. *See* mental health

APHA (American Public Health Association), 97

appropriations, federal, 10–12, 14

apps, and women's health, 367–68

Area Health Education Centers (AHECs), 448, 499*t*, 567. *See also* North Carolina Area Health Education Center

Arizona State MHI Program, 109*t*, 111*b*

ARPA (American Rescue Plan Act), 458, 467, 527, 529–30

assessment tools, implications of BPN for, 130

Association of American Medical Colleges (AAMC)

Anti-racism in Medicine Collection, 501–2

building community health systems, 478

supply and demand projections, 493

trustworthiness principles, 488

workforce diversity statistics, 494

Association of Black Women Physicians, 181*b*, *See also* African American Infant and Maternal Mortality Prevention Initiative

Association of Maternal and Child Health Programs (AMCHP), 417–18, 454

Association of State and Territorial Health Officials (ASTHO). *See also* Learning Community Model

best practices, 544–48, 545*b*, 546*b*

braiding and layering pilot, 541, 542*b*

development and support of public health leaders and agencies, 543–44

general discussion, 551–52

Local Enhancement Project, 417

MMM technical package, 550–51

overview, 415–16, 539–40

strategic priorities, 421–22

success stories, 548*b*, 548, 549*b*

Atlanta Healthy Start Initiative, 229

attorneys. *See* justice-conscious approach to reproductive health

B

backbone support

in collective impact framework, 141, 143*f*, 143, 143*t*

importance to success of IMPACT Collaborative, 160

LA County AAIMM Prevention Initiative, 169–70

back-loaded approach to prenatal care, 49–50

bad data, effect on maternal health outcomes, 301–6, 304*f*

Barr, W. B., 514–15

barrier analysis, 209–10

Basic Life Support in Obstetrics (BLSO®) program, AAFP, 520

BBF (Bootheel Babies and Families), 120–21, 122

Before and Beyond web site, 371–73

behavior, and infant and maternal mortality, 174*t*

Believe Her app, 386

Bellies to Babies Foundation, 430

Better Maternal Outcomes: Redesigning Systems with Black Women project
  codesigning and testing ideas, 231–32
  general discussion, 234–35
  lessons learned, 233–34
  overview, 188, 228–29
  pervasive health crisis leading to, 227–28
  process, 229–31, 230*f*
  rapid cycles amid rapidly changing world, 233

BHSC. *See* Broward Healthy Start Coalition

bias. *See also* racism
  addressed by MDMOM, 113*b*
  cultural competence training to decrease, 528–29
  in maternal health industry, 408–9
  misuse of race by maternal health data tools, 301–6, 304*f*
  and organization internals as zone of transformation, 85–86
  in perceptions of Indigenous people's health, 295–96

Big Springs Medical Association, 431*t*

Billings Clinic, 114*b*, 433–34

birth centers, Medicaid coverage for, 467–68

birth control provided through LHDs, 582

birth equity
  CHCF efforts to improve, 562–65, 563*f*
  defined, 354
  family physicians, role in striving for, 513–21, 516*b*
  role of community-based doulas in supporting, 391–402, 395*f*, 396*f*

Birthing Cultural Rigor, LLC, 24

birthing hospitals, in MDMOM Hospital Equity Initiative, 113*b*

birthing people, health of. *See* maternal health outcomes

BirthMatters, 397, 431*t*

birth weight, and community-based doula programs, 395*f*

Black Codes, 206–7

Black infant mortality, 166*f*, 166–67, 172, 174*t*

Black Mamas Matter Toolkit for Advancing the Human Right to Safe and Respectful Maternal Health Care, 223

Black Maternal Health Center of Excellence, 171

Black Maternal Health Momnibus Act of 2021 (Momnibus Act), 29, 196, 529–30

Black maternal health outcomes. *See also* African American Infant and Maternal Mortality Prevention Initiative; culturally responsive evaluation; equity; racial MCH disparities; racism; structural racism
  AMA strategic approaches to advance maternal health equity, 479–83, 482*f*
  Better Maternal Outcomes project, 227–35, 230*f*
  in BHSC HBWW initiative, 144–45, 146–47, 149
  California maternal mortality ratios, 562–63, 563*f*
  community-based doulas and birth equity, 391–402, 395*f*, 396*f*
  community-informed PRH models, 380–81
  family medicine and, 52
  in Harris County, Texas, 161–62
  legacy and impact of racism, 349–51
  in Los Angeles County, California, 166*f*, 166–67, 167*f*
  maternal environmental health, 247–56
  maternal mortality, 144, 167*f*, 191–92, 201–2, 213–14, 227–28, 513, 562–63, 563*f*
  and maternity care deserts, 579–81
  measuring structural racism using qualitative data, 274, 309–16, 314*b*
  and misuse of race by maternal health data tools, 301–6, 304*f*
  and need for diversity in maternal health workforce, 570–71
  perception versus facts about infant and maternal mortality, 172, 174*t*

perinatal mental health, bridging gap in, 409–11

policy and advocacy, employing to reduce inequities, 523–32

recognizing and uplifting community leadership, 386–87

reproductive justice as framework for well-being and health, 351–55, 353*f*

reproductive justice in incarcerated populations, 237–44

structural racism and, 191–98, 201–10, 203*f*

Black midwives, 349–51

Black Mothers Breastfeeding Association (BMBFA), 397

Black Mothers United (BMU), 407–8

Black Women for Wellness, 565

Black women/people

LQR research design example, 323*b*

need for and training in healthcare workforce, 483–84

up front and leading, in AAIMM Prevention Initiative, 172–76, 176*b*

blame game, AAIMM Prevention Initiative avoidance of, 178–80, 179*b*

BLC (Breastfeeding Learning Community), 545*b*

blended funding, 88, 541

blood pressure cuff kit project (Preeclampsia Foundation), 129

BLSO® (Basic Life Support in Obstetrics) program, AAFP, 520

BMBFA (Black Mothers Breastfeeding Association), 397

BMU (Black Mothers United), 407–8

Bodenheimer, T., 44

body mass index (BMI), 304–5

Bootheel Babies and Families (BBF), 120–21, 122

Bootheel Perinatal Network (BPN)

areas of success, 126*f*, 126–28, 128*b*, 129*b*

enhancing telehealth opportunities and technologies, 125

expansion of resources in Bootheel, 128–30

history of, 120–22

overview, 74, 120

partners, 122–23, 123*f*

program approach to care coordination, 124–25

RMOMS goals, 123–24, 124*f*

sustainable system, building, 125

BoRN platform (BPN), 127, 128

BPN Connect meetings, 129

braided funding, 88, 541, 542*b*

breast cancer risk, and personal care product use, 251–52

breastfeeding education, 384, 386, 397, 436–37

Breastfeeding Learning Community (BLC), 545*b*

Bridges, Khiara, 24, 31*b*

Briggs, L., 30*b*

broader structures and institutions, as maternal health zone of transformation, 80*f*, 80, 81–82, 83*t*, 87–89, 88*t*

Broomfield-Massey, Kimberley, 333*b*, 334*b*, 336*b*

Broward Healthy Start Coalition (BHSC)

collective impact framework, 141

Healthy Babies are Worth the Wait initiative, 140–41

ingredients for success, 149–51

integration of CI and RBA, 142, 143*f*, 143*t*

lessons learned, 149

operationalizing CI and RBA, 143–48, 148*f*

overview, 74–75, 139

results-based accountability, 141–42

Brown communities. *See* American Indian/Alaska Native women; Indigenous communities; Latina women; racial MCH disparities; racism; structural racism

budget, federal, 10–12

Bullard, Robert D., 250

C

California Assembly Bill 241, 530

California Dignity in Pregnancy and Childbirth Act, 85–86, 565

California Health Care Foundation (CHCF), 85–86

birth equity, 562–65, 563*f*

cesarean deliveries, 557–60, 561*f*

levers for advancing systemic change, 556*f*, 556–57

overview, 448, 555–57, 556*f*

perinatal mental health, 560–62

California Maternal Quality Care Collaborative (CMQCC), 530, 557–59, 563–64

California Rural Legal Assistance, Inc., 263

California Senate Bill 65 (California Momnibus bill), 565

capacity, enhancing in maternal health workforce, 496–505

carceral system. *See* incarcerated populations, reproductive justice in

Care Connections referral process, 157

care coordination
in Bootheel Perinatal Network, 124–25
in transformational maternal and child health, 43

career development work, by academic centers, 26

care interactions, in efforts to embed equity, 479–80

care models, integration of, 355–60, 356*f*

CARES (Coronavirus Aid, Relief, and Economic Security) Act, 458

caries, 93–94, 97–98. *See also* oral healthcare integration

Carolina Global Breastfeeding Institute (CGBI), 384, 436–37

categorization of maternal deaths by MMRCs, 279–80

CATs (community action teams), AAIMM Prevention Initiative, 168, 170, 180

causality, theory of in LA County AAIMM Prevention Initiative, 169*f*, 169

CBOs. *See* community-based organizations

CBPR (community-based participatory research), 209, 480–81, 485–86

CBWW (Center for Black Women's Wellness), 228–29, 230–31, 234–35. *See also* Better Maternal Outcomes: Redesigning Systems with Black Women project

CCHP (Center for Connected Health Policy), 435

CDC. *See* Centers for Disease Control and Prevention

Center for Antiracism Research for Health Equity, 29

Center for Black Women's Wellness (CBWW), 228–29, 230–31, 234–35. *See also* Better Maternal Outcomes: Redesigning Systems with Black Women project

Center for Connected Health Policy (CCHP), 435

Center for Global Healthy Cities, 28

Center for Maternal Health Equity, 214–15. *See also* Georgia Maternal

Health Research for Action Steering Committee

Center for Women's Health (CWH), 263–65

CenteringPregnancy prenatal program, 432–33, 468–69, 581–82, 585–86

Centers for Disease Control and Prevention (CDC)
community water fluoridation, 101
content of prenatal care, 49–50
ERASE MM program, 15–16, 278–79
federal partnerships, 15–16
Hear Her campaign, 383
Local Enhancement Project, 417
Maternal Mortality Review Information Application program, 278–79, 526
Model Surveillance Protocols, 282
Perinatal Quality Collaborative framework, 423*b*
preconception care, 50
Pregnancy Risk Assessment Monitoring System, 282–83, 546*b*

certified medical assistants (CMAs), 495

certified midwives (CMs), 493, 494

certified nurse midwives (CNMs), 492, 493, 494

certified nursing assistants (CNAs), 495

cesarean deliveries (C-sections), 303, 396*f*, 557–60, 561*f*

CGBI (Carolina Global Breastfeeding Institute), 384, 436–37

Chambers, Charis, 366–67, 368*f*

champion, in results-based accountability, 142, 143, 143*t*

CHAP (Community Health Access Project), 88–89

charity care, 21–22

Charles Drew University of Medicine and Science, 171

CHCC (Commonwealth Healthcare Corporation), 548b

CHCF. See California Health Care Foundation

Cheairs, Taneisha Gillyard, 411

chemical exposures due to personal care products, 251–52, 255, 256

Cherished Futures for Black Moms & Babies program (AAIMM), 171, 175

Chicago Doula Project, 394

Chicago Family Health Center, 431*t*

Chicago Health Connection. *See* HealthConnect One

childbirth complications, 3, 5, 9. *See also* maternal health outcomes

childbirth education, 429–31, 431*t*

child health, xiii–xiv. *See also* maternal and child health workforce; transformational maternal and child health

Children's Health Insurance Program (CHIP), 191–92, 527. *See also* Medicaid

Children's National Medical Center, 431*t*

CHN (cultural health navigator) model, 484–86

chronic illnesses, quality-improvement endeavors related to, 37–38

CHWPTP (Community Health Worker and Paraprofessional Training Program), 499*t*

CHWs (community health workers), 469–70, 495

CIE (Community Information Exchange), BPN, 122

CI framework. *See* collective impact framework

CILC (Collective Impact Learning Collaborative), 158–59

civil law and health. *See* justice-conscious approach to reproductive health

Cleveland Foundation, 26

clinical care. *See also* Bootheel Perinatal Network; healthcare; maternal health workforce

  at academic centers, 23–25

  clinical–community integration framework, 119–20, 126*f*, 126–28, 133–38

  and community-based doula programs, 398–99

  and community care team integration, 355–60, 356*f*

  standardization of postpartum, 383–84

Clinical Community Integration Roadmap (NHSA), 137–38

clinical models, CommonSpirit Health choice of, 64*b*

CMAs (certified medical assistants), 495

CMQCC (California Maternal Quality Care Collaborative), 530, 557–59, 563–64

CMs (certified midwives), 493, 494

CNAs (certified nursing assistants), 495

CNMI (Commonwealth of the Northern Mariana Islands), 548*b*

CNMs (certified nurse midwives), 492, 493, 494

codifying external partnerships, 65, 66*b*

co-leadership model, New Orleans AIM CCI, 136–37

collaboration. *See also* African American Infant and Maternal Mortality Prevention Initiative; Bootheel Perinatal Network; Broward Healthy Start Coalition; health system collaborations with external partners; maternal health zones of transformation model

  Angelica's story, 72

  in Better Maternal Outcomes project, 234

  to bridge gap in perinatal mental health, 411–13

  California Health Care Foundation emphasis on, 556–57

  community, in transformational MCH, 42–44, 44*f*, 45

  Georgia Maternal Health Research for Action Steering Committee, 214–23

  IMPACT Collaborative, 153–62, 154*f*, 162*f*

  improving maternal health through, 73–75

  National Healthy Start Association AIM CCI, 133–38

  oral healthcare integration, 93–102

  as retention strategy, 506–7

  State MHI Program, 107–10, 109*t*, 111*b*, 112*b*, 113*b*, 114*b*, 115*b*, 116*b*, 117*b*

Collaborative for Maternal and Infant Health (UNC), 372*b*, 382–83

collective impact (CI) framework

  academic centers and, 27

  in AIM CCIs, 137

  in Healthy Babies are Worth the Wait initiative, 140

  integration with results-based accountability, 142, 143*f*, 143*t*

  operationalizing in BHSC HBWW initiative, 143–48, 148*f*

  overview, 141

Collective Impact Learning Collaborative (CILC), 158–59

colleges. *See* academic centers, role in advancing maternal health

colonialism, 193, 206, 295–97. *See also* decolonizing maternal health research

colonias, drinking water in, 253–54
Committee Opinion Number 736
(ACOG), 381
Committee Opinion Number 832
(ACOG), 247
Committee Opinion on Informed
Consent and Shared Decision-
Making in Obstetrics and
Gynecology (ACOG), 357
common agenda, in collective impact
framework, 141, 143*f*, 143*t*, 144–45
CommonSpirit Health
general discussion, 68
overview, 59, 60
Step 1: understanding what to solve,
60*b*
Step 2: identifying and confirming
sponsors and stakeholders, 61
Step 4: developing criteria to select
partner, 62, 63*b*
Step 5: identifying partner, 62–63, 64*b*
Step 6: codifying partnership, 66*b*
Step 7: operationalizing partnership,
67*b*
Commonwealth Healthcare Corporation
(CHCC), 548*b*
Commonwealth of the Northern
Mariana Islands (CNMI), 548*b*
communication
about postpartum period, 384–86
LA County AAIMM Prevention
Initiative, 171
community. *See also* African American
Infant and Maternal Mortality
Prevention Initiative; Better
Maternal Outcomes: Redesigning
Systems with Black Women project;
Broward Healthy Start Coalition;
collaboration; culturally responsive
evaluation
academic medical centers and benefits
for, 21–22, 22*f*
access to relevant maternal health data,
328–30
in approach to maternal health crisis,
228–29
health and social challenges in context
of, 140–41
involvement in results-based
accountability, 141–42
involvement with data, in Indigenous
communities, 293–94
as maternal health zone of
transformation, 80*f*, 80, 81, 82, 83*t*,
86–87

MCHB support to advance maternal
health equity, 452–55
recognizing and uplifting to improve
postpartum care, 386–87
in socioecological model for role of
academic centers, 21*f*, 25–27
socio-ecological model of racism on
sexual, gender, and reproductive
health, 481–83, 482*f*
ties with Indigenous, when doing
research, 293
in transformational maternal and child
health, 42–44, 44*f*, 45
Community Action Network (Healthy
Start program), 229
community action teams (CATs),
AAIMM Prevention Initiative, 168,
170, 180
community asset mapping, 210
community-based doulas
future innovation and
recommendations, 401–2
HealthConnect One model, 394–97,
395*f*, 396*f*
Homeland Heart Birth & Wellness
Collective, 410
and hospital systems, 398–99
overview, 346, 391–93
reimbursement efforts, 399–401
versus traditional, non-community-
based, 392*b*
community-based education, NC AHEC
focus on, 574–76
community-based organizations (CBOs)
academic center partnerships with,
24–25
California Health Care Foundation
support for, 563–64
involvement in education of maternal
health workforce, 503–5
opportunities to use data and leverage
interventions, 285–86
community-based participatory research
(CBPR), 209, 480–81, 485–86
community-based utilization of data,
328–30. *See also* democratizing data
Community Birth Companion, 431*t*
community care
bridging gap in perinatal mental
health, 405–13
and clinical care team integration,
355–60, 356*f*
community-based maternal
healthcare, 87
postpartum care innovations, 381–83

Community Care Initiative. *See* Alliance for Innovation on Maternal Health Community Care Initiative

community-centered funding models for telehealth, 436–37

Community-Centered Health Home model, 39*f*, 39, 45

community-centered informed healthcare delivery models, 24

community-clinical-academic coalitions, 214–23

community–clinical integration framework, 119–20, 126*f*, 126–28, 133–38. *See also* Bootheel Perinatal Network

community culture, role in retaining maternal health workforce, 506–7

community engagement
  in academic health systems, 484–85
  and cross-sector collaborations, 73–75
  IMPACT Collaborative strategies for, 157–58

Community Health Access Project (CHAP), 88–89

community health centers, 98

community health systems, building, 478

Community Health Worker and Paraprofessional Training Program (CHWPTP), 499*t*

community health workers (CHWs), 469–70, 495

Community Information Exchange (CIE), BPN, 122

community-informed perinatal and reproductive healthcare (PRH) models, 380–81

community programs, IMPACT Collaborative, 157–58

community water fluoridation, 101

compensation, for community-based doulas, 399–401

comprehensive approach to maternal and child health, 40, 47–48, 49, 52–54. *See also* transformational maternal and child health

Comprehensive Health Home framework, 39*f*, 39–40, 42, 45. *See also* transformational maternal and child health

Congressional Budget Justification (President's budget), 12

Connecticut State Health Improvement Coalition, 549*b*

consent
  in clinical care and community care team integration, 357–58
  in longitudinal qualitative research, 321

content creation, for social media, 365–67

continuing education, 507

continuing professional development (CPD), 569, 572–74

continuous communication
  in collective impact framework, 141, 143*f*, 143*t*, 145–46
  importance to success of IMPACT Collaborative, 160

contraceptive counseling guidance (ACOG), 356

contraceptives provided through LHDs, 582

coordination, healthcare. *See* transformational maternal and child health

coordination of care, postpartum, 381–83, 384

Coronavirus Aid, Relief, and Economic Security (CARES) Act, 458

correctional institutions. *See* incarcerated populations, reproductive justice in

Council on Patient Safety in Women's Health Care, 227–28

Covered California marketplace, 559–60

COVID-19 pandemic
  Institute for Healthcare Improvement during, 233
  and New Orleans AIM CCI, 135–36
  and racial maternal health disparities, 201–2
  and state Title V programs, 457–58
  and transition to telehealth, 346, 428–29
  virtual care innovations in response to, 429–39

CPD (continuing professional development), 569, 572–74

crack baby panic, 30*b*

Cradle Cincinnati, 27, 387

CRE. *See* culturally responsive evaluation

credentialing for doulas, 498*b*

criminal legal system. *See* incarcerated populations, reproductive justice in

criminal violations, racial disparities in, 206–7

criteria to select external partner, 62, 63*b*

cross-sector collaborations. *See* collaboration

C-sections (cesarean deliveries), 303, 396*f*, 557–60, 561*f*

cuff kit project (Preeclampsia Foundation), 129

cultural competence
  defined, 330–31
  training in, 528–29

cultural congruence, 528

cultural context, defined, 330, 331

cultural health navigator (CHN) model, 484–86

culturally responsive evaluation (CRE)
  analyzing data, 337, 338*b*
  attention to culture and cultural context, 330
  collecting data, 336–37
  community access to relevant maternal health data, 328–30
  designing evaluation, 334–35
  disseminating and using results, 337–38
  engaging stakeholders, 333, 334*b*
  framing right questions, 334
  general discussion, 340
  identifying evaluation purpose, 333–34
  important concepts in, 330–31
  overview, 275, 327–28
  preparing for evaluation, 332, 333*b*
  selecting and adapting instrumentation, 335–36, 336*b*
  starting point for, 338–39, 339*t*
  steps in, overview of, 331, 332*f*

culture, defined, 330

cumulative pathways, in life-course theory, 204–5

CWH (Center for Women's Health), 263–65

Cycle to Respectful Care framework, 352–53, 353*f*, 380–81

D

data. *See also* culturally responsive evaluation
  Carrita's Story, 272
  in CHCF efforts to improve perinatal mental health, 561–62
  in CHCF efforts to reduce cesarean deliveries, 558–59
  decolonizing maternal health research, 289–98, 292*b*

democratizing, 277–86

ease of understanding, 275

ensuring equity in innovation related to, 481

gathering evidence of structural racism with, 274, 309–16, 314*b*

implications of BPN for utilization of, 131

importance to success of IMPACT Collaborative, 161

limitations as barrier to government-funded programs, 15

MCHB support to advance maternal health equity, 454

measures for racism and sexism, 275

missing, 275

misuse of race by maternal health data tools, 275, 301–6, 304*f*

modernization and interoperability, as ASTHO priority area, 422

narrative medicine and longitudinal qualitative research, 319–25, 323*b*, 325*f*

need for standardized collection system, 525–26

New Jersey MHI Program focus on analysis, 114*b*

sharing, in AIM CCIs, 137

using and improving to achieve equity, 273–75

data placemats, 338*b*

data sovereignty, Indigenous, 293–94

Davis, Dána-Ain, 31*b*

DC Health, 408

"Deadly Delivery" report (Amnesty International), 227

death, maternal. *See* maternal mortality

decision-making, in clinical care and community care team integration, 357–58

decolonizing maternal health research
  general discussion, 298
  historical abuses of Indigenous communities, 292*b*
  implementing decolonial framework for research, 294–98
  Indigenous research methods, 290–94
  overview, 274, 289–90

Decolonizing Methodologies (Tuhiwai Smith), 290, 292*b*

DEI (diversity, equity, and inclusion) curriculum, NC AHEC, 573–74

DELPH (Diverse Executives Leading in Public Health), 499*t*

Delphi consensus process, 215–16, 216*t*, 217*f*

demand projections, maternal health workforce, 493–94

democratizing data
federal data, 282–83
federal interventions to address maternal health, 284–85
opportunities for community-based organizations, 285–86
overview, 274, 277–78
state data, 278–82
state interventions to address maternal health, 283–84

dental caries, 93–94, 97–98

dental home, referral to, 98

dental–medical divide, 95–97. *See also* oral healthcare integration

Department of Health and Human Services (HHS), 477–78. *See also* Health Resources and Services Administration

Department of Public Health (DPH), Los Angeles County, 167–68, 181*b*. *See also* African American Infant and Maternal Mortality Prevention Initiative

Department of State Health Services (DSHS), Texas, 158

depression screenings, Medicaid coverage for, 470–71. *See also* mental health

design
of government-funded programs, 12
intentional, by AAIMM Prevention Initiative, 182

design teams, Better Maternal Outcomes project, 230–33

Detox Me app, 256

Detroit, Michigan, 397

Deutchman, M., 519

digital innovation in women's health, 365–69, 368*f. See also* telemedicine and telehealth; virtual care innovations

Dignity in Pregnancy and Childbirth Act (Senate Bill 464), 85–86, 565

Dignity in Pregnancy and Childbirth Project, 85–86, 565

disaggregated data use by BHSC, 150

disparities-based approach, 32

disseminating results of culturally responsive evaluation, 337–38

Diverse Executives Leading in Public Health (DELPH), 499*t*

diversity, equity, and inclusion (DEI) curriculum, NC AHEC, 573–74

diversity of maternal health workforce, 494–96, 497, 529, 531–32, 570–71

Diversity Science, 565

douches, vaginal, 252

Doula Learning Collaborative (DLC), New Jersey, 400–1

Doula Program (AAIMM), 171

doulas, 433*b*, 434*b*, *See also* Prison Birth Project
building workforce with credentialing, 498*b*
California Health Care Foundation support for, 565
in clinical care and community care team integration, 359
community-based versus traditional, 392*b*
"Doulas and Doctors and Mamas, Oh My!" training, 181*b*
future innovation and recommendations, 401–2
HealthConnect One model, 394–97, 395*f*, 396*f*
Homeland Heart Birth & Wellness Collective, 410
and hospital systems, 398–99
investing in to improve maternal health outcomes, 524–25
Medicaid coverage for services, 468
midwifery–doula clinical model, 64*b*, 66*b*
NC AHEC project related to, 571–72
overview, 346, 391–93
reimbursement efforts, 399–401
Tampa Bay Doula Program, 531
virtual care innovations, 429–31, 431*t*, 437*b*
and workforce diversity, 495–96

"Doulas and Doctors and Mamas, Oh My!" training, 181*b*

DPH (Department of Public Health), Los Angeles County, 167–68, 181*b*. *See also* African American Infant and Maternal Mortality Prevention Initiative

drinking water, access to safe, 253–54

DSHS (Department of State Health Services), Texas, 158

Duke University School of Nursing, 584–85

duty, tort law concept of, 260

E

Early and Periodic Screening, Diagnostic and Treatment (EPSDT) benefit, 49
early childhood care, 49
early childhood caries (ECC), 93–94, 97–98
early programming, in life-course theory, 204–5
Eat, Sleep, Console (ESC) model, 419
economic development, role of academic centers in, 26
ECU Health, 572–73
Eden, A. R., 519
education
   at academic centers, 25
   childbirth, virtual care innovations related to, 429–31, 431t
   on health equity for family physicians, 519
   in IHELP™ model, 262f
   and infant and maternal mortality, 174t
electronic health record (EHR) systems, 98–99
eligibility categories for Medicaid, 464, 464t, 465, 466–67
embedded researcher structure, at GVPH, 584–85
embedding equity, 479–80
embodiment, 311
EMBRACe (Equity for Moms and Babies Realized Across Chatham), 504b
Emergency Medical Treatment and Active Labor Act (EMTALA), 260
emergency preparedness, IMPACT Collaborative focus on, 159
employment, in IHELP™ model, 262f
endocrine-disrupting personal care products, 251, 252, 255, 256
Enhancing Reviews and Surveillance to Eliminate Maternal Mortality (ERASE MM) program, 15–16, 278
environment, defined, 248–49
Environmental Exposure Assessment, 255–56
environmental health, 248–49
environmental impacts on maternal health
   environmental justice, 250
   examples of maternal environmental health concerns, 250–54
   overview, 189, 247–48
   root of problem, getting to, 249
   strategies for improving maternal environmental health, 255–56
   understanding environmental health, 248–49
environmental justice, 250
episode-of-care approach, Medicaid, 472
EPSDT (Early and Periodic Screening, Diagnostic and Treatment) benefit, 49
equality, 19, 20f, 203f, 203
equity. See also birth equity; innovations to improve maternal health; maternal health equity; maternal health zones of transformation model; systems for maternal health equity; transformational maternal and child health
   academic center role in providing, 23–25, 27
   advancing in academic health systems, 479–83, 482f
   as ASTHO priority area, 421
   Better Maternal Outcomes project, 228–35
   centering, 187–89
   CommonSpirit Health criteria for external partners, 63b
   and culturally responsive evaluation, 327–28
   defined, 19, 20f, 203f, 203
   environmental impacts on maternal health, 247–56
   family physicians, role in striving for, 513–21, 516b
   fostering, as intentional value of AAIMM initiative, 173f, 177
   and innovations in women's health, 373–74, 374f
   justice-conscious approach to reproductive health, 259–68, 262f, 264f, 266f
   in maternal health workforce, centering, 496–505
   NC AHEC focus on, 573–74
   in NHSA AIM CCI, 134
   oral health, achieving, 94–95
   reproductive justice as centered on, 194–95
   reproductive justice in incarcerated populations, 243–44
   structural racism, 191–98, 201–10, 203f
   using and improving data to achieve, 273–75

Equity Action Lab model, 229–30, 234
Equity for Moms and Babies Realized
    Across Chatham (EMBRACe),
    504*b*
Equity-System Readiness tool, 173*f*, 177
ERASE MM (Enhancing Reviews and
    Surveillance to Eliminate Maternal
    Mortality) program, 15–16, 278
ESC (Eat, Sleep, Console) model, 419
Estelle v Gamble, 239–40
ethics
    of doing research in Indigenous
        communities, 291–94
    when applying novel qualitative
        methods, 321–22
ethnicity, in workforce diversity
    statistics, 494–96
ethnicity-based data, 280–81, 282
ethnic MCH disparities. *See* racial MCH
    disparities; racism; structural
    racism; transformational maternal
    and child health
ethnography, 314*b*, 314
eugenics movement, 193–94
European beauty norms, 252
evidence-based methods to decrease
    morbidity and mortality, 517
evidence-based public health practices,
    422
evidence-informed programs, 12–13
expanded care model. *See also*
        transformational maternal and
        child health
    overview, 38–39, 45
    Perinatal and Patient Safety
        Collaborative, 40–45
    related to doula care, 393
    staffing, 52–54
    transforming MCH scope of
        work, 49
expanded Medicaid coverage, 220–23,
    284–85, 464, 464*t*, 466–67, 527
experimentation, medical, 193–94, 206,
    292*b*
explore page, on social media, 365–66
external partners, health system
    collaborations with. *See* health
    system collaborations with external
    partners

F

Family Case Management, 84–85
family-centered care, 419

family physicians
    AAFP "Striving for Birth Equity"
        policy, 517–18
    AAFP Task Force on Maternal
        Morbidity and Mortality, 515–16,
        516*b*
    community-based education for in
        North Carolina, 575
    education and training for, 514–15
    education on obstetric emergencies,
        520
    evidence-based methods to decrease
        morbidity and mortality, 517
    expanded primary healthcare team
        approach, 51–54
    general discussion, 521
    health equity education, 519
    implicit bias training, 518–19
    OB Ready concept, 520
    overview, 448, 513–14
    rural disparities and opportunities,
        519
    supply and demand projections, 494
    UNC family medicine residency rural
        track, 502*b*
family planning (FP)
    local health departments, role in, 582
    Medicaid coverage for, 471
family stability, in IHELP™ model, 262*f*
Fatherhood Program (AAIMM), 171
federal budget and appropriations, 10–
    12, 14
federal funding for community-based
    doulas, 399–400
federal interventions to address maternal
    health, 284–85
federally qualified health centers
    (FQHCs), 37–38, 39–40, 42–43
federal maternal health data, 282–83
Federal Office of Rural Health Policy,
    119–20, 121, 123–24, 124*f*
federal partnerships
    additional considerations for, 16
    development of government-funded
        programs, 10–15, 13*f*
    example of strong, 15–16
    general discussion, 16–17
    overview and importance, 15, 17
    role of HRSA in promoting maternal
        health, 9–10, 11*t*
feedback loop, in BHSC HBWW
    initiative, 147–48, 148*f*
fee-for-service structures, Medicaid, 465
finance reform, 87–89, 88*t*

financial incentives
    for medical-legal partnerships, 266
    to work in underserved areas, 499*t*, 502*b*
Finger Lakes Performing Provider System (FLPPS), 398–99
First 5 LA. *See* African American Infant and Maternal Mortality Prevention Initiative
flawed data, effect on maternal health outcomes, 301–6, 304*f*
Flowers, Catherine Coleman, 247
fluoridated drinking water, 101
fluoride varnish, 99
focus group, in BHSC HBWW initiative, 146–47
forced sterilizations, 193–94, 292*b*
4th Trimester Project, 385–86
foundations, state-based. *See* California Health Care Foundation
FP. *See* family planning
FQHCs (federally qualified health centers), 37–38, 39–40, 42–43
fragmentation in maternal health industry, 408
Framework for Aligning Sectors, 78–79, 79*f*, 80*f*, 82, 87–88. *See also* maternal health zones of transformation model
Franklin, Melissa, 176
free-standing birth centers, Medicaid coverage for, 467–68
frontline staff
    data collection by for CRE, 336–37
    implications of BPN for, 130–31
front-loaded approach to prenatal care, 49–50
FSG consulting firm, 141
funders invested in women's health, 375
funding
    for community-based doulas, 399–401
    community-centered, for telehealth, 436–37
    IMPACT Collaborative, 158, 159, 161
    LA County AAIMM Prevention Initiative, 170–71
    leveraged by MCHB grantees, 455, 458, 459
    for maternal health programs, 13, 14
    for maternal health workforce development and diversifying, 499*t*
    reform of as form of systems transformation, 87–89, 88*t*

for state maternal health interventions, 540–41
for women's health in local health departments, 583–84, 584*f*
Future Forward National Convening of Equity-Centered Women's Wellness, 367, 368*f*, 370*f*, 370, 373–74, 374*f*

G

"garbage in, garbage out" concept, 301
geographic coverage, Medicaid, 467
geographic distribution of maternal health workforce, 492–93, 569–70, 579–81, 580*f*
Georgia Community Action Group, 215
Georgia Health Policy Center, 78–79, 79*f*
Georgia Maternal Health Research for Action Steering Committee
    calls to action, 221*t*
    Delphi consensus process, 215–16, 216*t*, 217*f*
    maternal health equity defined, 216–17, 218*f*, 219*t*
    overview, 214–15
    research priorities, 219–20, 221*t*
Georgia maternal mortality rate, 214
GI Bill, 206–7
GirlTrek nonprofit organization, 370–71
Giving Voice to Mothers Study, 227–28
goals
    collective, in AIM CCIs, 137
    importance to success of IMPACT Collaborative, 161
government-funded maternal health programs, 11*t*, 13*f*
    barriers and challenges, 14–15
    evidence-informed programs, 12–13
    federal budget and appropriations, 10–12
    performance measurement, 13–14
    program design, 12
    program funding, 13
    program purpose, 12
government funding for community-based doulas, 399–401
Graduate Medical Education service line, NC AHEC, 568, 574–76
graduate/residency programs, 497, 501
Granville Vance Public Health (GVPH), 579, 581–82, 583–87, 584*f*, 587*f*
Great Lakes Intertribal Council, 431*t*
group prenatal care, 24, 263–65, 468–69

H

handout, postpartum appointment, 384
Hanna, Linda M., 406–7
Hanna, Melissa, 406–7, 409
Hanna-Attisha, Mona, 28
Harper, Kimberly C., 31*b*
Harris County, Texas, 153–54, 154*f*, 161–62. *See also* Impacting Maternal and Prenatal Care Together Collaborative
hashtags, on social media, 365–66
Hayes, Crystal, 237–38, 240–43
HBWW initiative. *See* Healthy Babies are Worth the Wait® initiative
HCC (Health Career Connections), 499*t*
HCD (human-centered design), 209, 372*b*
HC One (HealthConnect One), 394–97, 395*f*, 396*f*, 398–99, 400–1
HDC (Health Disparities Collaboratives), 37–38
health. *See also* justice-conscious approach to reproductive health; maternal environmental health; maternal health outcomes
defined, 204
environmental, 248–49
and racial equity, as ASTHO priority area, 421
health agencies, ASTHO Learning Community Model strategies for, 421–22
health apps, 367–68
Health Belief Model, 255
healthcare. *See also* clinical care; family physicians; maternal health zones of transformation model; primary care; transformational maternal and child health
community-based maternal, 87
encouraging and promoting collaboration with, 150
experiences with, as theme in BHSC HBWW initiative, 147
and infant and maternal mortality, 174*t*
justice-conscious approach to reproductive health, 259–68, 262*f*, 264*f*, 266*f*
lack of access to high-quality, 4
MCHB essential services, 77, 78*f*

oral healthcare integration, 93–102
primary, for women, 51
prison maternal, reproductive justice and, 239–43
purchasers, in CHCF efforts to reduce cesarean deliveries, 559–60
reproductive justice, using to address structural change in, 195–96
and telemedicine, 433–35
training as critical to expanding telehealth services, 437–38
Healthcare Anchor Network, 26
Healthcare Effectiveness Data and Information Set (HEDIS) measures, 561–62
Health Career Connections (HCC), 499*t*
Health Careers service line, NC AHEC, 568
Healthcare Georgia Foundation, 235
HealthConnect One (HC One), 394–97, 395*f*, 396*f*, 398–99, 400–1
health departments. *See* local health departments
Health Disparities Collaboratives (HDC), 37–38
health equity. *See* equity
Health Equity Zone Initiative, 542*b*
health-harming legal needs, 261. *See also* medical-legal partnership model
health insurance coverage, 196. *See also* Medicaid
health justice lens, employing, 266–68
"health neighborhood" concept, 41–42
Health Resources and Services Administration (HRSA). *See also* Maternal and Child Health Bureau
development of government-funded programs, 10–15, 13*f*
federal partnerships, 15–16
general discussion, 16–17
healthcare quality-improvement endeavors, 37–38
Perinatal and Patient Safety Collaborative, 38, 39–44, 41*f*, 43*f*, 44*f*
role in promoting maternal health, 9–10
Rural Maternity and Obstetrics Management Strategies program, 119–20, 121, 123–24, 124*f*
women's preventive healthcare services, 371, 372*b*

health system collaborations with external partners. *See also* academic health systems
call to action, 67–68
overview, 57–59
Step 1: understanding what to solve, 60*b*, 60
Step 2: identifying and confirming sponsors and stakeholders, 61
Step 3: defining mission and vision, 61
Step 4: developing criteria to select partner, 62, 63*b*
Step 5: identifying partner, 62–63, 64*b*
Step 6: codifying partnership, 65, 66*b*
Step 7: operationalizing partnership, 65–66, 67*b*
Healthy Babies are Worth the Wait® (HBWW) initiative
lessons learned, 149
operationalizing CI and RBA, 143–48, 148*f*
overview, 140–41
Healthy Living App, 256
Healthy Start Initiative: Eliminating Disparities in Perinatal Health, 11*t*
Healthy Start program, 229, 451–52, 453
Hear Her campaign (CDC), 383
HEDIS (Healthcare Effectiveness Data and Information Set) measures, 561–62
helicopter research, 291
Her Health First, 407–8
HHS (Department of Health and Human Services), 477–78. *See also* Health Resources and Services Administration
High-Risk Pregnancy Program (UAMS), 508*b*
Hill, Marc Lamont, 202
Hispanic women, 193–94. *See also* equity; racial MCH disparities; racism; structural racism
historical context of structural racism, 188, 193–94, 205–8
holistic models of maternity care, 354–55
Homeland Heart Birth & Wellness Collective, 406, 409–11
home-visiting services, Medicaid coverage for, 469
Honikman, Jane, 412
HopkinsLocal (Johns Hopkins University), 26
hospital systems, doulas and, 398–99

housing, in IHELP™ model, 262*f*
HRSA. See Health Resources and Services Administration; Maternal and Child Health Bureau
human-centered design (HCD), 209, 372*b*
human resources for health equity at academic centers, 25
Hunter, E. L., 346, 347

I

Ibe, Chidiebere, 267
Icahn School of Medicine at Mount Sinai, 25
I Gave Birth project, 382–83
IHELP™ model, 261, 262*f*
IHI (Institute for Healthcare Improvement), 228–29, 230*f*, 230–31. *See also* Better Maternal Outcomes: Redesigning Systems with Black Women project
IHS (Indian Health Service), 291, 292*b*, 492
Illinois Department of Public Health (IDPH), 111*b*
Illinois Family Case Management, 84–85
Illinois Maternal Health Strategic Plan, 457
Illinois Maternal Health Task Force, 456–57
Illinois Title V MCH Services Block Grant program, 456–57
illness plots, 324
Immediate Postpartum Long-Acting Reversible Contraceptive project, 388
immigrant coverage, Medicaid, 467
IMPACT For Families program, 157
Impacting Maternal and Prenatal Care Together (IMPACT) Collaborative
action groups, 156–57
background, 153–54, 154*f*
collaborative structure, 155
community programs, 157–58
convening, 155
evolution of, 158–59
general discussion, 161–62, 162*f*
initial planning meetings, 154–55
lessons learned, 160–61
overview, 75
steering committee, 155–56
successes, 159–60
implementation science, 387–88

implementing external partnerships,
    65–66, 67*b*
implicit bias
    addressed by MDMOM, 113*b*
    CHCF support for addressing, 565
    cultural competence training to
        decrease, 528–29
    mandated training related to in
        California, 530
    and organization internals as zone of
        transformation, 85–86
    training for family physicians, 518–19
IMRI (Infant Mortality Reduction
    Initiative), 120–21
incarcerated populations, reproductive
        justice in
    general discussion, 243–44
    history of creation of reproductive
        justice, 238–39
    overview, 188–89, 237–38
    reproductive justice and prison
        maternal healthcare, 239–43
income, in IHELP™ model, 262*f*
income limits, for Medicaid, 464, 464*t*,
    465
Indian Health Service (IHS), 291, 292*b*,
    492
Indigenous communities. *See also*
        equity; racial MCH disparities;
        racism; structural racism
    AMA strategic approaches to maternal
        health equity, 479–83, 482*f*
    community-based doulas and birth
        equity, 391–402, 395*f*, 396*f*
    decolonization of research, 289–90
    disparities in maternal and child
        health, 297
    diversity of, 290
    ethics of doing research in, 291–94
    forced sterilization in, 292*b*
    historical abuses of, 292*b*
    historical context of structural racism,
        193–94
    implementing decolonial framework
        for research, 294–98
    Indigenous research methods, 290–94
    midwifery care in, 492
    need for and training in healthcare
        workforce, 483–84
    reproductive justice-focused
        approaches involving, 196
Indigenous data sovereignty, 293–94
Indigenous research methods (IRM),
    290–94

individuals
    health status, data measures used to
        inform, 275, 301–6, 304*f*
    and social services as zone of
        transformation, 84–85
    socioecological model for role of
        academic centers, 21*f*, 22–23
    socio-ecological model of racism,
        481–83, 482*f*
inequities. *See* equity; maternal health
        outcomes; maternal health zones
        of transformation model; racial
        MCH disparities; racism; structural
        racism; systems for maternal health
        equity
infant health, xiii–xiv
infant mortality
    collective impact work to reduce, 27
    in Los Angeles County, California,
        166*f*, 167, 178*f*
    need for standardized data collection
        system on, 525–26
    perception versus facts about Black,
        172, 174*t*
Infant Mortality Reduction Initiative
    (IMRI), 120–21
infertility in slave women, 193
informed consent
    in clinical care and community care
        team integration, 357–58
    in longitudinal qualitative research,
        321
infrastructure
    as ASTHO priority area, 421–22
    MCHB support to advance maternal
        health equity, 454
initial obstetric (OB) assessment
    provided through LHDs, 582–83
Innovation Hub, 454
innovations to improve maternal
        health. *See also* virtual care
        innovations
    ASTHO Learning Community Model,
        415–22, 423*b*
    call to action, 373–75
    clinical care and community care team
        integration, 355–60, 356*f*
    community-based doulas, 391–402,
        395*f*, 396*f*
    Cycle to Respectful Care framework,
        352–53, 353*f*
    digital innovation, 365–69, 368*f*
    ensuring equity in, 481
    general discussion, 360

innovations to improve maternal
health (*cont.*)

integrative models for maternity care
delivery, 354–55

legacy and impact of racism in
maternal health, 349–51

models for innovation, 355–60, 356*f*

overview, 345–48, 349

perinatal mental health, bridging gap
in, 405–13

postpartum care innovations, 379–88

Reproductive and Sexual Health
Equity Framework, 352

reproductive justice framework, 351–
55, 353*f*

social innovations, 369–73, 370*f*, 372*b*

through Medicaid, 466–71

women's health focus, 363–64

Innovations to ImPROve Maternal
OuTcomEs in Illinois (I
PROMOTE-IL) program, 111*b*,
456–57

Institute for Healthcare Improvement
(IHI), 228–29, 230*f*, 230–31. *See
also* Better Maternal Outcomes:
Redesigning Systems with Black
Women project

Institute of Medicine, 501–2

Institute of Women's and Ethnic Studies
(IWES), 136

institutional advocacy, advancing,
486–87

institutional racism, 482*f*, *See also*
structural racism

institutions, as maternal health zone of
transformation, 80*f*, 80, 81–82, 83*t*,
87–89, 88*t*

instrumentation, in culturally responsive
evaluation, 335–36, 336*b*

insurance coverage, 196. *See also*
Medicaid

integrative models for maternity care
delivery, 354–55

intentional values of AAIMM Prevention
Initiative

activities born of, 169–72

Black women/people up front and
leading, 172–76, 176*b*

fighting inequity while fostering
equity, 173*f*, 177

lessons of intentionality, 181–83

no blame game, 178–80, 179*b*

overview, 172

racism as root cause, 172, 173*f*, 174*t*

we are all pieces of the puzzle, 180–81,
181*b*

Intercultural Development Inventory,
130

interdisciplinary care teams, 111*b*

internalized racism, 482*f*

interoperability, data, 422

interpersonal health, socio-ecological
model of racism on, 481–83, 482*f*

interprofessional dental practice, 100–1

interprofessional education, NC AHEC
use of, 572–73

intersectionality, 247–48, 331, 479

INVU by Nuvo monitors, 434

Iowa Maternal Health Innovation
program (Iowa MHI), 109*t*, 112*b*

I PROMOTE-IL (Innovations to
ImPROve Maternal OuTcomEs in
Illinois) program, 111*b*, 456–57

IRM (Indigenous research methods),
290–94

Irth ("Birth, but we dropped the B for
Bias") platform, 25, 386–87

*Is My Evaluation Practice Culturally
Responsive?* tool, 338–39, 339*t*

IWES (Institute of Women's and Ethnic
Studies), 136

J

Jamaica Hospital Medical Center,
432–33

JJ Way® model of care, 354–55, 384

Johns Hopkins University, 26, 109*t*,
113*b*

Johnson & Johnson Health of Women
Team, 214–15. *See also* Georgia
Maternal Health Research for
Action Steering Committee

Jones, Adjoa, 166

jurisdictional successes, ASTHO
Learning Community Model,
420–21

justice, versus equality and equity, 19,
20*f*

justice-centered framework,
reproductive justice as, 194–95

justice-conscious approach to
reproductive health

case study 1: responding to a crisis,
263, 264*f*

case study 2: integrating structural
expertise into prenatal care,
263–65

health equity and social determinants, 259–61

overview, 189

reimagining care for pregnant persons, 265–68, 266f

unmet legal needs, 261–62, 262f

K

Kania, John, 27

Kentucky Perinatal Quality Collaborative (KyPQC), 423b

knowledge acquisition, as theme in BHSC HBWW initiative, 147

L

labor and delivery (L&D), 48

language

  intentional, AAIMM Prevention Initiative use of, 181–82

  as type of social innovation, 369–71, 370f

Latina women, 193–94. *See also* equity; racial MCH disparities; racism; structural racism

law and health. *See* justice-conscious approach to reproductive health

layering funding, 541, 542b

LCD (leading cause of death), in MMRC reports, 280

LCT. *See* life-course theory

leadership

  ASTHO development of, 543–44

  Black, in AAIMM Prevention Initiative, 172–76, 176b

  importance to success of IMPACT Collaborative, 160

  in NHSA AIM CCI, 134–37

lead exposure, 253, 254

leading cause of death (LCD), in MMRC reports, 280

Learning Community Model (ASTHO)

  general discussion, 422

  jurisdictional successes, 420–21

  Kentucky Perinatal Quality Collaborative, 423b

  key technical assistance themes, 418–19

  learning communities in action, 416–18

  overview, 346–47, 415–16

  standard components, 416

  strategies for state health agencies, 421–22

  supporting entire health agencies with, 544–48, 545b, 546b

learning opportunities for maternal health workforce, 507

legal advocacy, academic center role in providing, 28–29

legal checkup concept, 264–65

legal expertise. *See* justice-conscious approach to reproductive health

legal status, in IHELP™ model, 262f

legislative advocacy action group, IMPACT Collaborative, 156–57

legislative authority for maternal health programs, 14

LHDs. *See* local health departments

Library Services service line, NC AHEC, 569

life-course theory (LCT)

  overview, 10, 204–5

  perinatal MCH life course, 47–48

  and structural racism, 311, 312

  transformational maternal and child health, 40–42, 41f, 43f, 43–44

lifelong learning and equity, 501–5

Linking PRAMS and Clinical Outcomes Data Multi-Jurisdiction Learning Community, 546b

lived experiences

  importance in IMPACT Collaborative, 160

  qualitative evidence representing, 313

LMSW (local maternal safety workgroup), New Orleans, 135, 136

local businesses, academic center support for, 26

local communities, as maternal health zone of transformation, 80f, 80, 81, 82, 83t, 86–87, *See also* community

local data, limited availability of, 329

Local Enhancement Project, 417

local government, academic center partnerships with, 28

local health departments (LHDs)

  example of multidisciplinary team approach, 585–87, 587f

  funding women's health in, 583–84, 584f

  future of women's health, 587–88

  impact of health departments in women's health, 582–83

  overview, 448–49, 579–82, 580f

  systems in place to provide high-quality care, 584–85

local maternal safety workgroup (LMSW), New Orleans, 135, 136

logic model, in culturally responsive evaluation, 333

longitudinal approach to maternal and child health. *See* transformational maternal and child health

longitudinal qualitative research (LQR)
analysis in, 324–25
defined, 319–20
ethical considerations in application of, 321–22
fitting right research question to, 320–21
as pivotal tool in maternal health research, 320
recommendations for future action, 325*f*, 325
research design in, 322–24, 323*b*

long-term outcomes, and sustainability of academic health systems, 489

Los Angeles County, California. *See also* African American Infant and Maternal Mortality Prevention Initiative
Department of Health Services, 408
Department of Public Health, 167–68, 181*b*
maternal and child health outcomes in, 166*f*, 166–67, 167*f*, 170*f*, 178*f*

Louisiana Public Health Institute (LPHI), 136

LQR. *See* longitudinal qualitative research

M

Mahmee platform, 387, 406–9
Main, Elliott, 558
MAM (Mujeres Ayudando Madres), 431–32, 439*b*
Mama Certified initiative, 24
Mamas and Tatas, 432
MAMA's Neighborhood program, 408
Mamatoto Village, 432
managed care, Medicaid, 465–66, 471
Mandala Midwifery Care, 431
MAP (Maternal Action Project), 386
March of Dimes, 159. *See also* African American Infant and Maternal Mortality Prevention Initiative; Healthy Babies are Worth the Wait® initiative
Maryland Maternal Health Innovation Program (MDMOM), 113*b*

Massachusetts Medicaid, 471

mass incarceration, 30*b*, *See also* incarcerated populations, reproductive justice in

Maternal, Infant, and Early Childhood Home Visiting (MIECHV) Program, 11*t*, 451–52, 453

Maternal Action Project (MAP), 386

Maternal and Child Health (MCH) Coalition, 549*b*

maternal and child health (MCH) public health professionals, 496

maternal and child health (MCH) workforce. *See also* maternal health workforce
content of care, 48–49
numbers and scope of practice, 47–48
staffing expanded scope of care, 52–54
staffing present scope of care, 51–52
transforming MCH scope of work, 49–51

Maternal and Child Health Bureau (MCHB)
calls for innovation by, 345
development of government-funded programs, 10–15, 13*f*
examples of states leveraging programs, 455–58
federal partnerships, 15–16
general discussion, 16–17, 459
MCH essential services, 77, 78*f*
overview, 10, 11*t*, 447, 451–52
practical next steps for leveraging programs, 458–59
Rural Maternity and Obstetrics Management Strategies program, 119–20, 121, 123–24, 124*f*
support for states and communities to advance equity, 452–55
women's preventive healthcare services, 372*b*

Maternal and Family Wellness From an Indigenous Perspective training series, 111*b*

Maternal and Infant Assessment and Follow-up Plan, 383

Maternal Data Center (CMQCC), 558–59

maternal depression screenings, Medicaid coverage for, 470–71. *See also* mental health

maternal environmental health
and access to safe drinking water, 253–54

environmental justice, 250
examples of concerns, 250–54
overview, 247–48
and personal care products, 251–52, 255, 256
root of problem, getting to, 249
strategies for improving, 255–56
understanding environmental health, 248–49
maternal–fetal medicine (MFM) specialists, 127–28, 569–70
maternal health, working together to improve, xiii–xiv, 3–7
Maternal Health Committee (BHSC), 148
maternal health data. *See* data
maternal health equity. *See also* equity; systems for maternal health equity
advancing in academic health systems, 479–83, 482f
background, 213–14
calls to action, 220–23
case study overview, 214–15
defined, 216–17, 218f, 219t
Delphi consensus process, 215–16, 216t, 217f
overview, 188
research priorities, 219–20, 221t
Maternal Health Innovation (MHI) programs, 111b, 453–54
Maternal Health Learning and Innovation Center (MHLIC), 11t
maternal health organizations providing telemedicine, 431–33
maternal health outcomes. *See also* collaboration; data; equity; innovations to improve maternal health; maternal health equity; racial MCH disparities; systems for maternal health equity
AAFP Task Force on Maternal Morbidity and Mortality, 515–16, 516b
addressing inequities in NHSA AIM CCI, 133–38
Better Maternal Outcomes project, 228–35
and content of care, 48–49
current state of, 4–5, 9, 48, 73–74, 213–14
democratizing data, 277–86
environmental impacts on, 247–56
environmental justice and, 250
family physicians, role in, 513–21, 516b

in Harris County, Texas, 153–54, 154f, 161–62, 162f
Healthy Babies are Worth the Wait initiative, 140–41, 143f, 143–49, 148f
holistic view of, 77–78
HRSA role in improving, 9–10, 11t
impact of race on, 302
improving through collaboration, 73–75
journey forward, 593–94
misuse of race by maternal health data tools, 301–6, 304f
narrative medicine and longitudinal qualitative research on, 319–25, 323b, 325f
pervasive health crisis, 227–28
SCC efforts improving in Bootheel Perinatal Network, 129b
staffing expanded scope of MCH care to improve, 52–54
and structural racism, 188, 191–98, 201–10, 203f
transforming MCH scope of work, 49–51
and women's health, 363–64
maternal health research. *See* data; decolonizing maternal health research
maternal health task forces (MHTFs), 108–10, 115b
maternal health warning signs, 382–83
maternal health workforce
current state of, 492–96
diversity of, 494–96, 497, 529, 531–32, 570–71
expanded primary healthcare team approach, 47–54
general discussion, 509f, 509
geographic distribution, 492–93, 569–70, 579–81, 580f
graduate/residency programs, 497, 501
lifelong learning and equity, 501–5
NC AHEC focus on, 567–76
next generation of healthcare providers, 531–32
overview, 448, 491–92
retaining and supporting existing, 506–9
role of advocacy among healthcare providers, 531–32
strategic skills for, 505, 506b
strategies to enhance capacity and center equity, 496–505

maternal health workforce (*cont.*)
  supply and demand projections,
    493–94
  undergraduate programs, 497, 498–
    500, 499*t*
  youth programs, 497
maternal health zones of transformation
    model
  case examples, 82–89, 88*f*
  extending maternal health practice
    before, during, and after pregnancy,
    82, 83*t*
  extending reach of maternal health
    practitioners, 79–82, 80*f*
  Framework for Aligning Sectors, 78–
    79, 79*f*
  general discussion, 89
  overview, 74, 77–78, 78*f*
maternal morbidity, in MMRC reports,
    281. *See also* maternal health
    outcomes
maternal mortality
  in California, 167*f*, 555, 556*f*, 562–63,
    563*f*
  and collective impact framework, 144
  current problem related to, xiii, 4–5,
    9, 77
  democratizing data, 277–86
  disparities in, 213–14
  need for standardized data collection
    system on, 525–26
  perception versus facts about Black,
    172, 174*t*
  as pervasive health crisis, 227–28
  postpartum, 379
  Pregnancy Mortality Surveillance
    System, 283
  structural racism and, 191–92, 201–2
Maternal Mortality and Morbidity
    (MMM) Policy Statement, ASTHO,
    547–48
Maternal Mortality and Morbidity
    (MMM) technical package,
    ASTHO, 550–51
Maternal Mortality Review Committees
    (MMRCs)
  categorization of maternal deaths,
    279–80
  challenges of using data, 281–82
  contributing factors to maternal
    deaths, 213–14
  federal partnerships, 15–16
  identifying opportunities for system
    improvements through, 473

  improving data collection around
    maternal deaths, 526
  opportunities for community-based
    organizations to use data, 285
  other maternal health data available
    through reports, 280–81
  overview, 278, 279
  and Perinatal Quality Collaborative
    interventions, 283–84
  as state data source, 279–82
Maternal Mortality Review Information
    Application (MMRIA) program,
    CDC, 278–79, 526
Maternal Outreach through Telehealth
    for Rural Sites (MOTHeRS)
    program, 508*b*
maternal safety bundles (MSBs), in
    NHSA AIM CCI, 133–34
maternity care. *See also* perinatal mental
    health; postpartum care; prenatal care
  family physician training in, 514–17
  lack of access to high-quality, 4
  and telemedicine, 433–35
maternity care deserts, 4, 492–93, 519,
    579–81
maternity medical homes, 470, 472
MCH (Maternal and Child Health)
    Coalition, 549*b*
MCH (maternal and child health) public
    health professionals, 496
MCHB. *See* Maternal and Child Health
    Bureau
MCH workforce. *See* maternal and child
    health workforce; maternal health
    workforce
MDMOM (Maryland Maternal Health
    Innovation Program), 113*b*
meaning-making sessions, in culturally
    responsive evaluation, 337
measurement tools, IMPACT
    Collaborative, 161
MedEdPORTAL, 501–2
Medicaid
  access to prenatal care, 260
  care in academic centers for insured
    patients, 23–24
  EPSDT services, 49
  expanded coverage, 220–23, 284–85,
    464, 464*t*, 466–67, 527
  funding for community-based doulas,
    399–401
  general discussion, 472–73
  innovation in maternal and child
    health through, 466–71

need for further expansion of coverage, 285

overview, 448, 463–64

prenatal care under, 50

reimbursement for oral health services, 101

reproductive justice-focused approach to, 196

value-based payment programs, 471–72

variations in, 464–66, 464*t*

medical care and community care team integration, 355–60, 356*f*

medical experimentation, 193–94, 206, 292*b*

medical homes, 41–42, 472

medicalization, 313–14

medical-legal partnership (MLP) model
case study 1: responding to a crisis, 263
case study 2: integrating structural expertise into prenatal care, 263–65
as continuum, 263, 264*f*, 265
overview, 261–62
reimagining care for pregnant persons, 265–68

medical schools, pipeline programs in, 497*b*, 497–501, 499*t*

medication for opioid use disorder (MOUD), expanding access to, 418–19

Mejia, Kristin, 409–10, 411

mental health
ASTHO Learning Community Model addressing, 415–22, 423*b*
California Health Care Foundation focus on improving, 560–62
Kentucky Perinatal Quality Collaborative, 423*b*
local health department interest in, 586
Medicaid coverage for services, 470–71
overview, 346–47
perinatal, bridging gap in, 405–13
virtual care innovations, 429
and women's health, 364

mentorship, 532

messaging, as social innovation, 369–71, 370*f*

metrics, choosing for external partnerships, 65, 66*b*

MetroHealth, 26

MetroWest, 26

MFM (maternal–fetal medicine) specialists, 127–28, 569–70

MHI (Maternal Health Innovation) programs, 111*b*, 453–54

MHLIC (Maternal Health Learning and Innovation Center), 11*t*

MHTFs (maternal health task forces), 108–10, 115*b*

Michener, J., 31*b*, 346, 347

midwifery–doula clinical model, 64*b*, 66*b*

Midwifery Integrated Home Visitation Program (MI-Home), 434

midwives. *See also* doulas
Black, traditional, 349–51
California Health Care Foundation support for, 565
in clinical care and community care team integration, 358
Medicaid coverage for services, 467–68
virtual care innovations, 429–31, 431*t*, 437*b*

MIECHV (Maternal, Infant, and Early Childhood Home Visiting) Program, 11*t*, 451–52, 453

MI-Home (Midwifery Integrated Home Visitation Program), 434

mission, defining when creating external partnerships, 61

MLP model. *See* medical-legal partnership model

MMM (Maternal Mortality and Morbidity) Policy Statement, ASTHO, 547–48

MMM (Maternal Mortality and Morbidity) technical package, ASTHO, 550–51

MMRCs. *See* Maternal Mortality Review Committees

MMRIA (Maternal Mortality Review Information Application) program, CDC, 278–79, 526

mobile-friendly online resource centers, 368

mobile health apps, 367–68

Model Surveillance Protocols (CDC), 282

modernization, data, 422

MoMMA's Voices, 504–5

Momnibus Act (Black Maternal Health Momnibus Act of 2021), 29, 196, 529–30

Montana Obstetrics and Maternal Support (MOMS), 114*b*, 433–34

Montana State MHI Program, 109*t*, 114*b*

Monterey County Health Department, California, 263

mood disorders. *See* mental health

morbidity, maternal. *See* maternal health outcomes

Morehouse School of Medicine Center for Maternal Health Equity, 214–15. *See also* Georgia Maternal Health Research for Action Steering Committee

mortality. *See* infant mortality; maternal mortality

Morton, C., 57

MOTHER Lab, 532

MOTHeRS (Maternal Outreach through Telehealth for Rural Sites) program, 508*b*

Mothers Among Us program, 242

MOUD (medication for opioid use disorder), expanding access to, 418–19

MSBs (maternal safety bundles), in NHSA AIM CCI, 133–34

Mujeres Ayudando Madres (MAM), 431–32, 439*b*

multidisciplinary teams. *See also* collaboration
GVPH use of throughout pregnancy, 585–87, 587*f*
in postpartum care, 381–83

multigenerational mental wellness, 406

multimodal learning, NC AHEC focus on, 574

multisector partnerships, 487. *See also* collaboration; health system collaborations with external partners

municipal underbounding, 254

mutually reinforcing activities, in collective impact framework, 141, 143*f*, 143*t*, 146

"My Birth Matters" campaign (CHCF), 560

My Nursing Coach program, 406

N

narrative medicine
analysis in, 324–25
defined, 319
ethical considerations in application of, 321–22
fitting right research question to, 320–21
as pivotal tool in maternal health research, 320
recommendations for future action, 325*f*, 325
research design in, 322–24

NAS (Neonatal Abstinence Syndrome), 415, 422

NAS (Neonatal Abstinence Syndrome) Pilot Program, 420

Nashville Strong Babies program, 410

National Birth Equity Collaborative Cycle to Respectful Care, 352–53, 353*f*

National Center for Health Workforce Analysis (NCHWA), 493

National Center for Medical-Legal Partnership, 261, 265–66, 266*f*

National Committee for Quality Assurance, 561–62

National Consortium of Telehealth Resource Centers (NCTRC), 435

National Council of State Boards of Nursing, 495

National Forum of State Nursing Workforce Centers, 495

National Health Service Corps, 499*t*

National Healthy Start Association (NHSA) AIM CCI
general discussion, 137–38
lessons learned, 137
New Orleans case study, 134–36
overview, 133–34

National Institutes of Health (NIH), 50

National Interprofessional Initiative on Oral Health (NIIOH), 97

National Maternal Mental Health Hotline, 11*t*

national organizations, reaching out to, 504–5

National Partnership for Women & Families, 87

National Perinatal Association (NPA), 436

National Preconception Health and Health Care Initiative, 371–73

National Survey of Children's Health, 454, 459

National Vital Statistics System (NVSS), 283

NC AHEC. *See* North Carolina Area Health Education Center

NCHWA (National Center for Health Workforce Analysis), 493

NCTRC (National Consortium of Telehealth Resource Centers), 435

Nebraska Title V program, 458
neonatal abstinence syndrome (NAS), 415, 422
Neonatal Abstinence Syndrome (NAS) Pilot Program, 420
neonatal care, 48–49
networks, in transformational maternal and child health, 42–44, 44*f*, 45
Nevada PRISM team, 420–21
New Familia Health Support Services, 431*t*
New Jersey
  community doula care in, 400–1
  Maternal Health Innovation Program, 109*t*, 114*b*
  Title V program, 458
Newkirk, Vann R., II, 30*b*
NewMomHealth.com web site, 385
New Orleans AIM CCI collaborative, 134–36
New Orleans Health Department, 135–36
New York Title V Program, 457
NHSA AIM CCI. *See* National Healthy Start Association AIM CCI
NIH (National Institutes of Health), 50
NIIOH (National Interprofessional Initiative on Oral Health), 97
no blame game value, AAIMM Prevention Initiative, 178–80, 179*b*
nondental settings, oral healthcare integration in, 93–102
non-hospital-focused maternal safety bundles (MSBs), in NHSA AIM CCI, 133–34
nonprofit hospitals, community benefits of, 21–22, 22*f*
North Carolina
  local health departments, role of, 579–88, 580*f*, 584*f*, 587*f*
  Maternal Health Innovation program, 109*t*, 115*b*
  Title V program and Perinatal Health Strategic Plan, 455–56
North Carolina Area Health Education Center (NC AHEC)
  continual professional development, 572–74
  general discussion, 576
  graduate medical education, 574–76
  health workforce, 569–71
  overview, 567–69
  practice support, 571–72
North Dakota Medicaid, 470–71

NPA (National Perinatal Association), 436
Nurse–Family Partnership, 488–89
nurse practitioners (NPs), 493
nurses, and workforce diversity, 495
Nursing Workforce Diversity Program, 499*t*
Nurture NJ Maternal and Infant Health Strategic Plan, 400–1
NVSS (National Vital Statistics System), 283

O

obesity, 305
OB Ready concept (AAFP), 520
obstetric (OB) assessment through LHDs, 582–83, 585–86
obstetric (OB) care managers, at GVPH, 586
obstetric (OB) care, physicians providing in North Carolina, 570, 575
obstetric emergencies, education for family physicians on, 520
obstetrician/gynecologists (OB-GYNs). *See also* maternal and child health workforce; maternal health workforce
  Iowa MHI focus on, 112*b*
  legacy and impact of racism, 349–51
  shortage of, 47, 579–81, 580*f*
  staffing present scope of care, 51–52
  strategies to operationalize reproductive justice, 351–52
  supply and demand projections, 493, 494
O'Connor, Helen, 179–80
odor discrimination, 252
Ohio Council to Advance Maternal Health (OH-CAMH), 116*b*
Ohio Maternal Health Innovation program (Ohio MHI), 109*t*, 116*b*
Oklahoma Maternal Health Task Force (OMHTF), 117*b*
Oklahoma State MHI Program, 109*t*
OMNI (Opioid Use Disorder, Maternal Outcomes, and Neonatal Abstinence Syndrome Initiative) Learning Community, 416–17, 420, 423*b*
online care. *See* telemedicine and telehealth; virtual care innovations
online resource hubs, 368
Open Arms Perinatal Services, 396–97

operationalizing external partnerships, 65–66, 67b

opioid use disorder, expanding access to medication for, 418–19

Opioid Use Disorder, Maternal Outcomes, and Neonatal Abstinence Syndrome Initiative (OMNI) Learning Community, 416–17, 420, 423b

oral healthcare integration
  achieving oral health equity, 94–95
  current system design, 95–97
  general discussion, 101–2
  at local health departments, 586
  overview, 74, 93–94
  practical tips for medical professionals, 97–101

Oral Health Delivery Framework (NIIOH), 97

Oral Health in America surgeon general's report, 93

organizations
  as maternal health zone of transformation, 80f, 80–81, 82, 83t, 85–86
  in socioecological model for role of academic centers, 21f, 23–25

Ortiz, A. T., 30b

Othering & Belonging Institute, The, 29

P

paid family and medical leave, 549b

pan-disciplinary approach to maternal health, 29, 31b

Park, H., 32–33

partner engagement, and sustainability of academic health systems, 487–88

partnerships. *See also* collaboration; federal partnerships; health system collaborations with external partners
  for advocacy, involving academic health systems, 487
  importance to Montana Obstetrics and Maternal Support, 114b
  involving State Title V programs, 457–58
  when doing research in Indigenous communities, 293

PAs (physician assistants), 493, 494

Pathways Community HUB Institute (PCHI) model, 88, 89, 125

"Pathway to Equity, A" plan (Los Angeles County DPH), 167–68

patient-centered approach, 58–60, 354–55, 372b, *See also* health system collaborations with external partners; innovations to improve maternal health; reproductive justice

patient-centered contraceptive counseling guidance (ACOG), 356

Patient-Centered Medical Home (PCMH) model, 39f, 39

patient engagement
  in academic health systems, 484–85
  in CHCF efforts to reduce cesarean deliveries, 560

pay-for-performance model, Medicaid, 472

payments
  in CHCF efforts to reduce cesarean deliveries, 559–60
  and medical-legal partnerships, 266
  reform of, and oral healthcare in nondental settings, 101

PBGH (Purchaser Business Group on Health), 559

PBP. *See* incarcerated populations, reproductive justice in; Prison Birth Project

PCC (People's Community Clinic), 263–65

PCHI (Pathways Community HUB Institute) model, 88, 89, 125

PCMH (Patient-Centered Medical Home) model, 39f, 39

PDSA (Plan-Do-Study-Act) cycles, Better Maternal Outcomes project, 231, 233

pediatric care
  oral healthcare integration, 96–98
  telemedicine and telehealth in, 428

Peer Networks (ASTHO), 543–44

peer-recovery coaches and services, 419

people of color. *See* American Indian/Alaska Native women; Black maternal health outcomes; Indigenous communities; Latina women; racism; structural racism

People's Community Clinic (PCC), 263–65

performance measurement, government-funded maternal health programs, 13f, 13–14

Perigee Fund, 562

Perinatal and Patient Safety
Collaborative (PPSC), HRSA, 38,
39–44, 41f, 43f, 44f
perinatal and reproductive healthcare
(PRH) models, 380–81
Perinatal ECHO, 573
Perinatal Health Community Garden,
411
Perinatal Health Equity Collective,
North Carolina, 455–56
perinatal health outcomes, 48–49. *See
also* maternal health outcomes;
perinatal mental health; virtual care
innovations
Perinatal Health Strategic Plan (PHSP),
North Carolina, 455–56
perinatal mental health
ASTHO Learning Community Model
addressing, 415–22, 423b
California Health Care Foundation,
560–62
Homeland Heart Birth & Wellness
Collective, 409–11
Kentucky Perinatal Quality
Collaborative, 423b
local health department interest in,
586
Mahmee, 406–9
models of collaboration in competitive
world, 411–13
overview, 346–47, 405–6
virtual care innovations, 429
and women's health, 364
perinatal paradox, 48, 49
Perinatal Quality Collaboratives (PQCs),
283–84, 423b, 530
perinatal regionalization, 507
personal care products, and maternal
environmental health, 251–52, 255,
256
personalized maternity care, need for,
57–58. *See also* health system
collaborations with external
partners
personally mediated racism, 482f
personal stability, in IHELP™ model,
262f
person-first models of maternity care,
24, 380–81. *See also* health system
collaborations with external
partners
pesticide exposure, 263
PHSP (Perinatal Health Strategic Plan),
North Carolina, 455–56

phthalate exposure, 251–52, 255, 256
physician assistants (PAs), 493, 494
physician-centered healthcare delivery
models, 24
pilot phase of external partnerships, 65
pilot programs, 488–89
pipeline strategies, 497b, 497–501, 499t
Pizii, Marisa, 237–38, 240–43
placeandhealthwv.com website, 314b
place-based coverage, Medicaid, 467
place-based environmental exposures,
250–51, 253–54
Plan-Do-Study-Act (PDSA) cycles,
Better Maternal Outcomes project,
231, 233
plans of safe care, 419
playbook metaphor, 5
PMSS (Pregnancy Mortality Surveillance
System), 283
policy
CHCF support for changes in, 564–65
examples of successful
implementation, 529–31
to improve maternal health, 524–29
next generation of healthcare
providers, 531–32
overview, 448, 523–24
role of advocacy among healthcare
providers, 532
in socioecological model for role of
academic centers, 21f, 28–29
policy statements, ASTHO, 547–48
pooled funds, 88–89
population health
defined, 140
socio-ecological model of racism on,
481–83, 482f
and structural racism, 311
population level, and social services as
zone of transformation, 84–85
postpartum appointment handout, 384
postpartum care
general discussion, 388
implementing innovations, 387–88
innovation through meaningful
communication, 384–86
and local health departments, 586–87
measuring quality for accountability,
387
Medicaid coverage for, 284–85, 465,
467, 526–27
multidisciplinary teams, 381–83
need for renovation of, 380–81
overview, 346, 379–80

postpartum care *(cont.)*
  recognizing and uplifting community leadership, 386–87
  standardization of clinical practices, 383–84
Postpartum Support International (PSI), 412–13
Postpartum Visit (PPV) Quality Improvement Project, 530–31
Postpartum Visit Checklist, 385, 386
powell, john a., 29–32
power
  acknowledging in qualitative research, 321–22
  sharing to advance maternal health equity, 480–81
  sharing with Black women, 176*b*
PPSC (Perinatal and Patient Safety Collaborative), HRSA, 38, 39–44, 41*f*, 43*f*, 44*f*
PPV (Postpartum Visit) Quality Improvement Project, 530–31
PQCs (Perinatal Quality Collaboratives), 283–84, 423*b*, 530
Practical Playbook series, xiii–xiv, 5
Practice Support service line, NC AHEC, 569, 571–72
PRAMS (Pregnancy Risk Assessment Monitoring System), 282–83, 546*b*
PRAMS Learning Community, 546*b*
preconception care
  limited availability of, 364
  messaging and language around, 370*f*, 370
  transforming MCH scope of work, 50
  well woman primary care visits, 371–73, 372*b*
Preconception Collaborative Improvement and Innovation Network, 372*b*
Preeclampsia Foundation, 129
preeclampsia model, 49–50
pregnancy, extending maternal health practice before, during, and after, 82, 83*t*
pregnancy-associated deaths, 280. *See also* maternal mortality
Pregnancy Care ECHO, 508–9
pregnancy complications. *See* maternal health outcomes
Pregnancy Mortality Surveillance System (PMSS), 283
pregnancy-related deaths, 279–80. *See also* maternal mortality

Pregnancy Risk Assessment Monitoring System (PRAMS), 282–83, 546*b*
prenatal care. *See also* transformational maternal and child health
  content of care, 48
  group, 24, 263–65, 468–69
  local health departments, role in, 581–83, 585–87
  maternity medical homes, 470
  medical-legal partnerships and, 263–65
  oral healthcare integration, 96–97
  right to coverage, 260
  transforming MCH scope of work, 49–50
Prenatal Legal Checkup, 265
President's budget (Congressional Budget Justification), 12
presumptive eligibility, for Medicaid, 466–67
preterm births, 170*f*
preventability data, in MMRC reports, 280
Preventing Maternal Deaths Act, 31*b*, 526
preventive services guidelines from MCHB, 452, 454
PRH (perinatal and reproductive healthcare) models, 380–81
primary care
  building blocks of high-performing, 44
  expanded primary healthcare team approach, 52–54
  NC AHEC focus on improving, 567–76
  oral healthcare integration in, 93–102
  postpartum care innovations, 381–83
  social innovation in women's health, 371–73, 372*b*
  for women, 51
Principles of Trustworthiness (AAMC), 488
PRISM (Promoting Innovation in State and Territorial MCH Policymaking) Learning Community, 417–18, 420–21
Prison Birth Project (PBP). *See also* incarcerated populations, reproductive justice in
  overview, 237–38
  reproductive justice and prison maternal healthcare, 240–43

private partners. *See* collaboration; health system collaborations with external partners

product-based environmental exposures, 250–52

professional development, ongoing, 507

professional education strategies, 497*b*, 497–501, 499*t*

professional equity education, 503

program evaluation, 327–28. *See also* culturally responsive evaluation

programs, maternal health. *See* government-funded maternal health programs

Project ECHO (Extension for Community Health Outcomes), 433–34, 573

Promoting Innovation in State and Territorial MCH Policymaking (PRISM) Learning Community, 417–18, 420–21

provider–industry partner relationships. *See* health system collaborations with external partners

provider workforce. *See* maternal and child health workforce; maternal health workforce

PSI (Postpartum Support International), 412–13

public awareness action group, IMPACT Collaborative, 156

public health. *See also* Association of State and Territorial Health Officials; maternal health zones of transformation model; state health agencies

 as ASTHO priority area, 422

 community-centered funding models for telehealth in emergencies, 436–37. *see also* COVID-19 pandemic; virtual care innovations

 local health departments, role of, 579–88, 580*f*, 584*f*, 587*f*

 measuring structural racism using qualitative data, 309–16, 314*b*

 State MHI Program, 107–10, 109*t*, 111*b*, 112*b*, 113*b*, 114*b*, 115*b*, 116*b*, 117*b*

 workforce diversity, 496

Public Health AmeriCorps, 498–500, 499*t*

public-private-community partnership, AAIMM Prevention Initiative as, 166*f*, 166–69, 167*f*, 168*f*, 169*f*

Purchaser Business Group on Health (PBGH), 559

purchasers, in CHCF efforts to reduce cesarean deliveries, 559–60

purpose, intentional, of AAIMM Prevention Initiative, 182–83

pushing upstream to advance maternal health equity, 481–83, 482*f*

Q

qualitative analysis, in BHSC HBWW initiative, 146–47

qualitative data

 example of displaying, 314*b*

 measuring structural racism using, 309–10, 313–16, 314*b*

 narrative medicine and longitudinal qualitative research, 319–25, 323*b*, 325*f*

 overview, 274

quality, measuring for accountability in postpartum care, 387

quality improvement

 in CHCF efforts to reduce cesarean deliveries, 557–58

 CommonSpirit Health criteria for external partners, 63*b*

 frameworks for, 359

 through Medicaid, 471–72

quality of care action group, IMPACT Collaborative, 156

quantitative analysis, in BHSC HBWW initiative, 145

Queens Village initiative (Cradle Cincinnati), 27

Quetelet, Adolphe, 304–5

R

race, in workforce diversity statistics, 494–96

race-based data

 lack of in PRAMS, 282

 in MMRC reports, 280–81

race-based medicine, 302

racial equity. *See also* equity

 advancing in academic health systems, 479–89, 482*f*

 as ASTHO priority area, 421

 centering in maternal health workforce, 496–505

Racial Equity Learning Series (RELS), 134

racial healing, fostering, 483

racial MCH disparities. *See also* Alliance for Innovation on Maternal Health Community Care Initiative; Black maternal health outcomes; culturally responsive evaluation; innovations to improve maternal health; maternal health equity; transformational maternal and child health

AAFP "Striving for Birth Equity" policy, 517–18

Better Maternal Outcomes project, 228–35

community-based doulas and birth equity, 391–402, 395*f*, 396*f*

current state of, 4, 48, 144–45, 213–14

justice-conscious approach to reproductive health, 259–68, 262*f*, 264*f*, 266*f*

legacy and impact of racism, 349–51

maternal environmental health, 247–56

and maternity care deserts, 579–81

measuring structural racism using qualitative data, 274, 309–16, 314*b*

misuse of race by maternal health data tools, 275, 301–6, 304*f*

MMRIA as allowing for evaluation of, 278

overview, 213–14, 302

state interventions to address, 284

and structural racism, 188, 191–98, 201–10, 203*f*

racism. *See also* structural racism

CHCF support for addressing, 565

in clinical care in academic centers, 23–24

cultural competence training to decrease, 528–29

decolonizing maternal health research, 289–98, 292*b*

in LA County AAIMM Prevention Initiative theory of causality, 169*f*, 169

legacy and impact in maternal health, 349–51

in Los Angeles County "A Pathway to Equity" plan, 167–68

and maternal and child health outcomes, 48, 52

in medical education and training, 25

MMRIA as allowing for evaluation of, 278

need for standardized data collection system on, 525–26

and organization internals as zone of transformation, 85–86

professional equity education, 503

reproductive justice in incarcerated populations, 237–44

as root case, in AAIMM Prevention Initiative values, 172, 173*f*, 174*t*

socio-ecological model of impact on sexual, gender, and reproductive health in BIPOC communities, 481–83, 482*f*

teaching maternal health workforce about, 502–3

theories, models, and explanations of impact on MCH, 310–12

Raising Resilience, 431*t*

RBA. *See* results-based accountability

Reaching Our Sisters Everywhere (ROSE), 386, 436

Reach the Decision Makers program (UCSF), 28–29

Ready, Set, Baby curriculum (CGBI), 384

Ready, Set, Baby Live (CGBI), 436–37

reconciliation, fostering, 483

recurrent cross-sectional analysis, 324–25

Redesigning Systems with Black Women. *See* Better Maternal Outcomes: Redesigning Systems with Black Women project

redlining, 206–7, 254

Reduction in Peripartum Racial and Ethnic Disparities (RED) safety bundle, AIM, 284

referrals

to dental home, 98

implications of BPN for shared system for, 130

in Women With IMPACT program, 157

reflexivity, acknowledging in qualitative research, 321–22

Refugee Women's Health Clinic (RWHC), 484–86

Regional In Situ Obstetric and Neonatal Emergency Drills (ECU Health), 572–73

regionalization, perinatal, 507

Reiger, K., 57

reimbursement

for community-based doulas, 399–401

Medicaid structures for, 465–66

relationships
  importance to success of IMPACT
    Collaborative, 160
  in qualitative research, 322
  in socioecological model for role of
    academic centers, 21f, 23
  in transformational maternal and child
    health, 42
  when doing research in Indigenous
    communities, 293
RELS (Racial Equity Learning Series),
  134
Remikie, Sharetta, 147
remote maternal and infant care services.
  See virtual care innovations
Reproducing Race (Bridges), 24
Reproductive and Sexual Health Equity
  Framework, 352
reproductive health, justice-conscious
  approach to. *See* justice-conscious
  approach to reproductive health
reproductive justice (RJ)
  academic center role in providing,
    29–32
  clinical care and community care team
    integration, 355–60, 356f
  Cycle to Respectful Care framework,
    352–53, 353f
  defined, 351
  as equity-and justice-centered
    framework, 194–95
  history of creation of, 238–39
  in incarcerated populations, 237–44
  innovations to improve maternal
    health, 351–55, 353f
  integrative models for maternity care
    delivery, 354–55
  leveraging to increase maternal health
    workforce, 498b
  messaging and language centering, 369
  overview, 19
  Reproductive and Sexual Health
    Equity Framework, 352
  using to address structural change,
    195–96, 197–98
research, maternal health. *See* data;
  decolonizing maternal health
  research; Indigenous research
  methods; longitudinal qualitative
  research; narrative medicine
residency programs
  community-based education in North
    Carolina, 574–76
  family medicine, 514

residential segregation laws, 260–61
resource enrollment action group,
  IMPACT Collaborative, 156
resource hubs, online, 368
respectful care, 352–53, 353f, 357–58,
  380–81
Respectful Care team, Better Maternal
  Outcomes project, 231–32, 235
responsibility, shared, in AIM CCIs, 137
results-based accountability (RBA)
  in Healthy Babies are Worth the Wait
    initiative, 140–41
  integration with collective impact, 142,
    143f, 143t
  operationalizing in BHSC HBWW
    initiative, 143–48, 148f
  overview, 141–42
retaining maternal health workforce,
  506–9
Reynolds, Tina, 240–41
Rhode Island Health Equity Zone
  Initiative, 542b
Rhode Island OMNI team, 420
Richmond, California, 28
RJ. *See* reproductive justice
RMOMS program. *See* Bootheel
  Perinatal Network; Rural Maternity
  and Obstetrics Management
  Strategies program
Roberts, Dorothy, 31b
Robert Wood Johnson Foundation,
  78–79, 79f
robustness, as CommonSpirit Health
  criterion for external partners, 63b
Rochester, New York, 398–99
Ronik, Marci, 145–46, 147, 150
ROSE (Reaching Our Sisters
  Everywhere), 386, 436
Ross, Loretta, 31b
rural communities. *See also* Bootheel
  Perinatal Network; family
  physicians; telemedicine and
  telehealth; virtual care innovations
  access to dental care in, 94–95
  barriers to maternity care in, 119
  expanding virtual healthcare options
    and coverage, 528
  Iowa MHI focus on, 112b
  local health departments, role in, 579–
    88, 580f, 584f, 587f
  maternal health workforce in North
    Carolina, 569–70
  maternity care deserts in, 492, 493
  NC AHEC focus on, 573

Rural Maternity and Obstetrics
Management Strategies (RMOMS)
program, 11*t, See also* Bootheel
Perinatal Network
goals, 123–24, 124*f*
overview, 74, 119–20
purpose of, 121
rural track, family medicine residency,
502*b*
RWHC (Refugee Women's Health
Clinic), 484–86

S

Sacks, Tina, 31*b*
safe care, plans of, 419
safe drinking water, access to, 253–54
Safe Drinking Water Act (SDWA), 253
safety-net clinics, dental, 98
SaludMadre.com web site, 385
SAMHSA (Substance Abuse and Mental
Health Services Agency), 429
satisfaction surveys, by IMPACT
Collaborative, 161
SBHCs (school-based health centers),
98, 434–35
scaling up, implications of BPN for, 130
scaling up improvements in maternal
health equity, 448–49. *See also*
systems for maternal health equity
SCC (system care coordinator), BPN,
124–25, 127–28, 128*b*, 129*b*
scholarship, in socioecological model
for role of academic centers, 21*f*,
29–32, 30*b*, 31*b*
school-based health centers (SBHCs),
98, 434–35
Screening and Treatment for Maternal
Depression and Related Behavioral
Disorders, 11*t*
screenings, oral health, 97–98
SDF (silver diamine fluoride), 100
SDOH. *See* social determinants of
health
SDWA (Safe Drinking Water Act), 253
Secretary's Advisory Committee on
Infant and Maternal Mortality
(ACIMM), 11*t*
Section 1115 waivers, 466
segregation laws, racial, 260–61
segregation of clinical care in academic
centers, 23–24
self-care, as theme in BHSC HBWW
initiative, 147

Senate Bill 464 (Dignity in Pregnancy
and Childbirth Act), 85–86, 565
service delivery, reimagining, 507–9,
508*b*
service delivery action group, IMPACT
Collaborative, 156
service levels, in CommonSpirit Health
criteria for external partners, 63*b*
severe maternal morbidity (SMM), 162.
See also maternal health outcomes
sexual violence toward Indigenous
people, 296–97
Shahangian, J., 96–97
shared decision-making, in clinical
care and community care team
integration, 357–58
shared leadership, in New Orleans AIM
CCI, 136–37
Shared Leadership team, Better Maternal
Outcomes project, 232
shared measurement, in collective
impact framework, 141, 143*f*, 143*t*,
145
shared referral system, implications of
BPN for, 130
shared responsibility, in AIM CCIs, 137
sharing data, in AIM CCIs, 137
sharing power to advance maternal
health equity, 480–81
SHIP (State Health Improvement Plan)
structure, 549*b*
shortage in MCH workforce. *See*
maternal and child health
workforce; maternal health
workforce
Shower2Empower event, 146
Show Your Love Today web site, 371–73
Show Your Love wellness campaign,
366–67
silver diamine fluoride (SDF), 100
slavery, 193–94, 206, 350
Smart Care California, 559–60
smartphones, and women's health,
367–68
SMM (severe maternal morbidity), 162.
See also maternal health outcomes
social determinants of health (SDOH)
defined, 125
Indigenous-specific, 295–96
and maternal environmental health,
249
overview, 204–5
structural racism and, 192, 193
WHO definition of, 259

social innovations in women's health, 369–73, 370*f*, 372*b*

social media, and women's health, 365–67, 368*f*

Social Security Act, 260

social services, as maternal health zone of transformation, 80*f*, 80, 82, 83*t*, 84–85

social structures, as maternal health zone of transformation, 80*f*, 80, 81–82, 83*t*, 87–89, 88*t*

societal health, socio-ecological model of racism on, 481–83, 482*f*

socioecological model for role of academic centers
  community, 25–27
  individuals, 22–23
  organizations, 23–25
  overview, 19–20, 21*f*
  policy and advocacy, 28–29
  relationships, 23
  society and scholarship, 29–32, 30*b*, 31*b*

socio-ecological model of impact of racism on sexual, gender, and reproductive health in BIPOC communities, 481–83, 482*f*

socioeconomic status, 174*t*

Southeast Michigan IBCLCs of Color, 431*t*

Special Supplemental Nutrition Program for Women, Infants, and Children (WIC), 586

sponsors, identifying and confirming, 61

SPSN (Statewide Provider Support Network), North Carolina, 115*b*

SSDI (State Systems Development Initiative) program, 454

SSM Health, 128–29

staff, maternal health. *See* maternal and child health workforce; maternal health workforce

stakeholders
  aligning, 62
  engaging in culturally responsive evaluation, 333, 334*b*
  identifying and confirming, 61
  MCHB role in convening, 454–55
  relationships among in IMPACT Collaborative, 160

standardization of postpartum clinical practices, 383–84

standardized data-collection system on maternal and infant deaths, 525–26

start-up inertia, as CommonSpirit Health criterion for external partners, 63*b*

state-based foundations. *See* California Health Care Foundation

state health agencies
  ASTHO development and support, 543–44
  ASTHO Learning Community Model strategies for, 421–22
  ASTHO MMM technical package, 550–51
  best practices in supporting, 544–48, 545*b*, 546*b*
  funding for sustainability, 540–41, 542*b*
  general discussion, 551–52
  overview, 448
  success stories, 548*b*, 548, 549*b*

State Health Improvement Plan (SHIP) structure, 549*b*

State Loan Repayment Program, 499*t*

State Maternal Health Innovation Program (State MHI Program), 11*t*
  building collaborations, 108–10
  core components of collaboration, 111*b*, 112*b*, 113*b*, 114*b*, 115*b*, 116*b*, 117*b*
  federal partnerships, 15–16
  overview, 74, 107–8
  state awardees, 108, 109*t*

states
  examples of MCHB-funded programs, 455–58
  funding for community-based doulas, 400–1
  innovation in maternal and child health through Medicaid, 466–71
  interventions to address maternal health, 283–84
  maternal health data from, 278–82
  MCHB support to advance maternal health equity, 452–55
  variations in Medicaid, 463, 464–66, 464*t*

State Systems Development Initiative (SSDI) program, 454

Statewide Provider Support Network (SPSN), North Carolina, 115*b*

steering committee
  AAIMM Prevention Initiative, 168*f*, 168–69, 174–75
  IMPACT Collaborative, 155–56

sterilizations, forced, 193–94, 292*b*

strategic skills for maternal health workforce, 505, 506*b*

strengths, celebrating Indigenous people's, 297–98

stress
related to structural racism, 207–8
as theme in BHSC HBWW initiative, 147

"Striving for Birth Equity" policy (AAFP), 515–16, 516*b*, 517–18

structural competency, 261

structural determinants of health, 249

structural racism. *See also* Better Maternal Outcomes: Redesigning Systems with Black Women project
cultural competence training to decrease, 528–29
defined, 207
general discussion, 197–98, 210
historical context of, 193–94, 205–8
and impact of race on maternal health, 302
need for standardized data collection system on, 525–26
overview, 188, 191–92, 201, 350–51
path forward for maternal health, 208–10
policy and advocacy, employing to reduce, 523–32
qualitative data measuring and capturing, 274, 309–16, 314*b*
reproductive justice, addressing structural change with, 195–96, 197–98
reproductive justice as equity-and justice-centered framework, 194–95
reproductive justice in incarcerated populations, 237–44
seeing problem from different vantage point, 203*f*, 203–5
and social determinants of health, 192, 193
theories, models, and explanations of impact on MCH, 310–12

Student Services service line, NC AHEC, 568

Substance Abuse and Mental Health Services Agency (SAMHSA), 429

substance use
ASTHO Learning Community Model addressing, 415–22, 423*b*
Medicaid coverage for services, 471

success metrics, choosing for external partnerships, 65, 66*b*

supply projections, maternal health workforce, 493–94

Supporting Women Across Silos team (Better Maternal Outcomes project), 230, 232

sustainability
of academic health systems, 487–89
as ASTHO priority area, 421–22
in Bootheel Perinatal Network, 125
CommonSpirit Health criteria for external partners, 63*b*
of state maternal health interventions, 540–41

Sustaining Breastfeeding Innovations Through Policies and Programs initiative (BLC), 545*b*

system care coordinator (SCC), BPN, 124–25, 127–28, 128*b*, 129*b*

systemic approach to expanded care model, 38–39, 42, 45

systemic inequity. *See* racial MCH disparities; racism; structural racism

systemic racism. *See also* structural racism
in clinical care in academic centers, 23–24
in medical education and training, 25

systems, as maternal health zone of transformation, 80*f*, 80, 81–82, 83*t*, 87–89, 88*t*

systems for maternal health equity. *See also* Association of State and Territorial Health Officials; maternal health workforce
academic health systems, 477–89, 482*f*
Breanna's story, 444–45
California Health Care Foundation case study, 555–65, 556*f*, 561*f*, 563*f*
family physicians, role of, 513–21, 516*b*
local health departments, role of, 580*f*, 584*f*, 584–88, 587*f*
Maternal and Child Health Bureau, role of, 451–59
Medicaid, role of, 463–73
North Carolina Area Health Education Center example, 567–76
overview, 448–49
policy and advocacy, employing, 523–32

T

"Tackling Maternal Health Disparities"
(National Partnership for Woman
& Families), 87
Tampa Bay Doula Program, 531
targeted universalism, 29–32
Task Force on Maternal Morbidity and
Mortality (AAFP), 515–16, 516*b*
Teaching Health Center Graduate
Medical Education (THCGME)
Program, 499*t*
teaching hospitals. *See* academic centers,
role in advancing maternal health
technical assistance
in ASTHO Learning Community
Model, 418–19
from Maternal and Child Health
Bureau, 10
technology, using to increase medical–
dental integration, 98–99
telecommunications, using to bridge
gap in perinatal mental health,
405–13
teledentistry, 98–99
telehealth resource centers (TRCs), 435
Telehealth Technology Assessment
Resource Center (TTAC), 435, 436
telemedicine and telehealth
addressing inequities in, 437*b*
background, 427–29
in Bootheel Perinatal Network, 125,
128*b*
community-centered funding models,
436–37
doulas, childbirth education, and
midwifery care, 429–31, 431*t*
effect of COVID-19 pandemic on,
346, 428–29
expanding options and coverage,
527–28
future of, 438*b*
general discussion, 438–40
healthcare providers and, 433–35
high-risk pregnancy care via, 508*b*
maternal health organizations
providing, 431–33
maternal health services via, 508*b*
National Perinatal Association
courses, 436
resources and training materials,
435–36
training as critical to expanding
services, 437–38

and women's health, 369
and workforce retention, 507
territorial health agencies
ASTHO development and support,
543–44
ASTHO MMM technical package,
550–51
best practices in supporting, 544–48,
545*b*, 546*b*
funding for sustainability, 540–41,
542*b*
general discussion, 551–52
overview, 448
success stories, 548*b*, 548, 549*b*
Text4Baby mobile application, 530–31
THCGME (Teaching Health Center
Graduate Medical Education)
Program, 499*t*
theory of causality, LA County AAIMM
Prevention Initiative, 169*f*, 169
thick description, 314
Think Dirty app, 256
third-party vendors. *See* health system
collaborations with external
partners
time constraints, in government-funded
maternal health programs, 14
Title 19 of Social Security Act, 260
Title V Information System (TVIS),
458
Title V Maternal and Child Health
(MCH) Services Block Grants, 11*t*
and COVID-19 pandemic, 457–58
Illinois example, 456–57
North Carolina example, 455–56
overview, 451–52, 453
practical next steps for leveraging
programs, 458–59
Title V MCH Internship Program, 499*t*
Title V National Performance and
Outcome Measures, 454, 459
Title V Needs Assessment, 459
Toppin, Eloy, 29–32
tort law concept of duty, 260
trachoma experiments in Indigenous
communities, 292*b*
training
at academic centers, 25
in academic health systems, 483–84,
485–86
for community-based doulas, 394–95,
402
for doulas during COVID-19
pandemic, 430

training (*cont.*)
    implicit bias, for family physicians, 518–19
    programs addressing equity, 501–2
    telehealth, 435–36
    in underserved settings, 501
trajectory analyses, 324–25
trans-Atlantic slave trade, 193–94, 206
transformation, fostering, 483
transformational maternal and child health
    community collaboration, 42–44, 44*f*, 45
    Comprehensive Health Home framework, 39*f*, 39–40
    expanded care model, 38–39
    healthcare quality-improvement endeavors, 37–38
    key messages, 45–46
    life-course perspective, 40–42, 41*f*, 43*f*, 43–44
    overview, 37
    Perinatal and Patient Safety Collaborative, 39–44, 41*f*, 43*f*, 44*f*
    system implications, 45
    transforming MCH scope of work, 49–51
transformation zones. *See* maternal health zones of transformation model
transitions of care, postpartum, 381–83, 384
transparency, in CHCF efforts to reduce cesarean deliveries, 558–59
transportation, lack of, 260–61
trauma, and adverse birth outcomes, 311
TRCs (telehealth resource centers), 435
Tribal communities, co-creating projects with in Arizona, 111*b*, *See also* Indigenous communities; racial MCH disparities; racism; structural racism
Tribal research permits, 291
trustworthiness principles (AAMC), 488
truth, fostering, 483
TTAC (Telehealth Technology Assessment Resource Center), 435, 436
Tufts University School of Medicine, 497*b*, 532
Tuhiwai Smith, Linda, 290, 292*b*, 294–95
Turn the Curve (TTC) reports, 141–42, 148
TVIS (Title V Information System), 458
Two-Generation Clinic, 111*b*

U

UAMS (University of Arkansas for Medical Sciences), 508*b*
UIC (University of Illinois Chicago), 109*t*, 111*b*, 456–57
UNC. *See* University of North Carolina
underbound Black communities, 254
undergraduate programs, 497, 498–500, 499*t*
underrepresented in medicine (URiM) groups, 25, 494
underserved communities. *See also* rural communities
    financial incentives to work in, 499*t*, 502*b*
    NC AHEC focus on, 573
    training in, 501
unethical research in Indigenous communities, 292*b*
uninsured patients, care for, 21–22
United Way of Greater Atlanta, 235
universalism, targeted, 29–32
universities, importance to success of IMPACT Collaborative, 161. *See also* academic centers, role in advancing maternal health
University of Arkansas for Medical Sciences (UAMS), 508*b*
University of California, San Francisco, 28–29
University of Illinois Chicago (UIC), 109*t*, 111*b*, 456–57
University of Iowa, 112*b*
University of Minnesota, 29
University of Montana, 114*b*
University of North Carolina (UNC)
    Collaborative for Maternal and Infant Health, 372*b*, 382–83
    family medicine residency rural track, 502*b*
    4th Trimester Project, 385–86
    National Preconception Health and Health Care Initiative, 371–73
    partnership with GVPH, 584–85
    Preconception CoIIN, 372*b*
    teaching about racism at, 502–3
URiM (underrepresented in medicine) groups, 25, 494
usability, as CommonSpirit Health criterion for external partners, 63*b*

US Department of Health and Human Services (HHS), 477–78. *See also* Health Resources and Services Administration

user-generated content, on social media, 365–66

utilities, in IHELP™ model, 262*f*

V

vaginal birth after cesarean (VBAC) algorithm, 303, 304*f*

vaginal deliveries, 396*f*

vaginal douches, 252

Valleywise Health (VH), 484–85

value-based model of maternity care, 485–86

value-based payment (VBP) programs, Medicaid, 471–72

values, intentional. *See* intentional values of AAIMM Prevention Initiative

VBAC (vaginal birth after cesarean) algorithm, 303, 304*f*

vendors, partnerships with. *See* health system collaborations with external partners

venture capitalists (VCs) invested in women's health, 375

VH (Valleywise Health), 484–85

viability, as CommonSpirit Health criterion for external partners, 63*b*

Vidant Medical Center, 382–83, 508*b*

Village Fund (AAIMM), 171–72

Vinekar, Kavita, 23–24

violence toward Indigenous people, 296–97. *See also* racism

virtual care innovations
addressing inequities in telehealth, 437*b*
background, 427–29
community-centered funding models, 436–37
doulas, childbirth education, and midwifery care, 429–31, 431*t*
general discussion, 438–40
healthcare providers and telemedicine, 433–35
maternal health organizations providing telemedicine, 431–33
mental healthcare, 429
National Perinatal Association courses, 436

overview, 346
telehealth resources and training materials, 435–36
training as critical to expanding services, 437–38

vision, defining when creating external partnerships, 61

vulnerable populations, access for at CommonSpirit Health, 60*b*, 63*b*, 64*b*

W

WADRJ (Women of African Descent for Reproductive Justice), 238–39

Walia, Sunny, 407

warning signs, maternal health, 382–83

water, access to safe drinking, 253–54

water fluoridation, 101

we are all pieces of the puzzle value, AAIMM Prevention Initiative, 180–81, 181*b*

weathering hypothesis, 311–12

Wei, H., 412

wellness programs, messaging and language in, 370*f*, 370–71

well water, 253–54

well woman primary care visits, 371–73, 372*b*

We Still Here (Hill), 202

West Park, Florida, 145–46, 150

Wheeler, S., 28

WHO (World Health Organization), 204, 249, 259

WIC (Special Supplemental Nutrition Program for Women, Infants, and Children), 586

Wilkins, C. H., 21–22

Women of African Descent for Reproductive Justice (WADRJ), 238–39

Women of Color (WOC). *See* American Indian/Alaska Native women; Black maternal health outcomes; equity; Indigenous communities; Latina women; racial MCH disparities; racism; structural racism

women's health
background, 363–64
call to action, 373–75
digital innovation, 365–69, 368*f*
local health departments, role of, 579–88, 580*f*, 584*f*, 587*f*

women's health (*cont.*)
  overview, 347, 363
  primary healthcare for women, 51
  social innovations, 369–73, 370*f*,
    372*b*
  workforce supply and demand
    projections, 493
women's jail, Prison Birth Project in,
  240–43
Women's Preventive Services Initiative
  (ACOG), 371
Women With IMPACT (WWI)
  program, 157
workforce, maternal health. *See* maternal
  health workforce
workforce development, as ASTHO
  priority area, 421
World Health Organization (WHO),
  204, 249, 259

worry, as theme in BHSC HBWW
  initiative, 147
wraparound services
  at Granville Public Health, 585–87,
    587*f*
  postpartum, 381–83
WWI (Women With IMPACT)
  program, 157

Y

youth programs, 497

Z

ZOMA Foundation, 561–62
zones of transformation. *See* maternal
  health zones of transformation
  model